Mental Health and
Mental Disorders

Mental Health and Mental Disorders

AN ENCYCLOPEDIA OF CONDITIONS, TREATMENTS, AND WELL-BEING

Volume 1: A–E

LEN SPERRY
EDITOR-IN-CHIEF

Associate Editors
ALEXANDRA CUNNINGHAM
MELISSA A. MARIANI
MINDY PARSONS
STEVEN R. VENSEL

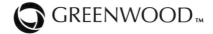

An Imprint of ABC-CLIO, LLC
Santa Barbara, California • Denver, Colorado

Library of Congress Cataloging-in-Publication Data

Names: Sperry, Len.
Title: Mental health and mental disorders : an encyclopedia of conditions,
    treatments, and well-being / Len Sperry, editor-in-chief.
Description: Santa Barbara, California : Greenwood, [2016] | Includes
    bibliographical references and index.
Identifiers: LCCN 2015018246 | ISBN 9781440803826 (hardback : acid-free paper)
    | ISBN 9781440803833 (ebook)
Subjects: LCSH: Psychiatry—Encyclopedias. | Mental health—Encyclopedias. |
    BISAC: PSYCHOLOGY / Mental Health. | PSYCHOLOGY / Psychopathology /
    Anxieties & Phobias.
Classification: LCC RC437 .M47 2016 | DDC 616.89003—dc23
LC record available at http://lccn.loc.gov/2015018246

ISBN: 978-1-4408-0382-6
EISBN: 978-1-4408-0383-3

20 19 18 17 16   1 2 3 4 5

This book is also available on the World Wide Web as an eBook.
Visit www.abc-clio.com for details.

Greenwood
An Imprint of ABC-CLIO, LLC

ABC-CLIO, LLC
130 Cremona Drive, P.O. Box 1911
Santa Barbara, California 93116-1911

This book is printed on acid-free paper ∞

Manufactured in the United States of America

This book discusses treatments (including types of medication and mental health therapies), diagnostic tests for various symptoms and mental health disorders, and organizations. The authors have made every effort to present accurate and up-to-date information. However, the information in this book is not intended to recommend or endorse particular treatments or organizations, or substitute for the care or medical advice of a qualified health professional, or used to alter any medical therapy without a medical doctor's advice. Specific situations may require specific therapeutic approaches not included in this book. For those reasons, we recommend that readers follow the advice of qualified health care professionals directly involved in their care. Readers who suspect they may have specific medical problems should consult a physician about any suggestions made in this book.

Contents

Alphabetical List of Entries

Guide to Related Topics

Following are the entries in this encyclopedia, arranged under broad topics for enhanced searching. Readers should also consult the index at the end of the encyclopedia for more specific subjects.

Books, Movies, Music, Internet, and Popular Culture

Archetypes and the Collective Unconscious, The (Book)

Authentic Happiness (Book)

Beyond Freedom and Dignity (Book)

Breakfast Club, The (Movie)

Chicken Soup for the Soul (Book)

Clockwork Orange, A (Movie)

Clueless (Movie)

Cobain, Kurt (1967–1994)

Conditioned Reflexes: An Investigation of the Physiological Activity of the Cerebral Cortex (Book)

Dahmer, Jeffrey (1960–1994)

Darkness Visible: A Memoir of Madness (Book)

Dead Poets Society (Movie)

Dictionary of Occupational Titles (Book)

Divided Self, The (Book)

Ego and the Mechanisms of Defense, The (Book)

Electronic Communication

Envy and Gratitude (Book)

Everything You Always Wanted to Know about Sex (but Were Afraid to Ask) (Book and Movie)

Facebooking

Feeling Good: The New Mood Therapy (Book)

Female Brain, The (Book)

Ferris Bueller's Day Off (Movie)

Frames of Mind: The Theory of Multiple Intelligences (Book)

Friday Night Lights (Movie)

Gifts Differing: Understanding Personality Types (Book)

Going Viral

Guide to Rational Living, A (Book)

Hip-Hop Music

Interpretation of Dreams, The (Book)

Juno (Movie)

Language and Thought of the Child, The (Book)

Love, Courtney (1964–)

Man Who Mistook His Wife for a Hat, The (Book)

Man's Search for Meaning (Book)

Marley, Bob (1945–1981)

Mean Girls (Movie)

Media Violence

Music, Influence of

"Nature of Love, The"

Occupational Information

On Becoming a Person (Book)

One Flew over the Cuckoo's Nest
(Book and Movie)

Our Inner Conflicts: A Constructive Theory of Neuroses (Book)

Phantoms in the Brain: Probing the Mysteries of the Human Mind (Book)

Principles of Psychology, The (Book)

Psychology of Self Esteem, The (Book)

Reality Television (TV)

Reggae Music

Risky Business (Movie)

Seven Principles for Making Marriage Work (Book)

Sexting

Sixteen Candles (Movie)

Sixth Sense, The (Movie)

Social Media

South Park (Television Program)

Sybil (Book and Movie)

Tattoo

Teen Pop Stars

Texting

Three Faces of Eve (Movie)

Twelve Traditions of Alcoholics Anonymous, The

Understanding Human Nature (Book)

Video Games

Working with Emotional Intelligence (Book)

Young Man Luther: A Study in Psychoanalysis and History (Book)

YouTube

Concepts

Abandonment

Abuse

Acculturation and Assimilation

Acculturative Stress

Adoption

Affect

Aggressive and Antisocial Behavior in Youth

Aging and Older Adults

Allostatic Load

Androgyny

Anger in Adults

Apathy

Attachment Styles

Baby Boomers

Bereavement

Biopsychosocial Model

Birth Order

Blended Families

Body Image

Body Piercing

Brain

Bystander Effect

Cancer, Psychological Aspects

Career Development

Caregivers

Cliques

Codependency

Cognitive Complexity

Cognitive Dissonance

Comorbidity

Compassion Fatigue

Competency and Competencies

Compliance

Coping

Crisis Housing

Cults

Culture

Paradoxical Intention

Parent, Loss of

Parenting Styles or Disciplinary Styles

Parents, Overinvolved

Pastoral Counselor

Peer Groups

Person–Environment Fit

Placebo Effect

Positive Psychology

Prejudice

Prescription Drug Abuse

Privilege and Privileged Communication

Profanity

Professional Identity

Prostitution

Psychodynamic

Psychopharmacology

Psychosexual Development, Stages of

Psychosocial Development, Stages of

Psychotherapist

Psychotherapy

Racial Identity Development

Rage

Reinforcement

Relapse and Relapse Prevention

Religion and Religiosity

Religious Coping

Resilience

Retirement

Retirement, Psychological Factors

Risk Management

Road Rage

School Phobia (School Refusal)

Secure Attachment

Self-Actualization

Self-Concept

Self-Esteem

Self-Fulfilling Prophecy

Self-Medication Hypothesis

Self-Mutilation/Self-Harm

Senior Mental Health

Sex and Gender

Sexual Abuse

Sexual Identity

Sexual Orientation

Shyness

Single-Parent Families

Sleep

Smoking Cessation

Social Learning Theory

Special Education

Spiritual Awakening

Spiritual Bypass

Spiritual Identity

Spirituality and Practices

Split Brain

Stigma

Stress

Suicide

Systems Biology

Tarasoff Decision

Temper Tantrum

Terminal Illness, Psychological Factors

Transgender

Trauma

Truancy

Well-Being

Willpower

Women's Mental Health Issues

Work Orientation

Worldview

Yoga

Zone of Proximal Development

Disorders

Abusive Personality

Acute Stress Disorder

Addiction

Addictive Personality

Adjustment Disorder

Adverse Childhood Experiences

Agoraphobia

Alcohol Use Disorder

Alexithymia

Alzheimer's Disease

Amnesia

Anorexia Nervosa

Anosognosia

Antisocial Personality Disorder

Anxiety Disorders in Adults

Anxiety Disorders in Youth

Anxious Personality Disorder

Aphasia

Asperger's Syndrome

Attention-Deficit Hyperactivity Disorder

Attention-Deficit Hyperactivity Disorder in Youth

Autism

Autism Spectrum Disorders

Avoidant Personality Disorder

Avoidant/Restrictive Food Intake Disorder

Binge Eating Disorder

Bipolar Disorder

Body Dysmorphic Disorder

Body Integrity Identity Disorder

Borderline Personality Disorder

Brief Psychotic Disorder

Bulimia Nervosa

Caffeine-Related Disorders

Cannabis Use Disorder

Capgras Syndrome

Catatonic Disorders

Childhood Disintegrative Disorder

Childhood Onset Fluency Disorder

Chronic Illness

Chronic Pain Syndrome

Circadian Rhythm Sleep–Wake Disorder

Cognitive Deficits

Compulsions

Conduct Disorder

Conversion Disorder

Counterdependent Personality Disorder

Counterphobic Personality Disorder

Cyclothymic Disorder

Delayed Ejaculation

Delirium

Delusional Disorder

Delusions

Dementia

Dependent Personality Disorder

Depersonalization/Derealization Disorder

Depression and Depressive Disorders

Depression in Youth

Depressive Personality Disorder

Developmental Coordination Disorder

Developmental Disabilities

Drugs, Natural Remedies, and Other Substances

Evening Primrose Oil

Focalin (Dexmethylphenidate)

GABA (Gamma-Aminobutyric Acid)

Geodon (Ziprasidone)

Ginkgo Biloba

Ginseng

Haldol (Haloperidol)

Hallucinogens

Inhalants

Kava Kava

Klonopin (Clonazepam)

Lavender

Lexapro (Escitalopram)

Lithium

Loxitane (Loxapine)

Luvox (Fluvoxamine)

Magnesium

Marijuana

Melatonin

Methadone

Naltrexone (Naltrexone Hydrochloride)

Namenda (Memantine)

Neurontin (Gabapentin)

Passionflower

Paxil (Paroxetine)

Pristiq (Desvenlafaxine)

Prozac (Fluoxetine)

Risperdal (Risperidone)

Ritalin (Methylphenidate)

SAMe (S-Adenosyl-Methionine)

Serotonin

St. John's Wort

Strattera (Atomoxetine)

Tegretol (Carbamazepine)

Thorazine (Chlorpromazine)

Tofranil (Imipramine)

Valerian

Valium (Diazepam)

Wellbutrin (Bupropion)

Xanax (Alprazolam)

Yohimbine

Zinc

Zoloft (Sertraline)

Zyprexa (Olanzapine)

Legislation and Legal Issues

Advance Directives

Affordable Care Act

Americans with Disabilities Act (ADA)

Custody and Custody Evaluations

Individualized Education Plan (IEP)

Insanity Defense

Mental Health Courts

Mental Health Laws

Tarasoff Decision

Mental Health Professionals, Positions, and Professional Topics

Caregivers

Case Management

Case Manager

Certified Addictions Professional (CAP)

Certified Rehabilitation Counselor (CRC)

Clinical Health Psychology

Clinical Mental Health Counseling

Clinical Psychology

Cognitive Behavior Analysis System of Psychotherapy (CBASP)

Cognitive Behavior Therapy

Common Factors in Psychotherapy

Community Mental Health

Contemplative Neuroscience

Counseling and Counseling Psychology

Cultural Competence

Culturally Sensitive Treatment

Diagnostic and Statistical Manual of Mental Disorders (DSM)

Ego Psychology

Emotionally Focused Psychotherapy

Ethics in Mental Health Practice

Evolutionary Psychology

Existential Psychotherapy

Expertise

Gerontological Counseling

Gestalt Psychotherapy

Group Counseling

Guidance Counselor

Impaired Professionals

Individual Psychology

Jungian Therapy

Logotherapy

Marriage and Family Therapist

Master Therapist

Mental Health Counselor

Mind-Body Psychotherapies

Mindfulness-Based Psychotherapies

Neo-Freudian Psychotherapies

Neuropsychiatry

Pastoral Counselor

Positive Psychotherapy

Privilege and Privileged Communication

Psychiatrist

Psychoanalysis

Psychologist

Psychopharmacology

Psychotherapist

Psychotherapy Skills and Competency

Publication Manual of the American Psychological Association

Rehabilitation Counseling

Risk Management

Social Workers

Spiritually Oriented Psychotherapy

Sports Psychology

Vocational Counseling

Organizations

Alcoholics Anonymous (AA)

American Academy of Child and Adolescent Psychiatry (AACAP)

American Counseling Association (ACA)

American Mental Health Counselors Association (AMHCA), The

American Psychiatric Association (APA)

American Psychological Association (APA)

American Rehabilitation Counseling Association (ARCA)

American School Counselor Association (ASCA)

American Society of Addiction Medicine (ASAM)

Child Protective Services

Commission on Rehabilitation Counselor Certification (CRCC)

Council for Accreditation of Counseling and Related Educational Programs (CACREP)

Drug Enforcement Administration (DEA)

National Institute of Mental Health (NIMH)

Substance Abuse and Mental Health Services Administration (SAMHSA)

People

Adler, Alfred (1870–1937)

Allport, Gordon (1897–1967)

Alzheimer, Alois (1864–1915)

Bandura, Albert (1925–)

Beattie, Melody (1948–)

Beck, Aaron T. (1921–)

de Shazer, Steve (1940–2005)

Dreikurs, Rudolf (1897–1972)

Ellis, Albert (1913–2007)

Erickson, Milton (1901–1980)

Erikson, Erik (1902–1994)

Frankl, Viktor (1905–1997)

Freud, Anna (1895–1982)

Freud, Sigmund (1856–1939)

Glasser, William (1925–2013)

Gottman, John (1942–)

Haley, Jay (1923–2007)

Harlow, Harry (1905–1981)

Hayes, Steven (1948–)

Holland, John Lewis (1919–2008)

Horney, Karen (1885–1952)

James, William (1842–1910)

Jung, Carl (1875–1961)

Kim Berg, Insoo (1934–2007)

Klein, Melanie (1882–1960)

Kohlberg, Lawrence (1927–1987)

Kübler-Ross, Elisabeth (1926–2004)

Lazarus, Arnold (1932–2013)

Linehan, Marsha (1943–)

Maslow, Abraham (1908–1970)

May, Rollo (1909–1994)

McGoldrick, Monica (1943–)

Meichenbaum, Donald (1940–)

Milgram, Stanley (1933–1984)

Millon, Theodore (1928–2014)

Minuchin, Salvador (1921–)

Moreno, Jacob (1889–1974)

Pavlov, Ivan (1849–1936)

Perls, Fritz (1893–1970)

Piaget, Jean (1896–1980)

Rogers, Carl R. (1902–1987)

Satir, Virginia (1916–1988)

Seligman, Martin (1942–)

Skinner, B. F. (1904–1990)

Vygotsky, Lev (1896–1934)

Watson, John B. (1878–1958)

Whitaker, Carl (1912–1995)

White, Michael (1948–2008)

Wilson, Bill. *See* Alcoholics Anonymous (AA)

Wolpe, Joseph (1915–1997)

Wundt, Wilhelm (1832–1920)

Zimbardo, Philip (1933–)

Social Issues

Adverse Childhood Experiences

Aggressive and Antisocial Behavior in Youth

Baby Boomers

Binge Drinking

Blended Families

Bullying and Peer Aggression

Child Abuse

Cliques

Columbine Shooting

Cults

Cyberbullying

Date Rape

Divorce

Domestic Violence

Drug Culture

Economic and Financial Stress

Elder Abuse

Ethnicity

Foster Care

Gangs

Hazing

Homelessness

Human Trafficking

Immigration, Psychological Factors of

Mass Shootings

Mental Health and Violence

Military Mental Health

Millennials

Parents, Overinvolved

Peer Groups

Performance-Enhancing Drugs

Poverty and Mental Illness

Prejudice

Prescription Drug Abuse

Profanity

Prostitution

Racial Identity Development

Road Rage

Single-Parent Families

Smoking Cessation

Social Justice Counseling

Socioeconomic Status

Temper Tantrum

Tests, Experiments, and Classifications

Beck Depression Inventory

Behavioral Assessment

Bender Gestalt Test

Brain Imaging

Children's Apperception Test (CAT)

Children's Depression Inventory

Computed Tomography (CT)

Conners Rating Scales

Diagnosis

Diagnostic and Statistical Manual of Mental Disorders (DSM)

Disability and Disability Evaluation

Early Recollections

Electroencephalography (EEG)

Executive Functions

Family Assessment

Hamilton Anxiety Scale (HAM-A)

Hamilton Depression Scale (HAM-D)

Hare Psychopathy Checklist-Revised (PCL-R)

Individualized Education Plan (IEP)

Insanity Defense

Intelligence Testing

International Classification of Diseases

Kaufman Adolescent and Adult Intelligence Test (KAIT)

Kaufman Assessment Battery for Children (K-ABC)

Magnetic Resonance Imaging (MRI)

Mental Competency Evaluation

Mental Measurements Yearbook, The

Mental Status Examination

Millon Clinical Multiaxial Inventory (MCMI)

Mini-Mental State Examination

Minnesota Multiphasic Personality Inventory (MMPI)

Neuropsychological Tests

Obedience to Authority: An Experimental View (Book)

Personality Tests

Polysomnography

Positron Emission Tomography (PET)

Psychodynamic Diagnostic Manual (PDM)

Qualitative Research

Quantitative Research

Rorschach Inkblot Test

Single-Photon Emission Computed Tomography (SPECT)

Special Education

Stanford Prison Experiment

Subjective Units of Distress Scale (SUDS)

Suicide Assessment

Thematic Apperception Test (TAT)

Wechsler Adult Intelligence Scale (WAIS)

Wechsler Intelligence Scale for Children (WISC)

Wide Range Achievement Test (WRAT)

Treatment

Acceptance and Commitment Therapy (ACT)

Acupressure

Acupuncture

Addiction Counseling

Adlerian Therapy

Advocacy Counseling

Anger Management

Animal-Assisted Therapy

Anxiety Reduction Techniques

Applied Behavior Analysis

Art Therapy

Assertiveness Training

Aversion Therapy

Behavior Therapy

Behavior Therapy with Children

Behavioral Activation

Behavioral Health

Behavioral Medicine

Bereavement Counseling

Best Practices

Bibliotherapy

Biofeedback

Biopsychosocial Therapy

Body Work Therapies

Bowen Family Systems Theory

Brief Dynamic Psychotherapy

Brief Therapy

Career Assessment

Career Counseling

Case Conceptualization

Case Management

Case Manager

Clinical Health Psychology

Clinical Mental Health Counseling

Clinical Psychology

Clinical Trial

Coaching

Cognitive Behavior Analysis System of Psychotherapy (CBASP)

Cognitive Behavior Therapy

Cognitive Behavioral Modification

Cognitive Problem-Solving Skills Training (CPSST)

Cognitive Remediation

Cognitive Retraining

Cognitive Therapies

College Counseling

Combined Treatment

Common Factors in Psychotherapy

Community Mental Health

Preface

The quest to understand mental health and its disorders is first noted in the writings of the ancient Greeks. With today's new technologies and constant research, scientists have uncovered many causes of mental disorders and conditions as well as new treatments to reduce symptoms as well as prevent these conditions. "Mental health" is a broad term that encompasses both dysfunction and well-being from conception through the life span.

The purpose of this encyclopedia is to provide a wide-ranging reference source on mental health and its disorders, written at a level accessible for upper high school and college students as well as for the layperson. The encyclopedia provides insights into the discipline of mental health and covers both healthy functioning and mental disorders or conditions, treatment methods, and factors that promote mental health and well-being.

Mental Health and Mental Disorders: An Encyclopedia of Conditions, Treatments, and Well-Being aims to open the door to mental health research for readers, as well as direct them to accurate and current resources for further investigation.

Scope

This encyclopedia helps the reader understand mental disorders and their treatment as well as normal development and prevention of mental illness. This reference work covers virtually every topic and consideration involving mental health. The reader will find that the 875 entries in this three-volume work comprise six areas of emphases:

- Mental disorders and conditions. These include both common and relatively rare disorders. Also included are diagnostic characterizations that follow the *Diagnostic and Statistical Manual of Mental Disorders, Fifth Edition*, commonly known as DSM-5.
- Treatment of these disorders. These include prescribed medications, psychological therapies, and herbs and other natural remedies.
- Tests and assessment methods used in evaluating or diagnosing mental conditions. These include standardized paper and pencil tests as well as biological and brain-imaging methods.
- Common psychological terms and concepts associated with mental and emotional well-being.

- Highly regarded individuals and organizations influential in researching disorders, developing treatments, or fostering professional development.
- Popular and classic books and films as well as high-profile individuals and culture-changing events. These have significantly influenced our understanding of mental health and illness and are also profiled.

To increase readability, technical terms are defined near the beginning of most entries. Terms are also included in the glossary at the end of volume three.

Contributors

The 13 contributors to this encyclopedia are all uniquely qualified to speak with authority regarding at least one aspect of mental health and its disorders. They have formal training and experience in psychiatry, clinical psychology, clinical mental health counseling, or child and adolescent development. Most have specialized in working with children, adolescents, and young adults and recognize the critical role of culture in mental health and illness. The collective expertise of these contributors allows a much broader understanding of mental health issues than a single author could ever provide.

User-Friendly Features

Mental Health and Mental Disorders: An Encyclopedia of Conditions, Treatments, and Well-Being is organized in the customary A–Z encyclopedia format. At the front of each volume is an alphabetical listing of all entry headings ("Alphabetical List of Entries"), allowing the reader to scan the list of all entries. A "Guide to Related Topics" is an additional aid, listing all the entries in the book under broad topics. Readers can look under topics such as "Disorders," "People," and "Social Issues" to quickly see all the entries included for that topic.

All entries have a "See also" section that connects the reader to other relevant topics. For example, in the entry "Anxiety Disorders in Adults" the connecting and cross-references will direct the reader to other entries that discuss similar disorder symptoms (Agoraphobia, Generalized Anxiety Disorder, Panic Attack, Panic Disorder, Social Phobia, Specific Phobia), and various treatment methods and approaches (Antianxiety Medication, Antidepressant Medication, Cognitive Therapy, Exposure Therapy).

Further Reading and Selected Resources

Each entry also includes current, reliable sources for additional statistics, research, or consumer-friendly education. Books, articles, and websites are included, allowing the reader to choose the level of detail and depth for further data and material. "Recommended Resources," a specially chosen short list of good books and online resources that are helpful to the layperson or student, is featured at the end of volume three. That volume also includes the "Glossary" of terms, with succinct definitions or descriptions of concepts, disorders, treatments, tests, and important people. The "List of

Organizations" features more than 120 groups and resource centers, ranging from the Albert Ellis Institute to the Association for Applied Sport Psychology to the Workplace Bullying Institute. The encyclopedia concludes with a comprehensive index.

Where to Start?

Obviously a reader's starting point is individually driven; however, if you are interested in a specific mental disorder, please read that entry first and follow it up with reading the "See also" selections. If you are using this reference for a research paper on a specific topic, simply start at the index or list of entries to guide you through the encyclopedia. Moreover, the further reading sections at the end of every work will provide you with additional references for your investigation. Finally, if you have an inquisitive mind and are a lifelong learner, allow yourself to be immersed in this ever-growing field of mental health as detailed in entries in these three volumes. You will find interesting and valuable information about this ever-developing field that may just pique your interest as it has mine.

Concluding Note

While this encyclopedia broadly overviews the expanding field of mental health in its extensive number of entries, it does not provide complete information on any one topic. The "Recommended Resources" section at the end of volume three provides readers with additional information to explore selected topics more fully. Furthermore, the material in this encyclopedia is not intended to be used for diagnostic purposes or for psychological treatment. While self-knowledge can be very helpful, it is not a substitute for professional help. Finally, because indications for psychological treatments continually change, readers are advised to seek updates from health professionals, professional literature, or authoritative websites.

Acknowledgments

This project was a joy to work on as it allowed me to share my passion about mental health and well-being with everyone. However, this project was enormous and could not have been completed without the help and devotion of my coeditors, Alexandra Cunningham, PhD, Melissa Mariani, PhD, Mindy Parsons, PhD, and Steven Vensel, PhD, and the other contributing authors.

Len Sperry, MD, PhD

Introduction: Mental Health

Mental health is a continuum, ranging from states of well-being to stressful life experiences to severe mental disorders. We hope that readers of *Mental Health and Mental Disorders: An Encyclopedia of Conditions, Treatments, and Well-Being* will find it a useful reference source for specific purposes like academic assignments, term papers, job reports, or, more generally, for better understanding themselves and others.

This three-volume encyclopedia is subtitled *An Encyclopedia of Conditions, Treatments, and Well-Being.* The following paragraphs will focus on these three concepts: conditions or mental disorders, treatments, and well-being. Before that let's first look at mental health.

Mental Health

So what is mental health? Mental health can be thought of as successful mental functioning that results in productive activities, fulfilling relationships, and the ability to cope with change and adversity. Another way of saying this is that mental health is indispensable to effective personal functioning, interpersonal and family relationships, and community life.

Change exerts a constant influence on mental health and can be a major source of anxiety for many in their personal and professional lives. Change, by itself, whether for good or not, can be a source of stress and can negatively influence mental health. For example, technological changes continue at an accelerating pace, and while they can be useful to many individuals, they pose a stressful challenge to others.

Advances in health care can positively or negatively affect mental health. For example, older adults today have increased their life and health expectancies compared with Americans 10 years ago. That means that those over the age of 65 have fewer physical health concerns. But a decline in mental faculties among an increasing number of aging adults can create significant mental health concerns. For instance, dementia and Alzheimer's disease were not major health and mental health concerns in the past because relatively few lived past the age of 60. In 1900 there were 120,000 Americans over age 85, while today there are more than 4 million older adults of that age, making them the fastest-growing age group. The U.S. Census Bureau estimates that by 2030 there will be 72 million adults over the age of 65, which represents 20% of the American population. Among those 85 and older it is estimated that 50% will be diagnosed with Alzheimer's disease (Vincent and Velkof, 2010). The point of these examples is that mental health and mental disorders are influenced by various factors.

Mental Disorders

Mental disorders are primarily disorders of the brain. These conditions usually have multiple causes and result from complex interactions between individuals' genes and their environment. Lifestyle factors and health behaviors, like smoking and exercise, and life experiences, such as severe and prolonged stress or a history of abuse, are such factors. Typically, such factors interact with an individual's genetic or biological predisposition to a mental disorder. For example, a traumatic brain injury or a mother's exposure to viruses or toxic chemicals while pregnant may play a part. Other factors that can increase the risk for mental illness are the use of illegal drugs or having a serious medical condition like cancer. Research on the causality of mental illness has convincingly replaced the now-disproved belief that mental illness is a moral failure.

Mental illnesses occur at similar rates around the world, in every culture and in all socioeconomic groups. Statistics reveal that one in five individuals suffer from a mental disorder. This represents at least 20% of Americans. However, only one-fourth of those individuals with disorders are receiving treatment (SAMHSA, 2014). And, currently, only about 4% of America's health-care budget is spent on mental health treatment and prevention.

The *Diagnostic and Statistical Manual of Mental Disorders, Fifth Edition* (called DSM-5), published by the American Psychiatric Association, provides a common language and standard criteria for the classification of mental disorders. It is the most commonly used clarification system in North America. It classifies mental disorders into categories. There are more than 20 categories of which the following are the most common.

- Anxiety disorders are disturbances in brain mechanisms designed to protect you from harm.
- Mood disorders are disturbances in usual mood states.
- Psychotic disorders are disturbances of thinking perception and behavior.
- Personality disorders are maladaptive personal characteristics.
- Eating disorders are disturbances of weight and feeding behavior.
- Substance-related and addiction disorders are disturbances of cravings.
- Neurodevelopmental disorders are early disturbances in usual brain development.
- Trauma- and stressor-related disorders are disturbances related to significant stressful events.

For example, post-traumatic stress disorder (PTSD) is one of the trauma- and stressor-related disorders. It is a common occurrence in those who witnessed or survived traumatic situations. Many veterans of the war in Iraq and Afghanistan suffer from PTSD and experience symptoms of flashbacks, nightmares, feelings of constant vigilance, and depression. But not all who were deployed to Iraq experience PTSD. Rather, it is most likely to occur in those with a biological predisposition.

Depression is a mental disorder experienced by more than 120 million American adults each year. Depression is a leading cause of drug and alcohol use. Sleep difficulties result in nearly 50 million prescriptions being written for sleep medications per year. Many individuals manage their anxieties by overeating or smoking. Over time, unhealthy ways of coping take their toll on physical as well as mental health, particularly in those who are predisposed to such conditions.

Treatment

Significant advances have been made in the treatment of mental disorders. This increased understanding of the causes of mental health disorders (at least some of them) and increasingly effective treatments allow clinicians to better tailor treatment to those disorders. As a result, many mental health disorders can now be treated almost as effectively as medical conditions.

Generally, treatment for mental health disorders is characterized as either somatic (biological) or psychological. Somatic treatments include drugs, electroconvulsive therapy, and other therapies that stimulate the brain. Psychological treatments include psychotherapy (individual, group, or family and marital), behavior therapy techniques (e.g., relaxation training or exposure therapy), and hypnotherapy. Research suggests that for major mental health disorders like major depressive disorder, a treatment approach involving both drugs and psychotherapy is more effective than either treatment method used alone.

Clinicians who treat mental disorders include psychiatrists, clinical psychologists, mental health counselors, social workers, and psychiatric nurse practitioners. However, in most states, psychiatrists and psychiatric nurse practitioners are the only mental health clinicians licensed to prescribe drugs. Other clinicians practice psychotherapy primarily. Many primary care doctors and other medical specialists also prescribe drugs to treat mental health disorders.

Well-Being

In the past, mental health treatments focused largely on reducing symptoms or returning the individuals to their previous level of functioning. Today, however, treatment may also focus on increasing individuals' functioning, resilience, and prevention. This focus is known as well-being. Well-being is defined as how individuals think about and experience their lives. It is an indicator of how well individuals perceive their lives to be going. It reflects several health, job, family, and social outcomes. Accordingly, higher levels of well-being are associated with decreased risk of disease, illness, and injury. It is associated with faster recovery for illness, better immunity, increased longevity, and better mental health. Those with high levels of well-being are more productive at work, tend to get along better with others, and are more likely to contribute to their communities.

While there is not yet consensus among researchers or clinicians on the definition of well-being, most agree that well-being involves the presence of positive emotions and the absence of negative emotions. Most would agree that it includes satisfaction with life, a sense of personal fulfillment, and positive functioning. In short, it is about judging life positively and feeling good. Furthermore, most agree that well-being is broader and more inclusive than mental health. In fact, several kinds of well-being can be described and are currently being researched. These are physical well-being, economic well-being, social well-being, emotional well-being, and psychological well-being. Depression, anxieties, addictive behaviors, and severe physical pain make it difficult to attain and maintain well-being. The reason is that these conditions interfere with the ability to see beyond one's immediate negative experience.

Further Reading

SAMSHA. November 20, 2014. "Nearly One in Five Adult Americans Experienced Mental Illness in 2013." Substance Abuse and Mental Health Services Administration (SAMSHA). http://www.samhsa.gov/newsroom/press-announcements/201411200815.

Vincent, Grayson K., and Virginia A. Velkof. "The Next Four Decades: The Older Population in the United States, 2010 to 2050." Current Population Reports, SP25–1138. Washington, DC: U.S. Census Bureau, 2010.

Abandonment

Abandonment is a psychological concept that defines a set of emotional reactions and behavioral responses to perceptions of rejection or loss in personal relationships.

Description

Abandonment, sometimes referred to as "abandonment issues," is a psychological concept related to the fear of rejection, loss, and helplessness in personal relationships. Abandonment issues develop in childhood, cause stress in relationship, and are treatable. Abandonment issues are associated with intense feelings of fear, sadness, loneliness, anger, and worry in response to perceived rejection and disapproval. Breaking up with a boyfriend or girlfriend, not being accepted by peers, someone not returning a phone call, or not being included in activities are examples of events that can cause feelings of abandonment. Abandonment dynamics are not identified as a specific psychological diagnosis but are included in the list of symptoms of various disorders such as borderline personality disorder and attachment disorders.

Abandonment dynamics involve how events are perceived and the intensity of feelings resulting from those perceptions. Perceptions are the thoughts and beliefs about the event. Feelings are the emotional reaction connected to the thoughts and beliefs. For example, it would be appropriate for an individual who was not asked to go to the movies with a group of friends to feel disappointed. If the person believes he or she was not included because friends thought the person was not available, even though available, the person perceives he or she was not included due to a misunderstanding about schedules. The person may feel disappointed or annoyed but is able to quickly get over it. A person with abandonment issues would perceive this as a personal rejection. The person would excessively worry over what he or she may have done to cause the rejection. The person may become enraged at being treated that way and spend days thinking about it and wondering why he or she was treated so unfairly. People with abandonment issues take things very personal and perceive events as extremely hurtful and are often overwhelmed by emotion.

Abandonment issues develop in childhood and are related to physical or emotional neglect and loss. Children need unconditional love and nurture. The loss of a parent through divorce, prolonged separation, or death can result in abandonment issues. A child who is emotionally abandoned may have one or both parents in the home but receive little love, guidance, warmth, approval, or emotional support from them. A child who is physically neglected by parents grows up alone, helpless, and rejected. Neglect and loss cause intense emotions, which become part of the child's personality. Neglect and loss in childhood can result in individuals who are always on the lookout for signs of being abandoned. Adults with abandonment issues are extremely insecure and sensitive.

Symptoms of abandonment include the following categories and examples:

- Clinging: desperation to remain close, needing constant reassurance of approval, an excessive need for affection and attention.
- Emotional blackmail: Use of threats of self-harm or rejection to continue the relationship.

- Low self-worth: personal value is determined by how others feel about you.
- Overreaction: excessive fear or panic reactions to small matters such as someone not answering a phone or not calling back right away.
- Submissive behaviors: doing things you do not want to do to keep others from rejecting you.

Current Status

Overcoming abandonment issues requires the help of mental health professionals. Talking therapies such as cognitive behavior therapy or dialectical behavior therapy can be effective in the treatment of abandonment issues. The focus of treatment is to decrease the emotional intensity and excessive behaviors associated with abandonment perceptions. Psychiatric medications are not prescribed in the direct treatment of abandonment issues but may be prescribed for individuals suffering from excessive anxiety and panic that is often associated with abandonment issues.

Steven R. Vensel, PhD

See also: Borderline Personality Disorder; Foster Care; Neglect

Further Reading

Lamay, Edward P., Jr., and Kari L. Dudley. "Caution: Fragile! Regulating the Interpersonal Security of Chronically Insecure Partners." *Journal of Personality and Social Psychology* 100, no. 4 (2011): 681–702.

Mikulincer, Mario, and Phillip R. Shaver. *Attachment in Adulthood: Structure, Dynamics, and Change.* New York, NY: The Guilford Press, 2007.

Abilify (Aripiprazole)

Abilify is an atypical antipsychotic medication useful in treating the symptoms of schizophrenia and bipolar disorder and agitation in dementia. Its generic name is aripiprazole.

Definitions

- **Atypical antipsychotics** are a newer group of antipsychotic medications that are useful in treating schizophrenia and other psychotic disorders.
- **Extrapyramidal symptoms** are side effects caused by certain antipsychotic drugs. They include repetitive, involuntary muscle movements, such as lip smacking, and the urge to be moving constantly.
- **Hallucinations** are false or distorted sensory perceptions that appear to be real perceptions. They are generated by the mind rather than by an external stimuli and can be caused by a medication, recreational drug, or mental disorder.

Description

Abilify is part of a class of drugs called atypical antipsychotics. They are called "atypical" because of their relatively lower risk of certain adverse side effects compared to traditional antipsychotic drugs. Abilify is useful in the short-term treatment of acute psychotic and acute manic states, as well as agitation in dementia. It is also used in the long-term treatment of chronic psychotic disorders. Abilify is thought to work by influencing dopamine, the neurotransmitter (chemical messengers) that affects movement and balance. Abilify appears to bind to dopamine receptors in the brain and prevent dopamine from fully activating them. This differs from traditional antipsychotics, which completely block dopamine receptors. Besides resulting in some relief of psychotic symptoms, these conventional drugs can cause severe movement side effects, called extrapyramidal symptoms, which Abilify does not.

Precautions and Side Effects

Abilify may increase the risk for diabetes, so those who are taking it and develop extreme thirst, frequent urination, or other diabetes symptoms should consult a physician. Women who are pregnant, intend to become pregnant, or are nursing should talk to their physician before beginning or discontinuing Abilify. There is increased risk for extrapyramidal symptoms, and withdrawal symptoms in newborns whose mothers took Abilify during their third trimester of pregnancy.

Because Abilify can cause drowsiness and impair judgment and motor skills, individuals are advised not to operate a motor vehicle or machinery. Since it has a sedative effect, alcohol use should be limited when taking Abilify. Because Abilify can affect the body's ability to regulate temperature, potentially leading to overheating and dehydration, those taking it should be cautious when exercising.

While Abilify tends to cause fewer neurological side effects than the traditional antipsychotic medications, it does have some side effects. The most common ones are anxiety, constipation, difficulty sleeping, dizziness, drowsiness, headache, nausea, nervousness, numbness, tremor, vomiting, and weight gain. Because it can cause significant weight gain and the development of metabolic syndrome (prediabetes), a practitioner may use Glucophage (metformin—the generic name for this diabetes drug) in patients who may be developing this syndrome, in an effort to avoid the development of diabetes and cardiovascular disease.

Len Sperry, MD, PhD

See also: Antipsychotic Medications; Dopamine; Tourette's Syndrome

Further Reading

Mondimore, Francis Mark. *Bipolar Disorder: A Guide for Patients and Families*, 2nd ed. Baltimore, MD: Johns Hopkins University Press, 2006.

Preston, John D., John H. O'Neal, and Mary C. Talaga. *Handbook of Clinical Psychopharmacology for Therapists*, 7th ed. Oakland, CA: New Harbinger, 2013.

Stahl, Stephen M. *The Prescriber's Guide: Antipsychotics and Mood Stabilizers. Stahl's Essential Psychopharmacology.* Cambridge, UK: Cambridge University Press, 2009.

Torrey, E. Fuller. *Surviving Schizophrenia: A Manual for Families, Patients, and Providers*, 5th ed. New York, NY: Harper Collins, 2006.

Abuse

Abuse is the intentional physical, psychological, or sexual maltreatment of an individual.

Definitions

- **Adverse childhood experience** is a traumatic experience in an individual's life that occurs before the age of 18 and is remembered as an adult. The three main types are abuse (e.g., sexual), neglect (e.g., emotional), and household dysfunction (e.g., divorce).

- **Child abuse** is the physical, sexual, or emotional abuse of a child or minor, usually under the age of 18.

- **Domestic abuse** is the abuse by one partner against the other in an intimate relationship. It can involve physical, sexual, and/or psychological abuse.

- **Elder abuse** is the physical, sexual, or emotional abuse of individuals, usually one who is disabled or frail.

- **Neglect** involves refusal or failure by those responsible to provide food, shelter, health care, or protection for a vulnerable elder.

- **Physical abuse** involves inflicting, or threatening to inflict, physical pain or injury on individuals or depriving them of a basic need.

- **Psychological abuse** involves inflicting mental pain, anguish, or distress on individuals through verbal or nonverbal acts. It is also called emotional abuse.

- **Sexual abuse** involves nonconsensual sexual contact of any kind, coercing an elder to witness sexual behaviors.

Description

Abuse is any action that intentionally harms or injures an individual. There are several types of abuse. These include neglect, physical abuse, sexual abuse, elder abuse, and psychological abuse. Substance abuse is another type of abuse. All forms of abuse in the United States are illegal and carry criminal penalties. A brief overview of the common forms of abuse across the lifespan follows.

Child abuse. Child abuse is a crime that all health and social service professionals are mandated to report. It takes various forms. The four main types are neglect, physical abuse, sexual abuse, and emotional abuse. The 2010 Child Maltreatment Report (NCANDS) found that neglect was the most common form of child abuse. It accounted for 78.3% of cases. By comparison, physical abuse accounted for 17.6% of cases. Sexual abuse accounted for 9.2% of cases, while psychological abuse accounted for 8.1% of cases. Adverse childhood experiences such as childhood sexual abuse may significantly impact the individual's health in adulthood.

Sexual abuse. "Sexual abuse" refers to nonconsensual sexual behavior between two adults, between an adult and child, or between two children, one of whom is forcefully dominant or significantly older. Sexual behaviors can include touching breasts, genitals, and buttocks while the victim is either dressed or undressed. Sexual abuse is also a reportable crime.

Domestic violence. Domestic violence involves abuse of an individual by another with whom the victim is living, has lived with, or is in a significant relationship. It is also known as domestic abuse, spousal abuse, battering, family violence, and intimate partner violence. It also includes rape. It can involve physical, psychological, and/or sexual abuse, including rape. The National Coalition Against Domestic Violence estimates that 1 in 5 women and 1 in 33 men will be the victim of a rape or an attempted rape during their lifetime.

Elder abuse. Like child abuse, elder abuse is also a reportable crime. It can also involve emotional abuse, neglect, physical abuse, or sexual abuse. Often, more than one type of abuse occurs. It is committed by caretakers and may occur in the home or in a residential facility. The National Center on Elder Abuse reported that in 2013 nearly 6 million cases of elder abuse were reported.

Len Sperry, MD, PhD

See also: Adverse Childhood Experience; Child Abuse; Elder Abuse; Neglect; Sexual Abuse

Further Reading

Crosson-Tower, Cynthia. *Understanding Child Abuse and Neglect*, 9th ed. New York, NY: Pearson, 2013.

Engel, Beverly. *The Emotionally Abusive Relationship: How to Stop Being Abused and How to Stop Abusing.* New York, NY: Wiley, 2002.

Evans, Patricia. *The Verbally Abusive Relationship: How to Recognize It and How to Respond*, 3rd ed. Avon, MA: Adams Media, 2013.

Payne, Brian K. *Crime and Elder Abuse: An Integrated Perspective*, 3rd ed. Springfield, IL: Charles C. Thomas Publishers, 2011.

Help Hotlines in the United States

Childhelp National Child Abuse Hotline 1-800-4-A-CHILD. TDD for the Deaf 1-800-2-A-Child. Help for children who are being abused or adults who are concerned that a child they know is being abused or neglected.

Elder Abuse Hotline 1-800-252-8966. Assistance in reporting and counseling about elder abuse.

National Domestic Violence Hotline 1-800-799-SAFE (7233). TTY for the Deaf: 1-800-787-3224. Help for both men and women who are victims of domestic violence.

Abusive Personality

"Abusive personality" is a term used to describe the personality of those who criticize, dominate, undermine, and physically harm their intimate partners (spouses).

Definitions

- **Abuse** is any behavior that intends to harm another's self-esteem or restrict autonomy (independence).

- **Antisocial personality disorder** is a mental disorder characterized by a pattern of disregarding and violating the rights of others.

- **Borderline personality disorder** is a mental disorder characterized by a pattern of instability in interpersonal relationships, self-image, affects, self-harm, and a high degree of impulsivity.

- **Domestic violence** is a form of abuse between intimate partners (spouses). It is also called domestic abuse.

- **DSM-5** stands for the *Diagnostic and Statistical Manual of Mental Disorders, Fifth Edition*, which is a diagnostic system used by professionals to identify mental disorders with specific diagnostic criteria.

- **Emotional abuse** is a form of abuse characterized by a person subjecting or exposing another to behavior that may result in anxiety, chronic depression, or post-traumatic stress disorder.

- **Intermittent explosive disorder** is mental disorder characterized by impulsive, aggressive, violent behavior or angry verbal outbursts.

- **Male privilege** is the belief in some societies that men have power which exempts them from certain responsibility which women are expected to perform because of their subordinate status.

- **Post-traumatic stress disorder** is a mental disorder characterized by nightmares, emotional numbing, and recurrent flashbacks of a traumatic event that an individual experienced or witnessed.

- **Spousal battering** is a type of domestic violence which involves a systematic pattern of intimidation, control, terror, and physical violence for the purpose of gaining total control over the partner.

- **Trauma symptoms** are any symptoms (anxiety, angry outburst, depression, etc.) that occur as a result of a severely distressing event.

Description

The abusive personality is a psychological profile of individuals (usually males) who engage in a pattern of criticism, domination, undermining, and physical harm to their intimate partners. This profile and pattern has been described in detail by the research of Canadian psychologist Donald Dutton (1943–). He found that these individuals tend to be jealous, easily threatened, and fearful. They also tend to mask these feeling with anger and controlling behavior. Dutton's research indicates that these individuals also show borderline personality or antisocial personality disorder behaviors. They are also likely to display chronic trauma symptoms. Most have a history of physical abuse, shaming, and rejection as children.

Dutton's research also found that this pattern of abusiveness is more than learned behavior. It is also the outgrowth of particular personality dynamics, typically the antisocial or borderline personalities. Among those with the abusive personality, the borderline personality is the more common. According to Dutton, the individual's abusive behavior results from the cyclical and unstable dynamics of this personality disorder. This abusiveness has a cyclic pattern: tension building, spousal battering, and contrition and the resolve to never hurt the partner again.

While this characterization of the abusive personality emphasizes personality dynamics and early life experiences, it is limited. It does not include other considerations such as biological factors, social factors, nor the feminist view, particularly of male privilege. In this view, domestic violence against women by men is "caused" by the misuse of power and control because of male privilege. DSM-5 does not have a specific diagnosis for abusive personality. However, if the diagnostic criteria for intermittent explosive disorder are met, this diagnosis can be used to identify this abusive pattern.

Len Sperry, MD, PhD

See also: Antisocial Personality Disorder; Borderline Personality Disorder; Domestic Violence

Further Reading

American Psychiatric Association. *Diagnostic and Statistical Manual of Mental Disorders* (DSM), 5th ed. Arlington, VA: American Psychiatric Association Press, 2013.

Dutton, Donald G. *The Abusive Personality: Violence and Control in Intimate Relationships*, 2nd ed. New York, NY: The Guilford Press, 2008.

Ellis, Albert, and Marcia Grad Powers. *The Secret of Overcoming Verbal Abuse: Getting Off the Emotional Roller Coaster and Regaining Control of Your Life.* Chatsworth, CA: Wilshire Book Co., 2001.

Acceptance and Commitment Therapy (ACT)

Acceptance and commitment therapy is a psychological treatment approach that assists individuals to accept what is outside their control and commit to action that enriches their lives. It is also known as ACT.

Definitions

- **Acceptance** is the process of opening up, making room, and dropping the struggle for painful feelings and sensations.

- **Cognitive defusion** is the process of stepping back or detaching from unhelpful thoughts, worries, and memories.

- **Committed action** is action guided by one's values.

- **Mindfulness** is conscious awareness of the present moment with openness and non-evaluation.

- **Observing self** is that part of the individual that is responsible for awareness and attention. It is separate from but aware of the thinking self.

- **Psychological flexibility** is the capacity to live in the present moment fully as a conscious human being.

- **Relational frame theory** is a framework for describing the relationship between two entities based on prior experience.

- **Third-wave approaches** are a type of behavior therapy that emphasizes acceptance and mindfulness.

Description

Acceptance and commitment therapy (ACT) is a form of behavior therapy that assists individuals to increase their acceptance of difficult and painful experiences and to increase their commitment to action that can improve and enrich their lives. ACT assumes that suffering results from the avoidance of emotional pain rather than the experience of it. It also assumes that language is at the root of most problems, particularly when it generates negative thoughts.

Instead of reducing symptoms like other treatment approaches, the goal of ACT is to learn how to accept and detach from them. When acceptance occurs, symptom reduction is a by-product. ACT treatment involves the use of metaphors, exercises, behavioral interventions, and mindfulness skills training. It uses mindfulness skills to develop psychological flexibility and clarify and foster values-based living.

Acceptance of situations without evaluation or attempts to change them is a skill that is developed through mindfulness exercises in and out of session. Instead of attempting to directly change or stop unwanted thoughts or feelings, ACT focuses on developing a mindful relationship with those experiences that can free an individual to be more receptive to take action that are life giving. ACT has proven effective with several clinical conditions. These include anxiety, depression, stress, chronic pain, anorexia (eating disorder), heroin and marijuana abuse, and schizophrenia.

ACT utilizes six basic principles and strategies to develop psychological flexibility in clients. (1) Acceptance is a strategy for allowing thoughts to come and go without struggling with them. (2) Cognitive defusion is a strategy for reducing the tendency to be dominated by negative or painful thoughts, images, emotions, and memories. (3) Contact with the present moment is a strategy for increasing awareness of the present moment and experiencing it with openness and receptiveness. (4) Observing the self is a strategy for accessing a continuity of consciousness which is unchanging. (5) Values is a strategy for discovering what is most important to the true self. (6) Committed action is a strategy for setting goals based on basic values and achieving them in a responsible manner.

Developments and Current Status

ACT was developed by psychologist Steven C. Hayes (1948–) in the 1980s. It is an outgrowth of behavioral therapy and cognitive behavior therapy (CBT). It is based on relational frame theory, which is its underlying theory of human language and cognition. ACT is also based on functional contextualism, which means that instead of viewing clients as damaged or flawed as many other approaches, it focuses instead on identifying the function and context of behavior. ACT is considered one of the new third-wave behavior therapies that build on older behavior therapies (first wave) and cognitive therapies (second wave). ACT is a therapeutic approach that is attracting attention and research support. It is increasingly being taught in graduate programs and practiced in various treatment settings. It also has garnered considerable research support. As of 2011 there were approximately 60 research studies that demonstrate the effectiveness of ACT.

Len Sperry, MD, PhD

See also: Behavior Therapy; Cognitive Behavior Therapy; Mindfulness

Further Reading

Eifert, Georg H., and John P. Forsyth. *Acceptance and Commitment Therapy for Anxiety Disorders: A Practitioner's Treatment Guide to Using Mindfulness, Acceptance, and Value-Guide Behavior Change Strategies.* Oakland, CA: New Harbinger, 2005.

Hayes, Steven, Victoria Follette, and Marsha Linehan, eds. *Mindfulness and Acceptance: Expanding the Cognitive-Behavioral Tradition.* New York, NY: Guilford Press, 2004.

Hayes, Steven C., and Spencer Smith. *Get Out of Your Mind and Into Your Life: The New Acceptance and Commitment Therapy.* Oakland, CA: New Harbinger, 2005.

Hayes, Steven C., and Kirk D. Strosahl. *A Practical Guide to Acceptance and Commitment Therapy.* New York, NY: Springer, 2004.

Hayes, Steven C., Kirk D. Strosahl, and Kelly G. Wilson. *Acceptance and Commitment Therapy: An Experiential Approach to Behavior Change.* New York, NY: Guilford Press, 2003.

Acculturation and Assimilation

Acculturation and assimilation are terms used to describe the process of adapting to cultural differences between the minority and majority group.

Definitions

- **Acculturative stress** defines the psychological, somatic, and social challenges that members of a racial or ethnic minority group experience as they adapt to the culture of the majority group.

- **Biculturalism** refers to the coexistence of two separate, distinct cultures.

- **Culture** defines the customary language, practices, attitudes, and traditions of a particular racial or ethnic group.

- **Enculturation** describes the process of first-culture learning typically experienced by infants or young children as they grow up and encounter their primary culture.

Description

"Acculturation" refers to the change process that one goes through when moving from one culture to another. This process is interactive and continuous. The terms "acculturation" and "assimilation" are often used interchangeably. *Enculturation* explains an individual's first-culture, or primary culture, learning experience. Acculturation would then be described as a second-culture learning experience. Several minority groups, immigrants, refugees, and indigenous peoples encounter assimilation issues when they come in contact with the dominant culture. Differences in language, food, and dress are often most apparent though varying beliefs, customs, and practices may also exist.

Anthropologists, psychologists, and sociologists have been investigating the concept of acculturation since the early 1900s and have focused primarily on the adaptations minority group members make in order to ease their transitions. John Wesley Powell first coined the term "acculturation" in an 1880 U.S. Bureau of American Ethnography report and subsequently used it to describe the psychological changes that resulted from cross-cultural imitation. A more widely used definition was proposed by Redfield, Linton, and Herskovits in 1936 defining acculturation as the process of change that happens when groups of individuals from different cultures come into contact with one another. Numerous variations of this definition have followed.

Multiple theories on acculturation have been developed. One of the most popular is a fourfold model that focuses on two dimensions. The first dimension relates to whether the individual retains or rejects his or her native culture and the second dimension relates to the individual's adoption or denial of the majority culture. Four strategies of acculturation can result: assimilation, separation, integration, or marginalization.

Individuals who assimilate adopt the cultural norms of the majority over their minority culture. If separation occurs, the individual rejects the majority culture and preserves his or her native customs. Group members who integrate adopt the norms of the dominant culture while still maintaining their original cultural identity. Those who are able to integrate the two are referred to as *bicultural*. Finally, marginalization is defined as when an individual rejects both the native culture and the culture of the majority group. Research suggests that while some individuals maintain one acculturation strategy, others may adopt different strategies in their public and private lives. Likewise, varying strategies may be applied to particular areas (religion, politics, education, and family values) depending on the value the individual places on them.

One's arrival to a new place can be coupled with positive and negative emotions. "Culture shock" is defined as the transitional anxiety one experiences on leaving familiar people and surroundings and replacing them with unfamiliar words, food, clothing, and customs. Pressure to conform to the dominant group's culture can also result in *acculturative stress* referring to the psychological, somatic, and social stress experienced by minority group members as they attempt to assimilate. Stress and anxiety can be compounded if either side lacks multicultural competence or if prejudicial/discriminatory views are held. Societal attitudes regarding multiculturalism can impact the acculturation process. Melting pot societies promote assimilation, group differences are respected, but blending among groups is expected. The opposite is seen in a segregationist society where various groups lack understanding and remain isolated from one another. In a multiculturalist society diversity is valued and members acculturate more gradually, slowly integrating the dominant culture into their lives. Simultaneously, members of the larger culture become exposed to and learn to respect aspects of the minority groups' culture.

Current Status and Impact (Psychological Influence)

Research regarding acculturation and assimilation continues to be conducted on immigrants, refugees, and indigenous peoples of all ages. Studies have examined various acculturation styles, resiliency factors, and similarities/differences across subgroups. Evidence suggests that certain protective factors are associated with positive outcomes, including the existence of social support and engaging in active coping styles. Findings also suggest that communication plays a central role in the acculturation process. Language development and fluency can facilitate or impede the rate at which one assimilates. Furthermore, effective communication between minority and majority group members has been associated with shorter transition periods, reduced levels of anxiety and stress, fewer conflicts, more personal connections, and positive emotions.

Melissa A. Mariani, PhD

See also: Acculturative Stress

Further Reading

Akhtar, Salman. *Immigration and Acculturation: Mourning, Adaptation, and the Next Generation*. Lanham, MD: Rowman & Littlefield, 2014.

Berry, John W., Jean S. Phinney, David L. Sam, and Paul Vedder. *Immigrant Youth in Cultural Transition: Acculturation, Identity, and Adaptation across National Contexts*. New York, NY: Psychology Press, 2012.

Sam, David L., and John W. Berry, eds. *The Cambridge Handbook of Acculturation Psychology*. Cambridge, UK: Cambridge University Press, 2006.

Acculturative Stress

"Acculturative stress" refers to the psychological, somatic, and social difficulties that members of a racial or ethnic minority group experience as they adapt to the culture of the majority group.

Definitions

- **Acculturation** describes the acclimation process people go through when moving from one culture to another.

- **Assimilation** refers to the gradual adaptation of a minority group member's customs, attitudes, and practices to those of the majority culture.

- **Culture** defines the customary language, practices, attitudes, and traditions of a particular racial or ethnic group.

Description

When an individual, family, or group moves from one place to another, they typically encounter differences between the cultures of their former residence and their new one. The process of reconciling cultural differences between the minority and majority group is known as *acculturation* or *assimilation*. Acculturation has been observed in most immigrants who relocate. Minority group members may feel self-imposed pressure to adjust or may perceive or experience pressure from the majority group to assimilate.

Adapting to a new culture can result in stress and anxiety. The term "acculturative stress" refers to the psychological, somatic, and emotional challenges that minority group members face as they attempt to adapt to the culture of the majority group. Changes in food, clothing, and surroundings may be more apparent while differences in attitudes, perceptions, traditions, and views may show up more gradually over time. Language proficiency of residents is often assumed, which can be a significant source of pressure and anxiety for immigrants. Lack of intercultural competence and discrimination can also contribute to challenges with acculturating. Families from foreign countries may immigrate in waves, meaning that all members may not be experiencing acculturation issues at the same time. In addition, children of immigrants tend to assimilate more quickly than parents/older minority group members providing another possible source of conflict.

Assimilation takes time and can be either a seamless process or a more difficult one depending on various factors. Protective factors that ease this transition include having positive relationships with others and healthy coping mechanisms. Social support can come from multiple sources such as family members, peers, mentors, and other significant individuals in one's life who can provide different levels and forms of ease. Active, rather than avoidant, coping strategies have also been linked to resiliency and more favorable outcomes. Active coping strategies include having realistic expectations, attempting to problem-solve, using humor, engaging in physical activity, and practicing calming/relaxation techniques.

Current Status and Impact (Psychological Influence)

Much research on the topic of acculturative stress has focused on college students who have immigrated in order to further their education in different countries. Moving away from one's support system while incurring financial, academic, and social pressure can be difficult for students. Acculturative stress has been associated with reduced academic performance, decreased levels of social engagement, and impaired physical health. Higher levels of depression and anxiety have also been noted in the literature for persons experiencing acculturative stress. Many studies have focused on the impact of acculturative stress on Latino, African American, and Asian families as traditionally these cultures have placed high value on familial relationships and a strong sense of interconnectedness.

Melissa A. Mariani, PhD

See also: Acculturation and Assimilation

Further Reading

Sam, David L., and John W. Berry, eds. *The Cambridge Handbook of Acculturation Psychology*. Cambridge, UK: Cambridge University Press, 2006.

Suarez-Morales, Lourdes, and Barbara Lopez. "The Impact of Acculturative Stress and Daily Hassles on Pre-adolescent Psychological Adjustment: Examining Anxiety Symptoms." *Journal of Primary Prevention* 30, no. 3 (2009): 335–349.

Ward, Colleen, Stephen Bochner, and Adrian Furnham. *The Psychology of Culture Shock*, 2nd ed. Philadelphia, PA: Routledge, 2001.

Wong, Paul T.P., and Lillian C.J. Wong. *Handbook of Multicultural Perspectives on Stress and Coping*. New York, NY: Springer, 2006.

Acetylcholine

Acetylcholine is a chemical messenger in the brain that is involved in learning and memory.

Definitions

- **Acetylcholine esterase inhibitors** are medications that block the action of acetylcholinesterase which is the enzyme that degrades

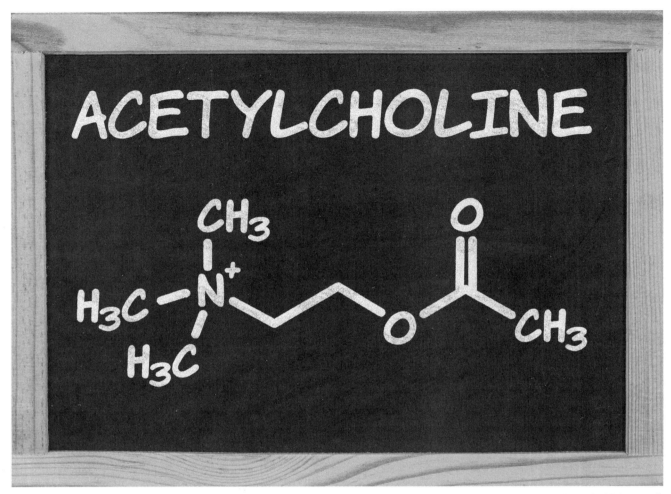

Acetylcholine is a neurotransmitter and among other functions is involved in learning and memory. People with Alzheimer's disease have greatly diminished amounts of acetylcholine. (Zerbor/Dreamstime.com)

(breaks down) acetylcholine and increases it in the brain.

- **Alzheimer's disease** is a progressive neurodegenerative disease in which dementia results from the degeneration and death of brain cells because of low levels of acetylcholine, plaques, and neurofibrillary tangles.

Description

Acetylcholine is a neurotransmitter (chemical messenger) in the brain. Acetylcholine was the first neurotransmitter to be discovered. It has various functions in both the peripheral and central nervous systems.

In the peripheral nervous system, it plays a vital role in activating muscles. In the central nervous system it acts as a major neurotransmitter for the autonomic nervous system, which controls heart, respiration, and secretion. Acetylcholine plays a vital role in maintaining all these functions.

It is also involved in learning and memory, and is greatly diminished in those with Alzheimer's disease. Some Alzheimer's medications work by inhibiting the action of acetylcholine esterase. Called acetylcholinesterase inhibitors, these medications increase acetylcholine levels in the brain. They appear to slow down the rate of cognitive decline in the early stages of Alzheimer's disease. These medications include Aricept, Reminyl, Cognex, and Exelon.

Acetylcholine is made from choline. Choline is similar to the B vitamins and is found in foods such as liver, muscle meats, fish, nuts, beans, peas, spinach, wheat germ, and eggs. Choline is also available as nutritional supplements. Like prescribed acetylcholinesterase inhibitors, choline supplementation is used for memory loss, Alzheimer's disease, and dementia. It is also used for depression, chronic hepatitis, cirrhosis, Huntington's chorea, Tourette's disease, certain types of seizures, and schizophrenia. Athletes use it for bodybuilding and delaying fatigue in endurance sports. Choline is taken by pregnant women to prevent neural tube defects, and it is used as a supplement in infant formulas. Other uses include preventing cancer, lowering cholesterol, and controlling asthma.

Precautions and Side Effects

Choline supplementation is considered safe when taken by mouth and used appropriately. Doses up to 3.5 grams daily appear to be safe for most pregnant and breast-feeding women and are not likely to cause unwanted side effects. There are relatively few side effects of taking choline supplements. These include sweating, a fishy body odor, stomach pain, diarrhea, and vomiting. Sweating (hyperhidrosis) can be bothersome. It involves abnormally increased perspiration on the hands, feet, armpits, and the back. There are no medications interactions reported with choline.

Len Sperry, MD, PhD

See also: Alzheimer's Disease

Further Reading

Doraiswamy, P. Murali, Lisa Gwyther, and Tina Adler. *The Alzheimer's Action Plan: What You Need to Know—and What You Can Do—about Memory Problems, from Prevention to Early Intervention and Care.* New York, NY: St. Martin's Press, 2009.

Mace, Nancy, and Peter V. Ravins. *The 36-Hour Day: A Family Guide to Caring for People with Alzheimer Disease, Other Dementias, and Memory Loss in Later Life,* 5th ed. Baltimore, MD: Johns Hopkins University Press, 2012.

Stargrove, Mitchell Bebel. *Herb, Nutrient, and Drug Interactions: Clinical Implications and Therapeutic Strategies.* St. Louis, MO: Mosby, 2007.

Ulbricht, Catherine E. *Davis's Pocket Guide to Herbs and Supplements.* Philadelphia, PA: F.A. Davis, 2011.

Acupressure

The practice of acupressure dates back 5,000 years in China by physicians who noted the healing benefits of applying pressure to certain locations on the body. This type of therapy, alone or in conjunction with other methods, has been used to alleviate nausea, pain, fatigue, and stress/anxiety.

Definition

- **Acupressure** is an ancient art of healing that uses tactile manipulation of pressure points on the body to relieve pain and promote wellness.

Description

Acupressure is an ancient healing art that applies tactile pressure to determined locations throughout the body in an attempt to stimulate healing, relieve pain, alleviate stress, and promote positive energy. Twelve channels, or meridians, have been identified along which these points lie. These points have a high electrical conductivity at the skin's surface, making them potent healing sites. Applying pressure to these sites releases tension and increases circulation of blood throughout the body. Relief at the site where pressure is applied, as well as added benefits to internal organs, has been discovered.

Acupressure is similar to acupuncture; however, acupuncture uses needles, while acupressure uses firm pressure from the fingers and thumbs. Acupressure has been used to treat many conditions, including nausea, muscular pain, chronic fatigue, stress, anxiety, addiction, learning issues, and mental disorders. This type of therapy has also been used in patients seeking to promote healing, detoxify the body, boost overall wellness, and even stimulate sexual reproduction.

Development (History and Application)

Discovered in Asia over 5,000 years ago, acupressure is a healing/therapeutic technique that employs the use of pressure to alleviate discomfort and illness in the body. The origins of this type of therapy date back to the early Chinese dynasties; soldiers would use stones and arrows in wartime. Physicians noted that wounded soldiers reported no longer experiencing chronic symptoms that they had suffered from years prior. A logical connection was then made between the ensued trauma and subsequent healing. These physicians then began developing healing techniques that incorporated making cuts or applying pressure to certain pressure points in the body. Over the years, physicians came to a consensus upon 12 trigger points lying along the meridians in the body. These meridians, invisible lines of energy, flow from the fingertips to the brain as well as to other vital organs and organ systems throughout the body. The application of pressure at these sites was shown to stimulate healing, permitting positive energy to flow freely throughout the body.

Terminology used in acupressure therapy can vary. The Chinese refer to healing energy as Qi or Chi. Japanese use the term "Ki," to refer to the life force, and "Reiki," to refer to the healing energy. Yogis use the word "prana" to describe this same life force and refer to pranic energy. However, all of these terms relate to the same universal energy that links all forms of life. By applying pressure to acupoints, blocked energy is released and able to flow to sites in need of healing.

Acupressure methods and styles also vary. Some methods incorporate different rhythms and pressures at the pressure points. Other styles use not only the fingers but also the hands, arms, legs, and feet. Shiatsu therapy is the traditional form of Japanese acupressure. This type of therapy uses deep pressure applied to each pressure site for three to five seconds. Jin Shin acupressure is different from Shiatsu because instead of one pressure site, two are focused on, and pressure is gently applied for a minute or longer. Tuina Chinese Massage and Thai Massage use acupressure techniques in combination with full body stretches and massage.

Current Status

Acupressure therapy can be used a standalone treatment or in conjunction with other treatments such as herbal/nutritional therapy, meditation, stretching, massage therapy, and counseling. Though this type of therapy is considered safe, it should be conducted only by a licensed or certified practitioner.

Western medicine does not endorse acupressure as a reliable treatment method. Many medical practitioners do not even believe that the meridians exist. Instead they attribute the healing qualities of acupressure to factors such as muscle manipulation, increased blood flow, and the stimulation of endorphins, all of which are natural sources of pain relief.

Melissa A. Mariani, PhD

See also: Acupuncture

Further Reading

Ezzo, Jeanette, Konrad Streitberger, and Antonius Schneider. "Cochrane Systematic Reviews Examine P6 Acupuncture-Point Stimulation for Nausea and Vomiting." *Journal of Alternative Complementary Medicine* 12, no. 5 (2006): 489–495.

Gach, Michael R. *Acupressure's Potent Points.* New York, NY: Bantam Books, 1990.

Xinnong, Cheng. *Chinese Acupuncture and Moxibustion*, 3rd ed. Beijing, China: Foreign Language Press, 2010.

Acupuncture

Acupuncture is a Chinese medical procedure that treats medical conditions with needles inserted at specified sites of the body.

Definitions

- **Acupressure** is a form of massage using acupuncture points.

- **Auricular acupuncture** is a form of acupuncture using only points found on the ears to stimulate and balance various internal organs.

- **Chi** is basic life energy.

- **Meridian** is a channel through which chi travels in the body.

- **Traditional Chinese medicine** is an ancient but still practiced form of healing based on the harmony and balance. It emphasizes diet and prevention and uses acupuncture and herbal to stimulate the body's own natural curative powers and reestablish balance.

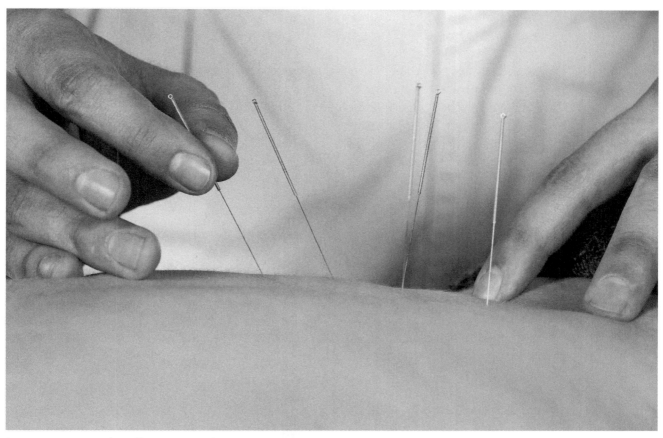

Acupuncture may be effective at reducing symptoms associated with certain mental disorders, such as depression, post-traumatic stress disorder, schizophrenia, bipolar disorder, and insomnia, but further research is needed. (Handmademedia/Dreamstime.com)

- **Yin and yang** are the two complementary forces in the universe. Life is better when there is a balance between yang (positive or masculine) and yin (negative or feminine).

Description

Acupuncture is a form of traditional Chinese medicine (TCM) in which sharp, thin needles are inserted in the skin at specific points of the body where the flow of energy is blocked. In TCM, disease is viewed as an imbalance in the organ system or chi meridians. The goal of treatment is to assist the body in reestablishing its balance. In TCM, disease can be caused by external factors such as the environmental stressors, by internal factors like emotional stressors, and other factors such as diet, injuries, or trauma. Infection is not viewed as a cause of disease but rather as weakness in the energy of

the body that permits illness. Acupuncture is believed to work by adjusting the flow of chi throughout the organ system, which strengthens the body and prompts it to physically or mentally heal itself.

Underlying the practice of TCM is a unique view of the world and of the human body that is very different from the scientific view of American medicine. A basic premise is that humans are microcosms of the larger, surrounding universe where everything is interconnected. The human body is made up various organs, tissues, and fluids which have distinct functions but are all interdependent. Health and disease involve degrees of balance or imbalance of these functions.

The theoretical framework of TCM has a number of key components. The first is yin-yang theory. Ying and yang are two opposing but complementary forces that shape the world and all life. The second is chi. It is the vital energy or life force that circulates in the body through a system of pathways called meridians. Health is an ongoing process of maintaining balance and harmony in the circulation of chi. The third is the eight principles that are used to analyze symptoms and categorize conditions. They are cold/heat, interior/exterior, excess/deficiency, and yin/yang. The fourth is the theory of five elements, which are fire, earth, metal, water, and wood. These elements help to explain how the body works and how these elements correspond to particular organs and tissues in the body. The *Yellow Emperor's Classic of Internal Medicine*, an ancient text written about 2,500 years ago, describes these components, principles, and elements.

In China, acupuncture is usually combined with herbal medicine. In Japan, acupuncture uses extremely thin needles and does not incorporate herbal medicine. Auricular acupuncture uses acupuncture points only on the ear, which are believed to stimulate and balance internal organs. In France, acupuncture is popular and widely accepted by the medical establishment. The medical establishment uses a system of acupuncture based on neuroendocrine theory rather than on TCM. Several forms of acupuncture are used in the United States with and without herbal medicine. Acupressure is also common.

Developments and Current Status

Acupuncture originated in China and has been practiced there for more than a thousand years. Acupuncture is also deeply embedded in the medical history of Japan, Korea, Vietnam, Taiwan, and other Asian regions. Although acupuncture had been used for hundreds of years ago in Europe, it was only during the second half of the 20th century that it began to spread rapidly in Western Europe, Canada, and the United States.

American medicine has been slow to accept acupuncture. Though many physicians use it, the American Medical Association does not recognize it as a specialty. Medical research in acupuncture is growing. The National Center for Complementary and Alternative Medicine of the National Institutes of Health funds research on acupuncture for medical conditions, such as chronic pain, anesthesia, and insomnia. When acupuncture is practiced by traditional medical professionals, its effectiveness to relieve pain is primarily believed to be due to acupuncture points being able

to stimulate muscles, nerves, and connective tissue, which act to increase the production of natural painkillers found within the body, and the increased flow of blood to these targeted locations. Some research has found that acupuncture is effective at reducing symptoms associated with other mental disorders, such as depression, post-traumatic stress disorder, schizophrenia, bipolar disorder, and insomnia. However, other medical studies do not support these findings, and further research into these applications is needed.

Nevertheless, the National Center for Complementary and Alternative Medicine, the American Medical Association, and other organizations from the United States have generally agreed that acupuncture is safe to be used when under the guidance of a trained practitioner who uses sterile needles. The World Health Organization recommends acupuncture as an effective treatment for over 40 medical problems, along with many mental disorders, and alcohol and substance abuse disorders.

Len Sperry, MD, PhD

See also: Acupressure

Further Reading

Filshie, Jacqueline. *Introduction to Medical Acupuncture*. Oxford, UK: Churchill Livingstone, 2008.

Gach, Michael R. *Acupressure's Potent Points: A Guide to Self-Care for Common Ailments*. New York, NY: Bantam Books, 2013.

Landgren, Kajsa. *Ear Acupuncture: A Practical Guide*. Oxford, UK: Churchill Livingstone, 2008.

Maciocia, Giovanni. *The Practice of Chinese Medicine: The Treatment of Diseases with Acupuncture and Chinese Herbs*. Oxford, UK: Churchill Livingstone, 2008.

Acute Stress Disorder

Acute stress disorder is a mental disorder characterized by recurrent and upsetting thoughts, inability to sleep or concentrate, or dissociation following a traumatic event.

Definitions

- **Cognitive behavior therapy** is a form of psychotherapy that focuses on changing maladaptive (faulty) behaviors, emotions, and thoughts. It is also known as CBT.

- **Cognitive restructuring** is a psychotherapy technique for identifying maladaptive (unhealthy) thoughts and changing them to present a more accurate view of a situation.

- **Dissociation** is a mental state in which the integrated functioning of an individual's identity is significantly disrupted or changed.

- **DSM-5** stands for the *Diagnostic and Statistical Manual of Mental Disorders, Fifth Edition*, which is a diagnostic system used by professionals to identify mental disorders with specific diagnostic criteria.

- **Exposure therapy** is a behavior therapy intervention (method) in which a client is exposed to a feared object or situation. It is also referred to as flooding.

- **Mood** is an individual's subjective emotional experience.

- **Pessimism** is a way of relating to one's world where the future is expected to hold more negative than positive outcomes.

- **Post-traumatic stress disorder** is a mental disorder characterized by nightmares, irritability, anxiety, emotional numbing, and recurrent flashbacks of a traumatic event that an individual experienced or witnessed. It is also referred to as PTSD.

- **Psychotherapy** is a psychological method for achieving desired changes in thinking, feeling, and behavior. It is also called therapeutic counseling.

- **Trauma** is a singular or recurrent event that is both extraordinary and severely distressing. It is also called traumatic event.

- **Trauma- and stressor-related disorders** are a group of mental disorders characterized by exposure to a traumatic or stressful event. These include post-traumatic stress disorder, reactive attachment disorder, and acute stress disorder.

Description and Diagnosis

Acute stress disorder is one of the DSM-5 trauma and stressor-related disorders. This disorder follows a traumatic event and is characterized by inability to experience positive emotions, recurrent and upsetting thoughts, inability to sleep or concentrate, avoidance of situations similar to the trauma, and dissociation. Traumatic events that cause this disorder include being subjected to attack, mugging, rape, robbery, murder, natural disaster, terrorism, war, or catastrophic accident. This disorder is similar to post-traumatic stress disorder and is often confused with it. Both disorders are distinguishable by the duration of symptoms, with the symptoms of acute stress disorder lasting less than one month.

Those with this disorder often reexperience the event with accompanying distressing symptoms. This trauma can include direct experience as well as witnessing trauma. Consequently, emergency responders and hospital staff often suffer from this disorder. The severity of the disorder increases if the event is a purposeful act that violates the individual directly and is further worsened by the degree of severity of the incident itself. Individuals who manifest this disorder are likely to experience intrusive and recurrent thoughts related to the traumatic event. These thoughts may also include guilt as a consequence of being unable to prevent trauma inflicted on another. These thoughts may also be expressed in dreams, including thematic elements from the event. Individuals may avoid places or things associated with the event. These individuals may be very reactive, irritable, or temperamental. They might also be anxious and hypervigilant of threats. The stress symptoms might be worsened by exposure to stimuli that is similar to those associated with the traumatic event.

The prevalence of this disorder is relatively high following traumatic events. In cases of trauma that do not involve personal violations, it is estimated that slightly less than one in every five individuals will experience acute stress disorder. In cases that do involve personal violation, the proportion increases to between 20% and 50% of individuals. Acute stress disorder is more common in females, probably because of the increased likelihood of physical violations such as rape. Other risk factors include a high level of worry, pessimism, and living or working in environments where trauma is likely to occur such as a war zone or emergency room (American Psychiatric Association, 2013).

According to the *Diagnostic and Statistical Manual of Mental Disorders, Fifth Edition*, individuals can be diagnosed with this disorder if they are exposed to a traumatic event and exhibit associated symptoms. These associated symptoms might include avoiding situation similar to that of the trauma, inability to experience positive emotions following the event, recurrent and upsetting thoughts about the event, inability to sleep or concentrate, and dissociation. When dissociation is present, symptoms may manifest as flashbacks where the individual relives the traumatic event or the inability to recall aspects of the event. These dissociative symptoms are also associated with post-traumatic stress disorder and are often confused. These two disorders are distinguishable by the duration of symptoms. If symptoms are present for less than one month, then acute stress disorder is applicable. Once symptoms have been present for one or more months, the appropriate diagnosis is post-traumatic stress disorder. It is also important to note that individuals cannot be diagnosed with acute stress disorder if they have only become aware of a trauma (e.g., reading a news article); they must have experienced or observed the trauma directly. Also, those with traumatic brain injury may exhibit symptoms of acute stress disorder (American Psychiatric Association, 2013).

The cause of this disorder is twofold. In part, it can be attributed to the traumatic event itself. However, certain attributes may play a role in the manifestation of this disorder in individuals who are more susceptible to this and other mental disorders. These attributes include having been exposed to past traumas, one's belief that one can influence outcome of one's life, and the unique meaning the individual gives to the traumatic event. As with most psychological disorders, research on the cause this disorder is ongoing.

Treatment

ASD is usually treated with psychotherapy. The most common form of therapy utilized is cognitive behavior therapy. Specific interventions (techniques) may include exposure techniques and cognitive restructuring. Prompt use of psychotherapy is critical to inhibit the development of the more severe and often chronic condition, post-traumatic stress disorder.

Jeremy Connelly, MEd, and Len Sperry, MD, PhD

See also: Cognitive Behavior Therapy; *Diagnostic and Statistical Manual of Mental Disorders* (DSM); Dissociative Disorders; Mood; Post-Traumatic Stress Disorder (PTSD); Psychotherapy; Trauma

Further Reading

American Psychiatric Association. *Diagnostic and Statistical Manual of Mental Disorders*, 5th ed. Arlington, VA: American Psychiatric Association, 2013.

Block, Stanley H., and Carolyn Bryant Block. *Mind-Body Workbook for PTSD: A 10-Week Program for Healing after Trauma*. Oakland, CA: New Harbinger, 2011.

Bryant, Richard, and Allison Harvey. *Acute Stress Disorder: A Handbooks of Theory, Assessment, and Treatment*. Washington, DC: American Psychological Association, 2000.

Williams, Mary Beth, and Soili Poijula. *The PTSD Workbook: Simple, Effective Techniques for Overcoming Traumatic Stress Symptoms*, 2nd ed. Oakland, CA: New Harbinger, 2013.

Addiction

Addiction is the compulsive use of a habit-forming substance or the irresistible urge to engage in a behavior despite harmful consequences.

Definitions

- **Addictive disorder** is a mental disorder that involves compulsive and uncontrolled pursuit of reward or relief with substance use or other compulsive behaviors.

- **Behavioral addiction** is a form of addiction caused by the compulsion to repeatedly engage in a behavior that causes harmful consequences. It is also referred to as process addiction or non-substance-related addiction.

- **Craving** is a strong desire for more of a substance or behavior (sex, shopping, Internet use) in order to experience a euphoric effect or to avoid withdrawal symptoms.

- **Dependence** is the need for a drug to function normally. Dependence can be psychological and/or physical. Psychological dependence is dependence on a psychoactive substance for the reward it provides. "Physical dependence" refers to the unpleasant physiological symptoms if the drug is stopped.

- **Detoxification** is a process of purging the body of the toxic effects of a drug or substance. During this process the symptoms of withdrawal are also treated. Also called detox, it is the first step in drug treatment program.

- **DSM-5** stands for the *Diagnostic and Statistical Manual of Mental Disorders, Fifth Edition*, which is a diagnostic system used by professionals to identify mental disorders with specific diagnostic criteria.

- **Psychoactive** refers to a drug or other substance that produces mood changes and distorted perceptions.

- **Relapse** is the recurrence of symptoms after a period of improvement or recovery.

- **Substance-related and addictive disorders** are a group of mental disorders that include substance disorders characterized by physiological dependence, drug-seeking behavior, tolerance, and social withdrawal. This group also includes the non-substance disorder of gambling.

- **Tolerance** refers to the need for higher doses of a substance or more frequent engagement in a behavior to achieve the same effect.

- **Twelve-Step group** is a self-help group whose members attempt recovery from various addictions and compulsions based on a plan called the Twelve Steps.

- **Withdrawal** is the unpleasant and potentially life-threatening physiological changes that occur due to the discontinuation of certain drugs after prolonged regular use.

Description

The American Society of Addiction Medicine (2013) offers the following definition of addiction. "Addiction is a primary, chronic disease of brain reward, motivation, memory, and related circuitry. Dysfunction in these circuits leads to characteristic biological, psychological, social, and spiritual manifestations. This is reflected in an individual pathologically pursuing reward and/or relief by substance use and other behaviors." This comprehensive definition emphasizes that addiction is a chronic brain disease that involves compulsiveness and which negatively impacts an individual's overall well-being. Persistent use typically leads to dependence and to tolerance. Discontinuation of the addiction can lead to withdrawal, increased cravings, and even relapse.

DSM-5 describes addiction and addictive disorders in the category called "substance-related and addictive disorders." It includes 10 classes of drugs: alcohol, caffeine, inhalants, opioids, hallucinogens, cannabis, sedatives-hypnotics and anxiolytics, stimulants, tobacco, and other substances. It also includes gambling disorder, which is a behavioral addiction. The behavioral addictions activate reward systems in the brain similar to drugs of abuse. They also produce behavioral symptoms comparable to symptoms produced by substance disorders. Assuming there is sufficient research to warrant their inclusion, other behavioral addictions are expected to be added in future DSM editions. These might include Internet addiction, sex addiction, exercise addiction, and shopping addiction (American Psychiatric Association, 2013).

Nicotine dependence is the most common type of addiction, while alcoholism is the most common addiction to a psychoactive substance. According to the National Survey on Drug Use and Health (NSDUH) in 2012, 23 million Americans age 12 or older had alcohol and drug addiction. Of these, more than 15 million were dependent on alcohol. Some 4 million were dependent on drugs, while the rest were dependent on both. Statistics from the National Drug Intelligence Center (2010) estimate the annual cost of addictions for the U.S. economy. It reports that abuse of tobacco, alcohol, and illicit drugs cost more than $600 billion annually in crime, lost work productivity, and health-care services.

Treatment

Treatment of addictions often requires a combination of medical, psychological, and social approaches.

Treatment often begins in specialized addiction treatment programs and clinics. These programs involve various treatment methods that focus on detoxification, reducing cravings, and preventing relapse. Common to many programs are Twelve-Step groups like Alcoholics Anonymous and Narcotics Anonymous. The prognosis for recovery from any addiction depends on the substance or behavior and the individual's personality and circumstances. Relapse is common, and those with addictions often make repeated attempts to quit before they are successful. Users of more than one drug typically have the more challenges in recovering from their addictions.

Len Sperry, MD, PhD

See also: Relapse and Relapse Prevention; Substance-Related and Addictive Disorders

Further Reading

American Psychiatric Association. *Diagnostic and Statistical Manual of Mental Disorders* (DSM), 5th ed. Arlington, VA: American Psychiatric Association Press, 2013.

American Society of Addiction Medicine. 2013. "Public Policy Statement: Definition of Addiction." http://www.asam.org/for-the-public/definition-of-addiction.

DiClemente, Carlo C. *Addiction and Change: How Addictions Develop and Addicted People Recover.* New York, NY: Guilford Press, 2006.

Hoffman, John, and Susan Froemke. *Addiction: Why Can't They Just Stop?* Emmaus, PA: Rodale Books, 2007.

National Drug Intelligence Center. *National Threat Assessment: The Economic Impact of Illicit Drug Use on American Society.* Washington, DC: United States Department of Justice, 2010.

National Survey on Drug Use and Health (NSDUH). "Results from the 2012 National Survey on Drug Use and Health: Mental Health Findings and Detailed Tables." http://samhsa.gov/data/NSDUH.aspx.

Prentiss, Chris. *The Alcoholism and Addiction Cure: A Holistic Approach to Total Recovery.* Malibu, CA: Power Press, 2007.

Addiction Counseling

Addiction counseling is therapy provided to people who are dependent on the use of one or more substances or activities.

Definitions

- **Addiction** is a chronic disease of the brain which involves compulsive and uncontrolled pursuit of reward or relief with substance use or other compulsive behaviors.

- **Addiction recovery** is the state of abstinence from addictive behaviors, usually achieved through self-reflection and spiritual exploration.

- **Relapse** is the recurrence of symptoms after a period of improvement or recovery.

- **Sober** means not consuming alcohol and drugs or engaging in other addictive activities.

Description

The American Medical Association defines addiction as a chronic disease with physical and emotional factors that impair control over the use of substances. Some examples of substances and activities people can become addicted to are alcohol, drugs, sex, gambling, and the Internet. For addiction counselors, working with people who are substance dependent or abusive is difficult because of a high rate of relapse, defensiveness, and a lack of research as how to best treat the conditions. The addiction counselor offers a different view and believes the problem of addiction is how you respond or fail to respond to substances and treatment. Addiction counseling rests on the idea that alcohol and drug problems become independent of their beginnings.

In counseling training, students have been taught to remove their own experience from the client's recovery processes. In addiction counseling there is more of a demand for personal involvement than seen in other counseling professions. Providing hope is a crucial dimension for addiction counselors as they offer themselves as "living proof" of hope. It is important to model the potential for long-term recovery through their own story and by guiding the client to a community of people in recovery.

Addiction counselors are exposed to many frustrations and losses. First, there is a high mortality rate of substance abusers. Many counselors use these experiences to deepen their understanding of the nature of addiction and to recommit themselves to finding new ways to reach their clients. Addiction counselors are aware that their clients are often involved in a life or death struggle for recovery. The stakes involved in this work are high and awareness brings its own burdens and rewards.

There are several rituals that are considered best practice for addiction counselors. These activities include rituals such as prayer, meditation, and self-reflection. Also included are mirroring rituals like reaching out to others for support and inspiration. Acts of self-care for the body and mind are also important for addiction counselors. Lastly, unpaid acts of service such as serving as a sponsor or giving back to the recovery community are valued.

Development

As early as 1774, the effects of alcohol abuse were known to be devastating. Substance-related problems in the United States began with the attack on Native Americans in the 18th and 19th centuries. Treatments for these problems at the time included use of native medicines, religion, and limiting its use and availability.

Addiction counseling started as a grassroots recovery community. Therapy with this population began in 1913 at a church in Boston with religious leaders called the Oxford Group. However, most laypeople believe that alcohol and drug treatment did not begin until the founding of Alcoholics Anonymous (AA) in 1935. Bill Wilson and Bob Smith used the Oxford Group as a model when they founded AA with a shift away from religion. AA viewed alcoholics as having an allergy to alcohol, which formed the basis of the disease or medical model. This was a change in the view of alcoholism, which had previously been viewed as a moral weakness. Soon after AA was founded, members began to be employed at substance abuse treatment centers.

In the early days alcoholics did not go to treatment centers through AA; they simply went through a detoxification process. This usually occurred in their local hospital, and from there most were referred to AA meetings. Supporters of AA and other Twelve-Step groups, believe it is the most effective way of treating addiction and should be the primary treatment program. Accordingly, it became the norm that clients needing help with alcoholism or substance abuse were referred to. This often was recommended instead of professional help or as an add-on to addiction counseling treatment.

In the 1940s it became clear that a definition and formalization of the addiction counselor should occur. The next major event in the treatment and counseling of alcoholics and other drug abusers was the opening of the Hazelden Treatment Center in Minnesota in 1949. Hazelden developed what later became known as the Minnesota Model. This model includes a combination of therapy, spirituality, group treatment, and the Twelve Steps. At Hazelden they integrated recovering, nonprofessionally trained counselors as part of the alcoholism treatment team. In 1954 addiction counselors were provided a professional role in Minnesota and other states later followed. The Substance Abuse and Mental Health Services Administration reports that today most residential treatment centers are a variation of the Minnesota Model.

Current Status

Currently, AA has over 115,000 independent groups throughout the world, with over 2,100,000 members (Alcoholics Anonymous, 2010). In the field of substance abuse there are three main approaches to addiction counseling. The traditional approach is the disease model which treats the addiction in the same medical model as other conditions. The research approach seeks the scientifically supported methods to treatment. And last, the managed care approach wants to identify the greatest benefit for the least cost.

These three movements conflict with one another, resulting in unrest among professional addiction counselors. The medical model believes in dependency where the research approach finds there is not enough evidence to support the claim. The managed care approach is unlikely to pay for anything that is highly disputed among professionals. Therefore, the conflicts in the field have led to difficulty in uniting and identifying common goals in addiction counseling.

Alexandra Cunningham, PhD

See also: Relapse and Relapse Prevention; Smoking Cessation; Substance Abuse and Mental Health Services and Administration (SAMHSA)

Further Reading

Alcoholics Anonymous World Services Inc. *Alcoholics Anonymous*. New York, NY: A.A. World Services Inc., 2010.

American Medical Association. "The Definition of Addiction." Last modified April 12, 2011. Accessed July 22, 2013. http://www.asam.org/advocacy/find-a-policy-statement/view-policy-statement/public-policy-statements/2011/12/15/the-definition-of-addiction.

Miller, Geri. *Learning the Language of Addiction Counseling*. Hoboken, NJ: John Wiley & Sons, Inc., 2010.

Addictive Personality

Addictive personality is the concept that addiction is the result of preexisting personality traits or defects.

Definitions

- **Addiction** is the persistent, compulsive dependence on a substance or a behavior for coping with unmanageable conflict and stress.

- **Antisocial personality** is a mental condition characterized by a pattern of disregarding and violating the rights of others.

- **Self-control** is the capacity for self-discipline. Some use this term interchangeably with willpower.

- **Willpower** is the ability to resist a short-term temptations in order to achieve a long-term goal. It also involves the ability to delay gratification. Some use this term interchangeably with self-control.

Description

Several factors influence the development of addiction. These include biological, environmental (social), and psychological factors. Of the psychological factors, personality traits are considered important in understanding why certain individuals seem to be more prone to developing an addiction than others. The question has been, why do some individuals develop a physical and psychological dependence on substances such as alcohol or drugs, or behaviors such as gambling or Internet use? For years there has been considerable debate over whether there is actually an "addictive personality." Several books and articles in newspapers and magazines suggest that there is, in fact, such a personality.

But research, to date, has yet to confirm the existence of the addictive personality. Notable is a study sponsored by the National Academy of Sciences by Lang (1983). It concluded that there is no single set of psychological traits that characterized proneness to the various addictions. However, the study did identify several common elements among those with various addictions. Individuals prone to addiction are more likely to engage in impulsive behavior and sensation (thrill) seeking and have difficulty with self-control, willpower, and delaying gratification. They tend to value nonconformity and have little commitment to socially value goals for achievement. They are also likely to be socially alienated, tolerate deviance, and have an antisocial personality. Finally, they commonly experience considerable stress but lack sufficient coping skills to deal with that stress. Lang suggested that this element helps to explain why drug and alcohol problems are highest during high periods of stress. For most individuals, adolescence and other stressful life transitions are the most stressful periods.

While there is insufficient research support for concept of the addictive personality, those with addiction seem to share certain commonalities. The value of identifying and further researching these common elements is twofold. First, they can help in predicting proneness to addiction. Second, they can help in devising better treatments for those with addiction.

Len Sperry, MD, PhD

See also: Addiction; Antisocial Personality Disorder; Willpower

Further Reading

American Psychiatric Association. *Diagnostic and Statistical Manual of Mental Disorders*, 5th ed. Arlington, VA: American Psychiatric Association Press, 2013.

Jampolsky, Lee L. *Healing the Addictive Personality: Freeing Yourself from Addictive Patterns and Relationships*. Berkeley, CA: Celestial Arts, 2008.

Lang, Alan R. "Addictive Personality: A Viable Construct?" In *Commonalities in Substance Abuse and Habitual Behavior*, edited by Peter K. Levison, Dean R. Gerstein, and Deborah R. Maloff, pp. 157–236. New York, NY: Lexington Books, 1983.

Nakken, Craig. *The Addictive Personality: Understanding the Addictive Process and Compulsive Behavior*, 2nd ed. Center City, MN: Hazleden, 1996.

Adjustment Disorder

Adjustment disorder is a mental disorder characterized by short-term emotional distress or behavioral problems following a stressful event.

Definitions

- **Acute stress disorder** is a mental disorder that affects individuals who have been exposed either directly or indirectly to a traumatic situation such as death, rape, or serious bodily harm. Those suffering from this disorder often reexperience the event with accompanying distressing symptoms.

- **Anxiety** is a negative emotional state characterized by feelings of nervousness, worry, and apprehension about an imagined danger.

- **Cognitive behavior therapy** is a type of psychotherapy that focuses on maladaptive (faulty) behaviors, emotions, and thoughts.

- **Culture** is the common beliefs, customs, and behaviors of a particular group, society, or nation.

- **Depression** is an emotional state characterized by feelings of sadness, low self-esteem, guilt, or reduced ability to enjoy life. It is not considered a mental disorder unless it significantly disrupts one's daily functioning.

- **DSM-5** stands for the *Diagnostic and Statistical Manual of Mental Disorders, Fifth Edition*, which is a diagnostic system used by professionals to identify mental disorders with specific diagnostic criteria.

- **Family therapy** is a type of psychotherapy for families that focuses on improving relationships and understanding between family members.

- **Mindfulness practices** are intentional activities that foster living in the present moment and awareness that is nonjudgmental and accepting.

- **Post-traumatic stress disorder** is a mental disorder characterized by nightmares, irritability, anxiety, emotional numbing, and recurrent flashbacks of a traumatic event that an individual experienced or witnessed. It is also referred to as PTSD.

- **Psychotherapy** is a psychological method for achieving desired changes in thinking, feeling, and behavior. It is also called therapeutic counseling.

- **Trauma- and stressor-related disorders** are a group of mental disorders characterized by exposure to a traumatic or stressful event. These include post-traumatic stress disorder, reactive attachment disorder, and disinhibited social engagement disorder.

Description and Diagnosis

Adjustment disorder is one of the trauma- and stress-related disorders as expressed in the DSM-5. This disorder is a common, short-term mental disorder characterized by difficulty coping with a significant but nontraumatic stressor. Individuals with this disorder are likely to experience emotional distress, difficulty in social or work settings, or both. An important aspect of this disorder is that the symptoms manifested are disproportionate to what might be normally expected following the stressful event. This may seem a simple task, but it can be a difficult assessment for a clinician to make. What qualifies for disproportionate varies significantly by a number of factors including culture, age, and personal history. Adjustment disorder is often associated with close personal relationships and financial, employment, or business issues. The symptoms of this disorder typically appear immediately following certain events such as news of a layoff. In contrast, this disorder may develop over the course of days or weeks following the finalization of a divorce. Adjustment disorder is most likely to manifest as psychological symptoms in adults and behavioral symptoms (e.g., defiance, fighting, and vandalism) in adolescents.

Adjustment disorder is common in mental health settings. It is estimated that adjustment disorder is present in 5%–20% of those treated in mental health settings but can be as high as 50%. This disorder is more likely to occur in individuals from lower socioeconomic backgrounds (American Psychiatric Association, 2013).

According to the *Diagnostic and Statistical Manual of Mental Disorders, Fifth Edition*, individuals can be diagnosed with this disorder if the following criteria are met. There must be an identifiable stressor followed by related symptoms. These symptoms must arise within three months. These symptoms must be related to a disproportionate level of emotional distress, disturbance in social or work-related functioning, or both. If the symptoms persist for longer than six months following the end of the stressor, then a different diagnosis is appropriate. Also, adjustment disorder is differentiated by the types of symptoms present; some individuals may indicate that they feel depressed, anxious, or both. Some individuals may have disturbances in conduct, while others may have conduct disturbance combined with depressed mood and/or anxiety (American Psychiatric Association, 2013). Adjustment disorder differs from both acute stress disorder and post-traumatic stress disorder in that the stressor does not involve threat of unnatural death, personal violation, or significant bodily harm. Specifically, adjustment disorder follows a life event that is in some way meaningful to the individual. Also, differing cultures maintain differing expectations pertaining to one's reactions to particular life events. Consequently, a clinician must carefully consider these expectations in his or her assessment of what reaction might be normally expected. For example, an individual from a collectivist (i.e., family-focused) culture may exhibit significantly more distress following a family crisis than someone from an individualistic (i.e., personal-focus) culture.

The cause of this disorder is a combination of the stressor and a number of personal factors. Like most mental disorders, the exact etiology (cause) is unclear, although it is believed to be a combination of genetics and environmental factors. However, the culture of the individual plays a significant role in the meaning given to the stressor by the individuals. Therefore, the cultural context in which this disorder occurs is very important to ascertain in each case.

Treatment

This disorder is usually treated with psychotherapy. Psychotherapy is most often aimed at reducing symptoms and improving any inhibited functioning that has resulted from this disorder. Specific forms of psychotherapy used in the treatment of this disorder may include family therapy, mindfulness practices, and cognitive behavior therapy. Individuals who develop depressive or anxiety symptoms may also be treated with medications, although this is not a preferred practice considering the short-term duration of symptoms. Self-help books and support groups are also common forms of informal treatment. Typically, these books and groups are specific to the stressor. For example, an individual suffering from adjustment disorder following divorce might read a self-help book about divorce or attend a support group with other divorcees.

Jeremy Connelly, MEd, and Len Sperry, MD, PhD

See also: Acute Stress Disorder; Cognitive Behavior Therapy; Culture; Depression and Depressive Disorders Depression; *Diagnostic and Statistical Manual of Mental Disorders* (DSM); Family Therapy; Mindfulness; Post-Traumatic Stress Disorder; Psychotherapy; Trauma- and Stressor-Related Disorders

Further Reading

American Psychiatric Association. *Diagnostic and Statistical Manual of Mental Disorders* (DSM), 5th ed. Arlington, VA: American Psychiatric Association, 2013.

Daitch, Carolyn. *Anxiety Disorders: The Go-to Guide for Clients and Therapists*. New York, NY: W.W. Norton, 2011.

Davis, Martha, Elizabeth Eshelman, and Mathew McKay. *The Relaxation and Stress Reduction Workbook*, 6th ed. Oakland, CA: New Harbinger Productions, 2008.

Forsyth, John, and Eifert, George. *The Mindfulness and Acceptance Workbook for Anxiety: A Guide to Breaking Free from Anxiety, Phobias, and Worry Using Acceptance and Commitment Therapy*. Oakland, CA: New Harbinger, 2007.

Adler, Alfred (1870–1937)

Adler was an Austrian medical doctor and psychotherapist who is best known as the founder of Individual Psychology, the theoretical approach which, in contrast to traditional psychoanalysis, offers a holistic, or more whole, view of the individual and stresses the importance of social factors.

Description

Alfred Adler was born on February 7, 1870, in Rudolfsheim, a suburb of Vienna, Austria, the second of seven children to a Jewish grain merchant and his wife. A sickly child, Alfred developed rickets which prevented him from walking until he was four and was later hospitalized with pneumonia. These early experiences inspired Alfred to pursue medical school at the University of Vienna where he also met his future wife, Raissa Timofeyewna Epstein, at a social political meeting. The couple went on to have four children together, Valentine, Alexandra, Kurt, and Cornelia. Adler graduated in 1895 and began practicing as an ophthalmologist, later moving into general practice, though his interest in psychology, sociology, and philosophy continued. In 1902, he was invited by Sigmund Freud to join a weekly discussion group at his home at which the foundations of the psychoanalytic movement were born. Freud respected Adler's ideas and considered him a colleague though the two were not friends. Adler remained an active member of the society for several years until his break from the group in 1911. The first dissenter from traditional psychoanalysis, he soon founded the Society for Individual Psychology in 1912 where he further honed his own theory and clinical approach.

Freud and Adler disagreed primarily about the impact of social factors on human development and behavior. While Freud stressed only internal dynamics (biological, sexual, and physiological), Adler emphasized the importance of external dynamics (social and environmental), adopting a more holistic view of the individual. Holism, or the holistic view, is a concept stressing the importance of all aspects of an individual or system (biological, chemical, emotional, physical, psychological, social) as equally whole parts that contribute to an entity's makeup and functioning.

Adlerian psychology thus contends that humans are social, creative beings whose behavior is purposeful and goal-oriented. Though Freud and Adler (as well as Carl Jung) studied how feelings of inferiority can impact psychological wellness, Adler further defined "inferiority complex" as a concept that stresses how feelings related to inadequacy, low self-esteem, and poor self-worth contribute significantly to an individual's personality, social development and relationships, and propensity for later mental health issues. According to Individual Psychology, experiences, both early and subsequent, impact one's personality and lifestyle; however, much depends on the person's subjective interpretation of these events. Birth order, family constellation, and early recollections can also affect the accomplishing of tasks

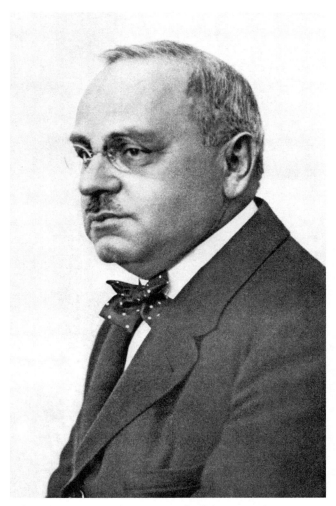

Alfred Adler was an Austrian medical doctor and prominent psychotherapist who is best known as the founder of Individual Psychology. (Bettmann/Corbis)

related to work, family, and friends. Those who learn to cooperate with others and contribute to the general welfare (social interest) achieve significance and become self-actualized. Social interest is one of Adler's key concepts (in German, "gemeinschaftsgefuhl"), which describes a feeling of community, when a person acts in the best interests of others, as opposed to being consumed by personal needs and concerns.

Impact (Psychological Influence)

The Individual Psychology movement gained considerable momentum during the early 1900s as Adler spoke internationally and opened clinics in his honor. In addition, he taught at Columbia University and later at the Long Island College of Medicine, which prompted him to move his family permanently to the United States. Adler influenced the works of Erich Fromm, Abraham Maslow, Rollo May, Karen Horney, and Carl Rogers and is revered as one of the top psychologists of the 20th century. His impact on modern-day psychology and counseling practice remains evident today in organizations such as the North American Society for Adlerian Psychology and educational institutions including The Adler School of Professional Psychology in Chicago, Illinois. Alfred Adler died of heart complications during a lecture tour in Aberdeen, Scotland, on May 28, 1937.

Melissa A. Mariani, PhD

See also: Adlerian Therapy; Freud, Sigmund (1856–1939); Individual Psychology

Further Reading

Adler, Alfred. *The Practice and Theory of Individual Psychology*. Eastford, CT: Martino Fine Books, 2011.

Adler, Alfred, and Colin Brett. *Understanding Life: An Introduction to the Psychology of Alfred Adler*. Center City, MN: Hazelden, 2009.

Hoffman, Edward. *The Drive for Self: Alfred Adler and the Founding of Individual Psychology*. New York, NY: Perseus Books, 1997.

Adlerian Therapy

Adlerian therapy is a psychotherapy approach that emphasizes the individual's lifestyle, belonging, and social interest.

Definitions

- **Family constellation** is the early developmental influences on an individual, including siblings, parents, peers, neighbors, and other key individuals like teachers.

- **Inferiority complex** is a behavioral manifestation of a subjective feeling of inferiority.

- **Inferiority feeling** is the emotional reaction to a self-appraisal of deficiency that is subjective, global, and judgmental.

- **Life style** refers to one's attitudes and convictions about belonging and finding a place in the world.

- **Lifestyle convictions** are the attitudes and beliefs that direct an individual's sense of belonging.

- **Life tasks** are the main challenges (work, love, and friendship) that life presents to all individuals.

- **Private logic** is convictions that run counter to social interest and fail to foster a constructive sense of belonging with others.

- **Projective technique** is a psychological test in which an individual's responses to ambiguous stimuli like are analyzed to determine underlying personality traits, feelings, or attitudes.

- **Safeguarding mechanisms** are the behaviors of attitudes that individuals select to evade responsibility and not meet the life tasks. It is called defense mechanism by other approaches.

- **Social interest** refers to the behaviors and attitudes that display an individual's sense of belonging, concern for, and contributions to the community.

Description

Adlerian therapy is a form of psychotherapy developed by Alfred Adler that emphasizes the individual's lifestyle, connectedness with others (belonging), meeting the life tasks, and contributions to society (social interest), which are considered the hallmarks of mental health. Adler considered all behavior as purposive and that individuals are motived to seek "belonging" or significance and meaning in their lives by the manner in which they functioned in social systems. He postulated that it was within the family constellation that individuals first learn how to belong and interact. Adler emphasized the unique and private beliefs which he called "private logic." This logic serves as a reference for attitudes, private views of self, others, and the world, and behavior which he called the "lifestyle" and "lifestyle convictions." Individuals form their lifestyle as they endeavor to relate to others, to overcome "feelings of inferiority," and to find a sense of belonging. Furthermore, Adler believed that healthy and productive individuals are characterized by "social interest," whereas those with poor adjustment or psychopathology show little social interest and tend to be self-focused.

Developments and Current Status

Adlerian therapy was developed by the Viennese physician Alfred Adler (1870–1937). Early in his professional career, Adler was invited by Freud to join the Viennese Psychoanalytic Society and remained friendly with Freud for some 10 years. As he came to view Freud as inflexible in his views and obsessed with sex and death, Adler broke with Freud in 1911 and continued to refine his own theory and psychotherapeutic approach. Subsequently, Adler influenced many others including Karen Horney, Gordon Allport, Aaron Beck, and Abraham Maslow. Maslow, Rollo May, and Viktor Frankl all studied under Adler, and credited him with influencing their own views.

Adlerian therapy fosters the process of change by stimulating cognitive, affective, and behavior changes. Although the individual is not always fully aware of his or her specific pattern and goal, through analysis of birth order, repeated coping patterns, and early memories, the psychotherapist infers the goal as a working hypothesis. Recognizing this pattern of limiting schemas and beliefs, the therapist helps the client to see life from another perspective. Change occurs when the client is able to see his or her problem from another view,

so he or she can explore and practice new behavior and a new philosophy of life.

Besides eliciting traditional intake material, for example, present concerns, mental status exam, and general social, occupational, and developmental history, the Adlerian psychotherapist collects and analyzes the client's family constellation and lifestyle convictions. The family constellation consists of the client birth order, identifications with parents and peers, family values, and family narrative. Lifestyle convictions are inferred from both habitual coping patterns and early recollections. Because a client's recollection of his or her earliest memories reflect past childhood events in light of current lifestyle convictions, early recollections are a powerful projective technique that quickly and accurately provides a working hypotheses of the way clients view themselves, others, and the world. The therapist elicits three or more memories, and the description of these memories are analyzed according to themes and developmental maturity and from these derives the client's lifestyle convictions which reflect the impact of the client's family constellation. Information from the family constellation and lifestyle convictions is useful in specifying a case formulation, including a diagnostic formulation and a clinical formulation, that is, an explanation of why and how the client perceives, feels, and acts in a patterned and predictable fashion.

Individuals develop three lifestyle convictions: a self-view—the convictions about who they are; a world view—convictions about how the world treats them and expects of them; and their ethical convictions—their personal moral code. When there is conflict between the self-concept and the ideal, inferiority feelings develop. It is important to point out that feelings of inferiority are not considered abnormal. However, when the individual begins to act inferior rather than feel inferior, the individual expresses an "inferiority complex." Thus, while the inferiority feeling is universal and normal, the inferiority complex reflects the discouragement of a limited segment of our society and is usually abnormal.

The goal of treatment is not merely symptom relief but the adoption of a contributing way of living. Adlerians view pain and suffering in a client's life as the result of choices made. This value-based theory of personality hypothesizes that the values a client holds and lives his or her life by are learned, and when they no longer work as evidenced by suffering or lack of happiness, the client can relearn values and lifestyles that work more "effectively." Some Adlerians believe that a client's lifestyle is best viewed as personal schemas or narratives. Because such maladaptive schemas or basic mistakes are believed to be true for the individual, the individual acts accordingly. Adler noted that these basic mistakes are over-generalizations, for example, "people are hostile," "life is dangerous," or misperceptions of life, "life doesn't give me any breaks," which are expressed in the client's physical behavior, language, dreams, values, and so on. The goal of intervention in Adlerian therapy is re-education and reorientation of the client to schemas that work "better." The actual techniques employed are used to this end. Adlerians tend to be action orientated. They believe the concept of insight is just a proxy for immobility. Insight is not a deep understanding that one must have before change can occur. For Adlerians, insight is understanding translated into action. It reflects the client's understanding of the purposeful nature of behavior.

Adlerian therapy is structured around four basic overlapping phases.

Relationship. In the relationship phase, the goal is to establish an empathic relationship between therapist and client in which the clients feels understood and accepted by the therapist. Establishing a mutual and collaborative relationship is essential for effective therapeutic outcomes to be achieved.

Assessment. In this phase, the purpose is to evaluate the client's concerns and objective and subjective circumstances. In addition to traditional initial assessment information, the Adlerian therapist elicits family constellation and lifestyle conviction material. This phase is described in more detail later.

Insight. In this phase the purpose is to explain the client to himself or herself, which is, to say, to develop insight into lifestyle convictions, mistaken goals, and self-defeating behavior patterns. While such a corrective cognitive experience is usually necessary for treatment to be effective, it is by no means sufficient to effect a corrective emotional experience or behavior change. Furthermore, insight does not always precede emotional and behavior change, which are the province of reorientation. Thus, while theoretically distinct, the insight and reorientation phases often overlap in clinical practice.

Reorientation. The purpose of this phase is to help clients to consider alternatives to the problems, behaviors, or situations and to commit to change. It involves strengthening the client's social interest. It attempts to bring each individual to an optimal level of personal, interpersonal, and occupational functioning. In so doing exaggerated self-protection, self-absorption, and self-indulgence are replaced with courageous social contribution. Therapeutic techniques include creative and dramatic approaches to treatment such as role-play, the empty chair technique, acting "as if," and psychodrama.

Overall, Adlerian therapy is a psychotherapy approach that reflects various psychodynamic, cognitive-behavioral, existential, constructivist, and humanistic principles. Yet it is unique in its focus on the lifestyle and its emphasis on belonging, meeting the life tasks, and social interest as the hallmarks of mental health.

Len Sperry, MD, PhD

See also: Adler, Alfred (1870–1937); Early Recollections

Further Reading

Carlson, Jon, Richard E. Watts, and Michael Maniacci. *Adlerian Therapy: Theory and Practice*. Washington, DC: American Psychological Association Books, 2006.

Dinkmeyer, Don, and Len Sperry. *Counseling and Psychotherapy: An Integrated Individual Psychology Approach*, 3rd ed. Columbus, OH: Prentice-Hall, 2000.

Mosak, Harold H., and Robert Di Pietro. *Early Recollections: Interpretative Method and Application*. New York, NY: Routledge, 2006.

Orgler, Hertha. *Alfred Adler: The Man and His Work*. New York, NY: Capricorn Books, 1963.

Adoption

Adoption is a process in which a child is legally raised by someone other than his or her biological parents (also sometimes referred to as birthparents). A child can be adopted by family members, such as aunts, uncles, and grandparents, or by unrelated individuals. Adoption fills a variety of societal needs, including providing parents for children given up by their birthparents, as well as for children whose parents are deceased or who have lost their parental rights, most often due to abuse or neglect.

Adoption also offers individuals and couples a way to create a family when they cannot become pregnant or carry a pregnancy to term. Adoption offers a legal relationship between an adult and a nonbiological child as a way of formally creating a parent–child relationship, such as in the case of a stepparent or grandparent raising a child.

Famous adoptees include Aristotle, Steve Jobs, Nelson Mandela, Babe Ruth, Moses, Jesse Jackson, Edgar Allan Poe, Marilyn Monroe, John Lennon, Malcolm X, and Bill Clinton.

Adoption is the legal process of establishing the parental rights for a child by an individual or couple who is not the child's biological parent(s) and raise the child as his or her own. In ancient times, adoption was used for political and economic reasons, usually to continue the male line of a family's lineage. These days, adoption is quite different; it is used as a means to create a family by both traditional and nontraditional families alike. This includes infertile couples and gay and lesbian couples, as well as those who choose adoption for altruistic reasons.

Adoptions peaked in 1970 most likely due to the stigma of being an unwed mother or single parent as well as more restricted access to birth control. Adoptions are fairly rare, with fewer than 3% of children in the United States being adopted.

Domestic adoption involves U.S. parents adopting U.S. children who are available due to a variety of reasons such as an unwed mother, financial instability, abandonment, abuse, neglect, placement in foster care, or the death of one or both parents. An estimated 18,000 infants are adopted each year in the United States, and in 2009 nearly 70,000 children were adopted from foster care. However, the number of adoptive families far exceeded demand as an additional 114,500 foster children were still waiting to be adopted at the end of 2009.

In addition to domestic adoptions, some prospective parents choose to adopt children from other countries. These are known as international adoptions, whereby U.S. citizens adopt orphans from countries, including Romania, China, Guatemala, and Ethiopia. The number of international adoptions has dropped by more than one-third from approximately 45,000 per year in 2004 to fewer than 29,000 in 2010. Through a variety of sources, including both domestic and international, more than 127,000 children are adopted each year in the United States.

There are several types of adoption, including open, closed, and semi-open. In closed adoptions, parents receive little or no information about their adopted child's biological parents. This is often done to protect the confidentiality of the biological parent(s). In contrast, open adoptions have become increasingly popular over the past 20 years, although those adults who had been adopted when they were babies or young children joined their new parents through closed adoptions.

An open adoption is one in which the biological parents and adoptive parents disclose information about themselves and, in many cases, the biological parents continue to have contact with the adopted child and his or her family. A combination of the two is known as semi-open adoptions. In these situations, non-identifying information is exchanged between birth parents and adoptive parents. This can include letters, photos, or e-mails and correspondence is handled by an agency or other third party.

The adoption process includes the use of an adoption agency or an attorney specializing in adoptions. All potential adoptive parents are required by federal law to complete a home study that prepares and educates the prospective adoptive parents, evaluates their ability to parent, and offers insight and information to the agency or attorney in order to make a proper placement. The home study includes background checks and interviews of the prospective parents and often extended family, as well as a visit to the home to make sure it is a safe environment for the child.

The psychological impact of adoption depends on a number of factors, including the age of the child, the parenting styles of the adoptive family, and circumstances surrounding the adoption, as well as cultural factors in both domestic and many international adoptions. Research has shown that most adoptees adjust well to their adoptive families; however, there are areas in which both adopted children and even adult adoptees can struggle.

Anxiety, depression, trust, relationship difficulties, and identity formation are noted challenges for adoptees. In some cases, more severe psychological disturbances have been reported. Notably, international adoptions from specific orphanages and from certain countries have shown to have a number of children who are later diagnosed with reactive attachment disorder. This often presents in children before the age of five as an inability to connect socially or to attach appropriately to caretakers.

Mindy Parsons, PhD

See also: Attachment Styles; Child Abuse; Child Neglect; Foster Care; Group Homes; Reactive Attachment Disorder

Further Reading

Brodzinsky, David M. *Being Adopted: The Lifelong Search for Self*. New York, NY: Knopf Doubleday Publishing Group, 1993.

Centers for Disease Control. 2008. "Adoption Experiences of Women and Men and Demand for Children to Adopt by Women 18–44 Years of Age in the United States, 2002." *Vital and Health Statistics*. Last modified August 2008. www.cdc.gov/nchs/data/series/sr_23/sr23_027.pdf.

Corder, Kate. "Counseling Adult Adoptees." *The Family Journal: Counseling and Therapy for Couples and Families* 20, no. 4 (2012): 448–452.

Eldridge, Sherrie. *Twenty Things Adopted Kids Wished Their Adoptive Parents Knew*. New York, NY: Random House Publishing Group, 2009.

Newton Varrier, Nancy. *Primal Wound: Understanding the Adoptive Child*. Louisville, KY: Gateway Press, 2003.

Selman, Peter. "The Global Decline of Intercountry Adoption: What Lies Ahead?" *Social Policy and Society* 11, no. 3 (2012): 381–397.

U.S. Census Bureau. 2012. "Statistical Abstract of the United States." 370. http://www.census.gov/prod/www/statistical_abstract.html.

U.S. Department of Health and Human Services. 2010. "The Adoption Home Study Process." https://www.childwelfare.gov/pubs/f_homstu.cfm.

Organization

National Council for Adoption
225 N. Washington Street
Alexandria, VA 22314
Telephone: (703) 299-6633
E-mail: ncfa@adoptioncouncil.org
Website: https://www.adoptioncouncil.org/

Adrenaline (Epinephrine)

Adrenaline is a neurotransmitter involved in the fight or flight response that increases heart rate, pulse rate, and blood pressure.

Definitions

- **Catecholamines** are a class of brain neurotransmitters released in the fight or flight response. They include epinephrine, norepinephrine, and dopamine.

- **Enzymes** are proteins that trigger chemical reactions in the body.

- **Glycogen** is a form of glucose (sugar) that is stored in the liver and muscles.

- **Norepinephrine** is a hormone produced by the adrenal gland, along with epinephrine, as part of the fight or flight response. It is also known as noradrenaline.

- **Tyrosine** is the amino acid from which epinephrine is made.

Descriptions

Adrenaline (also known as epinephrine) is a neurotransmitter (chemical messenger) released by the adrenal gland in response to stress. Adrenaline is made from noradrenaline (norepinephrine). It makes up about 80% of the catecholamines that are released as part of the body's stress response. When the body is confronted with a threat or stressful situation, the brain releases nerve signals to the adrenal gland to release adrenaline and noradrenaline. This is called the fight or flight response in which energy is diverted away from areas where it is not needed to those where it is most required, particularly the heart and muscles. When released, adrenaline circulates through the bloodstream until it reaches its target organs—the heart, blood vessels, liver, and fat cells. It binds to alpha-adrenergic and beta-adrenergic receptors. Each of these receptors triggers a different action within cells. Alpha receptors initiate smooth muscle contraction and blood vessel constriction, while beta receptors stimulate the heart

Structure of Adrenaline

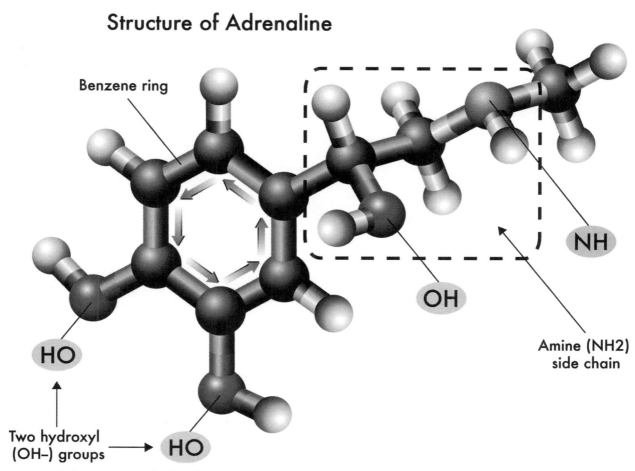

Benzene ring

NH

OH

Amine (NH2) side chain

HO

Two hydroxyl (OH–) groups → HO

Illustration of the structure of adrenaline. Adrenaline is a neurotransmitter involved in the fight-or-flight response that increases heart rate, pulse rate, and blood pressure. Some people can become addicted to the "adrenaline rush," which happens in extreme sports or in gambling. (Rob3000/Dreamstime.com)

muscle. The release of adrenaline prepares the body for action by causing an increase in blood and oxygen flow to the muscles, releases stored energy from the liver and fat cells, and constricts blood vessels raising the blood pressure.

Some experience a drug-like high from engaging in activities that trigger the fight or flight response. Called "adrenaline junkies" or "adrenaline addicts" these individuals skydive, mountain climb, or engage in extreme behaviors to experience a rush of adrenaline. Some compulsive gamblers attribute their addiction to the rush they get while gambling.

Adrenaline is used to treat life-threatening emergencies such as anaphylactic shock (severe allergic reaction) and cardiac arrest (heart stops beating). It has a very rapid effect on the heart, blood vessels, and the lungs. Administration of adrenaline by injection stimulates the heartbeat, makes the blood vessels narrower which raises blood pressure, and relaxes lung muscles which eases breathing. Adrenaline injections are also used for snake bites, bee stings, and other allergic reactions.

Precautions and Side Effects

Adverse reactions to adrenaline include palpitations, tachycardia (fast heart rate), arrhythmia, anxiety, headache, tremor, hypertension (high blood pressure), and acute pulmonary edema (fluid in the lungs).

Len Sperry, MD, PhD

See also: Anxiety

Further Reading

Church, Matt. *Adrenaline Junkies and Serotonin Seekers: Balance Your Brain Chemistry to Maximize Energy, Stamina, Mental Sharpness, and Emotional Well-Being.* Berkeley, CA: Ulysses Press, 2004.

Goldstein, David S. *Adrenaline and the Inner World: An Introduction to Scientific Integrative Medicine.* Baltimore, MD: Johns Hopkins University Press, 2006.

Meyer, Jerrold S., and Linda F. Quenzer. *Psychopharmacology: Drugs, the Brain and Behavior.* Sunderland, MA: Sinauer Associates, Inc., 2005.

Physician's Desk Reference. *PDR for Nonprescription Drugs, Dietary Supplements, and Herbs*, 30th ed. New York, NY: Physician's Desk Reference, 2008.

Advance Directives

"Advance directives" refers to a legal document that gives directions about what medical practices, procedures, and actions should be taken on a person's behalf if the person becomes incompetent or unable to communicate his or her health or mental health-care needs to caregivers and/or medical providers.

Description

In general, the term "advance directives" refers to a legal document that clearly outlines the actions a person would want carried out if his or her health became jeopardized. Caregivers must follow the steps listed in this document in order to fulfill the patient's wishes. Living wills and do-not-resuscitate orders are common types of advance directives. Mental health directives, or psychiatric advance directives (pads), specifically refer to measures that should be taken if a person becomes mentally incapable or loses the ability to make rational judgments for himself or herself. Pads come in two general forms: instructional directives and proxy directives. Instructional directives describe a person's

mental health treatment preferences, while proxy directives allow the person to name a health-care agent, or proxy, responsible for making treatment decisions if the person is unable to do so. A proxy must be a capable, competent adult (at least 18 years of age or older) who is not the person's current health-care provider. Most states include pads in general medical advance directives and require these documents to be witnessed, signed, and possibly notarized to ensure their legality. These papers should be kept on file along with a person's medical records and copies should also be given to caregivers.

Certain conditions must exist in order for a person to move forward with an advance directive. For one, the person must be considered mentally and physically competent at the time the document is created. Next, the language in the document must clearly communicate the person's wishes. In addition, once the directives are executed, steps must be taken to ensure that the items listed in the document are complied with.

History

The Cruzan case of 1990 had the most profound impact to date on the use of advance directives in providing end-of-life treatment decisions. Nancy Cruzan suffered life-threatening injuries after a serious automobile accident. She was hospitalized, in a vegetative state, and unable to communicate. Cruzan's parents, her caregivers, wanted to end Nancy's life knowing that she did not wish to be kept alive on life support. Nancy had told this to a friend of hers at an earlier point in time; however, these wishes were not formally documented. After much back-and-forth the courts finally ruled that it is a competent individual's constitutional right to control his or her medical care. More important, the courts extended this right to incompetent individuals provided that they had indicated their wishes before they become incapacitated. On December 1, 1991, as a direct result of the Cruzan case, Congress put into effect the Patient Self-Determination Act. This act mandated that health-care providers inform adult patients of their rights in end-of-life medical care decisions. Any health-care institution eligible to receive Medicare or Medicaid funds is now required to share information and engage in meaningful discussion with patients regarding their self-determination rights.

Current Status

All 50 states and the District of Columbia have laws that authorize certain forms of advance directives. Many of these laws though do not specifically reference mental health or psychiatric decision making. Minnesota was the first state to enact a law that clearly outlined psychiatric advance directives in 1991. Eleven states have followed, including Alaska, Hawaii, Idaho, Illinois, Maine, North Carolina, Oklahoma, Oregon, South Dakota, Texas, and Utah. These laws establish the rights of a mentally ill person. They permit ill persons to communicate their directives in writing when they are competent and outline their acceptance or refusal of psychiatric treatment.

Research indicates that opting for medical advance directives can be affected by factors such as individual attitudes, cultural beliefs, current state of health, and a patient's relationship with his or her health-care provider. The likelihood that a person will elect advance directives also increases with age. Though medical advance directives are more common, psychiatric advance directives are relatively new. Questions continue to be raised regarding their use. Research in this area is ongoing, and there are several pending court decisions on this topic. In the meantime, advance directives should be considered a viable way to empower people to take a more active role in their treatment. They can assist in the communication and execution of a person's wishes in the event of an unforeseen medical or psychiatric illness. Advance directives can also help to maintain a person's dignity and avoid conflicts among caregivers.

Melissa A. Mariani, PhD

See also: Caregivers

Further Reading

Cruzan v Director, Missouri Department of Health, 497 US 261, 110 S Ct 2841, 1990.

Fleischner, Robert. *An Analysis of Advance Directive Statues and Their Application to Mental Health Care and Treatment. Report to the National Association of Protection and Advocacy Systems*. Washington, DC: National Association of Protection and Advocacy Systems, 1998.

Jones, Adrienne L., Abigail J. Moss, and Lauren D. Harris-Kojetin. Use of Advance Directives in Long-Term Care Populations. NCHS Data Brief, no 54. Hyattsville, MD: National Center for Health Statistics, 2011.

Srebnik, Debra S., and John Q. La Fond. "Advance Directives for Mental Health Treatment." *Psychiatric Services* 50, no. 7 (1999): 919–925.

Adverse Childhood Experiences

Adverse childhood experience is a traumatic experience that occurs before the age of 18, is remembered as an adult, and negatively affects health.

Definitions

- **Child abuse** is the physical, sexual, or emotional abuse of a child or minor, usually under the age of 18.

- **Domestic abuse** is the abuse by one partner against the other in an intimate relationship. It can involve physical, sexual, and/or psychological abuse.

- **Household dysfunction** is a category or of adverse childhood experience that includes household substance abuse, household mental illness, and parental separation or divorce.

- **Neglect** involves refusal or failure by those responsible to provide food, shelter, health care, or protection for a vulnerable elder.

- **Physical abuse** involves inflicting, or threatening to inflict, physical pain or injury on individuals or depriving them of a basic need.

- **Psychological abuse** involves inflicting mental pain, anguish, or distress on individuals through verbal or nonverbal acts. It is also called emotional abuse.

- **Sexual abuse** involves nonconsensual sexual contact of any kind, coercing an elder to witness sexual behaviors.

- **Traumatic experience** is an event that causes physical or psychological distress or harm and is experienced as a threat to one's safety or the stability of one's world.

Description

Adverse childhood experiences are traumatic experiences that can significantly impact health in adult life. An important study of certain adverse childhood experiences has been ongoing by the Centers for Disease Control (CDC). The study grew from the 1980s when health-care professionals at the Kaiser Permanente managed care health system in San Diego were frustrated by a high dropout rate in their obesity prevention clinic. Kaiser Permanente eventually began a study of 17,000 participants, from 1995 to 1997, which looked at the effect of particular adverse childhood experiences on adults with serious health problems, comparing them with adults who did not report such early trauma. In 1997, the CDC joined and began its prospective research study called the Adverse Childhood Experiences (ACE) study. It included the 17,000 original participants and has tracked their health status ever since. The following is a brief description of the ACE study and its results.

For the ACE study, the three main types of adverse childhood experiences were abuse, neglect, and household dysfunction during the first 18 years of life. The category of neglect included emotional neglect and physical neglect. The experience of emotional neglect included not feeling special and not being loved, or that the person's family was not a source of strength, support, and protection. The experience of physical neglect included not having enough to eat, having to wear dirty clothes, not having someone to take the child to the doctor, or that his or her parents' drinking interfered with the child's care and upbringing. The category of household dysfunction included several factors. The first among these was the experience of having a mother or stepmother who often pushed, grabbed, slapped, threw something, kicked, bit, hit with a fist, or threatened or actually hurt the child with a knife or gun. It also included the experience of living with anyone who was a problem drinker or used street drugs. Also included was living with a household member who was depressed, mentally ill, or who had attempted suicide. The experience may have also included living with parents who were separated or divorced or a household member who went to prison.

Almost two-thirds of those studied reported at least one adverse childhood experience. More than one of five reported three or more of those early adverse experiences. The result of these childhood exposures was a multitude of medical and psychiatric conditions and health behavior problems. All of these appeared during adulthood, usually by the age of 35 or so. Medical conditions included a greater likelihood of having chronic obstructive pulmonary disease, heart disease, liver disease, sexually transmitted diseases, and reduced health-related quality of life. Substance abuse and psychiatric conditions included high levels of alcoholism and alcohol abuse, illicit drug use, depression, and suicide attempts. Problematic health behaviors included increased levels of early initiation of sexual activity, adolescent pregnancies, multiple sexual partners, and unintended pregnancies. It also included increased likelihood of being a smoker, early initiation of smoking, and the increased risk for domestic violence.

Len Sperry, MD, PhD

See also: Child Abuse; Domestic Violence; Neglect; Sexual Abuse; Trauma

Further Reading

Centers for Disease Control and Prevention (CDC). Injury Prevention and Control. Division of Violence Prevention, May 2014. Accessed March 30, 2015. http://www.cdc.gov/violenceprevention/acestudy/.

Karr-Morse, Robin, and Meredith S. Wiley. *Ghosts from the Nursery: Tracing the Roots of Violence*. New York, NY: Atlantic Monthly Press, 2014.

Karr-Morse, Robin, and Meredith S. Wiley. *Scared Sick: The Role of Childhood Trauma in Adult Disease*. New York, NY: Basic Books, 2013.

Advocacy Counseling

Advocacy counseling is a method in which a therapist and client work together to empower the client to get access to services they need. Counselors who promote advocacy within their clients assist them in seeking a way to change social or political systems that exist.

Definition

- **Advocacy** is a process in which an individual or group aims to influence decisions in political, economic, or social policy.

Description

The goal of advocacy counseling is to increase clients' feelings of empowerment and belonging. Usually these services are provided for individuals who are disadvantaged in different ways. A social justice approach to advocacy counseling involves advocating for clients within systems. By teaching clients how to access services and encouraging them to become self-advocates the counselor hopes to become obsolete. Specific techniques of advocacy counseling involve having client join self-help groups, speak out to others on client's rights, and consult with various groups. Counselors who are of the social justice model of counseling validate their clients' reality and empower them to take an active role in resolving their own issues.

The American Counseling Association (ACA) Advocacy Competencies are the basis for advocacy counseling. They provide guiding principles for counseling in three areas. These include client/student, school/community, and the public. Advocacy counselors help their clients respond to the challenges in the environment that prevent growth. They assist them in connecting with organizations and key people that seek social, economic, and political change. It is also important for advocacy counselors to share knowledge of their client's human development. This awareness through communication can help to alert the public about injustices. Lastly, it is important for advocacy counselors to act as change agents in their own systems that affect their clients. They can do this by getting involved in social justice movements.

Development

The history of advocacy in counseling began with Frank Parsons and Carl Rogers. These two inspired changes in social policy at individual and group levels. In addition to advocacy, people who strongly believed in ending oppression demonstrated advocacy through social justice. In the early 1900s, Clifford Beers advocated on behalf of the mentally ill and the reform of psychiatric hospitals.

The theme of counseling and social revolution was formally organized in 1971 when the American Personnel and Guidance Association (APGA) became the American Association for Counseling and Development (AACD). APGA and the AACD made advocacy a major focus. The focus called for social change through personal, professional, and political activities. Later in 1998 the former APGA, now the ACA, created the Council on Social Justice to implement social action to empower clients, students, and oppressed individuals and groups.

Current Status

Many professionals view advocacy counseling as being a philosophy and practice. To be an advocate in counseling one needs to hold strong beliefs about equality and act on behalf of those who are less powerful. This form of counseling addresses the personal issues of clients but also focuses on changing the environment of the client.

The history of advocacy in counseling provides a foundation for teaching advocacy skills from a social justice perspective. The awareness, knowledge, and skills model used in the multicultural competencies support advocacy-oriented counselors. Over the years advocacy counseling has not changed radically; it adjusts flexibly to the issues relevant to the time, place, and clients' needs.

Alexandra Cunningham, PhD

See also: Rehabilitation Counseling

Further Reading

American Counseling Association Advocacy Competencies. 2014. http://www.counseling.org/knowledge-center/competencies.

Cohen, D., R. de la Vega, and G. Watson. *Advocacy for Social Justice: A Global Action and Reflection Guide.* Bloomfield, CT: Kumarian Press, 2001.

Erford, Bradley T. *Orientation to the Counseling Profession: Advocacy, Ethics and Essential Professional Foundations*, 2nd ed. New York, NY: Pearson, 2013.

Toporek, R. L., L. H. Gerstein, N. A. Fouad, G. Roysircar, and T. Israel. *Handbook for Social Justice in Counseling Psychology: Leadership, Vision and Action.* Thousand Oaks, CA: Sage, 2006.

Affect

Affect is an observable pattern of behavior that describes an individual's prolonged emotional experience.

Definitions

- **Emotion** is a feeling state of consciousness (awareness) in which an emotion like joy, sorrow, and fear is experienced, as distinguished from cognitive (mental) states of consciousness. It is also referred to as emotional state.

- **Mental status exam** is an essential part of the initial assessment of an individual's status in the practice of counseling, psychology, and psychiatry.

- **Mood** describes an individual's subjective emotional experience.

- **Subjective** is the description of one's personal and distinct experience of an outer or inner event. It is the opposite of objective.

Description

"Affect" is a psychological term that describes the overt (observable) expression of one's emotion. It describes the immediate expression of an individual's emotional state, moment-to-moment. Affect is distinctly different from mood. Affect describes the observable characteristics of the individuals' emotional state. By contrast, mood describes individuals' subjective experience of their emotional state. It would be expected that if individuals describe their mood as "happy," then their affect would match. For example, a smiling and relaxed posture (indicators of affect) is consistent with a self-report of being happy (mood). Sometimes, there is a discrepancy between a self-reported mood and the observed affect.

A number of factors are used in the description of affect. These include congruence, intensity, range, reactivity, and appropriateness of emotional expressions. Affect is useful in understanding the degree of emotional functioning of individuals and their relationship to both their inner and outer conditions at any given moment. Affect is a key element of the mental status exam. Some of the possible affective states a clinician might use to describe an individual in the mental status exam include the following:

- **Blunted** is a severe lack or reduction of affective expression.
- **Euthymic** describes normal expression of affect.
- **Flat** indicates a lack of intensity of affect such as a monotone voice or blank face.
- **Inappropriate** is an affective expression inconsistent with the individual's statements or thoughts.
- **Labile** is a rapidly changing affective response.
- **Restricted** represents a mild reduction of affective expression.

As it pertains to the expression of certain emotions (happy, sad, angry, surprise, fear, disgust, and contempt), affect is considered universal across culture, regardless of geography. It follows that individuals from any nationality or culture are able to recognize these seven basic emotions in individuals.

Len Sperry, MD, PhD, and Jeremy Connelly, MEd

See also: Mental Status Examination; Mood

Further Reading

American Psychiatric Association. *Diagnostic and Statistical Manual of Mental Disorders*, 5th ed. Arlington, VA: American Psychiatric Association, 2013.

Ekman, Paul. *Emotions Revealed, Second Edition: Recognizing Faces to Improve Communications and Emotional Life*. New York, NY: Henry Holt and Company, 2003.

Wetherell, Margaret. *Affect and Emotion: A New Social Science Understanding*. Thousand Oaks, CA: Sage Publications, 2012.

The Affordable Care Act document. The Affordable Care Act, the law aiming to modify private and public health insurance so that all Americans can have health-care insurance by the year 2023, includes a number of requirements for mental health-care providers. (Redfinch/Dreamstime.com)

Affordable Care Act

The Affordable Care Act is the law that aims to modify private and public health insurance systems so that all Americans can have health-care insurance by the year 2023.

Definitions

- **Congress** is made of the individuals in the Senate and the House of Representatives responsible for creating the laws in the United States.

- **Evidence-based practice (EBP)** is the integration of research evidence, clinical expertise, and client values to provide quality health services that reflect the needs of the client.

EBPs serve to promote quality care and monitor client/patient outcomes.

- **Health reform** is the modification of the delivery of health care to offer insurance to uninsured people, improve access to health care, improve the quality of health care, and reduce the cost of health care.

- **Health-care disparities** refer to the difference between the occurrence of disease, type of health outcomes, access to medical care, and quality of medical care between particular populations, especially between racial and ethnic minority groups and nonminority groups.

- **Insurance exchanges (also known as insurance marketplaces)** are online sites where

Americans can go to compare and purchase health insurance, find answers to questions, and learn about health-care tax credits.

- **Interdisciplinary health care** is the collaboration of different types of health-care providers to deliver comprehensive care to individuals from a biological, psychological, and social perspective.

- **Mental health** refers to a person's psychological, emotional, and social well-being.

- **Outcomes research** is research that incorporates a client's experiences, values, and preferences as they relate to health services and treatment. Outcomes research is used by practitioners to make clinical decisions.

- **Summary of Benefits and Coverage (SBC)** is a universal health insurance form written in simple and easy-to-understand language that people can use to compare different health-care plans and types of coverage.

Description

The Affordable Care Act (ACA) is the health reform law passed by Congress and signed by President Barack Obama on March 23, 2010, that offers insurance exchanges online where Americans can go to find information on, and sign up for, affordable health insurance. The main goal of this law is not only to offer insurance coverage to uninsured people but also to increase the number of benefits individuals receive and lower the costs of health care. The law also removes limitations on preexisting conditions and extends the coverage of young adults under their parents' health insurance policy until the age of 26.

Goals of the ACA include reducing the high uninsured rate, stabilizing and decreasing health-care spending, emphasizing prevention, improving health outcomes, and reducing health inequalities. The ACA allows uninsured Americans, such as the 42 million uninsured people under the age of 65, access to health care at an affordable cost (HHS.gov/HealthCare). At the same time, the act is designed to begin reducing the total health-care spending in the United States. One

way costs can be reduced is by providing more funding for the prevention of diseases like diabetes, high blood pressure, obesity, heart disease, and cancer, which in many cases are avoidable. Prevention will also help improve people's long-term health and help them to live longer. Finally, the ACA aims to provide minorities with quality medical services in an effort to reduce and eliminate health-care disparities.

The ACA requires all insurance companies to offer customers health insurance information in simple language which is easy to understand so they can make comparisons among different insurance carriers and evaluate different types of coverage. All insurance companies must use what is called the Summary of Benefits and Coverage (SBC) form with plain language and a glossary of commonly used terms to help customers compare different health-care plans. Also under the ACA, insurance companies can no longer cancel policies when a person makes an honest mistake on an application or place a dollar limit on how much they will pay for medical services (on most of the covered benefits on an insurance policy).

Under the ACA, health insurance carriers on the insurance exchanges must provide benefits for mental health counseling and substance abuse services. Mental health services also include preventive care for depression, nutrition, weight loss, smoking cessation, and decreasing alcohol use. As with medical services, insurance companies cannot deny anyone mental health benefits due to a preexisting condition, charge more because of a preexisting condition, or place a dollar limit on necessary mental health care.

The ACA law has several implications for mental health training and practice. First, training and education models must be founded on evidence-based practices (EBPs) that are adaptable to different clinical settings and serve diverse populations. Second, training and education curricula must emphasize research methodology and the application of outcomes research to evaluate EBPs in prevention and treatment. Third, training and education programs must prepare graduate students for interdisciplinary, team-based health care in which the collective competencies of health and mental health professionals across disciplines combine to provide integrated quality treatment at a lower cost. Finally, the ACA requires mental health training and education programs to teach students how to conduct continuous assessments of client outcomes to measure the effectiveness of treatment (Chor, Olin, and Hoagwood, 2014, 96–100).

In terms of mental health practice, the ACA establishes practitioner accountability by creating networks of health-care providers, called accountable care organizations. Medical practitioners and specialty practitioners (such as mental health practitioners) merge together in a central location to better coordinate health and mental health services—improving health service quality, lowering costs, and making it easier for clients to access care. Network health-care providers are required to measure and track client outcomes, maintain credentialing and accreditation, and use the electronic medical record to coordinate care and report measurement data (Chor, Olin, and Hoagwood, 2014, 91–92).

Christina Ladd, PhD, and Len Sperry, MD, PhD

See also: Evidence-Based Practice

Further Reading

Cheng, Tina L., Paul H. Wise, and Neal Halfon. "Promise and Perils of the Affordable Care Act for Children." *Journal of the American Medical Association* 311, no. 17 (2014): 1733–1734.

Chor, Ka Ho B., Su-chin S. Olin, and Kimberly E. Hoagwood. "Training and Education in Clinical Psychology in the Context of the Patient Protection and Affordable Care Act." *Clinical Psychology Science and Practice* 21 (2014): 91–105.

HHS.gov/HealthCare. Accessed August 24, 2014. http://www.hhs.gov/healthcare/rights/.

McDonough, John E., and Eli Y. Adashi. "Realizing the Promise of the Affordable Care Act—January 1, 2014." *Journal of the American Medical Association* 311, no. 6 (2014): 569–570.

The 111th Congress. *The Patient Protection and Affordable Care Act: ObamaCare.* Washington, DC: One Hundred Eleventh Congress of the United States of America, 2010.

Aggressive and Antisocial Behavior in Youth

Aggressive and antisocial behaviors in youth represent a set of specific emotional states and behaviors that are severe enough to come to the attention of adults and authority figures.

Description

Aggressive behaviors are negative and hostile verbal and physical acts used to defy authority, get one's way, or express anger. Antisocial behaviors are acts that violate the rights of others. Losing one's temper and learning to control aggressive behaviors such as shouting, screaming, shoving, hitting, grabbing, and stealing are part of growing up. Aggressive behaviors in children and teens do not become a cause for counseling until they create significant problems in relationships, school, or work. Aggressive behaviors are also considered to be a problem when the behavior doesn't match a person's age. For instance, a teenager having a temper tantrum would be an example of behavior immature for the age. When behaviors go against the rights of others, they are called "antisocial" behaviors. Antisocial behaviors include harming others, breaking property on purpose, stealing, bullying, being cruel to animals, beating people up, selling drugs, defying authority, and breaking the law.

Causes and Symptoms

There are many causes for aggressive and antisocial behaviors. Researchers have identified conditions in the home, and the influence of others, as playing a large part in aggressive or antisocial behaviors. Researchers have also identified problems within a person, such as their ability to control themselves, how they feel about themselves, or their personality, to be at the root of bad behavior.

What happens in the home can play a significant part in causing aggressive behavior. Parents who are mean or abusive don't care about how a child performs in school, or their unloving attitude toward their child can result in aggressive behavior in children. Parents who do not discipline or correct their children nor teach them to control their aggressive behavior create an environment that fosters a sense of aggressiveness in their children. Parents' aggressive and hostile attitudes can result in a child learning to behave in aggressive and antisocial ways as a way of coping with life.

Being a part of the wrong crowd, such as a gang, can lead to the development of aggressive and antisocial behaviors. When people who are admired reward, or reinforce, bad behaviors, these behaviors can become part of the way a person lives. For instance, a "friend" who dares a person to shoplift and then goes on telling others about how great it was can result in more antisocial behaviors. Sometimes children who have learning disorders or have emotional problems act out aggressively and develop antisocial behaviors.

Diagnosis and Prognosis

When aggressive and antisocial behaviors become severe enough to require counseling, they are generally referred to as "behavior disorders" and include a number of specific disruptive, impulse-control, or conduct disorders, as described in the *Diagnostic and Statistical Manual of Mental Disorders, Fifth Edition*. People with behavior disorders have significant problems in relationships, school functioning, or work performance. To be diagnosed with a specific behavior disorder, the behaviors must be very disruptive to others and happen more often than is usual for a person of that age. There are two primary psychological conditions or disorders that are included in behavior disorders.

Oppositional defiant disorder (ODD) describes a person who is younger than 18 years and is very negative, purposefully annoying, and defiant of rules and adults. People with ODD often lose their temper, are very stubborn, argue a lot, and don't follow directions. They are angry, emotionally hurtful, and blame others for their problems. They are most likely to be verbally aggressive but are not usually physically aggressive.

Conduct disorder (CD) is a more severe form of behavior disorder. A person with CD is younger than 18 years and behaves in ways that violate other people's right to live safely and peacefully. Youth with CD cause harm to people, animals, and property. There are four types of behaviors that violate people's rights:

(1) Aggressive conduct that causes or threatens physical harm to other people or animals. This behavior includes threatening or causing harm and intimidating or bullying others. It also includes starting fights, forcing people to do things they do not want to do, including sexual acts, and taking other people's belongings by force or intimidation.

(2) Behaviors that cause property damage or loss such as starting fires or breaking other people's belongings on purpose.

(3) Theft and dishonest behaviors such as breaking into someone else's home, lying to get things, and stealing.

(4) Serious violation of rules. This behavior includes defying parental rules, running away from home, sneaking out at night, returning home very late or staying out all night, and skipping school.

Behavior disorders can be treated with psychotherapy. How much change can occur is related to the severity of the disorder, the home life of the child, and the psychological health of the child. Cognitive behavior therapy can be helpful in the development of problem-solving skills, social skills, and anger management. Counseling for children or adolescents who are diagnosed with ODD or CD is most effective when both the individual and the family are the focus of counseling. Family counseling focuses on helping parents develop appropriate expectations for their children and providing training in parenting, boundary setting, and positive discipline. Family counseling also focuses on establishing and maintaining a positive relationship among all family members. Individual counseling focuses on helping the child or adolescent improve his or her coping and problem-solving skills, learn how to appropriately express his or her feelings, and learn to identify and change his or her negative internal thoughts leading to disruptive behaviors.

Steven R. Vensel, PhD

See also: Conduct Disorder; Intermittent Explosive Disorder; Oppositional Defiant Disorder (ODD)

Further Reading

American Psychiatric Association. *Diagnostic and Statistical Manual of Mental Disorders*, 5th ed. Arlington, VA: American Psychiatric Association, 2013.

Kernberg, Paulina, and Saralea Chazan. *Children with Conduct Disorders: A Psychotherapy Manual*. New York: Basic Books, 1991.

Aging and Older Adults

"Aging and older adults" is the phrase used to describe the group of individuals aged 65 and older.

Definitions

- **Alzheimer's disease** is a form of dementia that affects thinking, memory, and behavior. It gradually worsens over time making it difficult, and eventually impossible, to communicate.

- **Baby boomers,** up until 2015 the largest generation of Americans, were born after World War II from 1946 to 1964.

- **Behavior disorders** are illnesses such as anxiety, emotional, and dissociative disorders.

- **Cerebrovascular disease** is a group of brain malfunctions that restrict or block blood flow to the brain.

- **Chronic obstructive pulmonary disease** is a disease that worsens over time because of obstructions in the lungs, which makes breathing difficult.

- **Dementia** is the loss of mental functions such as thinking, reasoning, memory, and language that is associated with diseases like Alzheimer's.

- **Hypochondriasis** is persistent fear and worry about having a particular physical or mental health illness even when health-care professionals cannot find evidence of any problem.

- **Socioeconomic status** is a person's social class standing that is determined by education level, income, occupation. The three levels of socioeconomic status are low, middle, and high.

- **Suicidality** is the likelihood an individual will intentionally kill himself or herself.

Description

Aging and older adults is the way we refer to people aged 65 and older. The number of these individuals in the United States has tripled over the last 100 years. The most significant increase occurred in January 2011 when the first group of baby boomers turned 65. By the year 2030, 20% of the American population will be 65 and older (Anderson et al., 2012). The aging of the baby boomers, coupled with an increase in life expectancy, has resulted in many more people living with chronic physical ailments. As people grow older, they begin to experience age-related changes that affect their ability to function. Common physical changes include hearing or vision loss, high blood pressure, heart disease, diabetes, and arthritis. Decreased cognitive functioning also becomes an issue. It takes older adults longer to learn new information and longer to recall information. With age, long-term memory declines significantly more than short-term memory (American Psychological Association, 2014).

The incidence of psychological problems also increases with age and interferes with normal functioning. Older adults may experience dementia, anxiety, depression, sexual dysfunction, substance abuse, suicidality, hypochondriasis, behavior disorders, and Alzheimer's disease (American Psychological Association, 2014). Furthermore, aging and older adults experience delayed and/or longer response times. They may require help with daily living activities such as housework, shopping, and yard work.

The aging and older adult population is becoming more racially, socially, and economically diverse as the number of older black and Hispanic minorities continues to increase. It is expected that the aging black population will increase from 8% to 10% and the aging Hispanic population will increase from 4% to 16% by the year 2050 (American Psychological Association, 2014). There are significant differences between older White adults and older minority adults. Minorities experience age-related illnesses earlier in life, have a higher occurrence of obesity and diabetes, less frequently report health issues to health-care workers, and put off obtaining health-care intervention. The increased rate of mental health problems among older minorities may be attributed to low socioeconomic status, dysfunctional communities, lack of education, unemployment, stereotyping, discrimination, and a lack of quality health care.

Health-care providers must be aware of the implications of aging. While most people are primarily concerned with physical health in later life, it is equally important to focus on mental health. The stress of coping with a physical illness can negatively impact mental well-being. The reverse is also true. The stress of a mental illness can negatively impact physical well-being. As people are living longer and as the baby boomers age, the number of adults aged 65 and over will rapidly increase. This is significant to note because the baby boom generation has a higher rate of mental health issues such as anxiety, depression, substance abuse, and dementia than the group of older adults before them. They are also more likely to seek mental health services than the aging cohort before them. However, these services must reflect the cultural differences of the population being served; therefore, it is imperative that practitioners develop the cultural competence necessary for effective treatment. Finally, as people age, the possibility of dementia increases. Therefore, the number of older adults living with dementia increases. As the baby boomers age and the incidence of mental illnesses increases, there is greater demand for culturally appropriate mental health services.

Health-care providers must consider the affordability and accessibility of quality health care. The primary source of income for people aged 65 and over is from Social Security benefits. Furthermore, 13% of older adults live in poverty (American Psychological Association, 2014). Economic factors significantly impact the ability of aging and older adults to access and pay for health care. The most efficient and cost-effective means of providing comprehensive health care to aging and older adults is through networks of health-care providers and centrally located practitioners who collaborate to offer a full range of quality services that are easily accessible at a reduced cost. As people live longer, the goal of health-care professionals is to help people maintain their physical and mental well-being over the years, regardless of age-related illnesses and challenges.

Christina Ladd, PhD, and Len Sperry, MD, PhD

See also: Alzheimer's Disease; Baby Boomers; Dementia

Further Reading

American Psychological Association. 2014. "Older Adults' Health and Age-Related Changes." Accessed August 28, 2014. http://www.apa.org/pi/aging/resources/guides/older.aspx?item=5.

Anderson, Lynda A., Richard A. Goodman, Deborah Holtzman, Samuel F. Posner, and Mary E. Northridge. "Aging in the United States: Opportunities and Challenges for Public Health." *American Journal of Public Health* 102, no. 3 (2012): 393–395.

Holtzman, D., and L. A. Anderson. "Aging and Health in America: A Tale from Two Boomers." *American Journal of Public Health* 102, no. 3 (2012): 392.

Lomranz, Jacob. *Handbook of Aging and Mental Health: An Integrative Approach.* New York, NY: Plenum Press, 1998.

Agoraphobia

Agoraphobia is extreme fear of public spaces, crowds, or areas from which escape may be difficult and results in intense anxiety.

Definitions

- **Antianxiety medications** are prescribed drugs that relieve anxiety symptoms. They are also called anxiolytics or tranquilizers.

- **Anxiety** is apprehension or worry about an imagined danger.

- **Anxiety disorders** are a group of mental disorders characterized by anxiety as a central or core symptom. The group includes agoraphobia, specific phobias, and social anxiety disorder.

- **Behavior therapy** is a form of psychotherapy that focuses on identifying and changing maladaptive behaviors.

- **Fear** is an emotional response to a known danger.

- **Panic attack** is an episode of sudden, intense, and debilitating sense of fear that is short lived.

- **Panic disorder** is an anxiety disorder characterized by severe panic attacks that occur so frequently as to produce significant distress and/or impaired functioning.

- **Phobia** is an intense fear of a person, place, or thing that significantly exceeds the actual danger posed.

Description and Diagnosis

Fear and anxiety are commonly used interchangeably in everyday conversation. However, these terms have different technical meanings. With disorders like agoraphobia it is useful to know and appreciate this distinction. In this disorder both are present in that the feared place or situation causes the symptoms of anxiety. Agoraphobia is a phobia in which individuals experience an intense fear of crowds, public places, open spaces, or places from which they believe that they cannot easily escape. Alternatively, the primary fear may also be embarrassment of being observed panicking by others in the public space. Those with this disorder commonly avoid exposure to such situations, while a minority tolerate their symptoms. Agoraphobia is classified as an anxiety disorder. In fact, agoraphobia is more likely to occur together with panic disorder than by itself.

Agoraphobia and its commonly co-occurring diagnosis can severely impact an individual's life. Those with disorder may become so fearful that they completely avoid leaving their home. In some cases, these individuals have lost their jobs and close relationships, as well as their independence. Agoraphobia is typically diagnosed in adolescence through early adulthood. The likelihood of developing this disorder is approximately 1.7% in adolescence and adulthood but is considerable less after the age of 65 (American Psychiatric Association, 2013).

According to the *Diagnostic and Statistical Manual of Mental Disorders, Fifth Edition*, an individual may be diagnosed with agoraphobia if he or she experiences extreme fear when either anticipating or directly being exposed to public transportation, open or closed public spaces, being present in large groups of individuals including lines, or being outside of his or her own home. Also, the panic symptoms must be the direct consequence of the agoraphobic situation, last at least six months, be out of proportion to the actual risk or danger, and be that escape would be difficult. The symptoms must also cause significant distress or result in significant level of impaired functioning. In addition, the disorder is not the result of a medical condition or another mental disorder. This disorder is to be diagnosed despite whether a panic disorder is present. If it is present both diagnoses should be made (American Psychiatric Association, 2013).

Like other mental disorders, agoraphobia have various causes, including genetic and environmental factors. Because it tends to run in families, genetic factors appear to contribute to its development. Various environmental factors may also trigger or predispose an individual to develop this disorder. These include other anxiety disorders, particularly panic disorder. A history of trauma or childhood abuse may be another factor.

Treatment

Treatment for agoraphobia may include therapy, medication, or a combination of both. Often, behavior therapy is used to reduce the fear and related anxiety. Antidepressant medications like Prozac or Zoloft may be prescribed to reduce the intensity of the chronic worry. Also, antianxiety medications, such as Ativan and Xanax, may be prescribed. Typically, treatment begins with medications that are used only until the fear and anxiety responses are reduced with behavior therapy. Since this disorder tends to co-occur with panic disorder, it is important that clinicians diagnose and treat both disorders simultaneously.

Len Sperry, MD, PhD, and Jeremy Connelly, MEd

See also: Ativan (Lorazepam); Behavior Therapy; Panic Attack; Panic Disorder; Phobic Disorder; Prozac (Fluoxetine); Social Anxiety Disorder; Xanax (Alprazolam); Zoloft (Sertraline)

Further Reading

American Psychiatric Association. *Diagnostic and Statistical Manual of Mental Disorders*, 5th ed. Arlington, VA: American Psychiatric Association, 2013.

Antony, Martin M., Michelle G. Craske, and David H. Barlow. *Mastering Your Fears and Phobias: Workbook.* New York, NY: Oxford University Press, 2007.

Pollard, Alec C., and Elke Zuercher-White. *The Agoraphobia Workbook: A Comprehensive Program to End Your Fear of Symptom Attacks.* Oakland, CA: New Harbinger, 2003.

Stahl, Bob, and Wendy Millstine. *Calming the Rush of Panic: A Mindfulness-Based Stress Reduction Guide to*

Freeing Yourself from Panic Attacks and Living a Vital Life. Oakland, CA: New Harbinger, 2013.

Alcohol Use Disorder

Alcohol use disorder is a mental disorder involving a pattern of alcohol use which leads to significant problems for the user.

Definitions

- **Addiction** is a chronic disease of the brain which involves compulsive and uncontrolled pursuit of reward or relief with substance use or other compulsive behaviors.

- **Alcoholism** is a general term for the compulsive and uncontrolled consumption of alcohol to the detriment of the drinker's health, relationships, and social standing.

- **American Society of Addiction Medicine** is an organization of physicians whose purpose is to improve the care and treatment of individuals with the disease of addiction and to advance the practice of Addiction Medicine. It is also referred to as ASAM.

- **DSM-5** is the abbreviation for the *Diagnostic and Statistical Manual of Mental Disorders, Fifth Edition*, which is the handbook mental health professionals use to diagnose mental disorders.

- **Substance-related and addictive disorders** are a group of DSM-5 mental disorders that include substance disorders characterized by physiological dependence, drug-seeking behavior, tolerance, and social withdrawal. This group also includes the non-substance disorder of gambling.

Description and Diagnosis

Alcohol use disorder is one of the substance-related and addictive disorders. It is characterized by the use of alcohol which results in significant distress or disrupted daily functioning. While drinking alcohol can be a pleasant way to relax and enjoy the company of others, individuals with alcohol use disorder drink to excess. As a result, they endanger themselves and others. "Alcohol use disorder" is the term used in DSM-5 to include the conditions of "alcohol abuse" and "alcohol dependence." In the past, these conditions were considered separate disorders. "Alcohol abuse" referred to short-term and less severe problems with alcohol, such as college students who binge drink. Alcohol dependence referred to long-term and more severe problems and was synonymous with alcoholism. Alcohol use disorder is a common disorder affecting approximately 16% of the adult population (American Psychiatric Association, 2013).

Alcohol use has both short- and long-term effects. Short-term effects include reduced coordination, decreased alertness, impaired ability to drive, clumsiness, slurred speech, and inability to walk without help. Other such effects include life-threatening unconsciousness and coma. Even with moderate use most drivers have slower reaction time and are a danger to themselves and others driving a vehicle. Long-term effects include various digestive and liver diseases such as alcoholic hepatitis, cirrhosis, gastritis, and pancreatitis; hypoglycemia; and other malnutrition-related problems. Long-term effects of alcohol also cause cardiovascular disease, nervous system problems including dementia, and death from lung and heart failure. Some of these long-term effects can occur in as little or less than 10 years of alcohol use.

According to the *Diagnostic and Statistical Manual of Mental Disorders, Fifth Edition*, individuals can be diagnosed with this disorder if they use alcohol in larger amounts than intended and have a persistent desire to cut back or control alcohol use. Craving (a strong desire or urge to use alcohol) is another criteria, as is tolerance (increasing amounts needed to become intoxicated) and withdrawal symptoms. The severity of this disorder can diagnosed or specified on a continuum of severity. Those presenting with two to three symptoms are classified as "mild," those with four to five symptoms are "moderate," and those with six or more are "severe" (American Psychiatric Association, 2013).

The cause of this disorder involves biological, psychological, and social-cultural factors. In addition to a strong neurological basis, psychological traits such as impulsiveness, low self-esteem, and a need for approval may be involved. Other factors include peer pressure, cultural acceptability, and the availability of alcohol. Early use of this drug is associated with impulsivity and lifelong problematic use. Alcohol is commonly used as a way of coping when other ways have failed or no longer work.

Treatment

The goal of treatment for this disorder is abstinence (no longer using alcohol). Treatment has three stages. The first is detoxification, which involves discontinuing alcohol use and treating withdrawal symptoms. The second is rehabilitation, which involves counseling and medications to give the recovering alcoholic the skills needed for maintaining abstinence. The third is maintenance, which includes the support of others to remain abstinent. This commonly involves regular Alcoholics Anonymous meetings and getting a sponsor. Effective treatment of this disorder involves determining the proper level of care for specific individuals. The American Society of Addiction Medicine has developed criteria for five levels of care assessed over six dimensions. The ASAM criteria are required in over 30 states and are considered the gold standard for determining the proper level of care.

Len Sperry, MD, PhD

See also: Addiction; Addictive Personality

Further Reading

American Psychiatric Association. *Diagnostic and Statistical Manual of Mental Disorders*, 5th ed. Arlington, VA: American Psychiatric Association, 2013.

Dodes, Lance. *Breaking Addiction: A 7-Step Handbook for Ending Any Addiction*. New York, NY: Harper Perennial, 2011.

Prentiss, Chris. *The Alcoholism and Addiction Cure: A Holistic Approach to Total Recovery*. Malibu, CA: Power Press, 2007.

Alcoholics Anonymous (AA)

Alcoholics Anonymous (AA) is a self-help fellowship that was founded by Bill Wilson and Dr. Bob Smith in 1935 to help people struggling with alcoholism.

Definitions

- **Addiction** is a chronic disease of the brain which involves compulsive and uncontrolled pursuit of reward or relief with substance use or other compulsive behaviors.

- **Alcoholism** is a general term for the compulsive and uncontrolled consumption of alcohol to the detriment of the drinker's health, relationships, and social standing.

- **Self-help fellowship** is a community in which individuals struggling with the same problem (e.g., alcoholism) help one another. It is also known as a mutual aid fellowship.

- **Temperance movement** was a national crusade that encouraged total abstinence from alcohol.

- **Twelve Steps** refer to the 12 guiding principles on which AA is based.

- **Twelve-Step Programs** are self-help groups whose members attempt recovery from various addictions based on a plan called the Twelve Steps.

- **Twelve Traditions** are the rules that govern how Twelve-Step Program groups operate.

Description

Alcoholics Anonymous is a mutual aid fellowship intended to help people with alcohol problems. AA is the first of many Twelve-Step Programs based on it. AA developed from an early 20th-century temperance movement called the Oxford Group. Members believed that alcoholism was a spiritual illness rather than the result of a weak will. They proposed a spiritual program that involved accepting a higher power and helping others. Many of these practices were carried over to AA.

AA members assist one another through sharing personal experiences, offering guidance, and sponsorship. This generally takes place during attendance at AA meetings, which may focus on members' stories, the Twelve Steps, or some other topic.

The AA fellowship is nonprofessional and does not employ doctors, counselors, or any other type of trained helper. A main principle of AA is that an alcoholic is best suited to understand and help another alcoholic. AA is not considered to be formal treatment but rather an additional method of support. AA groups operate independently from one another, though there is a small governing body based in New York. The organization does not take part in political, religious, or any other kind of debate. This is to protect its stated primary purpose of helping alcoholics achieve sobriety. AA claims that its current membership is nearly 2 million people worldwide. There are AA meetings in many different countries and those which cater to specific genders, age groups, and sexual orientations.

The core of AA is the Twelve Steps and Twelve Traditions. These have remained unchanged since their original format. The Twelve Steps focus on the process of addiction recovery. They include tasks such as admitting powerlessness, completing a moral inventory, making amends to those who were harmed, and helping other alcoholics. For example, Step 1 is "We admitted we were powerless over alcohol—that our lives had become unmanageable." The ultimate goal of the Twelve Steps is to achieve a spiritual awakening which will help the alcoholic remain sober. The Twelve Traditions focus on AA's organizational principles. They include maintaining anonymity in the press, staying out of public debates, and declining outside financial contributions. Both the Twelve Steps and Twelve Traditions are found in *Alcoholics Anonymous: The Story of How Many Thousands of Men and Women Have Recovered from Alcoholism*. This text is popularly called the "Big Book" by AA members. It is frequently read during AA meetings and contains chapters devoted to employers, unbelievers, and the family members of alcoholics.

Bill Wilson (1895–1971) was a founding member of AA. Born in East Dorset, Vermont, Wilson was a shy man who struggled with depression and anxiety throughout his young adult years. He served in the military during World War I and enrolled in law school on his return home. To deal with his increasing social anxiety in law school, Wilson drank excessively. The result was being dismissed from law school for drunkenness. After that he worked as a stock speculator and traveled the country with his wife, Lois. His drinking continued to worsen, resulting in financial failure and numerous hospitalizations at Towns Hospital in New York.

It was during one of these hospitalizations that he was reacquainted with Ebby Thatcher (1896–1966), an old friend who had stopped drinking with the help of the Oxford Group. Wilson continued to drink until he had what he described as a "spiritual experience" during another hospitalization. He reported that he saw a bright light and felt the presence of God. Wilson never drank again after this event. He joined the Oxford Group and helped another alcoholic, Dr. Bob Smith (1879–1950), during a business trip to Akron, Ohio, in 1935. The two began helping other alcoholics and promoting a spiritual program of recovery. They eventually split from the Oxford Group and started their own fellowship with the publication of *Alcoholics Anonymous*. Wilson was the primary author of this book, which contained the original Twelve Steps.

Bill Wilson continued to develop the AA program throughout his lifetime and remained a central figure in the movement. Some controversy surrounds his experimentation with lysergic acid diethylamide (LSD) in the 1950s and alleged infidelity. Wilson eventually died from emphysema in 1971 presumably because of long-term tobacco use.

George Stoupas, MS, and Len Sperry, MD, PhD

See also: Addiction; Addictive Disorder; Alcohol Use disorder; Twelve-Step Programs

Further Reading

Anonymous. *Alcoholics Anonymous: The Story of How Many Thousands of Men and Women Have Recovered from Alcoholism*. New York, NY: AA World Services, Inc., 2001.

Cheever, Susan. *My Name Is Bill: Bill Wilson: His Life and the Creation of Alcoholics Anonymous*. New York, NY: Washington Square Press, 2004.

Kurtz, Ernest. *Not God: A History of Alcoholics Anonymous*. Center City, MN: Hazelden, 1991.

Alexithymia

Alexithymia is the inability to identify or describe one's emotions.

Definitions

- **Autism spectrum disorder** is a mental disorder characterized by impaired social and communication skills, repetitive behaviors, and a restricted range of emotions and interests.

- **Cognitive behavior therapy** is a type of psychotherapy that focuses on maladaptive (problematic) behaviors, emotions, and thoughts. It is also called CBT.

- *Diagnostic and Statistical Manual of Mental Disorders* is the handbook mental health professionals use to diagnose mental disorders. The current edition (fifth) is known as DSM-5.

- **Emotion** is a complex physiological, cognitive, and behavioral reaction to a situation perceived to be personally significant. Happiness, sadness, surprise, disgust, anger, and fear are the six basic emotions recognized across cultures.

- **Emotional intelligence** is the ability to accurately identify and respond to emotions in oneself and others.

- **Feelings** are the subjective expression of emotion.

Description

The term "alexithymia" means "no words for feelings" in Greek. It was originally described by American psychiatrist Peter Sifneos (1920–2008) in 1973. Alexithymia is characterized by poor awareness of one's emotions, difficulty relating to others, confusing feelings with physical symptoms, lack of empathy, overly logical thinking, and lack of imagination or creativity. People may get lost in trivial details. These characteristics may differ from person to person. Those with alexithymia often lack insight and may appear robotic or detached to those around them. They may be able to identify basic emotions like "happy" or "sad" but cannot go into greater detail about their feelings. Rather than the complete absence of emotions, alexithymia is a problem of emotional expression. It often leads to interpersonal problems because these individuals tend to avoid intimate relationships or position themselves in either dependent or dominant roles. Those in romantic relationships with alexithymics are likely to find their relationships less than satisfying. It is not surprising that those with alexithymia have low levels of emotional intelligence.

Alexithymia is not a diagnosis included in the *Diagnostic and Statistical Manual of Mental Disorders, Fifth Edition*. However, it is often found in those with other mental disorders such as autism spectrum disorder. It is also linked with medical conditions such as migraine headaches, hypertension (high blood pressure), and lower back pain. It appears that unexpressed emotions somehow build up and are expressed indirectly in these medical conditions.

There are several theories about the cause of this disorder. These include genetic factors like neurological problems and environmental factors like childhood abuse. Problems in communication between the two hemispheres (sides) of the brain are believed to be its cause. Others believe that it is caused by an individual's fear of being overwhelmed by emotions and the decision to shut them out for protection. Alexithymia occurs in about 10% of adults.

Treatment

Traditional counseling may not be successful for those with alexithymia because they are not able to connect with their feelings. However, there are specialized cognitive behavior therapy interventions that have developed for those with this condition.

Len Sperry, MD, PhD, and George Stoupas, MS

See also: Diagnostic and Statistical Manual of Mental Disorders (DSM); Emotion; Emotional Intelligence

Further Reading

Barsky, Arthur J., and Emily C. Deans. *Stop Being Your Symptoms and Start Being Yourself*. New York, NY: HarperCollins Publishers, 2010.

Sifneos, Peter. "The Prevalence of 'Alexithymic' Characteristics in Psychosomatic Patients." *Psychotherapy and Psychosomatics* 22, no. 2 (1973): 255–262.

Taylor, Graeme J., R. M. Gabby, and James D. A. Parker. *Disorders of Affect Regulation: Alexithymia in Medical and Psychiatric Illness*. Cambridge, UK: Cambridge University Press, 1997.

Allostatic Load

Allostatic load is the by-product of chronic stress over time. It is a result of allostasis, which is the process of maintaining balance in the body through physiological (physical) changes.

Definitions

- **Adrenaline** is a neurotransmitter (chemical messenger) involved in the fight or flight response that increases heart rate, pulse rate, and blood pressure.

- **Brain** is the organ at the center of the nervous system. It is responsible for a wide range of functions, including learning, movement, and regulation of the body.

- **Dopamine** is the chemical messenger in the brain responsible for coordinating the movement of voluntary muscle groups. It also regulates attention, pleasure, and coping with stress.

- **Hormones** are chemicals in the body that are produced by glands to regulate physical functions like sleep, metabolism, and mood. Cortisol and testosterone are examples of hormones.

- **Neurotransmitters** are chemicals in the brain responsible for a variety of functions, including pleasure, motivation, and mood. Dopamine, serotonin, and gamma-aminobutyric acid are examples of neurotransmitters.

- **Stress** is the pattern of specific and nonspecific responses to events that tax or exceed an individual's ability to cope. Stress can be acute (short term) or chronic (long term).

- **Stress management** is a set of psychological techniques for increasing the capacity to better cope with psychological stress. It usually includes relaxation methods.

Description

Allostasis is the process of maintaining balance in an organism through physiological adjustments in response to environmental stimuli. The term literally means "maintaining stability through change." These changes are controlled by the brain through the release of hormones and neurotransmitters. They are intended to meet the expected demands of the individual. One example is epinephrine, also known as adrenaline. It is secreted by the adrenal gland when an individual perceives danger or experiences excitement. Adrenaline results in increased heart rate, respiration rate, and blood glucose levels. Cortisol is another stress hormone. It increases energy production in the body and suppresses the immune system. Neurotransmitters like dopamine are also released in response to stress. They act to increase concentration, motivation, and memory. All of these changes enhance performance and enable quick movements such as running or fighting. They involve many different regulatory systems in the body, such as the central nervous system and the inflammatory system. Once the perceived danger or excitement has passed, neurochemical levels decrease and the systems return to normal. This physiological process has clear short-term benefits. For example, being chased by a rabid dog would activate the stress response system and allow an individual to escape. Increased blood flow would enable faster movements and heightened awareness would lead to quick decision making. However, the long-term effects of stress can result in damage to the body and lead to disease.

The term "allostatic load" was originally used by biologist Bruce McEwen, PhD (1938–), and psychologist Eliot Stellar, PhD (1919–1993). They defined it as the by-product of chronic stress over time. It can be thought of as the price the body pays for constantly adapting to stress through allostasis. The neurochemical changes that accompany stress can negatively impact functioning if they occur frequently. While some stressful situations may happen on occasion, repeated activation of the stress response system may result from other environmental factors. For example, living in poverty can produce significant ongoing stress. Problems like insufficient food, large debt, and loss of a job can activate the body's stress response system. Unlike a chance encounter with a rabid dog, however, these environmental stressors do not quickly pass. Constant arousal leads to dysregulation (imbalance) of the body's stress response. An individual's allostatic load can be measured.

This measure includes factors such as cortisol levels, blood pressure, and cholesterol. High allostatic load scores have been associated with a number of mental and physical problems. These include increased risk of heart disease, impaired immune system, memory problems, and increased risk of death. Individuals who experience chronic stress are at risk for these conditions. An individual's response to stress depends on many factors like genetics, environment, and coping skills. There are ways to reduce the negative impact of stress through the use of techniques like stress management.

George Stoupas, MS, and Len Sperry, MD, PhD

See also: Adrenaline; Brain; Dopamine; Stress

Further Reading

McEwen, Bruce S., and Elizabeth Lasley. *The End of Stress as We Know It*. New York, NY: Dana Press, 2002.

McEwen, Bruce S., and Eliot Stellar. "Stress and the Individual: Mechanisms Leading to Disease." *Archives of Internal Medicine* 153, no. 18 (1993): 2093–2101.

Sapolsky, Robert M. *Why Zebras Don't Get Ulcers: The Acclaimed Guide to Stress, Stress-Related Diseases, and Coping*, 3rd ed. New York, NY: Holt Paperbacks, 2004.

Allport, Gordon (1897–1967)

Gordon Allport is regarded as one of the founding fathers of personality psychology. He developed his own eclectic theory based on traits, moving away from psychoanalytic and behavioral approaches that were popular views at the time. His life's work was devoted to cultivating his theory, examining the impact of social justice issues, and developing personality tests.

Description

Gordon Willard Allport was born on November 11, 1897, in Montezuma, Indiana, to John Edwards Allport and Nellie Edith (Wise) Allport, a country doctor and school teacher. Gordon was the youngest of four boys. The Allports were devout Protestants who believed in hard work, which led to educational and later professional success for Gordon and his siblings. The family moved to Cleveland, Ohio, when Gordon was six and the boys attended local public schools. In

his teenage years, Gordon ran his own printing business while serving as editor of the school newspaper. He graduated second in his class from Glenville High School, earning a scholarship to Harvard College. Gordon's brother, Floyd Allport, also a Harvard grad, went onto become an important social psychologist. Though the transition to college wasn't easy, Gordon soon acclimated, majoring in economics and philosophy and successfully earned his BA degree in 1919.

After graduating, Allport traveled to Istanbul, Turkey, to teach English and sociology at Robert College. He later returned to Harvard to pursue his master's degree and study under Herbert S. Langfeld. In 1921, he coauthored his first publication, *Personality Traits: Their Classification and Measurement*, with his brother Floyd. In 1922, he received his PhD in psychology. He then continued studying abroad, at places such as the University of Berlin, the Hamburg in Germany, and the University of Cambridge in England. In 1924, he returned to his alma mater and began teaching in the Department of Social Ethics. The remainder of his career was spent working on his Trait Theory from which came additional publications and personality assessments. He died in Cambridge, Massachusetts, on October 9, 1967.

A story always included in Allport's biographies surrounds his meeting the great Sigmund Freud in Vienna at the age of 22. The initial interaction consisted of complete silence, with Freud simply waiting for Gordon to begin talking, perhaps attempting to determine who could stand the silence longer. Gordon, feeling uncomfortable, blurted out an observation he made on the bus ride over to Freud's office. A little boy was very upset about having to sit in the seat where a dirty old man had previously sat. He hypothesized that the boy's behavior was likely the product of his apparently rigid, domineering mother. Rather than responding to Gordon's comments, Freud followed up with the question, "And was that little boy you?" Freud, of course, was referring to the unconscious process in Gordon's mind instead of the simplicity of the observation. This experience had a profound effect on Allport causing him to turn away from psychoanalytic theory, which he felt all too often sought reasons and answers where they did not exist. Allport did not believe it was necessary to look into a person's past in order to understand his or her present self. He even

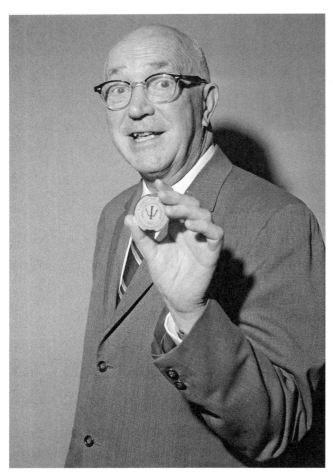

Gordon Allport is regarded as one of the founders of personality psychology, moving away from psychoanalytic and behavioral theories toward humanistic theories of psychology. (AP Photo/Bill Ingraham)

coined the term "functional autonomy," to highlight his view that one's current actions and motives are independent (autonomous) of past origins. Trait Theory posits that each person has a foundational self, composed of both phenomenological and functional components. The phenomenological part is our essential self and is made up of experiences we view as most central. The latter component comprises functions we undergo at different points throughout our life. Allport defined seven functions: (1) sense of body—develops in first two years of life, distinct boundaries between bodily self and outside world; (2) self-identity—first two years, sense of individuality and continuity; (3) self-esteem—develops between ages 2 and 4, sense of value to ourselves and others; (4) self-extension—ages 4 to 6, people, things, events that are essential to one's identity (5); self-image—also develops between ages

4 and 6, how others view us, the impression we make on them; (6) rational coping—learned during ages 6 to 12, ability to deal with problems in a rational, effective manner; and (7) appropriate striving—begins after the age of 12, sense of direction and purpose in life. These functions, though they reflect time periods similar to Freud's, should not be likened to stages, as they simply describe ways in which people develop.

While our functional selves are developing, one also develops personal traits or, as Allport named them, personal dispositions. Dispositions are concrete, distinct, and easily recognizable patterns in a person's behavior. Originally using the term "traits," Allport changed to the term "dispositions" to distinguish between things a person may see or perceive about another person when looking at another person versus characteristics that were unique to that individual. This distinction caused Allport to strongly encourage the use of idiographic methods of study. Idiographic methods, nowadays referred to as qualitative methods, focus on studying one person at a time in depth by way of interviews, observations, analysis of writings, and so on.

Allport compiled a list of over 4,500 different traits before collapsing them down into three categories: cardinal traits, central traits, and secondary traits. Cardinal traits are traits that dominate a person's entire personality. These types of traits are quite rare and often do not develop, if at all, until later in life. Central traits are more common and describe people's personalities. Examples of central traits are shy, kind, friendly, and smart. Allport estimated that most people have between 5 and 10 central traits. Secondary traits are more fluid and may be present only under certain conditions and circumstances. Personal preferences and situational attributes are examples of secondary traits (i.e., getting anxious during a flight).

Impact (Psychological Influence)

Gordon Allport's ideas have remained a part of mainstream psychological thought. His works went on to influence the views of other highly regarded theorists, including Abraham Maslow and Carl Rogers. He had a profound impact in shaping humanistic theory as a whole.

Melissa A. Mariani, PhD

See also: Humanistic Psychotherapy; Maslow, Abraham (1908–1970); Rogers, Carl (1902–1987)

Further Reading

Allport, Gordon W. *Becoming: Basic Considerations for a Psychology of Personality*. New Haven, CT: Yale University Press, 1955.

Allport, Gordon W. *Pattern and Growth in Personality*. New York, NY: Holt, Rinehart, & Winston, 1961.

Pettigrew, Thomas F. "Gordon Willard Allport: A Tribute." *Journal of Social Issues* (2009). Accessed January 7, 2013. http://findarticles.com/p/articles/mi_m0341/is_3_55/ai_58549253/.

Alzheimer, Alois (1864–1915)

Alois Alzheimer is known for his work with dementia, particularly dementia of the Alzheimer's type, more commonly referred to as Alzheimer's disease.

Alzheimer's disease is a medical and mental disorder that causes dementia usually, but not always, after age 65. It is the most common form of dementia, which is a disease associated with memory loss and decreased cognitive functioning. Alzheimer's is the most common type of dementia. In the *Diagnostic and Statistical Manual of Mental Disorders, Fifth Edition*, it is referred to as Neurocognitive Disorder Due to Alzheimer's Disease.

Description

Alois Alzheimer (1864–1915) was a Bavarian psychiatrist who published the first case of dementia, which was later identified as dementia of the Alzheimer's type. He was born in Marktbreit, Bavaria. He received his medical degree from Würzburg University in 1886. He was cofounder and copublisher of the journal *Zeitschrift für die gesamte Neurologie und Psychiatrie*. Throughout his professional career, Alzheimer published his finding in various scientific journals. Dr. Alzheimer worked with patients with mental illness early in his career. He eventually took a position in the Frankfurt's Asylum for Lunatics and Epileptics. There he became increasingly involved in the diagnosis and treatment of dementia. In 1901 Auguste Deter (1850–1906) became one of Dr. Alzheimer's patients. She presented with strange behavioral symptoms and loss of short-term memory. Dr. Alzheimer became particularly interested in her symptoms and continued to monitor her condition. She died in 1906 after

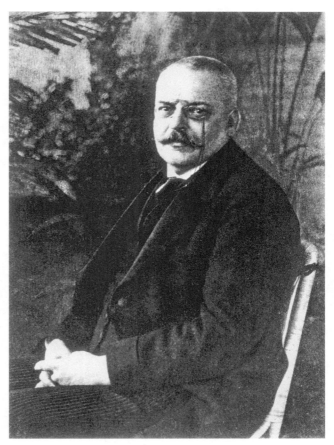

Alois Alzheimer from Bavaria was a psychiatrist who became known for his work with senile dementia, now more commonly known as Alzheimer's disease. (Corbis)

which Alzheimer had her medical records and brain sent to the lab of the famous German psychiatrist Emil Kraepelin (1856–1926) in Munich. The lab used special staining techniques and determined that Auguste Deter's brain contained amyloid plaques and neurofibrillary tangles. Amyloid plaques are protein fibers that are found in the brain of individuals with neurodegenerative disorders such as Alzheimer's, Parkinson's, and Huntington's disease. Neurofibrillary tangles are twisted masses of protein fibers in nerve cells which are found in the brains of individuals with Alzheimer's disease.

Afterward, Dr. Alzheimer gave several professional presentations about the pathology and symptoms of this form of senile dementia that differed from presenile dementia, which is a form of dementia that occurs in middle age (before 65 years) and progresses (worsens) rapidly, and other types of dementia. Kraepelin credited Alzheimer with the discovery of this form of dementia and called it Alzheimer's dementia in his definitive textbook of psychiatry. Since 1911, physicians in the United States and throughout the world have used Alzheimer's list of symptoms to diagnose their patients.

Dr. Alzheimer's research differentiated the senile form of dementia (eventually coined "Alzheimer's" in Kraepelin's textbook) from the other types of dementia. His years of work and research serve as the foundation for the search for a cure for Alzheimer's by the medical community today. In addition, Alzheimer's is considered one of the most disturbing diseases of old age today.

Len Sperry, MD, PhD, and Jon Sperry, PhD

See also: Alzheimer's Disease; *Diagnostic and Statistical Manual of Mental Disorders* (DSM)

Further Reading

American Psychiatric Association. *Diagnostic and Statistical Manual of Mental Disorders*, 5th ed. Arlington, VA: American Psychiatric Association Press, 2013.

Doraiswamy, P. Murali, Lisa Gwyther, and Tina Adler. *The Alzheimer's Action Plan: What You Need to Know—and What You Can Do—about Memory Problems, from Prevention to Early Intervention and Care.* New York, NY: St. Martin's Press, 2009.

Maurer, Konrad, and Maurer Ulrike. *Alzheimer: The Life of a Physician and Career of a Disease.* New York, NY: Columbia University Press, 2003.

Alzheimer's Disease

Alzheimer's disease is a medical and mental disorder that causes dementia, particularly late in life. It is also referred to as Neurocognitive Disorder Due to Alzheimer's Disease.

Definitions

- **Dementia** is a group of symptoms including loss of memory, judgment, language, and other intellectual (mental) function caused by the death of neurons (nerve cells) in the brain.

- The *Diagnostic and Statistical Manual of Mental Disorders, Fifth Edition,* is the handbook mental health professionals use to diagnose mental disorders.

- **Mild cognitive impairment** is a mental condition characterized by memory problems that do not significantly impact daily functioning. Commonly, the condition is hardly noticeable or troublesome to the individual. It is also known as MCI.

Description and Diagnosis

Alzheimer's disease is a progressive disease that destroys memory and other important mental functions and results in the loss of intellectual and social skills. It is the most common cause of dementia in individuals over the age of 65. Before the age of 70 about 10% of adults are diagnosed with the disorder. That figure rises to at least 25% after age 70. Women are more likely than are men to develop this disease, in part because they live longer (American Psychiatric Association, 2013).

The decline in mental functioning is progressive in terms of person, place, time, and situation. At first, individuals have trouble articulating why they are where they are ("situation"). Next, they have difficulty identifying where they are ("place"). Later, as the disease progresses, they have difficulty identifying what day or year it is ("time"). Finally, in advanced cases, they will lose a sense of who they are ("person"). New learning, such as the ability to listen to a story and repeat it, also declines. Genetic testing is essential in making the diagnosis of Alzheimer's disease.

Three stages of the disease are recognizable: early, middle, and late. In the early stage of Alzheimer's, specific signs and symptoms can be observed. These include short-term memory loss, difficulty performing familiar tasks, and increasing problems with planning and managing activities, like balancing a checkbook. It may also include trouble with language, such as difficulty recalling words for everyday things. In the middle stage of this disease, the individual may have difficulty completing everyday tasks, such as preparing meals or getting dressed. Individuals may experience intense feelings of paranoia and anger, and they may wander away or get lost. In the late stage of the disease, individuals are unable to care for themselves. They may be unable to communicate with or recognize others or to walk by themselves. They may have difficulty swallowing and be unable to smile.

According to the *Diagnostic and Statistical Manual of Mental Disorders, Fifth Edition*, individuals can be diagnosed with this disorder if they exhibit a steady progression of impairment of memory, learning, language, perception, or another cognitive domain. There must also be evidence of Alzheimer's disease from family history or genetic testing. In addition, there must be obvious evidence of decline in learning and memory, and this decline must be progressive. Furthermore, the absence of other neurological conditions is required (American Psychiatric Association, 2013).

Mild cognitive impairment (MCI) is an intermediate stage between the cognitive decline associated with normal aging and the more serious decline of dementia. MCI can involve problems with memory, language, thinking, and judgment. Individuals with MCI may recognized that their memory or mental function has "slipped." Family and close friends may also notice a change. However, these changes do not interfere with one's usual activities. For some, MCI may increase individuals' risk of progressing to dementia. Still, others with this condition experience no decline and may eventually get better.

The cause of this disorder is not yet well understood. However, brains affected by Alzheimer's disease have many fewer cells and many fewer connections than those with healthy brains. As brain cells die, significant brain shrinkage occurs. Two types of brain abnormalities are found in this disease. The first is plaques on the outside of brain cells. These plaques are clumps of a protein called beta-amyloid that interfere with cell-to-cell communication in the brain. Although the ultimate cause of brain-cell death in Alzheimer's isn't known, the collection of beta-amyloid on the outside of brain cells is a prime suspect. The second is tangles which are distortions in the cell's internal support and transport system involving a protein called tau. In this disorder, threads of tau protein twist into abnormal tangles inside brain cells.

Treatment

Because of the biological basis of this disorder, treatment is largely biological. Specific medications and management strategies may temporarily improve symptoms. Medications like Aricept can slow the progression of Alzheimer's symptoms for about half of those taking them for 6 to 12 months. Aricept is approved by the FDA (Food and Drug Administration) for all stages of Alzheimer's disease: early or mild stage, moderate or middle stage, and late or severe stage. It works by increasing levels of acetylcholine (a chemical) in the brain. Namenda is also FDA approved to treat moderate-to-severe Alzheimer's disease. It is thought to work in the brain by regulating the activity of glutamate (a chemical) in the brain.

While these medications may extend an individual's functioning and maintain his or her independence for a short time, there is no cure for this disorder. Therefore, it is important those with Alzheimer's and their caretakers seek supportive services and maintain a good support network. Family therapy can assist family members to understand, accept, and adjust to the individual's progressively deteriorating condition.

Len Sperry, MD, PhD

See also: Aricept (Donepezil); Dementia; Namenda (Memantine)

Further Reading

American Psychiatric Association. *Diagnostic and Statistical Manual of Mental Disorders*, 5th ed. Arlington, VA: American Psychiatric Association, 2013.
Burns, Alistair, and Bengt Winblad, eds. *Severe Dementia*. New York, NY: John Wiley & Sons, 2006.
Doraiswamy, P. Murali, Lisa Gwyther and Tina Adler. *The Alzheimer's Action Plan: What You Need to Know—and What You Can Do—about Memory Problems, from Prevention to Early Intervention and Care*. New York, NY: St. Martin's Press, 2009.
Mace, Nancy, and Peter V. Ravins. *The 36-Hour Day: A Family Guide to Caring for People with Alzheimer Disease, Other Dementias, and Memory Loss in Later Life*, 5th ed. Baltimore, MD: Johns Hopkins University Press, 2012.

Ambien (Zolpidem)

Ambien is a prescription medication used to treat sleep problems (insomnia) in adults. Its generic name is zolpidem.

Definitions

- **Gamma-aminobutyric acid** is a chemical messenger in the brain that leads to relaxation, calmness, and sleep by reducing nerve cell excitement.

- **Insomnia** is a chronic inability to fall asleep or to remain asleep throughout the night.

- **Sedative-hypnotics** are medications that induce calmness and sleep. Barbiturates and benzodiazepines are its main types. They are also called tranquilizers, sleeping pills, or sleepers.

Description

Ambien is in the class of medications known as sedative-hypnotics. Its primary use is in the treatment of insomnia. Ambien is believed to work by mimicking the neurotransmitter (chemical messenger) in the brain called gamma-aminobutyric acid which promotes relaxation and sleep. Unlike other sleeping medications, Ambien does not interfere with the quality of sleep or result in drowsiness on awakening. Instead, most who use Ambien awake feeling refreshed.

Precautions and Side Effects

Because Ambien is used to help individuals fall asleep, it should not be used with over-the-counter, herbal, or prescription medications, such as antihistamines or alcohol, which also cause drowsiness. Ambien should be used only with close medical supervision in people with liver disease and in the elderly, because these individuals are especially sensitive to the sedative properties of Ambien. Ambien should not be used before driving, operating machinery, or performing activities that require mental alertness. Those with a history of drug abuse, depression, or other mental disorders should be carefully monitored when using Ambien since it may worsen symptoms of some mental disorders.

Using Ambien can lead to sleep-related behaviors such as eating, talking, and driving while asleep, with no recollection of the events. More common side effects include headache, nausea, muscle aches, and daytime drowsiness. Such drowsiness may cause

individuals, particularly those over age 65, to be less coordinated and more susceptible to falls. Other less common side effects include anxiety, confusion, dizziness, and stomach upset.

Taking Ambien and other medications that causes drowsiness may result in substantially decreased mental alertness and impaired motor skills. Some examples include alcohol, antidepressants such as Tofranil or Paxil, antipsychotics such as Mellaril, and the antihistamines in many allergy and cold medications.

Len Sperry, MD, PhD

See also: Sleep Disorders

Further Reading

Doble, Adam, Ian Martin, and David J. Nutt. *Calming the Brain: Benzodiazepines and Related Drugs from Laboratory to Clinic.* London: Informa Healthcare, 2003.

Kryger, Meir H., Thomas Roth, and William C. Dement. *Principles and Practice of Sleep Medicine*, 5th ed. New York, NY: Saunders, 2011.

Preston, John D., John H. O'Neal, and Mary C. Talaga. *Handbook of Clinical Psychopharmacology for Therapists*, 7th ed. Oakland, CA: New Harbinger, 2013.

American Academy of Child and Adolescent Psychiatry (AACAP)

The American Academy of Child and Adolescent Psychiatry (AACAP) is a nonprofit group of psychiatrists and other related medical professionals created in 1953. It is a national organization with 7,500 members dedicated to helping children who have been diagnosed with psychiatric disorders.

Definition

- **Child and adolescent psychiatrists** are medical doctors with specialized training who assess, diagnose, and treat mental, behavioral, or developmental disorders in children and adolescents, usually by prescribing medication.

Description

The AACAP was organized to help improve the quality of life of the nearly 12 million U.S. youth who suffer from mental, behavioral, or developmental disorders. This group also offers information and support for the families of these youth.

The AACAP's mission is to "promote the healthy development of children, adolescents, and families through research, training, prevention, comprehensive diagnosis and treatment and to meet the professional needs of child and adolescent psychiatrists throughout their careers." Part of the work that the AACAP does includes setting guidelines for standards of care in treating children and adolescents who have been diagnosed with a mental illness.

Impact (Psychological Influence)

The organization offers many services to its members and to the families affected by mental illness. The AACAP provides information and support to parents and family members of affected children and adolescents. The group also is active in research that hopefully will lead to more effective treatments. The organization works to increase access to treatment and services for children and adolescents, and to reduce the stigma associated with mental illness. To do this, the organization provides a learning center for families who have a child diagnosed with a mental illness, behavioral or developmental disorder.

In an effort to support the families with information, the AACAP publishes a variety of informative guides for parents. For example, it publishes a *Parents' Medication Guide for Treating Childhood Depression* and the *Parents' Medication Guide for Bipolar Disorder*. These publications, as well as many prescription drug guides, are free and available at www.aacap.org.

The AACAP also is an advocate on behalf of the mental health of children and adolescents, focusing on access to services and improving national policies regarding mental health. Members are informed of upcoming legislation and regulatory actions so they can get involved in working with lawmakers on the importance of children's mental health.

The American Academy of Child and Adolescent Psychiatry is considered an Allied Assembly organization of the APA. The American Psychiatric Association (APA) was founded in 1844 and is considered the largest professional psychiatric organization.

Being an Allied Assembly organization of the APA means that the AACAP's mission and code of ethics are compatible with the APA's. A similar organization to AACAP is the International Association of Child and Adolescent Psychiatrists and Allied Professionals (IACAPAP), which was founded in 1935. IACAPAP pursues a similar mission to AACAP but has expanded membership that includes working with allied professionals, such as psychologists, social workers, pediatricians, and nurses.

Mindy Parsons, PhD

See also: American Psychiatric Association (APA)

Further Reading

The AACAP has published a quarterly journal since 1962. The publication is known as the *Journal of the American Academy of Child and Adolescent Psychiatry*. The journal is highly regarded for its leading psychiatric research and treatment, including a focus on the psychopharmacology of child and adolescent disorders.

Organization

The American Academy of Child and Adolescent Psychiatry
3615 Wisconsin Avenue, N.W.
Washington, DC, 20016-3007
Telephone: (202) 966-7300
Fax: (202) 966-2891
Website: http://www.aacap.org

American Counseling Association (ACA)

The American Counseling Association (ACA) is currently the world's largest nonprofit organization serving professional counselors working in various settings through education and professional development.

Definition

- **Professional counselors** are licensed/certified practitioners who work in educational or mental health settings and possess specialized skills that benefit clients in making progress emotionally, socially, behaviorally, or academically.

Description

The American Counseling Association is a not-for-profit organization responsible for the education, support, and development of professional counselors working in various settings (schools, mental health agencies, private practice, etc.). ACA was founded in 1952. It is currently the world's largest association exclusively representing professional counselors. It has a membership rate of more than 50,000. The mission of the ACA is "to enhance the quality of life in society by promoting the development of professional counselors, advancing the counseling profession, and using the profession and practice of counseling to promote respect for human dignity and diversity."

ACA provides valuable services to counselors by providing leadership training, making available up-to-date resources and publications, and offering continuing education opportunities. It has been instrumental in providing counselors the means by which to enhance their skills and expand their knowledge base. Establishing professional and ethical standards has also been a goal of the ACA. The organization has made a concerted effort to raise standards in terms of accreditation, licensure, and national certification. Advocacy is another part of the mission. Elected members represent the interests of the profession before Congress and federal agencies. In addition, they seek to recognize the accomplishments of professional counselors in public forums.

The formation of the association now referred to as ACA began in Los Angeles, California, in 1952. Four independent organizations, the National Vocational Guidance Association, the National Association of Guidance and Counselor Trainers, the Student Personnel Association for Teacher Education, and the American College Personnel Association, convened in hopes of unifying their professional efforts. The American Personnel and Guidance Association was established, but the name was later changed to the American Association of Counseling and Development in 1983. Then, on July 1, 1992, the association adopted its current name, the American Counseling Association. The new name was meant to reflect a common purpose between members no matter what setting they worked in.

The ACA is headquartered in Alexandria, Virginia, just outside Washington, D.C. It services professional counselors living in the United States as well as in 50 other countries. Some of these nations include Europe, Latin America, the Philippines, and the Virgin Islands. The ACA encompasses a comprehensive network with 19 chartered divisions and 56 branches itself. However, it also works with outside corporations in related fields to enhance services and benefits for its members. The various ACA divisions provide information, resources, and services specifically tailored to areas of specialized practice or principles of counseling. Divisions include the Association for Assessment in Counseling and Education, the Association for Adult Development and Aging, the Association for Creativity in Counseling, the American College Counseling Association, the Association for Counselors and Educators in Government, the Association for Counselor Education and Supervision, the Association for Humanistic Counseling, the American Mental Health Counselors Association, the Association for Lesbian, Gay, Bisexual, and Transgender Issues in Counseling, the Association for Multicultural Counseling and Development, the American Rehabilitation Counseling Association, the American School Counselor Association, the Association for Spiritual, Ethical, and Religious Values in Counseling, the Association for Specialists in Group Work, the Counselors for Social Justice, the International Association for Addictions and Offenders Counselors, the International Association of Marriage and Family Counselors, the National Career Development Association, and the National Employment Counseling Association. Members of ACA can enhance their professional identity and practice by joining one or more of these divisions. These divisions elect officers who govern their activities independently and are also permitted a say in national ACA governance. The Governing Council is the national governing body of the ACA. Nationally elected officers and representatives from each division and region serve terms of no longer than three years.

Impact (Psychological Influence)

The American Counseling Association has had a significant impact on professional counseling practice. It continues to set standards and make strides in the field. By 2009, ACA had enacted licensure in all 50 states. In 2010, ACA delegates announced their consensus on a definition of counseling to 20/20: A Vision for the Future of Counseling: "Counseling is a professional relationship that empowers diverse individuals, families, and groups to accomplish mental health, wellness, education, and career goals." By promoting public confidence and trust, the ACA provides a foundation of support for counseling professionals so that they can assist clients and students in dealing with life's challenges.

Melissa A. Mariani, PhD

See also: Counseling and Counseling Psychology

Further Reading

American Counseling Association. Alexandria, Virginia, 2013. "About Us: Our History." http://www.counseling.org/.

American Counseling Association. *The ACA Encyclopedia of Counseling*. Alexandria, Virginia, May 30, 2009.

American Mental Health Counselors Association (AMHCA), The

The American Mental Health Counselors Association (AMHCA) is a professional association of licensed clinical mental health counselors.

Description

The AMHCA is a professional organization with a membership of nearly 7,000 clinical mental health counselors. The mission of the AMHCA is to enhance the profession of clinical mental health counseling through licensing, advocacy, education, and professional development. The AMHCA sets standards of education, training, licensing, practice, advocacy, and ethics for the profession. Clinical membership in AMHCA requires a master's degree in counseling or a closely related mental health field and adherence to AMHCA's National Standards for Clinical Practice.

The AMHCA was founded in 1976 by a group of community mental health, community agency, and private practice counselors who identified their practice as "mental health counseling." The initial focus of the AMHCA was to establish a definition of mental health counseling, set education and training standards, create a national credentialing system, and establish a professional journal (*Journal of Mental Health Counseling*).

Impact (Psychological Influence)

The AMHCA defines the practice of clinical mental health counseling as the provision of professional counseling services involving the application of principles of psychotherapy, human development, learning theory, group dynamics, and the etiology (how it develops) of mental illness and dysfunctional behavior. Counselors provide services to individuals, couples, families, and groups, for the purpose of promoting optimal mental health, dealing with normal problems of living, and treating psychopathology. The practice of mental health counseling includes, but is not limited to, diagnosis and treatment of mental and emotional disorders, psychoeducational techniques aimed at the prevention of mental and emotional disorders, consultations to individuals, couples, families, groups, organizations, and communities, and clinical research into more effective psychotherapeutic treatment services.

In 1979 the AMHCA created the first educational and training standards for mental health counselors. In 1988 the Council for Accreditation of Counseling and Related Educational Programs adopted and adapted the AMHCA training standards and established the first accreditation standards for master's degree programs in Mental Health Counseling. Also in 1979 the AMHCA established the first credentialing body for mental health counselors: the National Academy of Certified Mental Health Counselors. In 1993 this certification was absorbed into the National Board for Certified Counselors.

The AMHCA provides national and state legislative advocacy services for members. Advocacy includes ensuring that counselors are recognized in federal and state laws; educating policy makers about the role of mental health counselors; increasing lawmakers' awareness about mental illness and its effects on people's lives; and enhancing public and private insurance plans so mental health benefits are offered similar medical and surgical benefits.

The AMHCA code of ethics defines and guides ethical behaviors and best practices for mental health counselors. The code identifies six key principles.

I. Commitment to Clients: guidelines regarding the counselor–client relationship; the counseling process; counselor responsibilities and integrity; assessment and diagnosis; record keeping, fee arrangements and bartering; other roles.

II. Commitment to Other Professionals: guidelines regarding relationships with colleagues and clinical consultations.

III. Commitment to Students, Supervisees, and Employee Relationships: guidelines for the integrity and welfare of supervisees, students, and employees.

IV. Commitment to the Profession: guidelines for teaching; research and publications; service on public or private boards and other organizations.

V. Commitment to the Public: guidelines for public statements and advertising.

VI. Resolution of Ethical Problems: guidelines resolve ethical dilemmas, which may arise in clinical practice.

Steven R. Vensel, PhD

See also: Council for Accreditation of Counseling and Related Educational Programs; Mental Health Counselor

Further Reading

American Mental Health Counselors Association. "AMHCA Code of Ethics." Accessed April 12, 2013. http://www .amhca.org/about/codetoc.aspx.

American Mental Health Counselors Association. "Standards for the Practice of Clinical Mental Health Counseling." Accessed April 12, 2013. http://www.amhca .org/about/default.aspx.

American Psychiatric Association (APA)

The American Psychiatric Association (APA) is the world's largest professional organization serving psychiatrists seeking to provide effective treatments for patients with mental health disorders.

Definition

• **Psychiatrists** are medical doctors who specialize in the diagnosis, treatment, and prevention of mental health disorders including intellectual disabilities and substance abuse issues.

Description

The American Psychiatric Association is a medical specialty organization that seeks to be the voice and conscience of modern psychiatry. It currently serves approximately 36,000 psychiatrists in the United States and throughout the world. APA's mission is to provide the highest quality of care to patients suffering with mental health issues, promote research and education related to psychiatric problems, advance the field of psychiatry, and provide proper service to its members. This mission is accomplished through services provided to patients, members, and the profession. Founded in 1844, APA has a long-standing record of providing psychiatrists at all career levels with professional support. Members advocate for available and accessible care for all persons suffering with mental illness.

In October 1844, the *Association of Medical Superintendents*, the foundations of APA, was formed of 13 superintendents from the then existing 24 mental health hospitals. Their purpose was to share ideas, communicate their experiences, and assist one another in providing proper treatment for those deemed mentally insane. In 1892, the association changed its name to the *American-Medico Psychological Association* and now opened membership to practitioners working in mental hospitals and private practice. Prompted by the work of Sigmund Freud and other leading psychoanalysts of the time, the National Committee for Mental Hygiene was in 1912 to shed further light on the issue of mental health. In 1917, the association adopted the first diagnostic and statistical manual. An official name change from the American Medico-Psychological Association to the American Psychiatric Association occurred in 1921. In 1946, the association adopted its first set of standards for psychiatric patients and an official first edition of the *Diagnostic and Statistical Manual of Mental Disorders* was then released until

1952. The first Assembly of APA's district branches, 16 at the time, was held on May 5, 1953, in Los Angeles, California. Prior to this date no unified mission or official representation existed. Since that time the association has progressed its cause and grown exponentially in membership comprising some 36,000 members to date.

The American Psychiatric Association is headquartered in Arlington, Virginia. APA is governed by a board of trustees of national and regional representatives who are elected by members with the authority to make policy changes to the Bylaws and act on behalf of the association. At present, the association has 74 district branches/state associations that work to streamline communication, offer educational programs and training opportunities, provide public outreach materials, and advance APA's mission through promotional advertising. These services assist in ongoing professional development for members, allowing them to continue to advance their clinical and diagnostic skill sets. The APA website houses information, resources, and training for professionals. The Continuing Medical Education and Lifelong Learning Center allows members to take continuing education credits online through various formats. Annual meetings are available through this site to provide members with the most up-to-date research and interventions for their patients. Members have the ability to get recertified through the site as well. APA also publishes four professional journals, the *American Journal of Psychiatry, Psychiatric Services, FOCUS: The Journal of Lifelong Learning*, and the *Journal of Neuropsychiatry and Clinical Neurosciences*. A philanthropic offshoot of APA, the American Psychiatric Foundation, works to promote mental health and wellness worldwide by providing public and professional education, funding, and recognition.

Impact (Psychological Influence)

APA provides valuable services to psychiatrists by providing a professional support network, making available current resources and publications, and offering continuing education, training, and grant opportunities. APA has established professional and ethical guidelines to direct clinical practice and advocates for the profession as a whole. Recent concerns for the profession including enhancing privacy laws, protecting scope of practice, and advocating for fair treatment, insurance coverage, and reimbursement for those suffering with mental health disorders and substance related issues are also being advanced through APA's efforts. APA released the most recent edition of the DSM (DSM-5) in May 2013.

Melissa A. Mariani, PhD

See also: Diagnostic and Statistical Manual of Mental Disorders (DSM); Psychiatrist

Further Reading

American Psychiatric Association. *Diagnostic and Statistical Manual of Mental Disorders*, Fifth Edition. Arlington, VA: American Psychiatric Association, 2013.

American Psychiatric Association. *History of the District Branches and of the District Branch Assembly*. Washington, DC: American Psychiatric Association, 1966.

Hales, Robert E., Stuart C. Yudofsky, and Laura Weiss Roberts. *The American Psychiatric Publishing Textbook of Psychiatry*, 6th ed. Arlington, VA: American Psychiatric Association, 2014.

American Psychological Association (APA)

The American Psychological Association (APA), the world's largest professional and scientific organization of psychologists, was established with the purpose of creating, communicating, and applying psychological knowledge to improve people's lives and to benefit the larger society.

Definition

- **Psychologists** are practitioners who hold doctoral-level degrees (PhD, PsyD, or EdD) in psychology and work in a variety of areas including education, research, private practice, health care, law, and business/industry to promote mental health and wellness.

Description

The American Psychological Association is comprised of over 134,000 members worldwide working in the psychology field to provide scientific research, education, treatment, and prevention care to people in need. As the largest professional association of psychologists, APA represents clinicians employed in diverse settings including schools, research labs, private practices, hospitals, courts, and businesses. Students pursuing degrees in psychology or other closely related fields are also eligible for membership. APA's mission is to "*to advance the creation, communication and application of psychological knowledge to benefit society and improve people's lives.*" This is accomplished through encouraging the broad development and application of psychology, promoting psychological research, improving current psychological practice by raising qualifications and establishing high standards, and disseminating psychological knowledge and research findings to those within the profession and outside community.

Founded in July 1892 at Clark University in Worcester, Massachusetts, APA was formed by a small group of men seeking to further a new field of psychology. Electing themselves and others, APA then consisted of only 31 members. Granville (G.) Stanley Hall (1844–1924), psychologist and educator credited with spawning the Child Study Movement, served as president. APA's first official meeting was held in December 1892 at the University of Pennsylvania with governance comprised of a council and executive committee. Membership grew modestly over the first 50 years; however, once a new category of nonvoting membership was opened in 1926, that of *associate members*, numbers increased from the hundreds to the thousands. APA reorganized during World War II, merging with other psychological associations to encompass a broader more flexible view of psychology. The greatest increase in membership resulted after World War II between 1945 and 1970 when numbers rose from some 4,000 to over 30,000. Several factors contributed to a growing interest in psychology, and this subsequent boom in APA membership included (a) returning servicemen who were in need of psychological care, (b) health benefits that were now provided to veterans through the GI Bill, (c) the inception of the Veterans Administration Clinical Psychology training program, and (d) the creation of the National Institute of Mental Health (NIMH), a U.S. agency dedicated to the focus, treatment, and prevention of mental health problems. A revised divisional structure also occurred post–World War II contributing to APA's growth. With only 19 approved divisions in 1944, APA presently has 54 divisions in various subdivisions of psychology.

The American Psychological Association is chartered in Washington, D.C., and is governed by a council of representatives with a board of directors. The council of representatives, made up of elected members from regional associations and APA divisions, is the sole legislative body responsible for determining policy and budgetary changes. The board of directors advises and offers recommendations to the council while an elected president executes matters related to the Bylaws. Several affiliate organizations are associated with APA, including the American Psychological Foundation responsible for philanthropic work, the APA Insurance Trust that oversees financial and insurance matters, Ethnic Minority Psychological Associations that support minority needs, such as the Society for the Psychological Study of Culture, Ethnicity, and Race, the APA Practice Organization and Education Advocacy Trust charged with promoting advocacy, education, and training efforts, and various state, regional, and international associations, as well as the honor societies of Psi Chi and Psi Beta.

Impact (Psychological Influence)

APA continues to provide services to its members by offering professional development and training, a forum for publishing psychological articles in peer-reviewed journals, access to up-to-date resources, and funding opportunities for scientific endeavors. The APA website hosts the *PsychInfo, PsychArticles*, and *PsychNet* databases, allowing members ready access to materials. The sixth edition of the *Publication Manual of the American Psychological Association* was released in 2009 to direct writers, editors, students, and educators in the APA writing style. The APA's *Ethical Principles of Psychologists and Code of Conduct*, now referred to as the *Ethics Code*, was amended in 2010 and is updated periodically to guide psychological practice and supervision. Supporting mental health for the general public is an additional goal of APA, furthered through advocating for federal policies and laws related to psychological wellness. The association also tracks current psychological trends in order to perpetuate knowledge, treatment, and prevention efforts.

Melissa A. Mariani, PhD

See also: Publication Manual of the American Psychological Association

Further Reading

American Psychological Association. "About APA." Washington, DC, 2014. http://www.apa.org/.

American Psychological Association. *Publication Manual of the American Psychological Association*. Washington, DC: American Psychological Association, 2009.

Dewsbury, Donald A. 1997. "On the Evolution of Divisions." *American Psychologist* 52: 733–741.

Evans, Rand B., Virginia Staudt Sexton, and Thomas C. Cadwallader, eds. *The American Psychological Association: A Historical Perspective*. Washington, DC: American Psychological Association, 1992.

American Rehabilitation Counseling Association (ARCA)

The American Rehabilitation Counseling Association (ARCA) is an organization of counselors, teachers, and students who want to improve the lives of people with disabilities.

Definitions

- **Rehabilitation counseling** is a type of counseling that focuses on helping individuals who have disabilities in order to achieve their career, personal, and independent living goals.

- **Rehabilitation counselors** are certified counseling professionals who help people with emotional and physical disabilities live independently.

- **Scope of practice** includes the procedures, processes, and acts which professionals can legally use in their jobs.

Description and History

ARCA was established in 1958 as a division of the American Counseling Association (ACA). ACA is an association for all professional counselors. Its mission is to enhance the lives of people with disabilities across their life span. In 1971, ARCA was identified as one of the five organizations that comprise the Council on Rehabilitation Education (CORE). CORE was created based on a need to give credit to educational programs for rehabilitation counselors. Currently, both ARCA and CORE are involved with the training, evaluation, and employment of rehabilitation counselors in the United States.

Impact (Psychological Influence)

ARCA has several goals. One goal is to organize members who encourage excellent practice, research, consultation, and learning. Another goal is to remove barriers for people with disabilities who want to access education, jobs, and community activities. ARCA also increases public awareness about disabilities and counseling through outreach and education. Finally, it offers counselors activities with government and other leadership.

ARCA also lists values for rehabilitation counselors. These values include the belief that people with disabilities should be included in the community. All people should be treated with dignity and worth. They are committed to giving equal rights to people with disabilities and to help empower their clients to achieve this. They emphasize that human functioning is universal and should focus on a person's strengths.

The work that rehabilitation counselors do with clients consists of different tasks. These tasks are considered within their scope of practice. ARCA lists what is within the scope of practice for rehabilitation counselors. This involves communication, setting goals, and empowering clients with disabilities. Counselors should be able to help people with physical, mental, developmental, cognitive, and emotional disabilities. They utilize some of the following processes in their work: assessment, diagnosis, career, individual and group counseling, case management, research, and more. These counselors can work with government systems to remove barriers and provide access to technology that might be helpful to the client.

Alexandra Cunningham, PhD

See also: American Counseling Association (ACA); Rehabilitation Counseling; Vocational Counseling

Further Reading

American Rehabilitation Counseling Association. "Welcome to ARCA." Last modified February 13, 2013. Accessed July 22, 2013. http://www.arcaweb.org.

U.S. Bureau of Labor Statistics. "Rehabilitation Counselors: Occupational Outlook Handbook." Last modified March 29, 2012. Accessed January 15, 2015. http://www.bls .gov/ooh/community-and-social-service/rehabilitation-counselors.htm.

American School Counselor Association (ASCA)

The American School Counselor Association (ASCA) is the school counseling division of the American Counseling Association (ACA) specifically developed to meet the needs of professional school counselors working in various educational settings.

Definition

- **Professional school counselors** are counseling practitioners employed in various educational settings who collaborate with parents and teachers to help students develop across academic, social, and career domains.

Description

Founded in 1952, the ASCA is an international nonprofit organization that was developed specifically to meet the needs of professional school counselors. ASCA welcomes school counselors with varying experience who work at different educational levels: elementary, middle, high school, and college. It believes in maintaining one vision and one voice for all counselors working in educational areas.

ASCA is the school counseling division of the ACA. Its current membership rate is over 31,000. ASCA provides professional development, guidance on best practices, and relevant resources to its members. Its vision statement reads, "The American School Counselor Association (ASCA) is the foundation that expands the image and influence of professional school counselors through advocacy, leadership, collaboration and systemic change. ASCA empowers professional school counselors with the knowledge, skills, linkages and resources to promote student success in the school, the home, the community and the world." The mission of the association is to represent professional school counselors and to promote professionalism and ethical practices. To date, ASCA's leadership board, the Delegate Assembly, has granted division charters to all 50 states and the District of Columbia.

Over the past two decades, ASCA has been at the forefront of driving policy and practice changes in the field of school counseling. The ASCA Ethical Standards for school counselors were adopted in 1984 and have been revised in 1992, 1998, 2004, and, most recently, 2010. In addition, ASCA and its parent organization, ACA, were influential in the passing of the Elementary School Counseling Demonstration Act of 1995. This piece of legislation provided funding for school counseling programs that proposed promising and innovative approaches. It also suggested a counselor to student ratio of 1:250 and that school counselors spend 80%–85% of their time engaged in direct services to students. Direct services include school counseling core curriculum, individual counseling and student planning, and responsive services. Indirect services refer to services provided on behalf of students after consulting with others (parents, teachers, other educators, community organizations). In 1997, after surveying more than 2,000 elementary, middle, and high school counselors working in K-12 settings, ASCA compiled a set of national standards for school counseling programs focused on the following key areas: (1) shifting the focus from counselors to counseling programs; (2) creating a framework for a national school counseling model; (3) establishing school counseling as an integral part of the academic mission of schools; (4) promoting equal access to school counseling services for all students; (5) emphasizing the key components of developmental school counseling; (6) identifying the knowledge and skills that all students should have access to as a part of a comprehensive school counseling program; and (7) providing for the systematic delivery of a school counseling program. Then in 2001, a group of experts in the field assembled to discuss the progress made in the profession during the previous 100 years. The group agreed that a model was needed to help school counselors add value to their school's mission. As a result, ASCA published the first edition of the ASCA National Model in 2003, which became a framework for comprehensive, development school counseling programs. Contributors included Trish Hatch, Judy Bowers, Norm Gysbers, Curly and Sharon Johnson, Robert Myrick, Carol Dahir, Cheri Campbell, Pat Martin, and Reese House. The purpose of this model was twofold: (1) to help move school counseling from a responsive service for some students to a program for every student and (2) to reestablish school counseling as a critical function to remove barriers to learning and help foster academic achievement and overall student success. The model called for school counseling programs to be comprehensive, developmental, and evidence based. School counseling programs are also based on standards in three domains: academic, personal/social, and career. By establishing policy and practice standards, ASCA seeks to ensure the viability of the school counseling profession.

Impact (Psychological Influence)

The American School Counselor Association established the RAMP (Recognized ASCA Model Program) program in 2003 in order to recognize model school counseling programs throughout the country. Schools apply for this designation and have to undergo a rigorous evaluation process. To date, over 400 schools have earned RAMP status. The National Model was revised in 2005 and the most recent edition was released in 2012. On January 1, 2006, the U.S. Congress declared the first week of February as National School Counseling Week, in response to advocacy from ASCA members. ASCA released School Counseling Competencies in 2008 in an effort to guide effective implementation of National Model programs. Though ASCA recommends a school counselor to student ratio of 1:250, the most recent reports, from the 2010 to 2011 school year, indicate a national average ratio of 1:471.

Melissa A. Mariani, PhD

See also: American Counseling Association (ACA); Guidance Counselor

Further Reading

American School Counselor Association. *The ASCA National Model: A Framework for School Counseling Programs*. Alexandria, VA: Author, 2005.

Campbell, C. A., and C. A. Dahir. *The National Standards for School Counseling Programs*. Alexandria, VA: American School Counselor Association, 1997.

American Society of Addiction Medicine (ASAM)

The American Society of Addiction Medicine (ASAM) is a professional organization whose purpose is to improve the treatment of addictions and to advance the practice of addiction medicine. It is also known as ASAM.

Addiction is a chronic disease of the brain, which involves compulsive and uncontrolled pursuit of reward or relief with substance use or other compulsive behaviors.

Addictions include alcoholism, a general term for the compulsive and uncontrolled consumption of alcohol to the detriment of the drinker's health, relationships, and social standing.

Description

The American Society of Addiction Medicine is a professional organization that represents over 3,000 physicians and related professionals whose focus is on addiction and treatment. The founder of ASAM was Ruth Fox, MD (1895–1989). The origin of ASAM was in the early 1950s when Dr. Fox held meetings with other physicians who were interested in alcoholism and treatment. In 1954, this group of physicians developed the New York City Medical Society on Alcoholism. As the membership grew, the society was named the American Medical Society on Alcoholism (AMSA). The American Academy of Addictionology was included in 1982, and efforts began to receive recognition for this specialty within the medical field. In 1983, AMSA formed a single national organization uniting all of these groups. In 1988, a house of delegates of the American Medical Association (AMA) accepted ASAM into membership as a national medical specialty society. The AMA is the largest association of physicians and medical students in the United States.

Impact (Psychological Influence)

ASAM's core motivation is to enhance the care and treatment of individuals with the disease of addiction while advancing the practice of addiction medicine. ASAM's mission is to improve the quality of addiction treatment and educate physicians, related professionals, and the public about addiction. In addition, ASAM advocates for research and prevention and promotes the proper role of physicians in the care of individuals with an addiction. ASAM has also established addiction medicine as a specialty recognized by purchasers and consumers of health-care services, physicians, governments, the general public, and professional organizations.

The values and goals of the framework of ASAM significantly contribute to the mental health field. These include leadership, integrity, respect, openness, advocacy, and connectedness. Some of these values and goals include having empathy and commitment for an individual with an addiction. In addition, ASAM promotes optimism for change, accepting the achievable, and determination for a healthy future. Furthermore, ASAM includes diversity of all medical specialists and treatments to assist individuals with an addiction.

Elizabeth Smith Kelsey, PhD, and
Len Sperry, MD, PhD

See also: Addiction; Addiction Counseling

Further Reading

Fishman, Marc J., and Gerald R. Shulman. *ASAM Patient Placement Criteria: Supplement on Pharmacotherapies for Alcohol Use Disorders*. Philadelphia, PA: Lippincott Williams & Wilkins Publishing, 2010.

Gastfriend, David R. *Addiction Treatment Matching: Research Foundations of the American Society of Addiction Medicine Criteria*. Binghamton, NY: Haworth Press, 2004.

Ries, Richard K. *Principles of Addiction Medicine*. Philadelphia, PA: Lippincott Williams & Wilkins Publishing, 2011.

Americans with Disabilities Act (ADA)

The Americans with Disabilities Act (ADA) is a civil rights law intended to protect against discrimination based on disability. It was originally adopted in 1990 and amended in 2008.

Definitions

- **Disability** is a physical or mental impairment that substantially limits one or more of the major life activities of an individual.

- **Disability evaluation** is a formal determination of the degree of a physical, mental, or emotional disability.

Description

The Americans with Disabilities Act is a civil rights law that was enacted by the U.S. Congress in 1990 and signed by President George H. W. Bush. It is considered a civil rights law because it safeguards the rights of citizens. This law extends the protections against discrimination introduced by the Civil Rights Act of 1964. This 1964 law applied to discrimination based on race, religion, sex, national origin, and other individual characteristics. The specific purpose of the ADA is to prohibit discrimination on the basis of disability. The ADA defines a disability as a physical or mental impairment that substantially limits one or more "major life activities" or bodily functions. This law also includes individuals with a history of such impairment and those who are perceived by others as having an impairment. Examples of major life activities are caring for oneself, eating, walking, and communicating. Major bodily functions described by the law include functions of the bowels, brain, and nervous system. The ADA does not list all of the impairments covered by the law. This is decided on a case-by-case basis. Some conditions are specifically excluded, such as current substance abuse or vision problems that can be corrected with glasses. A 2008 amendment to the law called the ADA Amendments Act extended protections introduced by the original law. It also made the law more specific by listing major life activities that qualified for protection.

The Americans with Disabilities Act is broken down into five sections, or "titles," that address different aspects of the law. Title I refers to employment. The ADA states that qualified individuals with disabilities may not be discriminated against in various situations. These include applying for jobs, advancement within a company, and training. An example of the type of discrimination that this law prohibits is denying employment to qualified applicants on the basis of their disability. Employers must also make reasonable accommodations for employees with disabilities. These include providing readers and interpreters. Title II covers public entities, like schools, and transportation. It prohibits disability-based discrimination in organizations at the local, state, and national levels. Title II also sets standards for handicapped accessible parking and "paratransit" services. Finally, this section sets the standard for public housing, housing assistance, and referrals. Title III refers to public accommodations and commercial facilities. These include public parks and swimming pools, restaurants, and shopping malls. This section prohibits any feature that might impede an individual's enjoyment or use of the area. Wheelchair ramps and handrails are examples of modifications intended to comply with this section of the law. Title IV of the ADA covers telecommunications. The law requires that all telecommunication companies provide equal services to disabled individuals. Telecommunications devices for the deaf, blind, and speech impaired are intended to aid in this goal. Title V is the final section of the ADA and addresses technical issues. It also includes a provision that protects individuals from retaliation for asserting their rights.

The ADA has been somewhat controversial. Before the law was passed by Congress, disability rights activists gathered in Washington, D.C., to protest. Many individuals with physical disabilities left their wheelchairs and other assistive devices behind and crawled up the steps to the Capitol Building. This event became known as the "Capitol Crawl." Some have criticized the law on the grounds that it requires businesses as well as any nonprofit organizations that receive any federal funding to pay for costly renovations to buildings. Others state that the ADA actually makes it less likely that employers will hire disabled individuals due to increased oversight. But many agree that the law has considerably reduced discrimination against those with disabilities.

Len Sperry, MD, PhD, and George Stoupas, MS

See also: Disability and Disability Evaluation

Further Reading

Davis, Lennard, ed. *The Disability Studies Reader*, 4th ed. New York, NY: Routledge, 2013.

Fleisher, Doris, and Frieda Zames, eds. *The Disability Rights Movement: From Charity to Confrontation*, 2nd ed. Philadelphia, PA: Temple University Press, 2011.

O'Brien, Ruth, ed. *Voices from the Edge: Narratives about the Americans with Disabilities Act*. New York, NY: Oxford University Press, 2004.

Amnesia

Amnesia is the inability to recall past events or retain new information. It usually occurs as a result of physical or psychological trauma.

Definitions

- **Alzheimer's disease** is a mental disorder characterized by amnesia and the decline of cognitive functions. It causes significant distress or impaired functioning in daily activities.

- **Anterograde amnesia** is the loss of memory that followed the causal event.

- **Cognitive** pertains to mental abilities and processes.

- **Dementia** is a loss of memory and mental ability that is sufficiently severe to interfere with normal activities of daily living.

- **Dissociative amnesia** is a mental disorder that involves amnesia and that causes significant distress or impaired functioning.

- **Retrograde amnesia** is the loss of memory that precedes the causal event.

- **Transient global amnesia** is a form of anterograde amnesia that is intense and short term and presents with no other symptoms.

- **Traumatic brain injury** is an insult or injury to the brain from an external force. In DSM-5, this disorder is known as Neurocognitive Disorder Due to Traumatic Brain Injury.

Description

Amnesia is the inability to recall important personal information that is different from ordinary forgetting (American Psychiatric Association, 2013). Individuals suffering from amnesia are likely to present firstly for the event that caused the amnesia. Consequently, they are likely to be encountered in a medical or crisis setting. In addition, amnesia can occur in other neurological or medical concerns and is not likely to be the primary diagnosis. Some individuals may exhibit a total inability to recall events leading up to the precipitating event. Others might exhibit profound forgetfulness or seem as if they very confused. Amnesia may last hours, weeks, years, or, in rare cases, a lifetime.

There are three kinds of amnesia: anterograde amnesia, retrograde amnesia, and transient global amnesia. Typically, retrograde amnesia does not involve a total loss of memory but is variable in regard to the period of memory loss preceding its onset. Transient global amnesia is often associated with physical or emotional stress. The isolated memory loss of amnesia does not affect an individual's awareness, general knowledge, intelligence, judgment, or personality. Those experiencing amnesia usually understand written and spoken words and can learn skills. They also understand that they have experienced some memory loss. Dissociative amnesia also involves amnesia. So too does dementia. However, in addition to the memory loss are other cognitive problems. Alzheimer's disease is common form of dementia.

Amnesia can be caused by damage to certain areas of the brain or through psychological means. The physical cause of amnesia is often traumatic brain injury that may result from car accidents, falls, or sport injuries. With psychological amnesia, the impairment is often attributed to assault, death of a loved one, or other disturbing event. Amnesia can also be caused by other medical conditions.

Treatment

Treatment begins with a thorough assessment to assess memory loss and identify likely causes. There is no direct treatment for amnesia. The primary goal of treatment is to resolve the underlying cause. That is to say if the amnesia is caused by traumatic brain injury, then it is the injury that is treated. Alternatively, if the cause is psychological trauma, then the psychological intervention will be aimed at helping the individual resolve the psychological issue directly in the hope that the amnesia will resolve as a consequence. A secondary goal is to increase the individual's capacity to better cope, enhance memory, and provide psychological support for these individuals and their families.

Jeremy Connelly, MEd, and Len Sperry, MD, PhD

See also: Alzheimer's Disease; Dementia; Dissociation; Dissociative Amnesia

Further Reading

American Psychiatric Association. *Diagnostic and Statistical Manual of Mental Disorders*, 5th ed. Arlington, VA: American Psychiatric Association, 2013.

Papanicolaou, Andrew C. *The Amnesias: A Clinical Textbook of Memory Disorders*. New York NY: Oxford University Press, 2006.

Amphetamines

Amphetamines are prescription medications that stimulate the nervous system and are used to treat depression and other conditions. They are also highly addictive.

Definitions

- **Anticonvulsants** are medications that relieve or prevent seizures.

- **Narcolepsy** is a disorder that causes individuals to fall asleep at inappropriate times during the day.

- **Tic** is a sudden involuntary behavior that is difficult or impossible for the person to suppress. Tics may be either motor (related to movement) or vocal (inappropriate language) and tend to be more pronounced under stress.

- **Tourette's syndrome** is a neurological disorder characterized by tics, including multiple involuntary movements and uncontrollable vocalizations.

Description

"Amphetamine" is the name of a class of drugs that stimulate the central nervous system. They produce their effects by altering chemicals that transmit nerve messages in the body. Amphetamines are used in the treatment of depression, obesity, attention-deficit hyperactivity disorder (ADHD), narcolepsy, and Tourette's syndrome. Brand names of commonly prescribed amphetamines are Biphetamine, Dexampex, Desoxyn, Ferndex, Methampex, Oxydess II, and Spancap. Generic names of amphetamines include amphetamine, dextroamphetamine, and methamphetamine. Stimulants used in the treatment of ADHD are methylphenidate (trade name: Ritalin), mixed amphetamine salts (trade name: Adderall), and dextroamphetamine (trade name: Dexedrine). Since most of these drugs tend to be short-acting, it is usually necessary to take several doses a day to maintain the therapeutic effect. Longer-acting versions of these drugs, such as Ritalin LA and Adderall XR, permit once or twice a day dosing. Amphetamines are usually given orally and their effects can last up to 20 hours.

Precautions and Side Effects

Because they are highly addictive, they should be prescribed only after other therapeutic approaches have failed. They should be used with great caution in children under three years of age and for anyone with a history of elevated blood pressure and those with tics and Tourette's syndrome. Also, those with a history of an overactive thyroid should not take amphetamines, nor should those with moderate-to-severe high blood pressure, glaucoma, or psychotic symptoms such as hallucinations and delusions. Also, those with a history of

drug abuse, psychomotor agitation, or cardiovascular disease should not use amphetamines.

Caution is needed in the use of amphetamines in young children because of concerns about the possibility of sudden death or retarded growth. A small number of deaths have been reported, and some studies indicate that taking stimulants can slow growth rate in children. As a result some physicians recommend drug holidays in which the drug is temporarily stopped during times that require less focus or self-discipline, such as weekends or a summer vacation. Studies indicate that the adverse effects on growth rate are eliminated by these drug holidays.

For adults, amphetamine use should not be discontinued suddenly. Rather, the dose should be lowered gradually and then discontinued under the supervision of a physician. Generally these drugs should be taken early in the day so as not to interfere with sleep at night. Hazardous activities should be avoided until the person's condition has been stabilized with medication. The use of amphetamines during pregnancy has been associated with fetal growth retardation, premature birth, and heart and brain abnormalities.

Amphetamines can cause considerable side effects and may be toxic in large doses. The most common side effects associated with amphetamines are irregular heartbeat, increased heart rate or blood pressure, dizziness, insomnia, restlessness, headache, shakiness, dry mouth, metallic taste, diarrhea, constipation, and weight loss. Other side effects can include changes in sexual drive, nausea, vomiting, allergic reactions, chills, depression, irritability, and indigestion. High doses, whether for medical purposes or illicit ones, can cause addiction, dependence, increased aggression, and, in some cases, psychotic episodes.

Len Sperry, MD, PhD

See also: Narcolepsy; Tourette's Syndrome

Further Reading

Erickson, Carlton K. *Addiction Essentials: The Go-to Guide for Clinicians and Patients.* New York, NY: W.W. Norton, 2011.

Galanter, Marc, and Herbert D. Kleber, eds. *The American Psychiatric Publishing Textbook of Substance Abuse*

Treatment, 4th ed. Washington, DC: American Psychiatric Press, Inc., 2008.

Iversen, Leslie. *Speed, Ecstasy, Ritalin: The Science of Amphetamines.* Oxford, UK: Oxford University Press, 2006.

Preston, John D., John H. O'Neal, and Mary C. Talaga. *Handbook of Clinical Psychopharmacology for Therapists*, 7th ed. Oakland, CA: New Harbinger, 2013.

Anafranil (Clomipramine)

Anafranil is an antidepressant medication used primarily to treat obsessive-compulsive disorder. It is also used in treating depression and other medical and psychiatric conditions. Its generic name is clomipramine.

Definitions

- **Obsessive-compulsive disorder** is a mental disorder characterized by problematic obsessions (repetitive thoughts and impulses) and compulsions (repetitive behaviors).

- **Serotonin** is a neurotransmitter (chemical messenger) found throughout the body, including the digestive tract and the brain. It contracts smooth muscle and affects with mood, attention, and sleep. Low levels of Serotonin are associated with depression.

Description

Anafranil is a tricyclic antidepressant, a class of drugs with a three-ring chemical structure. Its primary use is the treatment of the obsessions and compulsions of obsessive-compulsive disorder when these symptoms greatly disrupt an individual's daily activities. It is also used in panic disorder, pain management, sleep problems like narcolepsy (uncontrollable attacks during deep sleep), and anorexia nervosa. It is also helpful in reducing other compulsive behaviors such as hair pulling, nail biting, Tourette's syndrome (tics and vocalizations), and childhood autism.

The first tricyclic, imipramine (trade name: Tofranil), was found to decrease depressive symptoms, presumably by increasing serotonin in the brain. Because Anafranil significantly increases serotonin levels in the brain, it is most effective in reducing compulsions.

Precautions and Side Effects

Seizures are the most important risk associated with Anafranil. The risk of seizure increases with larger doses and after abrupt discontinuation of it. Care must be taken in the use of Anafranil in those with a history of epilepsy or condition associated with seizures, such as brain damage or alcoholism. Anafranil may worsen glaucoma and adversely affect heart rhythm in those with cardiac disease. Because some studies associate antidepressants with increased suicidal thoughts in children and adults up to age 24, the use of Anafranil should be carefully monitored. The safety of Anafranil use during pregnancy has not been fully determined. However, it is known that tricyclic antidepressants pass into breast milk and may cause sedation and depress breathing in nursing infants.

Anafranil may cause several side effects. Like other tricyclic antidepressants its side effect may initially be more pronounced but decrease with continued treatment. Common side effects are headache, confusion, nervousness, restlessness, sleep difficulties, numbness, tingling sensations, tremors, nausea, loss of appetite, constipation, blurred vision, difficulty urinating, menstrual pain, impotence, decreased sex drive, fatigue, and weight gain.

Len Sperry, MD, PhD

See also: Depression; Obsessive-Compulsive Disorder (OCD); Serotonin; Tofranil (Imipramine)

Further Reading

Maina, Giuseppe, Umberto Albert, and Filippo Bogetto. "Obsessive-Compulsive Disorder Resistant to Pharmacological Treatment." In *Obsessive-Compulsive Disorder Research*, edited by B.E. Ling, pp. 171–199. Hauppauge, NY: Nova Science Publishers, 2005.

Preston, John D., John H. O'Neal, and Mary C. Talaga. *Handbook of Clinical Psychopharmacology for Therapists*, 7th ed. Oakland, CA: New Harbinger, 2013.

Simpson, H. Blair, and Michael R. Liebowitz. "Combining Pharmacotherapy and Cognitive-Behavioral Therapy in the Treatment of OCD." In *Concepts and Controversies in Obsessive-Compulsive Disorder*, edited by Jonathan Abramowitz and Arthur C. Houts, pp. 359–376. New York, NY: Springer Science, 2005.

Stahl, Stephen M. *Antidepressants*. New York: Cambridge University Press, 2009.

Androgyny

One way in which society defines men and women is in terms of how masculine or how feminine they are based on their appearance, personality, and mannerisms. Femininity is often associated with someone who is nurturing, warm, sympathetic, sensitive, affectionate, and emotional. Masculinity is associated with being aggressive, dominant, strong, competitive, and independent. However, men and women can also be viewed in terms of how androgynous they are. This third concept looks at how some people are a combination of masculinity and femininity, meaning that they have high levels of both masculine and feminine traits.

Definition

- **Androgyny** is the combination of personality traits that are both feminine and masculine. An androgynous individual is sometimes hard to identify as either distinctly male or female—whether it is in appearance, dressing, or behavior. This type of person is known as an androgyne.

Stereotypes about men and women have changed significantly over the past three to four decades. Most social scientists now believe that men are not completely masculine and women are not completely feminine. In fact, men and women both have traits of each. To a certain extent, this illustrates the concept of androgyny, meaning that a person possesses both masculine and feminine traits in varying degrees. Someone who exhibits high levels of both masculine and feminine traits would be defined as androgynous.

Androgyny can be a controversial issue. Some categorize it as a deviant form of sexuality, while others

look at it as an idealized form of oneness. The term "androgynous" has also been used to describe a hermaphrodite, which is someone who is born with both male and female sex organs.

One of the leading researchers of androgyny was Sandra Bern who, in the 1970s, developed the Bern Sex-Role Inventory. It is among the most popular gender measurements with results classifying individuals into one of four gender orientations: masculine, feminine, androgynous, or undifferentiated.

Beginning in the 1970s and continuing to present day there has been an emergence of nontraditional males in pop culture that embodied more androgynous traits. Some of the most notable changes began in music with Robert Plant, Mick Jagger, Prince, Boy George, David Bowie, Dee Snider, Michael Jackson, and Marilyn Manson, to name a few.

Mindy Parsons, PhD

See also: Gender Identity Development; Sexual Identity

Further Reading
American Counseling Association. *The ACA Encyclopedia of Counseling*. Alexandria, VA, 2009, p. 483.

DiDonato, Matthew D., and Sheri A. Berenbaum. "The Benefits and Drawbacks of Gender Typing: How Different Dimensions Are Related to Psychological Adjustment." *Archives of Sexual Behavior* 40 (2011): 457–463.

Maheshwari, N., and V. Kumar. "Personal Effectiveness as a Function of Psychological Androgyny." *Industrial Psychiatry* 17 (2008): 39–45.

Prakash, Jyoti, A. S. M. Kotwal, V. S. S. R. Ryali, K. Srivastava, P. Bhat, and R. Shashikumar. "Does Androgyny Have Psychoprotective Attributes? A Cross-Sectional Community Based Study." *Industrial Psychiatry* 19 (2010): 119–124.

Singer, June K. *Androgyny: The Opposites Within*. Lake Worth, FL: Nicholas-Hayes Publishing, 2000.

Vorster, Johannes N. "Androgyny and Early Christianity." *Religion & Theology* 15 (2008): 97–132.

Anger in Adults

"Anger" refers to the external behaviors and internal emotional, physiological, and cognitive processes a person experiences when feeling angry.

Description

Anger is one of the most common human emotions and is a combination of a person's thoughts, feelings, and behaviors in response to a stimulus. Anger serves the purpose of enabling an individual to recognize problems and take action.

Anger is considered an adaptive and constructive emotion when it is employed to maintain positive relationships, assert appropriate authority, or promote change. For example, if someone sees a student being bullied, the observer will first become aware of the problem by the emotional feelings, physical sensations, and thoughts associated with anger. The observer's heart rate increases and muscles tense; the observer may feel a sense of heat flushing his or her face. The observer has the thought of how unfair or hurtful the bullying is and that he or she must stop it. Emotionally the observer feels compassion and anger. This experience is often referred to as "righteous indignation." "Righteous indignation" refers to anger resulting from a perception of mistreatment, injustice, or malice. These feelings may lead to a behavioral response that is used to stop the bullying.

Causes and Symptoms

Physical sensations of anger included muscle tension such as fist clenching or teeth grinding, body temperature change, and sweating. When cartoon characters are depicted as angry, they turn red, steam begins shooting out of their ears, and they clench their fist and grimace. Although these depictions are cartoonish they do illustrate some of the physical body responses to anger. Common verbal expressions of anger include "it makes my blood boil,, "I wanted to explode," and "I went off on somebody."

Anger encompasses a wide range of emotional experiences from being mildly annoyed to intense rage. The emotional state of anger is highly associated with thoughts and behaviors. There are three components of anger that are used to determine if a person has an anger problem: frequency, intensity, and duration. Frequency refers to how often a person is angered, intensity refers to how angry a person becomes, and duration refers to how long the anger lasts.

Anger is considered dysfunctional when behaviors become malicious or spiteful and the individual seeks to hurt the offender or get revenge. Verbal abusiveness such as yelling, screaming, name-calling, and making threats are examples of verbal anger behaviors. Pushing, blocking, hitting, and breaking things are examples of physically abusive behaviors. Other anger behaviors include hand gestures, facial expressions, spitting, and other body language expressions. Functional or healthy anger expression is related to the psychological capacity of emotional regulation. Being able to regulate one's emotions is positively associated with health outcomes, relationships, academic performance, and successful problem solving.

How we think about an event determines how we feel about it. How we think about an event is called an "appraisal." Appraisals determine the initial intensity and general positive or negative functionality of the emotion. Repetitive or constant thinking about a negative event is called "rumination." People who ruminate can't "let it go"; they "stew over it" and are unable to "get over it." "Reappraisal" is actively changing the way in which one thinks about an event.

Researchers who study anger have determined that how a person appraises, or thinks about an event, determines the person's emotional response to the event. People who ruminate and do not change or modify how they think about the event stay angry or increase their anger and aggressive behaviors. People who reappraise events, thus changing how they think about the event, decrease both the intensity of the experience and the duration of the emotional upset.

Diagnosis and Prognosis

Because there is such a wide range of anger experience and expression, including appropriate expressions of anger such as frustration or annoyance, anger in and of itself is not a diagnosable disorder. Anger is included as a symptom in several disorders listed by the *Diagnostic and Statistical Manual of Mental Disorders, Fifth Edition* (DSM-5), including oppositional defiant, post-traumatic stress, and some personality disorders. There is a recognized disorder titled "intermittent explosive disorder" in which the central feature is repeated behavioral anger-based aggressive outburst. Diagnosis is made depending on the intensity of the verbal and physical aggression and frequency of the aggressive outburst. These outbursts are impulsive (not planned) and are grossly out of proportion to the stressing event. The outbursts are recurrent and cause either considerable distress in the individual or significant problems at work and with his or her personal relationships. The core feature of the disorder is failure to control impulsive aggressive behaviors in response to events that would not typically result in aggressive outburst.

Individuals who have experienced physical and emotional trauma, alcoholism, and domestic violence while growing up are at increased risk for intermittent explosive disorder. Treatments are available, including individual and group talking therapies. Although there are no medications directly prescribed for anger control, some drug therapies have beneficial effects in treating underlying mood disorders.

Anger is one of the most common of human emotions. When unregulated, the emotional and behaviors components of anger can lead to significant problems in maintaining healthy relationships and social functioning. When managed by reappraisals, anger can become a healthy and productive emotion leading to positive relationships and social change.

Steven R. Vensel, PhD

See also: Aggressive and Antisocial Behavior in Youth; Conduct Disorder; Oppositional Defiant Disorder (ODD)

Further Reading

American Psychiatric Association. *Diagnostic and Statistical Manual of Mental Disorders*, 5th ed. Arlington, VA: American Psychiatric Association Press, 2013.

Digiuseppe, Raymond, and Raymond Chip Tafrate. "A Comprehensive Treatment Model for Anger Disorders." *Psychotherapy* 38, no. 3 (2011): 262–271.

Ray, Rebecca, Frank Wilhelm, and James Gross. "All in the Mind's Eye? Anger Rumination and Reappraisal." *Journal of Personality and Social Psychology* 94, no. 1 (2008): 133–145.

Anger Management

Anger management describes the process of acquiring skills to recognize signs that one is becoming angry and take action to deal with the emotion in a productive, healthy way.

Description

"Anger management" refers to a set of psychological, therapeutic techniques and exercises that a person can use to deal with anger in an effective manner. This process involves recognizing triggers and calming oneself down before the situation escalates. Anger management is suggested for people who are unable to control their anger or manage anger appropriately once it surfaces. The purpose of an anger management strategy is to learn to deal with anger in a positive, healthy way. These skills can be taught to oneself through the use of books or other resources or be learned in an anger management class taught by a mental health professional.

Development

Anger is a natural human emotion. Everyone experiences anger at one time or another. Physical well-being can be negatively impacted by anger. Research indicates that anger can increase a person's chances of developing heart disease. This risk is higher for men than women. Anger is linked to other physical problems as well, such as insomnia, digestive issues, and headaches. However, anger can also have survival benefits—it serves as part of our brain's *fight or flight* response to perceived threat or harm. Anger should be expressed, though, in appropriate ways. An anger management approach teaches a person to cope with anger rather than suppress it. Acceptance, acknowledgment, and truth are an important part of an anger management approach. One must also be taught to recognize signs of anger. These include physical symptoms that signify that anger may be building. Examples may include increased heart rate, increased body temperature, reddening of the face, clenched fists, tightening of the jaw, and quickening of the breath. Identifying stressors is another integral piece in this process as stress can be caused by different factors such as work, family, or health.

A person may himself or herself recognize that he or she has anger management issues, or this may be suggested to the person by a family member or friend. In more severe cases, a person may be mandated to attend anger management classes by the legal system, often resulting from the inability to control one's anger in a previous situation. Anger management strategies can be practiced alone, one on one, in a small group, or in a class setting. These sessions are typically led by a psychologist or other trained mental health professional. Depending on a person's needs and the circumstances and severity of the problem, these sessions can last from weeks to months to even longer. If a person has other mental health issues, this can also adversely affect treatment. Some of these conditions include a history of substance abuse, depression, anxiety, and/or social disorders such as Asperger's syndrome. Other factors that can impact success are lack of self-care (nutrition, sleep, exercise) and stress. Common techniques employed in anger management training include relaxation, guided imagery, deep-breathing, stress management, problem solving, conflict resolution, cognitive behavior therapy, and solution-focused strategies.

Certain steps encompass most anger management programs. One, the participant learns his or her anger triggers and notes situations where these are likely to cause anger to arise. Two, the participant recognizes physical signs and symptoms that signify that anger is building. Three, the participant employs anger management strategies in order to calm down and control his or her anger. Last, the participant learns to deal with the situation in a positive, healthy way and express feelings and needs in order to solve the problem effectively.

Current Status

No anger disorders are listed in the DSM-5. Most research conducted on anger management surround its use with persons who suffer from anxiety and depression. These strategies are related to psychological treatment for these disorders. Effective interventions for anger management support a cognitive behavioral approach. Accepting personal responsibility and being conscious and in control of negative thought patters are key aspects of this type of therapy.

Melissa A. Mariani, PhD

See also: Anger in Adults; *Diagnostic and Statistical Manual of Mental Disorders* (DSM)

Further Reading

Beck, Richard, and Ephrem Fernandez. "Cognitive-Behavioral Therapy in the Treatment of Anger: A Meta-analysis." *Cognitive Therapy and Research* 22 (1998): 63–74.

Enright, Robert D. *Forgiveness Is a Choice: A Step-by-Step Process for Resolving Anger and Restoring Hope.* Washington, DC: American Psychological Association, 2001.

Kassinove, Howard, and Raymond Chip Tafrate. *Anger Management: The Complete Treatment Guidebook for Practitioners.* Atascadero, CA: Impact, 2002.

Potegal, Michael, Gerhard Stemmlar, and Charles Spielberger, eds. "*International Handbook of Anger.*" Springer Science Media. Accessed 2010. doi:10.1007/97803879676229.

Animal-Assisted Therapy

Animal-assisted therapy is a goal-directed therapy that involves the presence of or interaction with an animal as a fundamental part of a client's treatment.

Description

Animal-assisted therapy is used for a number of different conditions. These can range from problems involving emotional distress to anxiety-related symptoms and disorders. Therapy dogs are the most common although a wide variety of animals are now being used. Other animals involved in these types of interventions include horses and dolphins.

There are references in history to the therapeutic presence of animals for medical problems, especially psychological ones. After World War II, animal-assisted therapy began to be a subject of serious consideration, especially with medical professionals who were working with children. It was found that animals could serve as catalysts or mediators of human social interaction. It can expedite both the process of socialization and learning as well as helping with building rapport between patients and therapists.

There are two things that distinguish animal-assisted therapy from the simple presence of animals in therapy. First, the intervention involves the intentional presence or use of an animal and a psychological or medical professional delivers the therapy. This professional is required to practice within the scope of his or her professional training and expertise. In order to be successful, animal-assisted therapy must be carefully directed and the animals must be carefully chosen and often trained to be able to participate in treatment.

Development

Ancient literature and tradition stated that being licked by a dog was curative. Since then the use of comfort or support animals has been recognized for some time. Florence Nightingale, for example, made the first mention of it in the 1800s. But it is only more recently that the value of such animal-assisted therapy for treatment of conditions like mental health disorders has been acknowledged.

Sigmund Freud, one of the fathers of psychology, noticed the calming effect his dog had on his patients when his dog was in the room during sessions. In modern times Boris Levinson introduced the practice of animal-assisted therapy and the first complete work in the field through his book. In 1977, Sam and Elizabeth Corson opened the first pet-assisted therapy program at a psychiatric unit at Ohio State University.

Alan Beck and Aaron Katcher began their work documenting the direct changes in the physical responses of patients in the presence of a friendly dog. They found that patient's breathing became more regular, heartbeat slowed, and muscles relaxed. These symptoms suggest lowering of the nervous system and therefore stress. Animal-assisted therapy began with dogs but has grown to popularly include equine, or horse, and dolphin-assisted therapies.

Current Status

The popularity of animal-assisted therapies is growing. New programs emerge frequently, and an increasing variety of animals are being used for this therapy. Use of therapy animals has highlighted the positive benefits of touch in counseling. Therapy animals provide a nonjudgmental space for individuals to work out their problems in a way that can include nonthreatening touch.

From a therapeutic perspective, there has been a lot of work done in order to agree on methodological standards and strategies that help establish the scientific evidence base for the efficacy of animal-assisted therapies. In the early 2000s handbooks and research articles began to be published on this topic. As best practices emerge, the practice of animal-assisted therapy has gained more credibility among other more traditional treatments in counseling and therapy.

Alexandra Cunningham, PhD, and William M. Cunningham, MA

See also: Freud, Sigmund (1856–1939); Psychotherapy

Further Reading

Chandler, Cynthia K. *Animal Assisted Therapy in Counseling.* New York, NY: Routledge, 2011.

Fine, Aubrey H., ed. *Handbook on Animal Assisted Therapy: Theoretical Foundations and Guidelines for Practice.* St. Louis, MI: Elsevier Science, 2011.

Ristol, Frances, and Eva Domenec. *Animal Assisted Therapy: Techniques and Exercises for Dog Assisted Interventions.* Coral Gables, FL: SMILES CTAC, 2012.

Anorexia Nervosa

Anorexia nervosa is a mental disorder characterized by refusal to maintain minimal normal body weight along with a fear of weight gain and a distorted body image.

Definitions

- **Binge eating** is a pattern of disordered eating consisting of episodes of uncontrolled intake of food.

- **Bulimia nervosa** is a mental disorder characterized by recurrent binge eating with loss of control over one's eating and compensation for eating.

- **Eating disorder** is a class of mental disorders that are characterized by difficulties with too much, too little, or unhealthy food intake, and may include distorted body image.

Description and Diagnosis

Anorexia nervosa is an eating disorder that is diagnosed when an individual displays a body weight significantly below what is normal or expected for the individual's current age and height. The individual is preoccupied with self-image and appears to be in denial regarding the severity of weight loss. The individual presents with distorted perceptions regarding his or her body (distorted body image). The individual believes he or she has "fat thighs" or a "fat stomach" when he or she actually lacks appropriate body mass, meaning that the individual is too thin. The extreme weight loss in anorexia nervosa is due to the individual's fear of gaining weight. The body mass index (BMI) is used to indicate the severity of the disorder with ranges from mild to extreme. There are two subtype patterns of anorexia nervosa; one is restricting food intake, while the other is bingeing and purging. The subtypes involve patterns of food restriction, and patterns of bingeing, that is, eating followed by purging through vomiting and/or use of laxatives. The binge eating/purging subtype can be distinguished from bulimia nervosa. While both engage in binge eating and purging, the bulimia nervosa maintains body weight that is minimally normal or above normal level (American Psychiatric Association, 2013).

Some facts about the prevalence (extent) of the disorder are as follows: Anorexia nervosa is more common in females with a 10 to 1 ratio. It is more common in economically advantaged countries like the United States, Australia, and Japan. It is less common in low- and middle-income countries. In the United States, the prevalence is lower among Latinos and African Americans (American Psychiatric Association, 2013). The disorder often presents in adolescence or young adulthood. The disorder is found more often in settings that value thinness, such as modeling, acting, cheerleading, and athletics.

According to the *Diagnostic and Statistical Manual of Mental Disorders, Fifth Edition*, individuals can be diagnosed with this disorder if they are significantly below normal levels in body weight, have an intense fear of gaining weight, and exhibit practices of food restriction. The diagnosis also depends on displaying undue preoccupation with body weight or denial of current low body weight. Anorexia nervosa can be either restricting type or binge eating/purging type. Severity of mild, moderate, severe, and extreme forms of this disorder can be specified based on body weight (American Psychiatric Association, 2013).

The causes and course of this disorder are many and complex. Anorexia nervosa runs in families and it takes a considerable toll on health requiring both medical and dental examinations to determine the level of biological treatment required. In addition, there are often significant neurological ramifications especially to an extended practice of anorexia nervosa. Social aspects of this disease involve consideration of the family dynamics and the role played by the anorexic individual in the family. Within this social context the anorexic develops psychological beliefs about perfectionism or the desire to remain a child. These beliefs are reflected in their everyday behavior, which focuses on excessive food restriction and preoccupation with their body image while largely ignoring other areas of life such as intimacy, work or school, and friendships. While anorexic individuals may initially be able to function adequately in school or work, cognitive performance deteriorates over time as a result of the disorder.

Treatment

Because of the multifaceted nature of this disorder, its clinical treatment must include medical, dental, and psychological evaluations and interventions. Because this is one of the few mental disorders that can be life threatening, medical evaluation and treatment are required for any individual presenting with an extremely low BMI. Time spent in states of semi-starvation results in loss of bone density, loss of menses (periods), digestion problems, and cardiac arrhythmia (abnormal heart rhythms). Depression and social relation issues as well as obsessive-compulsive behaviors around eating and exercise are also common. Individual and group therapy are common psychological interventions. Because suicide rates among anorexics are very high, assessment of suicidal thoughts and behaviors is essential (American Psychiatric Association, 2013).

Len Sperry, MD, PhD

See also: Binge Eating Disorder; Bulimia Nervosa

Further Reading

American Psychiatric Association. *Diagnostic and Statistical Manual of Mental Disorders*, 5th ed. Arlington, VA: American Psychiatric Association, 2013.

Costin, Carolyn, Gwen Schubert Grabb, and Babette Rothschild. *8 Keys to Recovery from an Eating Disorder: Effective Strategies from Therapeutic Practice and Personal Experience*. New York, NY: W.W. Norton, 2012.

Siegel, Michele, Judith Brisman, and Margot Weinshel. *Surviving an Eating Disorder: Strategies for Family and Friends*, 3rd ed. New York, NY: Harper Perennial, 2009.

Anosognosia

Anosognosia is a condition in which individuals have no awareness that they have a medical disease or disability.

Definitions

- **Bipolar disorder** is a mental health disorder characterized by a history of manic episodes (bipolar I disorder), mixed, or hypomanic episodes (bipolar II disorder), usually with one or more depressive episodes.

- **Delusions** are fixed false beliefs that persist despite contrary evidence.

- **Dementia** is a group of symptoms, including loss of memory, judgment, language, and other intellectual (mental) function caused by the death of neurons (nerve cells) in the brain.

- **Hallucinations** are false or distorted sensory perceptions that appear to be real perceptions that are generated by the mind rather than external stimuli.

- **Hemiplegia** is a condition resulting from an illness, injury, or stroke that causes total or partial paralysis of one side of the body.

- **Schizophrenia** is a chronic and mental disorder that affects behavior, thinking, and emotion, which make distinguishing between real and unreal experiences difficult.

Description

Anosognosia is described as a deficit of self-awareness of an impairment or medical condition. Individuals with anosognosia do not realize that they are ill. It can create a tremendous challenge for the individual, family members, and caregivers. Many individuals who are diagnosed with bipolar disorder, Alzheimer's disease, dementia, and schizophrenia have this condition. Having this lack of awareness increases the risk of treatment failure because many individuals are noncompliant with taking their medications. This may result in the reappearance of various symptoms including hallucinations and delusions. Other features of anosognosia include the failure to acknowledge one's hemiplegia or other disabilities, such as blindness or paralysis.

Anosognosia is not the same as denial of illness. Anosognosia has a biological basis. It is caused by damage to the right side of the brain. In contrast, there is more likely to be a psychological (mental) basis involved in those in denial of their medical condition. Nearly half of individuals with schizophrenia have moderate or severe impairment in their awareness of illness. It is particularly common for those with bipolar disorder to experience hallucinations and/or delusions. Yet nearly 40% of individuals with bipolar disorder also have impaired awareness of illness (American Psychiatric Association, 2013). Not surprisingly, anosognosia is one of the main reasons why those with schizophrenia and bipolar disorder do not take their medications.

Len Sperry, MD, PhD, and Elizabeth Smith Kelsey, PhD

See also: Alzheimer's Disease; Bipolar Disorder; Dementia; Hallucinations; Schizophrenia

Further Reading

Amador, Xavier, and Anna-Lica Johanson. *I Am Not Sick I Don't Need Help*. Peconic, NY: Vida Press, 2000.

American Psychiatric Association. *Diagnostic and Statistical Manual of Mental Disorders*, 5th ed. Arlington, VA: American Psychiatric Association, 2013.

Lorenzo, Pia, and Paul M. Conway. "Anosognosia and Alzheimer's Disease." *Brain Impairment* 9 (May 2008): 22–27.

Prigatano, George P. *The Study of Anosognosia.* New York, NY: Oxford University Press, 2010.

Antabuse (Disulfiram)

Antabuse is a prescription medication used in the treatment of chronic alcoholism. Its generic name is disulfiram.

Description

Antabuse is used as a conditioning treatment for alcohol dependence. When taken with alcohol, Antabuse causes unwanted and unpleasant effects, and the fear of these effects negatively conditions the individual to avoid subsequent alcohol use. So how does Antabuse work? When alcohol is ingested, the body metabolizes or breaks it down into acetaldehyde, the toxic substance that causes the hangover symptoms experienced after heavy drinking. Normally, the body continues to break down acetaldehyde into acetic acid, a harmless substance. Antabuse interferes with this metabolic process by preventing the breakdown of acetaldehyde into acetic acid. The result is that acetaldehyde levels increase up to 10 times greater than normally occur when drinking alcohol. These very high levels of acetaldehyde cause reactions that range from mild to severe, depending on how much Antabuse and how much alcohol is consumed. In other words, Antabuse serves as physical and psychological deterrent to an individual trying to stop drinking. It does not reduce the individual's craving for alcohol, nor does it treat alcohol withdrawal symptoms. For these reasons, Antabuse should be used in conjunction with counseling and other treatment methods.

Precautions and Side Effects

Those with a history of diabetes, severe myocardial disease, coronary occlusion, or psychosis should not take Antabuse. Neither should those with advanced or severe liver disease take Antabuse. Those with a history of seizures, hypothyroidism, or nephritis need close monitoring if Antabuse is used. Besides avoiding alcohol, individuals should also avoid any products containing alcohol, such as cough and cold preparations and mouthwashes. They should also avoid topical preparations that contain alcohol, such as aftershave lotion and perfume.

The common mild side effects of Antabuse includes drowsiness and fatigue. Others include nausea, vomiting, sweating, flushing, throbbing in the head and neck, headache, thirst, chest pain, palpitations, dyspnea, hyperventilation, and confusion. More severe reactions include respiratory depression, cardiovascular collapse, heart attack, acute congestive heart failure, unconsciousness, arrhythmias, and convulsions. Antabuse is also associated with impotence.

Len Sperry, MD, PhD

See also: Addiction; Alcoholism; Substance Abuse Treatment

Further Reading

Benton, Sarah Allen. *Understanding the High-Functioning Alcoholic: Professional Views and Personal Insights.* Westport, CT: Praeger Publishers, 2009.
Hedblom, Jack H. *Last Call: Alcoholism and Recovery.* Baltimore, MD: Johns Hopkins University Press, 2007.
Maltzman, Irving. *Alcoholism: Its Treatments and Mistreatments.* Hackensack, NJ: World Scientific Publishing Co., 2008.
MedlinePlus. "Alcoholism." U.S. National Library of Medicine, National Institutes of Health. Accessed November 7, 2014. http://www.nlm.nih.gov.ezproxy.fau.edu/medlineplus/alcoholism.html.
Substance Abuse and Mental Health Services Administration. "Faces of Change: Do I Have a Problem with Alcohol or Drugs?" U.S. Department of Health and Human Services. Accessed November 7, 2014. http://www.kap.samhsa.gov/products/brochures/pdfs/TIP35.pdf.

Antianxiety Medications

Antianxiety medications are a class of central nervous system depressants that slow normal brain function. Also known as anxiolytics and sedatives, these drugs are prescribed to reduce anxiety and tension and to induce sleep. Prolonged use or abuse of these drugs can result in substance dependence and withdrawal symptoms. Antianxiety medications are among the most abused drugs in the United States, whether obtained legally by prescription or illegally through the black market.

Definitions

- **Anxiolytic** refers to a substance that relieves anxiety and any of a group of medications prescribed to induce a feeling of calm and relaxation and relieve anxiety; it is also called tranquilizers.

- **Benzodiazepines** is a group of central nervous system depressants that are used to relieve anxiety or to induce sleep.

- **Intoxication** is a state in which significant behavioral or psychological changes follow ingestion of a substance.

- **Sedative** is any medication that induces relaxation and sleep.

- **Substance abuse** is a milder form of addiction than substance dependence wherein the user does experience tolerance or withdrawal symptoms.

- **Substance dependence** is the state in which an individual requires the ongoing use of a particular substance to avoid withdrawal symptoms.

- **Tranquilizer** is another name for anxiolytic.

- **Withdrawal symptoms** are a group of physical and/or psychological symptoms that are experienced when a drug or other substance is discontinued after prolonged use.

Description

Antianxiety medications, or "anxiolytics," are powerful central nervous system depressants that are prescribed to reduce feelings of tension and anxiety, as well as to induce sleep. Antianxiety medications are usually taken orally, and although these drugs work differently, they all produce a pleasant drowsy or calming effect. When used over a prolonged period, tolerance develops. This means that larger doses are needed to achieve the initial effects. Continued use can lead to physical dependence, and withdrawal symptoms result when the dosage is reduced or stopped. When combined with other anxiolytics or other central nervous system depressants, such as alcohol, the effects are additive.

The drugs associated with this class of substance-related disorders are benzodiazepines that include Valium, Librium, Xanax, Halcion, and ProSom; barbiturates that include Seconal and Nembutal; and barbiturate-like substances that include Quaalude, Equanil, and Doriden. Each of these antianxiety drugs is capable of producing wakeful relief from tension or inducing sleep, depending on dosage. Other legal uses of antianxiety medications include medical treatment and prevention of seizures, and these antianxiety medications are used as muscle relaxants and anesthetics and to make other anesthetics work more effectively.

Precautions and Side Effects

Even when these depressants are prescribed for medical reasons, an individual taking central nervous system depressants usually feels sleepy and uncoordinated during the first few days of treatment. As the body adjusts to the effects of the drug, these feelings begin to disappear. If the medication is used long term, the body develops tolerance, and increasing doses are needed to obtain the desired effect of general calming or drowsiness.

The use of antianxiety medications can pose extreme danger when taken along with other medications that cause central nervous system depression, such as prescription pain medicines, some over-the-counter cold and allergy medications, and alcohol. Use of additional depressants can slow breathing and respiration and can lead to death. Withdrawal from antianxiety medications can be dangerous and should be done under medical supervision. The safest method of withdrawal involves a gradual reduction of dosage. Abrupt withdrawal from these medications can lead to seizures due to the sudden increase in brain activity.

Antianxiety Medication Addiction and Treatment

Abuse of antianxiety medication can develop with prolonged use, as tolerance grows relatively quickly. Increasing amounts of the drug are then needed to produce the initial effect. It is not uncommon for individuals to become addicted to antianxiety medications even when they are medically prescribed.

The most common pattern of abuse and dependence to antianxiety medications involves use among teens and young adults, which escalates to abuse or dependence. Dependence may begin with occasional use at social gatherings and then eventually to daily use and high levels of tolerance. A somewhat less common pattern of abuse and dependence to antianxiety medications involves individuals who initially obtain medications by prescription, usually for treatment of anxiety or insomnia. Though the vast majority of those who use medications as prescribed do not develop substance dependence problems, a significant number develop tolerance and withdrawal symptoms.

Substance dependence, the more severe form of addiction, involves various cognitive, behavioral, and physiological symptoms associated with continued use of the substance. It always includes both tolerance and withdrawal symptoms. Abuse is a less severe form of addiction that may involve risky behavior, such as driving while under the influence. For example, individuals with an abuse disorder may miss work or school or get into arguments with relatives or friends about their substance use. These problems can easily escalate into full-blown dependence. Progression to full-blown dependence begins with intoxication. Intoxication involves significant problematic behaviors or psychological changes, including inappropriate sexual or aggressive behavior, mood swings, impaired judgment, and impaired work functioning, that develop during or shortly after use of the antianxiety medication. As with alcohol dependence, these behaviors may be accompanied by slurred speech, unsteady gait, memory or attention problems, poor coordination, and stupor or coma. Memory impairment is not uncommon, especially anterograde amnesia where, like in an alcoholic blackout, the individual does not remember anything that occurs after use of the drug.

Withdrawal is a characteristic syndrome that develops when use of the antianxiety medication is significantly reduced or discontinued abruptly. Abrupt discontinuation of an anxiolytic is similar to the abrupt discontinuation or "going cold turkey" in to heavy alcohol use. Symptoms may include increased heart rate, respiratory rate, blood pressure and body temperature,

sweating, hand tremor, insomnia, anxiety, nausea, and restlessness. Seizures are likely to occur in one out of four individuals undergoing untreated withdrawal. In the most severe forms of withdrawal, hallucinations and delirium can occur. Withdrawal symptoms are generally the opposite of the acute effects experienced by first-time users of the drugs. The length of time of the withdrawal period varies depending on the drug and may last as short as 10 hours or as long as three to four weeks. The longer the substance has been taken and the higher the dosage, the more likely that withdrawal will be severe and prolonged.

Successful treatment for antianxiety medication addiction typically incorporates several treatment modalities. Psychotherapy or counseling, particularly cognitive behavior therapy, focuses on helping addicted individuals identify and change the behaviors, attitudes, and beliefs that contributed to their drug usage. Combined with prescribed medications to make withdrawal safer and easier, therapy can help the addicted individual in making a full recovery. It may require multiple courses of treatment before full recovery can be achieved. Narcotics Anonymous is an important and necessary part of ongoing recovery support.

Len Sperry, MD, PhD

See also: Benzodiazepines; Substance-Related and Addictive Disorders

Further Reading

Erickson, Carlton K. *Addiction Essentials: The Go-to Guide for Clinicians and Patients.* New York, NY: W.W. Norton, 2011.

Galanter, Marc, and Herbert D. Kleber, eds. *Textbook of Substance Abuse Treatment*, 2nd ed. Washington, DC: American Psychiatric Press, 2008.

Preston, John D., John H. O'Neal, and Mary C. Talaga. *Handbook of Clinical Psychopharmacology for Therapists*, 7th ed. Oakland, CA: New Harbinger, 2013.

Toufexis, Donna. *Anti-Anxiety Drugs.* New York, NY: Chelsea House Publishers, 2006.

Antidepressant Medications

Antidepressants are prescribed medications that are primarily used to treat depression and depressive disorders.

Definition

- **Depressive disorders** are medical conditions that interfere with daily life and normal functioning, and involve symptoms such as excessive sadness, altered sleep or eating patterns, and lack of energy. Common depressive disorders are major depression, dysthymic disorder, dysthymia, major depressive disorder, and bipolar disorder with periods of mania and depression.

Description

Antidepressant medications are used primarily to reduce symptoms of depression and in the treatment of anxiety disorders, seasonal affective disorder, some eating disorders, some pain syndromes, migraine headache, smoking cessation, fibromyalgia, and some sleep disorders. The type of antidepressant medication prescribed depends on the particular array of symptoms a patient displays or reports. There are several different types of antidepressant drugs. All of them work by altering the level or activity of neurotransmitters (chemical messengers) in the brain.

The main classes of antidepressant medications are tricyclic antidepressants, monoamine oxidase inhibitors (MAOIs), selective serotonin reuptake inhibitors (SSRIs), serotonin-norepinephrine reuptake inhibitors (SNRIs), and atypical antidepressants. Those who do not improve with one type of antidepressant drug may sometimes be helped by another type of antidepressant, because different classes of medication work somewhat differently.

Tricyclic antidepressants. These were the first class of medications found to be useful in treating depression and related conditions. These medications work by preventing neurons (nerve cells) from reabsorbing the neurotransmitters serotonin, dopamine, and norepinephrine after they are released. Tricyclic antidepressants tend to have more side effects than other types of antidepressants. Specific tricyclic antidepressants include Tofranil, Elavil, Anafranil, Sinequan, Norpramin, Pamelor, Vivactil, and Surmontil.

Monoamine oxidase inhibitors. Monoamine oxidase inhibitors (MAOIs) are medications that prevent neurotransmitters such as dopamine, serotonin, and norepinephrine from being broken down into inactive chemicals. This means that when MAOIs are used, more of these neurotransmitters are available to send messages in the brain. MAOIs can have potentially serious side effects since they prevent the tyramine (an amino acid) from being broken down. Tyramine is found in foods like aged cheese, smoked meats and fish, and raisins. If tyramine cannot be broken down, it can accumulate in the body, causing increased blood pressure and possibly stroke. Specific MAOIs include Marplan, Nardil, and Parnate.

Selective serotonin reuptake inhibitors. The selective serotonin reuptake inhibitors (SSRIs) are a class of antidepressants that work by preventing neurons from reabsorbing serotonin after it is released. The effect of serotonin on adjoining neurons is prolonged. The SSRIs include Celexa, Lexapro, Prozac, Luvox, Paxil, and Zoloft.

Serotonin-norepinephrine reuptake inhibitors. Serotonin-norepinephrine reuptake inhibitors are a class of antidepressants that work similar to SSRIs. But instead of blocking serotonin only, they block the absorption of both serotonin and norepinephrine. Effexor, Pristiq, and Cymbalta are commonly prescribed SNRIs.

Atypical antidepressants. The atypical antidepressants are a collection of medications with different chemical makeups than the other classes of antidepressants. Examples of atypical antidepressants include Wellbutrin, Remeron, and Desyrel.

Precautions and Side Effects

Use of antidepressant medications may increase suicidal thoughts in children, adolescents, and adults through the age of 24. Antidepressants can precipitate mania in those who are susceptible to bipolar disorder. Various medical conditions may affect the efficacy or risks of antidepressants. These conditions include headaches, epilepsy, recent heart attacks or stroke, kidney disease, and diabetes. The use of antidepressants in pregnancy and breast-feeding can be problematic and if used must be done under close medical supervision. Those who abruptly stop taking most antidepressants may experience withdrawal symptoms.

Antidepressant use often involves side effects. Specific effects depend on the specific medication and the individual's characteristics. Possible side effects include dry mouth, constipation, nausea, bladder problems, sexual problems, blurred vision, dizziness, drowsiness, insomnia, increased heart rate, headache, nervousness, and agitation. Newer antidepressants, such as the SSRIs and SNRIs, are considered to have fewer and less troublesome side effects than the tricyclic antidepressants and the MAOIs. Antidepressants can interact with other medications, so individuals should inform their doctor about all medications and herbal supplements. Alcohol and recreational drugs can decrease the effectiveness of antidepressants and should not be combined with these medication.

Len Sperry, MD, PhD

See also: Depression

Further Reading

Dunbar, Katherine Read, ed. *Antidepressants.* Farmington Hills, MI: Greenhaven Press, 2006.

O'Connor, Richard. *Undoing Depression: What Therapy Doesn't Teach You and Medication Can't Give You,* 2nd ed. New York, NY: Little, Brown, 2010.

Preston, John D., John H. O'Neal, and Mary C. Talaga. *Handbook of Clinical Psychopharmacology for Therapists,* 7th ed. Oakland, CA: New Harbinger, 2013.

Stahl, Stephen M. *Antidepressants.* New York, NY: Cambridge University Press, 2009.

Antipsychotic Medications

Antipsychotics are prescription medications used to treat psychotic disorders, including schizophrenia, schizoaffective disorder, and psychotic depression.

Definitions

- **Extrapyramidal symptoms** are side effects of certain antipsychotic drugs. They include repetitive, involuntary muscle movements, such as lip smacking, and the urge to move constantly.

- **Neuroleptic malignant syndrome** is a potentially fatal condition resulting from antipsychotic use characterized by severe muscle rigidity (stiffening), fever, sweating, high blood pressure, delirium, and sometimes coma.

- **Psychosis** is a severe mental condition in which an individual loses touch with reality. Symptoms include hallucinations (hearing or seeing things that are not there), delusions (fixed false beliefs that persist despite contrary evidence), and disordered thinking.

- **Schizophrenia** is a mental disorder in which it is difficult to distinguish real from unreal experiences. Symptoms include hallucinations, delusions, thought and communication disturbances, and withdrawal from others.

- **Schizoaffective disorder** is a severe mental disorder in which an individual exhibits signs of both schizophrenia and a mood disorder.

- **Tardive dyskinesia** are involuntary movements caused by certain antipsychotic medications. They include tongue thrusting, repetitive chewing, jaw swinging, and facial grimacing.

Description

Antipsychotic medications are used to treat psychotic disorders, ranging from schizophrenia, schizoaffective disorder, delusional disorder, brief psychotic disorder, substance-induced psychotic disorder, and psychotic depression. They are also used to treat the psychosis associated with other medical conditions, such as dementia. Antipsychotics are thought to work by blocking dopamine receptors in the brain and interfering with dopamine transmission.

There are two classes of antipsychotic medications: older or "typical" antipsychotics (also known as first-generation antipsychotics) and newer, "atypical" antipsychotics (also known as second-generation antipsychotics). The typical antipsychotics have been in use since the 1950s. They are effective in treating "positive" symptoms of schizophrenia (abnormal thoughts and perceptions, such as delusions, hallucinations, or disordered thinking).

The "atypical" antipsychotics have been in use since the 1990s. They tend to be effective in treating both positive and "negative symptoms" (lack of speech, "flat" facial expressions, apathy, lack of pleasure in normally pleasurable activities). Clozaril was the first of this class. It proved to be effective in treating disorders that had not responded well to typical antipsychotics. Several other atypical antipsychotics were introduced after Clozaril. These include Risperdal, Zyprexa, Seroquel, and Geodon. There are side effects associated with each of these, but they are generally better tolerated than the conventional types of antipsychotics.

Precautions and Side Effects

The atypical antipsychotic medications have largely replaced the older medications, presumably because of lower risk of side effects. Choosing which class of antipsychotic medications to use is challenging for the prescriber. On one hand, atypical antipsychotics are more expensive and more likely to cause weight gain and diabetes. On the other hand, they may be more effective than older medications in treating psychotic symptoms.

The typical antipsychotics were believed to produce a number of unpleasant side effects, the worst of which were extrapyramidal symptoms, neuroleptic malignant syndrome, and tardive dyskinesia. In contrast, the risk of tardive dyskinesia was presumed to be lower with the atypical antipsychotics, particularly Clozaril. However, Clozaril can cause agranulocytosis (a loss of the white blood cells that fight infection). To avoid this, those taking Clozaril must have their white blood cell counts monitored every week or two. The inconvenience and cost of blood tests and the cost of the medication have made treatment with Clozaril difficult for many. This is unfortunate since Clozaril may be the most effective of all the antipsychotic medication. A major research study (the CATIE trial) suggests that the typical antipsychotics may be just as safe and as well tolerated as the atypicals. In the past, these older medications were often used at much higher doses than are used currently. This may explain why they appeared to cause more side effects.

Len Sperry, MD, PhD

See also: Clozaril (Clozapine); Schizoaffective Disorder; Schizophrenia

Further Reading

Mondimore, Francis Mark. *Bipolar Disorder: A Guide for Patients and Families,* 2nd ed. Baltimore, MD: Johns Hopkins University Press, 2006.

Stahl, Stephen M. *The Prescriber's Guide: Antipsychotics and Mood Stabilizers. Stahl's Essential Psychopharmacology.* Cambridge, UK: Cambridge University Press, 2009.

Torrey, E. Fuller. *Surviving Schizophrenia: A Manual for Families, Patients, and Providers,* 5th ed. New York, NY: Harper Collins, 2006.

Antisocial Personality Disorder

Antisocial personality disorder is a mental disorder characterized by a persistent pattern of disregarding and violating the rights of others.

Definitions

- ***Diagnostic and Statistical Manual of Mental Disorders*** is the handbook mental health professionals use to diagnose mental disorders. The current edition (fifth) is known as DSM-5.

- **Personality disorder** is a long-standing pattern of maladaptive (problematic) behavior, thoughts, and emotions that deviates from the accepted norms of an individual's culture.

- **Psychopathic personality** is a mental disorder characterized as amoral behavior, inability to love and understand another's feelings (empathy), extreme self-centeredness, and failure to learn from experience. It is also known as psychopathy and psychopath.

- **Psychotherapy** is a psychological method for achieving desired changes in thinking, feeling, and behavior. It is also called therapeutic counseling.

- **Sociopathic personality** is a mental disorder characterized by amoral and criminal behavior and lacks a sense of moral responsibility. It is also known as sociopathy and sociopath.

Description and Diagnosis

Antisocial personality disorder is a personality disorder characterized by a pattern of antisocial behavior. Such behavior begins in childhood or early adolescence and is characterized by aggressiveness, fighting, hyperactivity, poor peer relationships, irresponsibility, lying, theft, truancy, poor school performance, runaway behavior, and inappropriate sexual activity, as well as drug and alcohol abuse. As adults, assaultiveness, self-defeating impulsivity, hedonism, promiscuity, unreliability, and continued drug and alcohol abuse may be present. Criminality may be involved. These individuals fail at work, change jobs frequently, tend to receive dishonorable discharges from the military, are abusing parents and neglectful spouses, have difficulty maintaining intimate relationships, and may be convicted and spend time in prison. Antisocial behavior often peaks in late adolescence and early 20s and lessens in late 30s. This disorder is four times more common in males than in females.

In the past this disorder was known as psychopathic personality and sociopathic personality. While there are some similarities among these disorders and antisocial personality disorder, there are differences. The first and second editions of the *Diagnostic and Statistical Manual of Mental Disorders* provided descriptions of the psychopathic personality or the sociopathic personality. However, starting with DSM-III, the designation "antisocial personality disorder" has been used along with specific diagnostic criteria.

The clinical presentation of the antisocial personality disorder can be described in terms of behavioral style, interpersonal style, thinking style, and feeling style. The behavioral style of this disorder is characterized by poor job performance, repeated substance abuse, irresponsible parenting, persistent lying, delinquency, truancy, and violations of others' rights. These individuals can also be impulsive, angry, hostile, and cunning. Even though they may engage in rule-breaking behavior, they can be successful in business, politics, and other professions. They are forceful individuals who regularly engage in risk-seeking and thrill-seeking behavior. Their interpersonal style is characterized by antagonism and belligerence. They also tend to be highly competitive and distrustful of others and thus poor losers. Their relationships may at times appear to be "slick" as well as calculating. Their relationships are characteristically shallow and superficial, and often involve no lasting emotional ties or commitments. Their thinking style tends to be impulsive and rigid or inflexible as well as externally oriented. Because they are contemptuous of authority, rules, and social expectations, they easily rationalize their own behavior. Their feeling style of this disorder is characterized by the avoidance of "softer" emotions such as warmth and intimacy because they regard these as signs of weakness. The need to be powerful and the fear of being abused and humiliated lead to a denial of the "softer" emotions as well as their uncooperativeness. Guilt is seldom, if ever, experienced. They also find it difficult to tolerate boredom, depression, or frustration and subsequently are sensation-seekers. In addition, they tend to be callous toward the pain and suffering of others, and show little shame for their own deviant actions.

The cause of the antisocial personality disorder is not well understood. The parenting style these individuals experienced growing up often was hostile, abusive, or neglectful. Their parents and siblings may have engaged in and modeled antisocial behavior. In addition, these individuals have a characteristic view of themselves, the world, and others, and a basic life strategy. They tend to view themselves as cunning and entitled to take whatever they want. They are also likely to view themselves as strong, competitive, energetic, and tough. They tend to view others as abusive and devious or as easy prey to be used and abused. They tend to view life as hostile and rules as keeping them from fulfilling their needs. Accordingly, their basic life strategy and pattern is to take what they want and break rules and defend themselves against efforts to be controlled or abused by others.

According to the *Diagnostic and Statistical Manual of Mental Disorders, Fifth Edition*, individuals can be diagnosed with this disorder if they exhibit a pervasive pattern of disregarding and violating the rights of others. They disrespect and disregard laws and social norms, and regularly engage in acts that are grounds for arrest. These individuals lie, are deceitful, and will take advantage of others for pleasure or for personal profit. They are impulsive and fail to plan ahead. They are also irritable and aggressive, which results in physical fights or assaults. It is not surprising that these individuals disregard the safety of others as well as themselves. Their irresponsibility is demonstrated by their failure to engage in consistent work behavior and failure to meet financial obligations. Furthermore, their lack of remorse is shown by their indifference in having hurt, mistreated, or stolen from others (American Psychiatric Association, 2013).

Treatment

Unlike other personality disorders in which psychotherapy can be effective, the antisocial personality disorder is less amenable to such treatment. Typically, these individuals are usually not interested in making life changes. When treatment is required by the courts, employers, or other agencies, these individuals are likely to resist treatment efforts. However, special residential treatment programs have shown some promise. There appears to be at least one exception to receptivity to psychotherapeutic treatment. When the antisocial personality disordered individual experiences a moderate degree of depression, he or she may be willing to engage in psychotherapy in order to reduce depressive symptoms.

Len Sperry, MD, PhD

See also: Personality Disorders; Psychopathic Personality; Psychotherapy

Further Reading

American Psychiatric Association. *Diagnostic and Statistical Manual of Mental Disorders*, 5th ed. Arlington, VA: American Psychiatric Association Press, 2013.

Babiak, Paul, and Robert Hare. *Snakes in Suits: When Psychopaths Go to Work.* New York, NY: Harper, 2007.

Hare, Robert D. *Without Conscience: The Disturbing World of Psychopaths among Us.* New York, NY: Pocket Books, 1993.

Schouten, Ronald, and James Silver. *Almost a Psychopath: Do I (or Does Someone I Know) Have a Problem with Manipulation and Lack of Empathy?* Center City, MN: Hazelden Publishing, 2012.

Sperry, Len. *Handbook of Diagnosis and Treatment of the DSM-5 Personality Disorders*, 3rd ed. New York, NY: Routledge, 2016.

Anxiety Disorders in Adults

Anxiety disorders in adults are a group of mental disorders characterized by anxiety as a central or core symptom.

Definitions

- **Antianxiety medications** are prescribed drugs that relieve anxiety symptoms. They are also called anxiolytics or tranquilizers.

- **Anxiety** is apprehension or worry about an imagined danger.

- **Behavior therapy** is a form of psychotherapy that focuses on identifying and changing maladaptive behaviors.

- **Cognitive therapy** is a type of cognitive behavior therapy that focuses on identifying and changing automatic thoughts and maladaptive beliefs.

- **Exposure therapy** is a behavior therapy intervention (method) in which a client is exposed to a feared object or situation.

- **Fear** is an emotional response to a known danger.

- **Panic** is an intense sense of fear.

- **Panic attack** is an episode of sudden, intense, and debilitating sense of fear that is short lived.

- **Phobia** is an intense fear of a person, place, or thing that significantly exceeds the actual danger posed.

- **Selective mutism** is a mental disorder in which children or adolescents fail to speak in some social situations although they have the ability to talk normally at other times.

- **Separation anxiety disorder** is an anxiety disorder characterized by excessive anxiety resulting from separation from those to whom a child is attached.

Description and Presentation

This group of disorders includes specific phobia, social anxiety disorder, panic disorder, agoraphobia, and generalized anxiety disorder that are common in adults. It does not include anxiety disorder that is common in children or adolescents like separation anxiety disorder or selective mutism. Children and/or adolescents can also experience specific phobia. But since they are also common in adults, they are described here. Anxiety disorders in adults share the primary feature of anxiety, anxiety that is not caused by medication or recreational drugs. Adults typically refer to their experience of anxiety as fear, nervousness, worry, tension, or something similar. Many experience anxiety numerous times in their lives, but what separates anxiety disorders from normal experience is that symptoms last for at least six months. In addition, they must cause clinically significant distress or must disrupt the individual's daily functioning.

Certain characteristics have been associated with a risk of developing anxiety disorders in adulthood. First, there may be genetic factors that increase the likelihood of developing an anxiety disorder. Abuse or neglect in childhood may also be a risk factor in the development of anxiety disorders in adulthood.

Here is a brief description of five anxiety disorders commonly diagnosed in adults.

Specific phobia. Is a phobia related to a specific fear such as being a passenger on an airplane, blood, closed spaces, or spiders? What separates a specific phobia from a fear is that the experience of fear far exceeds the actual dangers posed, or they may experience anxiety. In addition, they are likely to avoid the feared object(s). Although this condition is primarily concerned with the fear evoked by the phobic object, there is often an element of anxiety leading up to an imminent or likely exposure to it.

Approximately 8% of the U.S. population has a specific phobia. Furthermore, like most of the anxiety disorders, they tend to occur twice as often in women than men (American Psychiatric Association, 2013). Depending on the circumstances, individuals may be prescribed antianxiety medication for situations in which they will have to endure their phobic object (e.g., for a plane flight). For long-term change, treatment for specific phobia most commonly includes exposure therapy. As the name suggests, individuals are gradually exposed to what they fear while maintaining a relaxed and calm state.

Social anxiety disorder. Also referred to as social phobia, this disorder is characterized by excessive fear of being critically evaluated by others in a social situation. Often, fear revolves around some sort of performance such as a presentation, dance, or speech. In more severe cases, simply attending a party or having a conversation with a stranger may be sufficient to induce significant fear. Infrequent anxiety or fear related to social circumstances is a common occurrence. What characterizes this disorder from normal social functioning is that the anxiety or fear almost always occurs as opposed to occasionally. Social anxiety can cause someone to become isolated or, in severe cases, unable to maintain relationships and/or be employed.

Approximately 7% of the U.S. population experiences this disorder. It is notable that this disorder is far less prevalent in some cultures than in the United States. Also, this tends to occur twice as often in women than men (American Psychiatric Association, 2013). This disorder is commonly treated with exposure therapy or cognitive therapy.

Panic disorder. Individuals with this disorder experience both recurring panic attacks and anxiety in regard to experiencing future attacks. These attacks may include physical symptoms such as heart palpitations (pounding heart), sweaty palms, shortness of breath, and tingling in the fingers. Individuals experiencing a panic attack may also sense that they are in some way detached from their experience (called derealization). In addition, they may have a sense that they are dying or going crazy.

An important component of panic attack is that there is no realistic, plausible cause of their acute fear. For example, an individual experiencing a panic attack may think that he or she will choke while having no physical obstruction of the airway. It is important to note that this condition, like other anxiety disorders, is not caused by medication, drugs, or illness. Panic attack is also different from panic in that normal panic results from a realistic concern. Individuals who experience this disorder may also experience agoraphobia.

Panic disorder is less prevalent than other anxiety disorders. Approximately 2.5% of the U.S. population experiences panic disorder. Unlike the other anxiety disorders, it seems that panic disorder occurs in similar proportions to both sexes (American Psychiatric Association, 2013). This disorder is commonly treated with both drugs and behavior therapy. Antidepressant medications may be prescribed to reduce the anxiety about future attacks, while antianxiety medications may be used to reduce the intensity of the actual attack. Behavior therapy is used to reduce the fear and related anxiety and ultimately resolve the disorder. Treatment often begins with medications that are used only until the fear and anxiety responses are reduced with behavior therapy. Without treatment, this condition will likely become chronic.

Agoraphobia. Agoraphobia is a phobia in which individuals experience an intense fear of crowds, public places, open spaces, or places from which they believe that they cannot easily escape. Alternatively, the primary fear may also be embarrassment of being observed panicking by others in the public space. Like other phobias, individuals with this disorder commonly avoid exposure to what they fear. The likelihood of developing this disorder is approximately 1.7% in adolescence and adulthood. Also, it is likely to occur with panic disorder. Agoraphobia is usually treated the same as panic disorder and is treated and simultaneously with it (American Psychiatric Association, 2013).

Generalized anxiety disorder. Generalized anxiety disorder is a constant uncontrollable worry that both is excessive and causes individuals distress. The worries may focus on multiple concerns about their children, their health, or their job. Or, the worries may be very broad so that the individual literally worries

about worrying. Those who experience this disorder often have sleeping difficulties and feel fatigued and/or irritable. Also, they may experience mild physical symptoms such as trembling, muscle tension, or sweating.

The likelihood that at individual will experience this disorder at some point in his or her lifetime is 9%. It occurs more frequently in those of European descent than non-European descent. Also, it occurs far more frequently in first-world nations than in the developing nations (American Psychiatric Association, 2013). Treatment includes a wide range of options, including antidepressants medication, antianxiety medications, cognitive therapies, and behavioral therapies.

Jeremy Connelly, MEd, and Len Sperry, MD, PhD

See also: Antianxiety Medications; Antidepressant Medications; Agoraphobia; Cognitive Therapies; Exposure Therapy; Generalized Anxiety Disorder; Panic Attack; Panic Disorder; Social Anxiety Disorder; Specific Phobia

Further Reading

American Psychiatric Association. *Diagnostic and Statistical Manual of Mental Disorders*, 5th ed. Arlington, VA: American Psychiatric Association, 2013.

Antony, Martin M., Michelle G. Craske, and David H. Barlow. *Mastering Your Fears and Phobias: Workbook.* New York, NY: Oxford University Press, 2007.

Bandelow, Borwin, Katharina Domschke, and David Baldwin. *Panic Disorder and Agoraphobia.* New York, NY: Oxford University Press, 2014.

Bourne, Edmund. *The Anxiety and Phobia Workbook*, 5th ed. Oakland, CA: New Harbinger, 2010.

Butler, Gillian. *Overcoming Social Anxiety and Shyness: A Self-Help Guide Using Cognitive Behavioral Techniques.* New York, NY: Basic Books, 2008.

Daitch, Carolyn. *Anxiety Disorders: The Go-to Guide for Clients and Therapists.* New York, NY: W.W. Norton, 2011.

Forsyth, John, and George Eifert. *The Mindfulness and Acceptance Workbook for Anxiety: A Guide to Breaking Free from Anxiety, Phobias, and Worry Using Acceptance and Commitment Therapy.* Oakland, CA: New Harbinger, 2007.

Anxiety Disorders in Youth

Anxiety disorders in youth describe conditions of excessive anxiety and worry that occur in children and manifest in different ways.

Definitions

- **Anxiety** is a negative emotional state characterized by feelings of nervousness, worry, and apprehension about an imagined danger.

- **Anxiety disorders** cause people to feel excessively scared, distressed, and uneasy during situations in which others would not experience these symptoms.

Description

Anxiety disorders are the most common mental illnesses in America. Sometimes these disorders are often difficult to recognize because people attempt to hide them or they get confused for other issues. Anxiety disorders are especially common in children and adolescents. There are several disorders that fall under the category of anxiety disorders. Among the most common anxiety disorders for youth are phobias, panic disorders, obsessive-compulsive disorder, and post-traumatic stress disorder.

Phobias are a fear of something that poses little or no actual danger. The fear leads many to completely avoid objects or situations that can cause feelings of terror, dread, and panic. Phobias can substantially restrict a child's ability to socialize with others, go to school, or participate in family outings. Separation anxiety is a kind of phobia that is common among some children. This anxiety specifically presents when a child is removed from a person or object he or she is attached to. Children and adolescents with phobias or separation anxiety usually anticipate the worst and often complain of fatigue, tension, headaches, and nausea.

Panic disorder can often result in panic attacks. It is characterized by sudden feelings of terror that strike repeatedly and without warning. Physical symptoms can include chest pain, heart palpitations, shortness of breath, dizziness, abdominal discomfort, feelings of unreality, and fear of dying. Children and teens with this disorder may experience unrealistic worry, self-consciousness, and tension.

Obsessive-compulsive disorder describes those who have frequent, unwanted thoughts, behaviors, or feelings. Many times obsessive thoughts or worries lead youth to engage in a pattern of behavior they find difficult to control. Common compulsions may include counting, checking, organizing objects, and excessive hand washing.

Post-traumatic stress disorder: persistent symptoms of this disorder occur after a child or teen has experienced a trauma. This can include traumatic events such as physical or emotional abuse, natural disasters, or witnessing extreme violence. Usually these children experience nightmares, flashbacks, lack of feeling, sadness, rage, and difficulty focusing.

Causes and Symptoms

As with many other psychological disorders, it is still unclear whether the causes of anxiety disorder in young people are more biological or environmental. Some professionals consider anxiety disorders to have both neurological and environmental causes. Researchers indicate that children and adolescents are more likely to have anxiety disorders if their parents or caregivers also have anxiety issues.

Diagnosis and Prognosis

In order to properly identify anxiety disorders in youth, it is important to consider physical, cognitive, and emotional characteristics. Anxiety is part of a child's flight or fight response. Experiencing anxiety helps a child learn how to determine fighting for or fleeing a situation. This is part of normal development and is important to have for balance and mental health. Multiple assessments exist to try to prevent a mistaken diagnosis.

Mental health professionals must take into account the individual's general medical condition. Anxiety can often be associated with the experience of certain illnesses or as a side effect of medications. Left untreated, anxiety disorders can debilitate the lives of young people. How well any individual does with treatment depends on the severity of the condition.

Most patients can be helped through a combination of medication and therapy to gain a better quality of life.

Treatment

Among the range of effective treatments for anxiety disorders are medications, individual therapy, family therapy, or a combination of these. Cognitive behavior therapy in combination with medication is the most effective treatment for youth and adults with anxiety disorders. Therapy can help teach children and adolescents how to deal with their fears by modifying and practicing new behaviors, which can lead to positive change.

For parents and caregivers it is important to learn about anxiety disorders so that they can understand and help their child with an anxiety disorder. Psychoeducation, support groups, and seeking individual counseling can be helpful for parents who have a child with anxiety disorder. In providing treatment to the youth with anxiety disorders, parents and caregivers should involve the child or adolescent in the process of decision making and problem solving to enhance their success later in life.

Alexandra Cunningham, PhD, and
William M. Cunningham, MA

See also: Adverse Childhood Experiences; Antianxiety Drugs; Anxiety Disorders in Adults; Anxiety Reduction Techniques; Obsessive-Compulsive Disorder (OCD); Panic Attack; Panic Disorder; Phobias; Post-Traumatic Stress Disorder (PTSD) in Youth; Separation Anxiety Disorder

Further Reading

American Psychiatric Association. *Diagnostic and Statistical Manual of Mental Disorders, DSM-IV-TR*. Washington, DC: American Psychiatric Association, 2000.
American Psychiatric Association. *Diagnostic and Statistical Manual of Mental Disorders*, 5th ed. Alexandria, VA: American Psychiatric Association, 2013.
Kendall, Philip C., and Cynthia Suveg. "Treating Anxiety Disorders in Youth." In *Child and Adolescent Therapy: Cognitive-Behavioral Procedures*, Edited by Philip C. Kendall, 3rd ed., pp. 243–294. New York, NY: Guilford Press, 2006.
National Alliance on Mental Illness. "Anxiety Disorders in Children and Adolescents." NAMI, National Alliance on Mental Illness. Accessed October 8, 2013. http://www.nami.org/Content/ContentGroups/Helpline1/Anxiety_Disorders_in_Children_and_Adolescents.htm.

Anxiety Reduction Techniques

Anxiety reduction techniques are skills that an individual can learn, which will help handle or overcome the causes, symptoms, and effects of anxiety, stress, and tension. These techniques are divided into two categories, physical and mental, because of the strong connection between the two for people dealing with anxiety.

Definitions

- **Anxiety** is a negative emotional state characterized by feelings of nervousness, worry, and apprehension about an imagined danger.

- **Stress** is the pattern of specific and nonspecific responses to events that tax or exceed an individual's ability to cope.

- **Stress management** is a set of psychological techniques for increasing the capacity to better cope with psychological stress. It usually includes relaxation methods.

Description

Anxiety reduction techniques can be both physical and psychological and help those who suffer from anxiety, tension and stress. Usually the suffering is strong enough that individuals often find it difficult to engage in and enjoy daily living. Sometimes the symptoms are so severe that the person will do just about anything to find relief.

People who experience anxiety undergo psychological problems that create stress and tension. This mental stress is often related to physical problems as well and leads to chronic anxiety and stress. This long-term anxiety can lower the immune system, increase blood pressure, and increase muscle tension. All of these symptoms can eventually lead to serious life-threatening illnesses. Health-care professionals therefore have sought to treat the causes and symptoms of anxiety, stress, and tension in a variety of ways.

Medical interventions for anxiety reduction include the use of prescription drugs and have been used for decades. This approach, however, has some problems and can prevent effective long-term resolutions for the problem causing the stress. In addition to that stress, the medication could contribute to addictive behaviors and is a reality when using medication as treatment. Some individuals who use medication to relieve anxiety experience negative side effects and dependency, which leads to more stress and anxiety.

This vicious cycle led many health-care professionals to explore and begin using other anxiety reduction techniques. Some of these techniques include psychotherapy in the form of relaxation and cognitive behavioral strategies. Research also provides a rationale for the use of physical to reduce anxiety. Both of these techniques can be helpful for professionals working with individuals with anxiety so they can be taught through professional help and continue practicing these techniques outside of therapy.

Development

One of the first modern investigators of the effects of alternative methods on stress was Dr. Herbert Benson, who published the book *The Relaxation Response* (1975). His approach challenged the medication approach to encourage more psychological and physical activities that reduce stress. Since then the field has rapidly expanded with both traditional medical and alternative approaches multiplying over the years.

There are a variety of options available for relieving anxiety and stress. Among the most common are physical activities such as diaphragmatic breathing (as in yoga), massage, exercise and relaxation. Common mental relaxation techniques include visualization and imagery, hypnosis, and meditation.

The clinical basis for the success of these techniques lies in the fact that they stimulate the production of natural opiates in the brain. These brain chemicals have been found to block pain and to create a feeling of euphoria or a "high" much like the medications prescribed for anxiety. Through the natural release of this chemical, individuals with anxiety are less likely to utilize medication and experience side effects or dependence.

Current Status

Recently, the field of biofeedback to treat anxiety has been introduced. Biofeedback relies on the use of a machine that measures brain waves, cardiac rhythm, pulse, breathing, muscle tension, or conduction of electricity by the skin. It is a conditioning process. When a more internally tranquil state is recorded by the equipment, the patient is rewarded by a pleasant tone or colored light. The procedure then aims at helping the patient concentrate on maintaining the positive changes that have occurred in the body.

Other more recently popular anxiety reducing techniques include cognitive restructuring. This approach is based on becoming aware of the chronic stressors in life and learning how to reappraise them. This is a kind of cognitive restructuring activity that can lessen the stress of uncertainty and the anxiety about loss of control through identifying and practicing healthy coping mechanisms. In general, the work on optimistic thinking and positive psychology and cognitive restructuring attests to the power of the mind to promote health and well-being.

Alexandra Cunningham, PhD, and
William M. Cunningham, MA

See also: Anxiety Disorders in Adults; Anxiety Disorders in Youth; Mindfulness

Further Reading

Benson, Herbert. *The Relaxation Response.* New York: Morrow, 1975.

McKay, Matthew, Martha Davis, Elizabeth Robbins Eshelman, and Patrick Fanning. *The Relaxation and Stress Reduction Workbook.* Oakland, CA: New Harbinger, 2008.

Paul, Gordon L. *Insight versus Systematic Desensitization in Psychotherapy: An Experiment in Anxiety Reduction.* Palo Alto, CA: Stanford University Press, 1966.

Stahl, Bob, and Wendy Millstine. *Calming the Rush of Panic: A Mindfulness-Based Stress Reduction Guide to Freeing Yourself from Panic Attacks and Living a Vital Life.* Oakland, CA: New Harbinger, 2013.

Anxious Personality Disorder

Anxious personality disorder is a personality disorder characterized by a persistent, continuous pattern of anxiety.

Definitions

- **Antianxiety medications** are prescribed drugs that relieve anxiety symptoms. They are also called anxiolytics or tranquilizers.

- **Anxiety** is a negative emotional state characterized by feelings of nervousness, worry, and apprehension about an imagined danger.

- **Anxiety disorders** are a group of mental disorders characterized by anxiety which tends to be intermittent instead of persistent. The group includes panic disorder, phobias, and generalized anxiety disorder.

- **Characterological anxiety** is a persistent pattern or trait of anxiety which reflects an individual's general level of distress. It contrasts with state (situational) anxiety which reflects an individual's distress in a given situation.

- **Cognitive behavior therapy** is a type of psychotherapy that focuses on maladaptive (problematic) behaviors, emotions, and thoughts. It is also called CBT.

- **Defense mechanisms** are strategies for self-protection against anxiety and other negative emotions that accompany stress.

- **DSM-5** stands for the *Diagnostic and Statistical Manual of Mental Disorders, Fifth Edition*, which is a diagnostic system used by professionals to identify mental disorders with specific diagnostic criteria.

- **Exposure therapy** is an intervention (method) in which a client is exposed to a feared object or situation. It is also referred to as flooding.

- **Generalized anxiety disorder** is an anxiety disorder characterized by chronic anxiety and multiple exaggerated worries even when there is little or nothing to provoke it.

- **Mindfulness practices** are intentional activities that foster living in the present moment and awareness that is nonjudgmental and accepting.

- **Personality disorder** is a long-standing pattern of maladaptive (problematic) behavior, thoughts, and emotions that deviates from the accepted norms of an individual's culture. Personality disorder reflects an individual's unique personality structure.

- **Psychoanalytic theory** is a psychological theory that explains behaviors and perceptions as the result of unconscious, sexual, and biological instincts. It was originally developed by Sigmund Freud.

- *Psychodynamic Diagnostic Manual* (**PDM**) is a diagnostic system based on psychoanalytic theory that is used by professionals to identify mental disorders with specific diagnostic criteria.

Description and Diagnosis

Anxious personality disorder is a personality disorder that overlaps considerably with the DSM-5 diagnosis of generalized anxiety disorder. While anxiety is the psychologically organizing experience in anxious personality disorder, it differs from the anxiety disorders. In most anxiety disorders, the anxieties involve specific objects or situations. For example, with a spider phobia, the anxiety involve spiders, which is a specific object. In contrast, anxious personality disorder involves characterological anxiety, which is a "free-floating" or global sense of anxiety with no object or situation.

Those with this disorder have failed to develop adequate coping strategies for dealing with the common stresses and fears of everyday life. They typically report having had a parent, who because of that parent's own anxiety could not adequately comfort them or provide a sense of security or support.

Two or more of the following types of anxiety are common among those with this personality disorder:

signal anxiety (emotional cues that a specific situation was previously considered dangerous), moral anxiety (dread of violating one's core values), separation anxiety (fear of loss of a relationship), and annihilation anxiety (terror of loss of a sense of self). This contrasts with the various anxiety disorders in which only one of these tends to predominate.

Many are surprised to learn that the anxious personality disorder is not included in DSM-5. However, it is described in the *Psychodynamic Diagnostic Manual* (PDM). According to the PDM (2006), the anxious personality disorder is diagnosable by the following criteria. Individuals exhibit an anxious or timid temperament (inborn personality characteristics). They are preoccupied with being safe amid perceived dangers. Their basic emotion is fear. Their basic belief or view of themselves is that they are in constant danger from unknown forces. Their basic belief or view of others is that others are the sources of either danger or protection. Furthermore, they are unable to adequately shield themselves from such danger because their defense mechanisms are inadequate.

Treatment

Treatment of the anxious personality disorder tends to be long term and challenging. Therapists do well to demonstrate an attitude of confidence in the individual's own capacities to tolerate and reduce anxiety. It is also important to develop and maintain a strong therapeutic relationship since these individuals tend to become discouraged because of their long-standing symptoms. Exposure therapy and mindfulness practices can be very useful in anxiety reduction. Other cognitive behavior therapy techniques can be helpful in understanding and mastering this disorder. Antianxiety medications can also be considered in reducing anxiety symptoms. However, because of the risk of addiction, these medications should be prescribed with caution for individuals with this personality disorder.

Len Sperry, MD, PhD

See also: Anxiety Disorders in Adults; *Diagnostic and Statistical Manual of Mental Disorders* (DSM); Exposure Therapy; Mindfulness; Personality Disorders; Psychoanalysis; *Psychodynamic Diagnostic Manual* (PDM)

Further Reading

PDM Task Force. *Psychodynamic Diagnostic Manual (PDM)*. Silver Spring, MD: Alliance of Psychoanalytic Organizations, 2006.

Apathy

Apathy is a state of emotional indifference; it is the absence of interest, concern, or enthusiasm in things most people enjoy about life.

Description

"Apathy" is a term used to describe an emotional state of indifference and lack of passion. It is most often a temporary feeling that is experienced by most people. Apathy is frequently a symptom of various psychological and emotional disorders. Apathy is a lack of passion and enthusiasm for life. There is a suppression of emotion or feelings. Apathetic people live with a lack of concern, excitement, or interest in relationships, current events, and meaning in life. They are numb to the excitement and wonder of life.

Apathy is described as a lack of motivation. It is characterized by a decrease in three key categories of functioning. There is a decrease in goal-oriented behavior in which there is a lack of effort to engage in activities or an overreliance on others to structure activities. There is also a decrease in goal-directed thinking characterized by a lack of interest in learning, a lack of interest in new experiences, and a lack of concern about one's personal problems. The third category is a decrease in emotion and emotional responsiveness.

Apathy is most often transient, meaning it is a phase that people go through but do not stay in. Apathy is not depression and is not considered a separate mental health disorder. People suffering from depression are debilitated or incapacitated in some fashion. Depressed people often lack the ability to fully function or engage in life. Apathetic individuals, who are not suffering from a mental health disorder, are able to fully function in life. They just do so with little enthusiasm and passion. A common phrase used by apathetic people is "Who cares?"

Current Status

Apathy is a common experience in medical and mental health conditions. Apathy is common in depression and in individuals suffering from adjustment disorder and other mood disorders such as persistent depressive disorder. Apathy is also associated with disorders such as Asperger's syndrome and Alzheimer's disease. It is also associated with some medical conditions such as hypothyroidism and hyperthyroidism. Because apathy is not a separate mental health disorder, there is no specific treatment for it. Periods of apathy are considered a normal part of life. When apathy persists over a longer period of time, the individual is more likely to be suffering from a medical or mental health condition.

Everyone experiences periods of apathy. Apathy is often a coping response after a highly emotional experience takes place. During these times emotional energy is spent and sometimes exhausted; people just run out of emotional energy. Apathy is the experience people have while they recharge or recover emotionally. For instance, consider a senior in high school who has worked very hard to get into a top college. The university has very competitive entrance requirements and the student has studied and worked very hard to get in. She has participated in extracurricular activities and has volunteered in service projects to enhance her chances of getting into this highly regarded university. She has also spent countless hours on the Internet exploring all of the facets of the school and city it is located in. She has followed its football games on television and has a sweatshirt with the school mascot on it. She worked hard on the application, received excellent recommendations from teachers, and submitted the application well before the deadline. But she didn't get in and is extremely disappointed. We can predict that she will go through a period of time where she doesn't seem to care about college or where she attends. Because of the intense emotional energy spent in the pursuit of the college, she feels numb and tells her best friend she "couldn't care less" about college. She declines an invitation to a party and stays home that weekend and mopes around the house. However, after a brief period of time she begins to recover and begins to think about other colleges. She remembers that her best friend talked about her favorite college and she decides to check it out on the Internet.

She is back on track and is excited by the different options she has.

Apathy is an emotional state that most individuals experience in their lifetime. Short periods of apathy are not cause for alarm and are considered normal. When apathy is longer lasting, it may be a sign of emotional struggle and be of concern if the individual is not functioning well.

Steven R. Vensel, PhD

See also: Adjustment Disorder; Persistent Depressive Disorder

Further Reading

American Psychiatric Association. *Diagnostic and Statistical Manual of Mental Disorders*, 5th ed. Arlington, VA: American Psychiatric Association Press, 2013.

Burns, David D. *The Feeling Good Handbook*. New York, NY: Penguin, 1999.

Starkstein, Sergio. "Apathy in Parkinson's Disease: Diagnostic and Etiological Dilemmas." *Movement Disorders* 27, no. 2 (2012): 174–178.

Aphasia

Aphasia is the impaired ability to understand words, signs, or gestures caused by a brain injury or disease.

Definitions

- **Alzheimer's disease** is a medical and mental disorder that causes dementia particularly late in life. It is also referred to as Neurocognitive Disorder Due to Alzheimer's Disease.

- **Dementia** is a group of symptoms including loss of memory, judgment, language, and other intellectual (mental) function caused by the death of neurons (nerve cells) in the brain.

- **Depression** is an emotional state characterized by feelings of sadness, low self-esteem, guilt, or the reduced ability to enjoy life. It is not considered a disorder unless it significantly disrupts one's daily functioning.

- **Epilepsy** is a medical condition when seizures reoccur. It is also known as seizure disorder.

- **Seizure** is an episode of abnormal electrical activity in the brain that results in physical findings and changes in behavior.

- **Stroke** is a medical condition when there is deprivation of oxygen to the brain due to a lack of blood flow.

Description

Aphasia is an impairment or disturbance in the comprehension and expression of language. The degree of impairment can range from having difficulty remembering words to having the inability to speak, read, or write. Symptoms can be mild or severe. When the symptoms are severe, communication may be nearly impossible. Some signs and symptoms of aphasia include the inability to form words, inability to repeat a phrase, or inability to pronounce words. Other symptoms may involve the inability to comprehend language, persistent repetition of phrases, inability to name objects, and the inability to write sentences that make sense. Aphasia does not affect intelligence.

Individuals with cancer, seizures, epilepsy, Alzheimer's disease, or other brain diseases may experience aphasia. Those who have had a stroke or head injury are likely to experience severe aphasia. There are also progressive forms of aphasia that develop slowly. These types of aphasia include brain tumor, dementia, or infection. The more extensive the brain damage, the greater the likelihood of severe and lasting disability.

Aphasia can cause a number of problems in one's life due to lack of communication. Often, good quality of life is significantly reduced. Aphasia can also cause problems in relationships, jobs, education, and day-to-day functioning. It can also lead to depression, frustration, and humiliation. Some individuals with aphasia are very aware of their difficulties. Others are not so aware of when there is a breakdown in communication. Individuals with aphasia claim the worst part of their disorder is the rejection they receive from others who do not understand what aphasia is.

Len Sperry, MD, PhD, and Elizabeth Smith Kelsey, PhD

See also: Alzheimer's Disease; Dementia; Depression; Seizures; Stroke

Further Reading

Davis, Albyn G. *Aphasia and Related Cognitive-Communicative Disorders.* New York, NY: Pearson, 2013.

Mesulam, M. M. "Primary Progressive Aphasia." *Annals of Neurology* 49, no. 4 (April 2001): 425–432.

Papathanasiou, Ilias, Patrick Coppens, and Constantin Potagas. *Aphasia and Related Neurogenic Communication Disorders.* Burlington, MA: Jones & Bartlett Learning, 2013.

Applied Behavior Analysis

Applied behavior analysis is a science that aims to understand and improve human behavior.

Description

Applied behavior analysis (ABA) differs from other approaches to understanding behavior in its focus, goals, and methods. The focus of ABA is to understand behaviors you can observe. These are defined as specifically and objectively as possible. Treatment is then focused on improving the behaviors that are identified in a systematic way. It explores what environmental factors influence the way people act. The way ABA trained therapists do this is by gathering information and tracking data and by making sure that treatment is effective.

There are three major beliefs of ABA that originate from behavioral theory. The first is that behavioral philosophy is scientific. The next is that research and analyzing behavior is required for experimentation. Last, ABA requires the development of techniques and technology for the goal of improving behavior.

Therapists work with young children and older adults. Early intervention involves trained therapists directing treatment. There are a wide variety of techniques available in ABA. Usually it involves a structured environment but can be done in the home, school, or community. ABA sessions have historically focused on individual therapy between a behavior analyst and client. But group instruction using ABA techniques is useful as well.

Development

The field of psychology began with the study of conscious states. In the early 1900s a shift to focus on behavior started with John B. Watson. He wanted to focus psychology on observable events that can predict and control behavior. These experiments officially began with B. F. Skinner through research and publications. Skinner established the field of experimental analysis of behavior. He was able to provide a guideline for breaking down behaviors into smaller parts and understanding specific influences on behavior. He revolutionized the field of ABA and in some ways made it radical and controversial.

Another important figure in the development of ABA was Don Baer. He believed the key point of behaviorism is to understand what people do. He was known for being able to break down the process of behaviorism and ABA in a way that students and others could truly understand. He was also involved in studying the effects of punishment, escape, and avoidance on young children.

In 1959 one of the most important papers that established ABA was released, *The Psychiatric Nurse as a Behavioral Engineer.* The publication of this paper and others allowed professionals to start thinking of ABA beyond trained therapists. The principles of ABA began being used and published in schools, hospitals, and beyond. In the early 1960s and 1970s university programs began to offer programs in ABA. Then in 1968, an important year for ABA, the *Journal of Applied Behavior Analysis (JABA)* came into existence. In this first volume various psychologists, including Don Baer, published articles and helped several become known as the founding fathers of ABA.

Current Status

During the 1990s and 2000s the field of applied behavior analysis grew with the formation of organizations and publications of books and journals on the subject. On a practical level, ABA has helped many different kinds of learners to improve. These areas of improvement can range from academic to language to lifestyle. Today it is widely recognized as effective and safe for various conditions including developmental disorders like autism.

Effective ABA practices currently involve an individualized approach to each client. The therapist tailors treatment to the needs and abilities of the person he or she works with. The common elements of ABA therapy include a planning or assessment phase and then applying proven techniques.

In recent decades, the provision of a training program for those who can provide ABA therapy was established. The Behavior Analyst Certification Board was created to ensure that ABA therapy is being provided at a high standard of care. Those seeking to use behavior therapy or ABA should find a certified professional in the form of a Board Certified Behavior Analyst. These professionals are known as BCBA or BCaBA professionals.

Alexandra Cunningham, PhD

See also: Behavior Therapy; Behavior Therapy with Children; Skinner, B. F. (1904–1990); Watson, John B. (1878–1958)

Further Reading

Cooper, John O., Timothy E. Heron, and William L. Heward. *Applied Behavior Analysis*, 2nd ed. New York, NY: Pearson, 2007.

Kearney, Albert. K. *Understanding Applied Behavior Analysis: An Introduction to ABA for Parents, Teachers and Other Professionals.* London, UK: Jessica Kingsley Publishing, 2007.

Archetypes and the Collective Unconscious, The (Book)

The Archetypes and the Collective Unconscious by Swiss psychiatrist Carl Gustav Jung was originally published in 1959. This book is Jung's explanation of a universal unconscious of mankind, which he believed was impersonal in nature and expressed as instinct. In the book, Jung states that the universal unconsciousness is not anything that has been blocked from our consciousness but instead is a preconscious experience that has always existed. As he explains it, "Thinking existed long before man was able to say, 'I am conscious of thinking.'"

Definitions

- **Anima** is the female image that is part of the male psyche.

- **Animus** is the male image that is part of the female psyche.

- **Archetype** is a pattern of behavior used to organize, understand, and interpret how we experience life. Archetypes can be fluid, meaning they can change over time.

Jung was a great influence on the field of psychology. Freud personally selected Jung in 1910 as the first president of the International Psychoanalytic Association. However, in 1914, Jung rejected Freud's theories and founded his own system of Analytical Psychology, which was based on archetypal and symbolic theory.

In his book, Jung introduces archetypes as symbols of preconscious thinking. He identifies the following archetypes: the anima in men, the animus in women, the persona, the self, the mother archetype, the child archetype, the hero, and the trickster. In addition to these conscious archetypes, there is an archetype for the unconscious, which Jung calls the shadow. The shadow is made up of what is suppressed from the consciousness and is at a more superficial level than the other archetypes. The shadow is considered a darker element, comprised of chaos, wildness, sex, and life instincts.

According to Jung, everyone's consciousness evolves in stages. When an agreement is reached between the universal (archetypical) unconscious and the individual ego (consciousness), a person reaches individuation. Both the reason of consciousness and the chaos of the unconscious should continue to be expressed, because this conflict and collaboration is what makes us human.

Throughout his career as a scientist and practicing clinician, Jung focused on religion and spirituality. He believed religion was important to the human psyche, and he chose to focus on it in the context of his work. He focused on Christianity and spirituality in his work, and in this book Jung examines the change in a person's psychic state as a result of Christianity. Jung looks at Christ as a symbol of wholeness, along with symbols from Gnosticism and alchemy. He also examines Gnostic symbols of self and how the

Quaternity is used in alchemy as a way to organize wholeness.

Using a series of 24 mandalas, Jung describes both the history of our psychological development as humans and a patient's progress toward individuation. The mandala, a symbol from Tibetan Buddhism, was used by Jung to represent the totality of self. The mandala symbol helps reduce mental confusion and restore balance.

Jung explores the archetype of the self, representing the person as a whole. Jung saw the self as a psychological union of the conscious, or masculine, and the unconscious, or feminine. When the conscious and unconscious are together, they stand for psychic totality.

From Jung's work, many terms today are in common use, including archetype, introvert, extrovert, synchronicity, anima, and New Age spirituality. His work has influenced many fields, including psychology, medicine, art, religion, and literature. *The Archetypes and the Collective Unconscious* shows a unique insight into his efforts to combine Christian teachings with other examples of thought and expression.

Mindy Parsons, PhD

See also: Jung, Carl (1875–1961); Jungian Therapy

Further Reading

Levinson, Martin H. "Books: Deirdre Bair, Jung: A Biography, 2003." *ProQuest Social Sciences Premium Collection* 62 (2005): 1.

Muncie, Wendell. "New Biological Books: The Archetypes and the Collective Unconscious, The Collected Works of C. G. Jung." *The Quarterly Review of Biology* 36, no. 2 (1961): 149–150.

Aricept (Donepezil)

Aricept is a prescribed medication used to treat Alzheimer's disease. Its generic name is donepezil.

Definitions

- **Acetylcholine** is a chemical messenger that transmits nerve impulses from cell to cell.

It causes blood vessels to dilate, lowers blood pressure, and slows the heartbeat. A sufficient level of acetylcholine is associated with mental focus and attention.

- **Alzheimer's disease** is a progressive neurodegenerative disease in which dementia results from the degeneration and death of brain cells because of low levels of acetylcholine, plaques, and neurofibrillary tangles.

- **Dementia** is a group of symptoms (syndrome) associated with a progressive loss of memory and other intellectual functions that interfere with one's ability to perform the tasks of daily life. It impairs memory and reasoning ability, causes disorientation, and alters personality.

Description

Aricept is used to treat symptoms of dementia associated with Alzheimer's disease. While it can result in small improvements in dementia for a short period of time, Aricept cannot stop the progression of Alzheimer's disease. Aricept is in a class of medications called cholinesterase inhibitors. Such medications prevent the breakdown of acetylcholine, a chemical messenger (neurotransmitter) that facilitates nerve impulses within the brain. An adequate level of acetylcholine is associated with mental focus and attention. As brain cells die, they can no longer transmit nerve impulses. In certain regions of the brain, cell death results in symptoms of dementia. By maintaining sufficient acetylcholine levels in the brain, Aricept facilitates the transmission of nerve impulses.

Precautions and Side Effects

Individuals with heart conditions, stomach ulcers, bladder obstruction, asthma, chronic obstructive lung disease, or a history of seizures should use Aricept only under close medical supervision. Aricept should not be used during pregnancy nor by nursing women unless the benefits outweigh the risks.

Side effects reported with the use of Aricept include sleep difficulties, dizziness, nausea, diarrhea, muscle cramps, and headache. These side effects are usually mild, short lived, and usually subside when Aricept is stopped. Other less common side effects include depression, drowsiness, fainting, loss of appetite, unusual dreams, weight loss, frequent urination, arthritis, and easy bruising.

Research has found that the effects of Aricept on Alzheimer's disease can be enhanced when Aricept is combined with Namenda, another Alzheimer's medication. Clinical trials have shown that the combination of Aricept and Namenda is more effective than the use of Aricept alone in the treatment of moderate to severe Alzheimer's disease. This combination appears to be safe as well as effective. Aricept does interact with some medications and can increase the side effects associated with use of Luvox, an antidepressant.

Len Sperry, MD, PhD

See also: Alzheimer's Disease; Namenda (Memantine)

Further Reading

Burns, Alistair, and Bengt Winblad, eds. *Severe Dementia.* New York, NY: John Wiley & Sons, 2006.

Doraiswamy, P. Murali, Lisa Gwyther, and Tina Adler. *The Alzheimer's Action Plan: What You Need to Know—and What You Can Do—about Memory Problems, from Prevention to Early Intervention and Care.* New York, NY: St. Martin's Press, 2009.

Mace, Nancy, and Peter V. Ravins. *The 36-Hour Day: A Family Guide to Caring for People with Alzheimer Disease, Other Dementias, and Memory Loss in Later Life,* 5th ed. Baltimore, MD: Johns Hopkins University Press, 2012.

Art Therapy

Human expression through art dates back more than 40,000 years to Paleolithic cave paintings of hunting expeditions and large wild animals. Since prehistoric times, art expression has proven to be one of mankind's most powerful means of communicating experience. Through artistic expression there is much to be learned about ourselves and one another, especially in therapeutic settings. As a profession, art therapy, which emerged in the mid-20th century, is focused on better understanding the human condition and the inner workings of the psyche as revealed through art expression.

Definition

- **Art therapy** is a mental health specialty used by specially trained therapists working with clients using a variety of art media. The process of creating art is a form of therapy that helps clients to explore their feelings, improve personal insight, resolve emotional conflicts, and address a variety of challenges, including addictions, social skills, anxiety, and depression.

As a mental health area of specialization, art therapy is used in a variety of clinical settings and with a wide array of diverse populations. Art therapy is also used in nonclinical settings, including art studios and various workshops that focus on developing creativity. Art therapists require specific and extensive training to receive certification and use this form of therapy in working with clients of all ages, including children, adolescents, adults, and the elderly.

This form of therapy can be used by itself, or it can be used in combination with other forms of therapy, such as cognitive behavior therapy or group therapy. Art therapy can be used in working with individuals, couples, families, and groups and for a variety of mental health challenges, from post-traumatic stress disorder (PTSD) in war veterans to schizophrenia, and from depression to sexual abuse in childhood.

Art therapy is considered a form of expressive therapy in which a client can use a wide variety of art materials and mediums. This includes pottery, clay, chalk, paint, crayons, markers, collages, mandalas, and other art materials. Art therapy can also use digital media, such as painting and drawing programs on computers and tablets. Unlike like a typical art class that focuses on learning skills or techniques, art therapy sessions are looking at the client's inner experience—how he or she feels, perceives, and imagines.

One example of an art therapy technique is coloring a mandala, which has been proven to reduce anxiety because it induces a meditative state, which in turn lowers a person's blood pressure and pulse rate and slows breathing and metabolism. Famed psychoanalyst Carl Jung referred to mandalas as a representation of the unconscious self. The process of creating a mandala is both therapeutic and symbolic. Creating mandalas, like most art therapy, has little to do with the final product, but rather the therapeutic value in the journey of the process.

The use of art therapy is based on using the creative process for self-expression as a way for clients to resolve conflicts, solve problems, improve behavior, strengthen interpersonal skills, reduce stress and anxiety, improve self-esteem, and improve personal awareness. In short, this type of therapy uses the creative process to develop a better understanding and insight into the individual client, and it is backed by traditional psychotherapeutic theories and techniques. When those theories and techniques are combined with an in-depth understanding of the psychological forces that play into the creative process, the results can be highly therapeutic for the client. Around the mid-1900s, doctors started to notice people frequently used various forms of art to express their mental health challenges. This, in turn, led to therapists using the artwork as a way of healing. It can be used as part of their treatment or to assess clients—for example, having a client do a Kinetic Family Drawing or House-Tree-Person Test.

The research on art therapy continues to show a generally positive response for the therapeutic effects on a variety of populations. Art therapy has proven particularly effective with returning war veterans who suffer from PTSD, and it also has shown tremendous benefits both psychologically and physically with older adults who are confined to hospitals or nursing homes. Several studies focusing on institutionalized older adults reveal that art therapy increases creativity and generally improves the patient's level of happiness, peacefulness, and calmness, while reducing depression and sense of despair.

Art therapy works in a variety of populations by helping the individual verbalize his or her feelings and past experiences. Community mental health agencies, schools, private counseling offices, hospitals, and nursing homes are all potential settings where art therapy services may be available.

Becoming an art therapist requires training in both therapy and art, including studying psychology and human development. Art therapists often have a clinical practice of some kind and use art therapy as treatment for mental health issues. Through the art created by clients, art therapists discern nonverbal symbols and metaphors expressed through the art and the creative process itself—information that may not otherwise be expressed verbally.

Mindy Parsons, PhD

See also: Expressive Arts Therapy; Figure Drawing; House-Tree-Person Test

Further Reading

Farokhi, Masoumeh. "Art Therapy in Humanistic Psychiatry." *Procedia—Social and Behavioral Sciences* 30 (2011): 2088–2092.

Kapitan, Lynn. "Does Art Therapy Work? Identifying the Active Ingredients of Art Therapy Efficacy." *Art Therapy: Journal of the American Art Therapy Association* 29, no. 2 (2012): 48–49.

Loesl, Susan. "Introduction to the Special Issue on Art Therapy in the Schools: Art Therapy + Schools + Students = ?" *Art Therapy: Journal of the American Art Therapy Association* 27, no. 2 (2010): 54–55.

Malchiodi, Cathy. *The Art Therapy Sourcebook*, 2nd ed. New York, NY: McGraw-Hill, 2006.

Perry Magniant, Rebecca C. *Art Therapy with Older Adults: A Sourcebook*. Springfield, IL: Charles C. Thomas Publisher, Ltd., 2004.

Wadeson, Harriet. "National Art Education Association. Art Therapy Research." *Art Education, Art Therapy and Art Education* 33, no. 4 (April, 1980): 31–34.

Organization

American Art Therapy Association, Inc. (AATA)
4875 Eisenhower Avenue, Suite 240
Alexandria, VA 22301
Telephone: (888) 290-0878
E-mail: info@ar1ttherapy.org
Website: http://www.arttherapy.org/

The AATA states that its mission is "to serve its members and the general public by providing standards of professional competence, and developing and promoting knowledge in, and of, the field of art therapy." http://www.arttherapy.org/.

Asperger's Syndrome

Asperger's syndrome, also called Asperger's disorder, is a diagnosis on the autism spectrum where people have good verbal skills but noticeable social problems.

Definitions

- **Asperger's disorder** is a neurological condition marked by challenges in socializing and restricted interests or repetitive behaviors.

- **Autism spectrum disorders** are developmental disabilities that affect a person's ability to communicate, socialize, and behave like most others.

Description

Asperger's disorder or syndrome (AS) is commonly described as a high-functioning form of autism due to normal language development and intelligence. Those who are diagnosed with it exhibit difficulty interacting socially and behave differently than others. They usually have problems such as poor one-on-one conversations, obsessive interest in a limited range of subjects, and repetitive patterns of behavior.

The disorder is named after Dr. Hans Asperger (1906–1980), an Austrian physician, who first described the particular behaviors that mark people with this syndrome in a paper published in 1944. He observed a group of boys with good language skills but poor communication and motor skills. Dr. Asperger called the group of boys who had marked social problems but good language and cognitive skills the "little professors." Their limited and all-consuming interests led them to be highly verbal yet seemingly unaware of interest displayed by others. These boys also had awkward motor skills. He also noted that their fathers had experienced similar problems in their lives. A translation of Dr. Asperger's original paper is provided by Dr. Uta Frith in her book *Autism and Asperger Syndrome* (1991).

Although people with AS have good verbal skills, they do have trouble relating socially with the overall effectiveness of their communication. Because of this people with AS are often characterized by what is seen as weird behaviors and experience social isolation in childhood. They have difficulty with two-way and nonverbal communication. When you add in clumsiness with gross motor movement, they often find it difficult to establish common bonds with their peers. These characteristics can have an ongoing and lifelong impact on their ability to live independently and to hold a job or on other important areas of daily life functioning.

Causes and Symptoms

Currently, there is not a single cause or group of causes for Asperger's syndrome nor any of the diagnoses on the autism spectrum. While no specific genes have been found to relate to Asperger's, some researchers have noted structural differences in specific areas of the brain that do not occur in unaffected children.

Although we are not sure of the reasons for this, Asperger's disorder does affect a greater number of males than females, sometimes estimated at four to one ratio. It has often been identified as occurring in families across generations which may indicate that environmental factors also play a role in its development. Those who manifest the characteristics of AS often are of normal to high intelligence. Their limited ability to exhibit age-appropriate social interaction often leads to overcompensation on their limited areas of intellectual interest. This misguided attempt to engage others is often seen as overwhelming them with facts and repetition, which can lead to rejection by their circle of acquaintances. Their inability to read the emotional reactions of others can result in poor judgments about the motives and intents of the people they encounter. The worst result is that they can be victimized and deceived by others.

People with AS often have impairments with theory of mind. Theory of mind is the mental ability of people to take the perspective of others. This can often lead to social confusion and awkwardness among those with AS and their peers.

Often teachers and adults responsible for educating and supporting individuals with AS are impressed by their intelligence and verbal skills and can forget or ignore the sometimes less obvious social skill difficulties. People with AS can often be overlooked because their deficits aren't as obvious as those with more moderate or severe autism spectrum disorders.

Diagnosis and Prognosis

Asperger's disorder is marked by four diagnostic criteria. This includes a limited ability to recognize and use social interaction skills and lack of success in building relationships with their peers. This is due to limited social turn taking and an overemphasis on their own restricted interests.

Repetitive patterns of behavior especially around an intense focus on one or a few areas of interest are also present for people with AS. A rigid adherence to routines and need for sameness is characteristic of the diagnosis. In addition, small or whole-body tics like finger flapping or hand twisting are commonly occurring. Many people with AS have ongoing preoccupations with aspects or parts of objects. In order to receive a diagnosis there should be no noticeable delay in language acquisition or learning skills. Yet significant challenges in interpersonal, work, and other areas of social relationships should be present.

Asperger's syndrome is considered a chronic or lifelong condition. The prognosis appears significantly better for those with AS than for many others on the autism spectrum. Researchers suggest that as they mature, many people can learn to be self-sufficient and are capable of high-level employment.

Treatment

While there is no cure for Asperger's disorder, there are many ways that people can progress. One way to do this involves recognizing and adjusting their behaviors to be more effective communicators in social situations. This can be done through individual and group therapy, behavior modification, and social skills training. People with AS commonly receive behavior, occupational, and language therapy. Education for parents, siblings, and close friends also helps them to limit those with Asperger's disorder and to recognize and limit any problematic behaviors.

Alexandra Cunningham, PhD

See also: Autism; Autism Spectrum Disorders; Pervasive Developmental Disorders

Further Reading

American Psychiatric Association. *Diagnostic and Statistical Manual of Mental Disorders*, 5th ed. Arlington, VA: American Psychiatric Association, 2013.
Firth, Uta. *Autism and Asperger Syndrome*. Cambridge, UK: Cambridge University Press, 1991.

National Autism Society. "Autism and Asperger Syndrome: An Introduction." Last modified January 28, 2013. Accessed July 22, 2013. http://www.autism.org.uk/about-autism/autism-and-asperger-syndrome-an-introduction.aspx.

Assertiveness Training

Assertiveness training (AT) is a therapeutic procedure designed to help people improve their sense of self-esteem as well as their ability to communicate more clearly with others.

Definition

- **Assertiveness** is the quality of being self-assured and confident without being aggressive.

Description

In the history of modern American self-help and personal development movements, AT became a popular intervention designed to promote self-respect and self-expression. Assertiveness has been seen not only as a way to express ourselves clearly and act in our own best interests but also as a means of combating social fears and discomfort by standing up for ourselves without undue anxiety. From the beginning assertiveness was identified as a key behavioral skill that could enhance self-esteem and which could be learned and improved through awareness and practice. AT also aims to help people overcome many socially debilitating conditions such as depression, social anxiety, and problems resulting from unexpressed anger. Because of this it came to be part of the teaching and therapeutic practice of many personal development experts, behavior therapists, and cognitive behavioral therapists.

Although they exhibit individual differences, the various ATs tend to have some objectives in common. Chief among them is to increase awareness of personal dignity and rights. As such, AT fit nicely into the 1960s and 1970s, a period that saw both the civil rights struggle and the rising demand for equal rights for women. Other commonalities among the trainings include the importance of making the distinction between the three key ideas of passivity, assertiveness, and aggressiveness, whether these are expressed verbally or nonverbally. Respect for personal boundaries has been another key concept.

Development

Assertiveness training was introduced by Andrew Salter in the early 1960s and popularized by Joseph Wolpe. The term and concept was popularized among the general public by books such as *Your Perfect Right: A Guide to Assertive Behavior* (1970) by Robert E. Alberti and *When I Say No, I Feel Guilty: How to Cope Using the Skills of Systematic Assertiveness Therapy* (1975) by Manuel J. Smith.

The heyday of AT in its initial forms came in the late 1970s and early 1980s. Some self-proclaimed gurus used extreme techniques in an effort to help people break through perceived social barriers. As a result some people acted out in socially inappropriate and obnoxious ways in the name of empowerment and assertiveness. When used poorly and with bad intentions, so-called assertiveness techniques could be psychological tools that led readily to psychological damage or abuse.

Current Status

Assertive behavior continues to be identified as especially valuable in several areas of psychological health. In health care, which remains a complex and confusing system often controlled by medical experts, it is good to know how to request clearly what you need. It is also important, especially for men, to learn how to be assertive emotionally and clear in their expressions of intimacy. Finally, it can be a great help in being able to know how to say "no" to peer pressures to use drugs or, especially in the case of children and adolescents, to resist unwanted sexual advances.

Alexandra Cunningham, PhD, and William M. Cunningham, MA

See also: Social Skills Training

Further Reading

Bishop, Sue. *Develop Your Assertiveness*. Philadelphia, PA: Kogan Page, 2006.
Bolton, Robert. *People Skills: How to Assert Yourself, Listen to Others, and Resolve Conflicts*. New York, NY: Simon & Schuster, 1986.

Bower, Sharon Anthony, and Gorden E. Bower. *Asserting Yourself-Updated Edition: A Practical Guide for Positive Change*. Reading, MA: Perseus Books, 2004.

Ativan (Lorazepam)

Ativan is a prescribed antianxiety medication used to treat anxiety disorders and anxiety associated with depression. Its generic name is lorazepam.

Definitions

- **Anterograde amnesia** is a type of memory problem (amnesia) in which new memories cannot be formed while existing memories remain intact.

- **Benzodiazepines** are a group of central nervous system depressants that are used to relieve anxiety or to induce sleep.

- **Sedative-hypnotics** are medications that induce calmness and sleep. Barbiturates and benzodiazepines are its main types. These are also called tranquilizers, sleeping pills, or sleepers.

Description

Ativan is a sedating (causes drowsiness) medication that is classified as a benzodiazepines. Like other benzodiazepines, Ativan is believed to work by increasing gamma-aminobutyric acid (GABA), a chemical messenger in the brain. GABA inhibits the transmission of nervous impulses in the brain and spinal cord and decreases symptoms associated with anxiety. Ativan's primary use is to treat anxiety disorders and anxiety associated with depression. Secondary uses include the management of nausea and vomiting, insomnia, and seizures. Ativan is also used prior to surgery to produce sedation, sleepiness, drowsiness, relief of anxiety, and a decreased ability to recall the events surrounding the surgery. Ativan differs from drugs such as Valium and Librium in that it is shorter acting and does not accumulate in the body after repeated doses.

Precautions and Side Effects

Ativan can cause physical and psychological dependence, so it should be used with caution in those with a history of drug abuse. Its dosage should not be changed nor should it be suddenly discontinued. Instead, when stopping this medication, the dosage should gradually be decreased and then discontinued. If Ativan is stopped abruptly, individuals may experience withdrawal symptoms such as agitation, irritability, difficulty sleeping, and convulsions. Those with narrow-angle glaucoma, severe uncontrolled pain, or severe low blood pressure should not take Ativan. It has been associated with birth defects when taken during the first three months of pregnancy. Women taking this drug should not breast-feed. Ativan has also been reported to cause anterograde amnesia.

Common side effects of Ativan include drowsiness and sleepiness. Because of this, individuals exercise caution in driving, operating machinery, or performing activities that require mental alertness. Less common side effects include dizziness, reduced sex drive, weakness, unsteadiness, disorientation, nausea, agitation. Some individuals experience headache, difficulty sleeping, rash, yellowing of the eyes, vision changes, and hallucinations.

Alcohol and other central nervous system depressants can increase the drowsiness associated with this medication. Herbal remedies kava kava and valerian may increase the effects of Ativan. Individuals should not drink alcohol when taking Ativan and for 24 to 48 hours before receiving an injection prior to surgery.

Len Sperry, MD, PhD

See also: Benzodiazepines; Sedative, Hypnotic, or Anxiolytic Use Disorder

Further Reading

Doble, Adam, Ian Martin, and David J. Nutt. *Calming the Brain: Benzodiazepines and Related Drugs from Laboratory to Clinic*. London, UK: Informa Healthcare, 2003.

Preston, John D., John H. O'Neal, and Mary C. Talaga. *Handbook of Clinical Psychopharmacology for Therapists*, 7th ed. Oakland, CA: New Harbinger, 2013.

Toufexis, Donna. *Anti-anxiety Drugs*. New York, NY: Chelsea House Publishers, 2006.

Attachment Styles

The theory behind attachment styles was first developed by John Bowlby (1907–1990), with significant contributions that later came from Mary Ainsworth (1913–1999). Attachment styles are generally classified as either secure or insecure attachments; however, there are three subtypes of insecure attachments that include anxious-ambivalent, avoidant, and disorganized-disoriented. Attachment styles are considered important because the ability to create secure or insecure attachments with others impacts an individual throughout his or her lifespan.

Definition

- **Attachment styles** refer to the way in which an individual cognitively and emotionally interacts with others. Attachment styles are important since human relationships are central and connect into all areas of a person's life.

Description

The development of attachment theory is credited to John Bowlby. Bowlby initially worked with the World Health Organization on the area of juvenile delinquency. His work with juvenile delinquents led to his discovery of attachment as an evolutionary adaptation. Bowlby believed that a child's attachment to his or her mother served as a model for the child's later relationships and, in part, determined his or her ability to be emotionally stable. Bowlby held that it was not the perceived relationship between a caregiver and child but the actual interactions that create the blueprint for how an individual relates to others throughout his or her lifetime.

In the 1960s, Mary Ainsworth joined with Bowlby and became a major theoretical contributor to attachment theory. She used a measurement technique called the Strange Situation Test to explore the different kinds of attachments infants have to their primary caregivers. Twelve-month-old babies and their mothers were brought into a room and the baby was subjected to a series of eight, three-minute episodes whereby there were changes to the social situation.

Some of these episodes were likely to be stressful to the baby. Initially, the baby and mother were left alone in the room; then the mother and a stranger (one of the researchers) would enter and leave the room in varying patterns. The baby's reactions were recorded as well as the baby's exploration of the room and response to the return of the mother after she had left the room.

Ainsworth and her colleagues identified three patterns of response correlating to attachment styles and a fourth was added in later research. The four types of attachment styles are securely attached; anxious-ambivalent—insecurely attached; avoidant—insecurely attached; and disorganized-disoriented—insecurely attached. It is believed that attachment styles originate from the type of caregiving received in the baby's first year of life.

In studies on attachment, the majority of babies are found to be securely attached. These babies display distress when separated from their mother, which results in crying and attempts to go after her. Upon the return of the mother they greet her happily and will reach for her. Once they feel reassured by their mother's presence, they are comfortable in exploring the room. Ainsworth felt that babies in this category used their mother as a secure base. In Ainsworth's study, 65% of the babies showed this response style, and this figure has been replicated through many subsequent studies.

Babies identified as anxious-ambivalent—insecurely attached display high levels of anxiety, struggling to gain security even with the presence of their mother. These babies are often stressed and distressed when separated from their mother. The defining characteristic of these babies is that upon the return of the mother they greet her angrily and resist their mother or respond listlessly to her efforts to comfort the child. These babies rarely go off and explore the room after their mother's return. This style accounted for about 10% of the babies.

Avoidant babies account for about 20% of most samples. These babies fail to cry when separated from their mothers. They also avoid or ignore her when she returns. These babies often are unemotional during the separation and reunification with their mother. These babies will direct attention toward toys or other things present in the room. It has been suggested by researchers that this is done as a way of defending themselves against anxiety.

Disorganized-disorientated babies account for about 5%. These babies were initially difficult to identify and categorize. These infants display contradictory behaviors. They show an inclination to approach their mother when stressed as well as avoid her when she approaches.

Attachment research initially looked at life disruptions but has since moved toward focusing on parent–child interactions. Research has found that those with insecure attachments have related to numerous difficulties later in life. Unresolved attachment can also be connected to past trauma and rejection. In childhood, the goal of attachment is protection given by the parent. In adulthood it is survival and emotional caregiving. When the needs are not met, there is an increase in anxiety and the person becomes dismissive and preoccupied or feels unresolved.

When a child is securely attached, he or she is able to be separate from parents, seek comfort from them when frightened, greet them with positive emotions, and prefer them to strangers. When an adult is securely attached, he or she is able to have trusting lasting relationships and higher self-esteem, is comfortable sharing his or her feelings with others, and seeks out social support.

When a child is ambivalently attached, he or she may be wary of strangers, may become greatly distressed when his or her parents leave, and does not appear to be comforted when they return. As adults, these children are reluctant to become close to others, worry that their partner doesn't love them, and become very distraught at the end of relationships. Children who are avoidant will avoid parents; they do not seek contact or comfort and show little to no preference for parents over strangers. As adults, they have problems with intimacy, invest little emotion into relationships, and are unwilling or unable to share their thoughts and feelings.

Mindy Parsons, PhD

See also: Insecure Attachment; Reactive Attachment Disorder; Secure Attachment

Further Reading

Ainsworth, Mary Dinsmore Salter. "Attachments beyond Infancy." *American Psychologist* 44 (1989): 709–716.

Broderick, Patricia C., and Pamela Blewitt. *The Life Span: Human Development for Helping Professionals*, 3rd ed. Upper Saddle River, NJ: Pearson, 2010.

Spangler, G., and K. E. Grossman. "Biobehavioral Organization in Securely and Insecurely Attached Infants." *Child Development* 64 (1993): 1439–1450.

Van Ecke, Yolanda, Robert C. Chope, and Paul M. Emmelkamp. "Bowlby and Bowen: Attachment Theory and Family Therapy." *Counseling and Clinical Psychology Journal* 3 (2006): 81–108.

Weizmann, Frederic. "Edward John Mostyn Bowlby (1907–1990)." *The Psychologist* 14 (2001): 465.

Attention-Deficit Hyperactivity Disorder

Attention-deficit hyperactivity disorder (ADHD) is characterized by a persistent pattern of inattention and a compulsive activity level that is more severe than those exhibited by other individuals at a comparable level of psychological development.

Definition

- **Hyperactivity** means more active than is usual or desirable.

Description

Attention-deficit hyperactivity disorder is one of the most commonly identified, and misidentified, neurobehavioral disorders. The average age of ADHD onset is about seven years of age although it can continue or arise in adolescence and adulthood. Symptoms include problems staying focused and paying attention, difficulty controlling behavior, and being over active.

ADHD affects about 4.1% of American adults aged 18 years and older. It has been estimated that the disorder affects 9.0% of American children aged 13 to 18 years (National Institutes of Health). Men are four times more likely to exhibit signs of ADHD than women. While, as with those on the autism spectrum, studies show that the number of people being diagnosed with ADHD is increasing, it is still unclear how much of this increase is due to the existence of the label to describe dysfunctional behaviors that in the past would only have been seen as deliberately annoying or impolite behaviors. In order to be classified as ADHD, the questionable behavior patterns that the individual exhibits must clearly interfere with social, academic and/or occupation functioning at the expected developmentally appropriate level.

Causes and Symptoms

As with many other conditions, research has not led to a clear conclusion as what causes ADHD, although many studies suggest that genes play a large role. Like many other disorders, ADHD probably results from a combination of factors. In addition to genetics, researchers are considering possible environmental factors as well as how brain injuries, nutrition, and the social environment might contribute to ADHD.

Recently, the idea that refined sugar causes ADHD or makes symptoms worse is popular, but ongoing research tends to discount this theory, not support it. Inattention, hyperactivity, and impulsivity are the key behaviors of ADHD. While it is normal for people to be inattentive, hyperactive, or impulsive at times, for those who suffer with ADHD, these behaviors are more severe and occur much more frequently. To be diagnosed with the disorder, a person must exhibit symptoms for six or more months and to a degree that is markedly greater than other people of the same age.

Recognizing ADHD symptoms and seeking help will lead to better outcomes for those affected children, their families, and/or their coworkers. Key symptoms are difficulty sustaining attention and the ability to persist in completing tasks; failure to give sufficient attention to details so that careless mistakes are common; appearing to be distracted or just not hearing instructions; frequent distractions and going from one activity to another without completing any one of them; difficulty organizing work, work space, schedules, or activities; and dislike for activities that demand sustained attention or effort and easy distraction by stimuli irrelevant to the task or activity at hand.

It is important to remember that other possible causes of these behaviors must be examined and dismissed before it is proper to consider a diagnosis of ADHD.

Diagnosis and Prognosis

Most people get distracted, act impulsively, and struggle to concentrate at one time or another. Sometimes, these normal factors may be mistaken for ADHD. Coming to the reasoned conclusion that a person has ADHD is a several-step process. There is no single test to diagnose ADHD, and many other problems, like anxiety, depression, and certain types of learning disabilities, can exhibit similar symptoms. It is important that the person be medically examined, including hearing and vision tests, to rule out other problems that have similar symptoms to ADHD. It can also be helpful to consult a checklist that rates ADHD symptoms and get a comprehensive picture of the person's circumstances and developmental history from family and acquaintances.

Treatment

Currently available treatments focus on reducing the symptoms of ADHD and improving functioning. Treatments include medication, various types of psychotherapy, education or training, or a combination of treatments. Treatments can relieve many of the disorder's symptoms, but there is no cure. With treatment, most people with ADHD can be successful at work and lead productive lives.

Alexandra Cunningham, PhD, and William M. Cunningham, MA

See also: Attention-Deficit Hyperactivity Disorder in Youth

Further Reading

American Psychiatric Association. *Diagnostic and Statistical Manual of Mental Disorders*, 5th ed. Alexandria, VA: American Psychiatric Association, 2013.

National Institute of Mental Health (NIMH). "What Is Attention Deficit Hyperactivity Disorder (ADHD, ADD)?" Accessed January 10, 2014. http://www.nimh.nih.gov/health/topics/attention-deficit-hyperactivity-disorder-adhd/index.shtml.

Weiss, Margaret, Lily Trokenberg Hechtman, and Gabrielle Weiss. *ADHD in Adulthood: A Guide to Current Theory, Diagnosis, and Treatment*. Baltimore, MD: Johns Hopkins University Press, 2001.

Attention-Deficit Hyperactivity Disorder in Youth

Attention-deficit hyperactivity disorder (ADHD) in youth is when a child or adolescent has problems with controlling overactive behaviors and attending to and focusing on tasks.

Definition

- **Hyperactivity** means more active than is usual or desirable.

Description

While ADHD does affect about 4.1% of American adults aged 18 years and older, the rate is much higher in children. It has been estimated that the disorder affects 9.0% of American children aged 13 to 18 years. Boys are four times more likely to exhibit signs of ADHD than girls (Centers for Disease Control, 2012). ADHD is one of the most commonly identified neurobehavioral disorders that affect young children. The average age of ADHD onset is about seven years although it can continue or arise in adolescence and even into adulthood. Symptoms include difficulty staying focused and paying attention, difficulty controlling behavior, and hyperactivity.

Researchers and mental health professionals show that the number of children being diagnosed with ADHD is increasing. It is still unclear why this is occurring; in 1970 only 1% of children were diagnosed with ADHD. How much of this increase is due to the existence of the label to describe dysfunctional behaviors that in the past would only have been seen as deliberately annoying or impolite behaviors is unclear.

In order to be classified as ADHD, the questionable behavior patterns that the individual exhibits must clearly interfere with social, academic, and/or occupational functioning at the expected developmentally appropriate level. In the past few years there has often been a "rush to judgment" that a child may have ADHD where in given situations it may be some level of incompetency in the adult lead (such as a teacher) who is responsible by giving inconsistent, unclear, or contradictory information or instructions.

Causes and Symptoms

As with many other conditions, research has not led to a clear conclusion as what causes ADHD, although many studies suggest that genes play a large role. Like many other disorders, ADHD probably results from a combination of factors. In addition to genetics, researchers are considering possible environmental factors as well as how brain injuries, nutrition, and the social environment might contribute to ADHD. Recently, the idea that refined sugar causes ADHD or makes symptoms worse is popular, but ongoing research tends to discount this theory not support it.

Inattention, hyperactivity, and impulsivity are the key behaviors of ADHD. While it is normal for all children to be inattentive, hyperactive, or impulsive at times, for children with ADHD, these behaviors are more severe and occur much more frequently. To be diagnosed with the disorder, a child must exhibit symptoms for six or more months and to a degree that is markedly greater than other children of the same age.

Some children with ADHD also have other illnesses or conditions. For example, they may have one or more of the following: a learning disability, oppositional defiant disorder, conduct disorder, anxiety/depression, and bipolar disorder. ADHD also may coexist with sleep problems, bed-wetting, substance abuse, or other disorders or illnesses.

Recognizing ADHD symptoms and seeking help early will lead to better outcomes for both affected children and their families. Some key symptoms include difficulty sustaining attention and the ability to persist in completing tasks; failure to give sufficient attention to details so that careless mistakes are common; appearing to be distracted or just not hearing instructions; frequent distractions and going from one activity to another without completing any one of them; difficulty organizing work, work space, schedules, or activities; dislike for activities that demand sustained attention or effort and easy distraction by stimuli irrelevant to the task or activity at hand. It is important to remember that other possible causes of these behaviors must be examined and dismissed before it is proper to consider a diagnosis of ADHD.

Diagnosis and Prognosis

Children are diverse in development and personality; they mature at different rates and have different interests, temperaments, and energy levels. Most children get distracted, act impulsively, and struggle to concentrate at one time or another. Sometimes, these normal factors may be mistaken for ADHD.

ADHD symptoms can appear early in life, often between the ages of three and six, and because symptoms vary from child to child, the disorder can be hard to diagnose. Parents may first notice that their child loses interest in things sooner than other children or seems constantly "out of control." Often, teachers notice the symptoms first, when a child has trouble following rules or frequently "spaces out" in the classroom or on the playground.

Coming to the reasoned conclusion that a child has ADHD is a several-step process. There is no single test to diagnose ADHD, and many other problems, like anxiety, depression, and certain types of learning disabilities, can exhibit similar symptoms. It is important that the child be medically examined, including hearing and vision tests, to rule out other problems that have similar symptoms to ADHD. It can also be helpful to consult a checklist that rates ADHD symptoms and get a comprehensive picture of the child's developmental history from parents, teachers, and, sometimes, the child himself or herself. It is also important to remember that certain situations, events, or health conditions may cause temporary maturational delays in behavior in a child that seem like ADHD.

Treatment

Currently available treatments focus on reducing the symptoms of ADHD and improving functioning. Treatments include medication, various types of psychotherapy, education or training, or a combination of treatments. Treatments can relieve many of the disorder's symptoms, but there is no cure. With treatment, most people with ADHD can be successful in school and lead productive lives.

Alexandra Cunningham, PhD, and
William M. Cunningham, MA

See also: Attention-Deficit Hyperactivity Disorder

Further Reading

American Psychiatric Association. *Diagnostic and Statistical Manual of Mental Disorders*, 5th ed. Alexandria, VA: American Psychiatric Association, 2013.

Centers for Disease Control. "Attention-Deficit/Hyperactivity Disorder." Accessed January 10, 2014. http://www.cdc.gov/ncbddd/adhd/.

Gnaulati, Enrico. *Back to Normal: Why Ordinary Childhood Behavior Is Mistaken for ADHD, Bipolar Disorder, and Autism Spectrum Disorder*. Boston, MA: Beacon Press, 2013.

National Institute of Mental Health (NIMH). "What Is Attention Deficit Hyperactivity Disorder (ADHD, ADD)?" Accessed January 10, 2014. http://www.nimh.nih.gov/health/topics/attention-deficit-hyperactivity-disorder-adhd/index.shtml.

Authentic Happiness (Book)

Authentic Happiness: Using the New Positive Psychology to Realize Your Potential for Lasting Fulfillment is a best-selling book about the science of positive psychology and finding real happiness.

Definitions

- **Positive psychology** is the science about the best things in life with a focus on positive emotions, traits, and institutions.

- **Well-being** is the state of being happy, healthy, or successful.

Description

Martin P. Seligman (1942–) is the director of Positive Psychology Center at the University of Pennsylvania. He is a leading figure and founder of the Positive Psychology movement. He became world famous when he developed the theory of learned helplessness in the 1960s. His first best-selling book *Learned Optimism* was published in 1990. It is the first book about positive psychology. After receiving funding and conducting more research on positive psychology, Seligman published *Authentic Happiness* 2002.

In a departure from other psychological approaches, Seligman focuses on building positive emotions and strengths in therapy. He states that real, lasting happiness comes from focusing on one's personal strengths to improve all aspects of one's life. Using practical exercises, brief tests, and a website program, Seligman shows readers how to identify their highest virtues and use them in ways they haven't yet considered. The book is divided into three sections: positive emotions, positive traits, and positive institutions.

The section on positive emotions is the longest section of the book and focuses on what psychologists know about positive emotions. Seligman uses the terms "happiness" and "well-being" as synonyms throughout the book. He discusses the positive results involved in nurturing positive emotions and experiencing life optimally. The scientific research to support the positive effects of positive emotions is highlighted in this section.

The second section describes character strengths and the idea of signature strengths, which are a person's primary positive traits. Seligman lists 24 strengths and virtues that people identify with. Some examples of signature strengths are to be curious, loving, kind, or spiritual. In order for a trait to become a signature strength, the person must own and enjoy it purposefully.

The last section of *Authentic Happiness* discusses the influence of positive institutions or "Mansions of Life." It discusses how the ideas of positive psychology apply to many systems in life, including work, family, and education. Seligman focuses on the importance that things in our environment have in influencing our psychological state. Therefore, places like schools and government agencies need to adopt the principles of optimism and positive emotions in order to generate psychologically healthy people.

As Seligman concludes this book, he recommends ways to achieve happiness or well-being. Achieving happiness is the desired goal in using positive psychology. Happiness and well-being can come by using signature strengths in work, relationships, and finding life's purpose. Seligman states that happiness is about experiencing life positively and optimistically to achieve this ultimate goal.

Impact (Psychological Influence)

The movement of positive psychology, led by Seligman and others, has created a shift in thinking about psychological well-being. The theories and techniques proposed by positive psychologists challenge the medical model of psychology, which tends to focus on illness and decreasing the negative. The proposition that counseling and therapy should shift from the mind-set of reducing bad symptoms to increasing positive traits and emotions was initially seen as radical.

Positive psychology has not only influenced clients seeking therapy to improve but has also been recommended for counselor well-being. Mental health professionals are vulnerable to burnout and compassion fatigue, which can lead to difficulties in providing effective counseling to clients. Researchers show that students, counselors, and therapists who utilize tools from positive psychology themselves can prevent early burnout and fatigue.

Since this new wave of psychology was introduced into the field, there has been extensive research and effort put forth. The research and practice of positive psychology has been supported through traditional methods for testing the effectiveness of therapy. The pursuit of authentic happiness and well-being through the use of positive psychology is now supported by mental health professionals around the world. The publication of *Authentic Happiness* and many other books since has impacted the field greatly with its presentation of a different and easily applicable way of approaching counseling.

Alexandra Cunningham, PhD

See also: Positive Psychology; Seligman, Martin (1942–); Well-Being; Well-Being Therapy

Further Reading

Peterson, Christopher. "Positive Social Science." *The ANNALS of the American Academy of Political and Social Science* 591 (2004): 186–201.

Peterson, Christopher. *A Primer in Positive Psychology.* New York, NY: Oxford University Press, 2006.

Seligman, Martin E. P. *Authentic Happiness: Using Positive Psychology to Realize Your Potential for Lasting Fulfillment.* New York, NY: The Free Press, 2002.

University of Pennsylvania. "Authentic Happiness." Accessed July 22, 2013. www.authentichappiness.com.

Autism

Autism is a developmental disability that affects the brain's ability to help an individual socialize, communicate, and behave like most others.

Definitions

- **Autism spectrum disorders** are developmental disabilities that affect the brain and impact a person's ability to communicate, socialize, and behave like most others.

- **Asperger's syndrome,** also called Asperger's disorder, is a diagnosis on the autism spectrum where people have good verbal skills but noticeable social problems.

Description

Autism spectrum disorders (ASDs) include the diagnoses of autistic disorder, Asperger's disorder, and pervasive developmental disorder-not otherwise specified (PDD-NOS). Two other diagnoses that are sometimes considered in the category are Rett syndrome and childhood disintegrative disorder, which are rare, regressive genetic conditions.

In 1943 Leo Kanner, an American psychiatrist, was the first doctor in the world to publish a paper about children with ASDs. Dr. Kanner gave children the label of autism, based on the term created by Dr. Eugen Blueler in 1912 as he described patients who were trying to escape from reality. In Austria, Dr. Hans Asperger also identified children with high-functioning ASDs and worked with Dr. Kanner to write the first medical papers on the subject.

People with ASDs can be very mildly to severely disabled. In the United States, 1 in 88 children is diagnosed with an ASD. People with ASDs have problems with social, communication, and behavior skills. They can repeat behaviors and might not like change in their routines. These people have different ways of reacting to things, learning, and paying attention.

Causes and Symptoms

ASDs have no single cause. Some studies strongly suggest that people are predisposed to having ASDs. In some cases, parents and other family members show mild behaviors that can be linked to autism. Researchers believe that genes and factors in the environment contribute to the disorders.

There are several signs that help identify that a person might have an ASD. This includes problems with his or her speech. Individuals with ASD also have the ability and tendency to repeat things. There is likelihood they will avoid eye contact or have atypical facial expressions. People with autism appear to be unaware or uninterested in other people and have trouble understanding other's feelings. At a young age, children with autism don't tend to play pretend, such as acting like an animal or feeding a doll. They also don't typically point to show interest, which is a typical behavior of young children. Many times people with autism react unusually to sensory input, like the way things smell, taste, look, feel, or sound.

A few main challenges exist for people with ASD. These challenges are in social communication and behaving like their peers. There are ranges of abilities and challenges within these categories. For example, one person with ASD might not be able to talk at all, while another can talk too much without much purpose. Also, one person with ASD might have a few close friends, while another doesn't know how to socialize at all. Therefore, every person with ASD will act a little bit differently than the other. The most common diagnoses among the ASDs are autistic disorder, Asperger's disorder, and PDD-NOS.

Diagnosis and Prognosis

Autistic disorder is usually diagnosed between the ages of 18 and 36 months. This diagnosis includes speech delay or loss of speech during early childhood. It also includes challenges in self-care like using the toilet and keeping clean. In some cases, people with autistic disorder can have lower intellectual levels than other people. Because of these things, people with autistic disorder are more severely disabled than some other people with ASDs. Children diagnosed at an early age will benefit from therapy or intervention in order to help build their skills. If they learn to speak and behave with progress, they can be less disabled and considered high functioning.

Asperger's disorder and PDD-NOS is usually diagnosed between the ages of seven and eight years. People diagnosed with Asperger's disorder are always able to speak but might not do it well. This means they can communicate but usually not to get their needs met. They also have average or above-average intellect, meaning they are as smart as or smarter than most other people. Because of this, people diagnosed with Asperger's disorder or PDD-NOS are considered high functioning.

Treatment

Autism is a lifelong condition that can be helped but not cured. Some people with autism can lead normal or near-normal lives. The best-studied therapies include behavioral, educational, and medical treatments. These include, but are not limited to, applied behavior analysis, special education, and drug therapy. Counseling and educating families affected by autism can help them cope, get treatment, and find support. Therefore, parent and caregiver treatment and involvement is an essential part of treating the person with autism.

Alexandra Cunningham, PhD

See also: Asperger's Syndrome; Autism Spectrum Disorders; Pervasive Developmental Disorders

Further Reading

American Psychiatric Association. *Diagnostic and Statistical Manual of Mental Disorders*, 4th ed., text revision. Washington, DC: American Psychiatric Association, 2000.

American Psychiatric Association. *Diagnostic and Statistical Manual of Mental Disorders*, 5th ed. Arlington, VA: American Psychiatric Association, 2013.

Centers for Disease Control. "Autism Spectrum Disorders (ASDs): Data & Statistics." Last modified March 29, 2012. Accessed January 10, 2015. http://www.cdc.gov/ncbddd/autism/data.html.

Kanner, Leo. "Autistic Disturbances of Affective Contact." *Acta Paedopsychiatr* 4 (1943): 36–100.

Sicile- Kira, Chantal, and Temple Grandin. *Autism Spectrum Disorders: The Complete Guide*. New York, NY: The Berkley Publishing Group.

Autism Spectrum Disorders

Autism spectrum disorders (ASD) are developmental disabilities that affect a person's ability to communicate, socialize, and behave like most others.

Definition

- **Behavior** is an observable action demonstrated by a human or animal caused by either internal or external occurrences.

Description

Autism spectrum disorders and related conditions impact the neurodevelopment of a person from a young age. Those diagnosed with ASD usually have social and behavioral challenges. These challenges range from mild to severe. In the mildest forms, a person can have trouble making friends and can hyperfocus on areas of interest that are considered odd to others. In severe forms of ASD a person might not be able to speak and might engage in behaviors that result in serious injury. Therefore, people with this diagnosis are different in how they seem to others but overall have problems socializing and acting like their same-aged peers.

In 1943 Leo Kanner, an American psychiatrist, was the first doctor in the world to publish a paper about children with ASDs. Dr. Kanner gave children the label of autism, based on the term created by Dr. Eugen Blueler in 1912 as he described patients who were trying to "escape from reality." In Austria, Dr. Hans Asperger also identified children with high-functioning ASDs and worked with Dr. Kanner to write the first medical papers on the subject.

Causes and Symptoms

Autism spectrum disorders have no single cause. Some studies strongly suggest that people are predisposed to having ASDs. In some cases, parents and other family members show mild behaviors that can be linked to autism. Researchers believe that genes and factors in the environment contribute to the disorders.

People with ASDs can be very mildly to severely disabled. In the United States, 1 in 88 children is diagnosed with an ASD. People with ASDs have problems with social, communication, and behavior skills. They can repeat behaviors and might not like change in their routines. These people have different ways of reacting to things, learning, and paying attention.

There are several signs that help identify that a person might have an ASD, including lack of or delay in speech; repeats things; avoids eye contact; appears to be unaware or uninterested in other people; has trouble understanding other's feelings; doesn't pretend play (act like an animal or feed a baby doll); doesn't gesture or point to show interest; reacts unusually to the way things smell, taste, look, feel, or sound and has trouble expressing their needs.

Three main challenges exist for people with ASD. These challenges are in communicating, socializing, and behaving like most others. There are ranges of abilities and challenges within these three categories. For example, one person with ASD might not be able to talk at all, while another can talk too much without making sense. Also, one person with ASD might have many friends, while another doesn't know how to socialize at all. Therefore, every person with ASD will act a little bit differently than the other. The most common diagnoses among the ASDs are autistic disorder, Asperger's disorder, and pervasive developmental disorder-not otherwise specified (PDD-NOS).

Diagnosis and Prognosis

Currently ASD identifies people of different abilities on a range of mild, moderate, or severe. In past years, ASDs have included the diagnoses of autistic disorder, Asperger's disorder, and PDD-NOS. Two other diagnoses that are sometimes considered in the category are Rett syndrome and childhood disintegrative disorder, which are rare, regressive genetic conditions. These labels are no longer used medically but could still be used in common language.

Severe forms of ASD, like the former autistic disorder, are usually diagnosed between the ages of 18 and 36 months. This diagnosis includes a speech delay or loss of speech during early childhood. It also includes challenges in taking care of oneself, like using the toilet and keeping clean. In some cases, people with autistic disorder can have lower intellectual levels than other people. Because of these things, people with autistic disorder are more severely disabled than some other people with ASDs. Children diagnosed at an early age will benefit from therapy or intervention in order to help build their skills. If they learn to speak and behave with progress, they can be less disabled and considered high functioning.

Milder forms of ASD, the former Asperger's disorder and PDD-NOS, are usually diagnosed between the ages of seven and eight years. People diagnosed with Asperger's disorder are always able to speak but might not do it well. This means they can communicate but usually not to get their needs met. They also have average or above-average intellect, meaning they are as smart as or smarter than most other people. Because of this, people diagnosed with Asperger's disorder or PDD-NOS are considered high functioning.

Treatment

ASDs are lifelong conditions that can be helped but not cured. Some people with ASDs can lead normal or near-normal lives. The best-studied therapies include behavioral, educational, and medical treatments. These include, but are not limited to, applied behavior analysis, special education, and drugs. Many treatments for ASDs exist, but few are supported by scientific evidence. Counseling families affected by ASDs can help them cope, get treatment, and find support.

Alexandra Cunningham, PhD

See also: Asperger's Syndrome; Autism; Pervasive Developmental Disorders

Further Reading

American Psychiatric Association. *Diagnostic and Statistical Manual of Mental Disorders*, 5th ed. Arlington, VA: American Psychiatric Association, 2013.

Centers for Disease Control. "Autism Spectrum Disorders (ASDs): Data & Statistics." Last modified March 29, 2012. Accessed January 10, 2015. http://www.cdc.gov/ncbddd/autism/data.html.

Sicile-Kira, Chantal, and Temple Grandin. *Autism Spectrum Disorders: The Complete Guide*. New York, NY: The Berkley Publishing Group, 2006.

Aversion Therapy

Aversion therapy is used to deter people from engaging in certain behaviors by exposing them to negative consequences to those actions.

Definitions

- **Aversion therapy** is a treatment in which the patient is discouraged from a behavior being subjected to a punishing stimulus when he or she engages in that behavior.

- **Desensitization techniques** are behavior change methods for reducing an individual's oversensitivity to fearful situations by intentionally and gradually exposing the individual to various emotionally distressing events.

Description

The purpose of aversion therapy is to decrease or stop certain behaviors by having a client associate unpleasant or painful experiences with doing the activity. For example, a bad-tasting substance might be placed on the tips of a person's fingers to discourage nail-biting or skin-chewing behaviors. Aversion therapy is a form of behavioral conditioning as it influences actions or behaviors through punishment. For much of its history, aversion therapy was dependent on the use of either chemical reactions or electric shock.

Aversion therapy has been widely used to help people stop the use of alcohol or other addictive drugs, from cigarettes (nicotine) to heroin (opioids). A specific example of chemical aversion therapy was the use of drugs like lithium with alcoholic clients. These chemicals induce nausea in those abusing alcohol so that they would associate the drinking of alcoholic beverages with the negative experience of vomiting.

In the case of electric shock aversion therapy, a patient who exhibits violent behavior might be made to watch images of violent crime while some kind of electrical shock is administered. The aim is that the association of engaging in the behavior with the negative experience of the electrical shock will help prevent the violent behaviors. Many behaviorists believe that the use of chemicals, electric shock, and other aversion therapies should only be used when the behaviors are more dangerous than the use of the aversive techniques.

Development

Aversion therapy began to be used in the 1930s to treat alcohol and drug-addicted patients. Later, it was extended to purely psychological conditions, such as homosexuality under the idea that homosexuality was freely chosen. During these years homosexuality was clinically classified as a mental health disorder. Any psychologically deviant behavior, like homosexuality, was subject to change through aversion therapy.

Aversion therapy with its strong connection to discomfort, pain, and punishment began to fall out of favor in the 1970s. Its controversial use with psychiatric patients and people diagnosed with homosexuality created problems among helping professionals. In 1973 the American Psychiatric Association removed homosexuality from the list of disorders in its *Diagnostic and Statistical Manual of Mental Disorders*. After this, aversion therapy began to be rejected as a valid approach to the treatment of homosexuality although it still persists in certain isolated pockets of society. Its association with abusive treatment of homosexuality has especially led to its being discredited and rejected.

Current Status

Currently, aversion therapy is still used especially for drug and alcohol treatment and among certain behavioral specialists. Aversion therapy is an unpleasant experience, by design, and such methods have often been judged to fall into the category of cruel or unusual punishment. Therefore, today it is usually based on the use of the imagination and the association of unpleasant images or memories with the undesirable behavior. This approach is called desensitization.

Covert desensitization is an approach that was elaborated by American psychologist Joseph Cautela. Using visual imagery techniques, he paired images of undesirable behavior, like smoking, with vivid pictures of aversive stimuli, like vomiting. This system is designed to counteract the positive responses that had been associated with the patient's previous behavior.

Alexandra Cunningham, PhD

See also: Covert Sensitization

Further Reading

Kraft, Tom, and David Kraft. "Covert Sensitization Revisited: Six Case Studies." *Contemporary Hypnosis* 22 (1990): 202–209.

Rachman, S., and J. Teasdale. *Aversion Therapy and Behaviour Disorders: An Analysis.* Coral Gables, FL: University of Miami Press, 1969.

Spiegler, Michael D., and David C. Guevremont. *Contemporary Behavior Therapy*. Belmont, CA: Wadsworth Cengage Learning, 2010.

Avoidant Personality Disorder

Avoidant personality disorder is a mental disorder characterized by a pattern of social withdrawal, feelings of inadequacy, and oversensitivity to negative evaluation.

Definitions

- **Assertiveness training** is a behavior change method for increasing self-esteem and self-expression in intimidating interpersonal situations.

- **Desensitization techniques** are behavior change methods for reducing an individual's oversensitivity to fearful situations by intentionally and gradually exposing the individual to various emotionally distressing events.

- *Diagnostic and Statistical Manual of Mental Disorders* **(DSM)** is the handbook mental health professionals use to diagnose mental disorders. The current edition (fifth) is known as DSM-5.

- **Personality disorder** is a long-standing pattern of maladaptive (problematic) behavior, thoughts, and emotions that deviates from the accepted norms of an individual's culture.

- **Psychotherapy** is a psychological method for achieving desired changes in thinking, feeling, and behavior. It is also called therapeutic counseling.

Description and Diagnosis

The avoidant personality disorder is a personality disorder characterized by a pervasive pattern of social isolation, fearfulness, nonassertiveness, feelings of inadequacy, social awkwardness, and extreme sensitivity to criticism and rejection. Because individuals with this disorder believe they are socially inept, unappealing, or inferior, they fear being embarrassed, criticized, or rejected. So, when faced with the prospect of making new social contacts, they predictably say a quick "no" to new work or social relationships that may threaten their otherwise safe and controlled life space. The only exception is when they are certain of being liked and accepted by another. Both the avoidant personality disorder and the schizoid personality disorder are socially isolative. However, unlike those with schizoid personality disorder, avoidant individuals actually crave relationships and often have some friends with whom they feel safe. Those with avoidant personalities share some features with the dependent personality disorder. These include feelings of inadequacy and a lack of assertiveness.

The avoidant personality disorder is characterized by the following behavioral style, interpersonal style, thinking style, and feeling style. The behavioral style of avoidant personalities is characterized by social withdrawal, shyness, distrustfulness, and aloofness. Their behavior and speech is both controlled and inactive, and they appear nervous and awkward. Interpersonally, they are overly sensitive to rejection. Even though they desire acceptance by others, they keep distance from others and require unconditional approval before being willing to "open up." They often "test" others to determine who can be trusted to like them. Their thinking style is one of heightened alertness and self-doubt as they scan their emotional environment searching for clues of potential criticalness or rejection. Their feeling style is marked by shyness and nervousness. Since they have often experienced criticism, disapproval, and nonacceptance by others, they often experience feelings of sadness, tenseness, and loneliness.

The cause of this disorder is not well understood. Avoidant personality disorder is strongly associated with anxiety disorders and is associated with actual or perceived rejection by parents or peers during childhood. Furthermore, these individuals tend to have characteristic view of themselves, the world, and others, and a basic life strategy. They view themselves as adequate and frightened of rejection. They tend to view the world as unfair, demanding, critical, and rejecting. Accordingly, their basic life strategy and pattern is to be vigilant, demand reassurance, and fantasize and daydream about being involved in safe and affirming relationships. So, it is not surprising that those with avoidant personalities are attracted to virtual relationships in romance novels and soap operas.

According to the *Diagnostic and Statistical Manual of Mental Disorders, Fifth Edition*, individuals can be diagnosed with this disorder if they exhibit a pervasive pattern of being socially inhibited, feeling inadequate, and overly sensitive to the negative evaluations of others. This is typically because they view themselves as socially inept, unappealing, or inferior to others. They consistently avoid work activities that require close interpersonal contact for fear of being criticized or rejected. They will not get involved with others unless they are certain of being accepted. Fearing they will be shamed or ridiculed, they are uncomfortable and act with restraint in intimate relationships. In anticipation of shame or ridicule, they are uncomfortable and are hesitant in intimate relationships. Similarly, they experience feelings of inadequacy and inhibition in new interpersonal situations. Commonly, these individuals will refuse to take personal risks or engage in activities that may prove embarrassing.

Treatment

The clinical treatment of this disorder usually involves psychotherapy. A primary goal of therapy is to desensitize the individual to the criticism of others. Desensitization techniques are useful and effective in this regard. A related goal is to increase the individual's self-esteem, self-confidence, and assertiveness. Assertiveness training can also be effective in reversing an individual's avoidant and isolative pattern.

Len Sperry, MD, PhD

See also: Dependent Personality Disorder; Personality Disorders; Psychotherapy; Schizoid Personality Disorder

Further Reading

American Psychiatric Association. *Diagnostic and Statistical Manual of Mental Disorders*, 5th ed. Arlington, VA: American Psychiatric Association Press, 2013.

Butler, Gillian. *Overcoming Social Anxiety and Shyness: A Self-Help Guide Using Cognitive Behavioral Techniques*. New York, NY: Basic Books, 2008.

Dobbert, Duane L. *Understanding Personality Disorders: An Introduction*. Lanham, MD: Rowman & Littlefield, 2011.

Kantor, Martin. *The Essential Guide to Overcoming Avoidant Personality Disorder*. Santa Barbara, CA: Praeger, 2010.

Sperry, Len. *Handbook of Diagnosis and Treatment of the DSM-5 Personality Disorders*, 3rd ed. New York, NY: Routledge, 2016.

Avoidant/Restrictive Food Intake Disorder

Avoidant/restrictive food intake disorder is a mental disorder characterized by avoiding or restricting food intake.

Definitions

- **Anorexia nervosa** is n mental disorder characterized by refusal to maintain minimal normal body weight along with a fear of weight gain and a distorted body image.

- **Behavior therapy** is a form of psychotherapy that focuses on identifying and changing maladaptive (faulty) behaviors.

- **Bulimia nervosa** is a mental disorder characterized by recurrent binge eating with loss of control over one's eating and compensation for eating.

- **Cognitive behavior therapy** is a form of psychotherapy that focuses on changing maladaptive (faulty) behaviors, emotions, and thoughts.

- **DSM-5** stands for the *Diagnostic and Statistical Manual of Mental Disorders, Fifth Edition*, which is a diagnostic system used by professionals to identify mental disorders with specific diagnostic criteria.

- **Feeding and eating disorders** are a class of DSM-5 mental disorders characterized by a persistent disturbance of eating that significantly impairs physical health or everyday functioning. They include anorexia nervosa and avoidant/restrictive food intake disorder.

- **Psychotherapy** is a psychological method for achieving desired changes in thinking, feeling, and behavior. It is also called therapy and therapeutic counseling.

- **Specifiers** are extensions to a diagnosis that further clarifies the course, severity, or type of features of a disorder or illness.

- **Systemic desensitization** is a behavioral technique in which an individual is gradually exposed to an object, place, or event that triggers anxiety, while engaging in some type of relaxation at the same time to reduce the symptoms of anxiety.

Description and Diagnosis

Avoidant/restrictive food intake disorder is one of the DSM-5 feeding and eating disorders. It is characterized by avoiding or restricting food intake. Common symptoms include not being able to eat certain foods based on their texture or aroma. Some individuals with this disorder may only like hot or cold foods or hard or soft foods. Others will refuse foods based solely on color. For example, an individual may not eat strawberries because he or she does not like the color red. In some cases, individuals will refuse entire food groups like vegetables and fruits. Individuals with this disorder may even limit certain food types based on specific brands (e.g., store brand name of a cereal versus Kellogg's brand cereal). Other symptoms include unfavorable reactions to foods, such as vomiting or gagging. Infants with this disorder may show signs of irritability and difficulty consoling during feeding times, and may appear uninterested or withdrawn.

The name of this disorder was replaced in the DSM-5. It was previously known as "Feeding Disorder of Infancy or Early Childhood" in the previous edition (American Psychiatric Association, 2013). DSM-5 has expanded the disorder to include adults as well as infants and children.

According to the *Diagnostic and Statistical Manual of Mental Disorders, Fifth Edition*, individuals can be diagnosed with this disorder if an individual is avoiding or restricting the intake of food and fail to meet the necessary requirements for nutrition or sufficient energy. One of the following criteria is also needed for the diagnosis. The criteria are significant loss of weight, significant deficiency in nutrition, dependence on oral supplements, use of a feeding tube, or noticeable interference with psychosocial functioning. The disturbance does not occur solely in anorexia nervosa or bulimia nervosa. The diagnosis cannot be made if symptoms are the result of a medical condition or another mental disorder. The diagnosis must include the specifier, "in remission" if none of the criteria have not been met for an extended period (American Psychiatric Association, 2013).

The occurrence of this disorder most commonly occurs in early infancy or early adolescence but may persist into adulthood. Furthermore, avoiding or restricting foods may be based on sensory characteristics of foods introduced in the first decade of life but may occur as well into adulthood. In some cases, parent–child interaction may contribute to the infant's and adolescents' feeding problems (American Psychiatric Association, 2013). For example, presenting food to the child inappropriately or a parent interpreting a child's behavior as an act of regression or rejection may contribute to this disorder. Inadequate nutritional intake may worsen irritability and developmental delays for infants, adolescents, and adults. If child abuse or neglect is suspected as a cause of this disorder, changing caregivers has been shown to improve this disorder. No matter the age of an individual with this disorder, social functioning tends to be negatively affected.

Treatment

Psychotherapy is often effective in the treatment of individuals with this disorder. Cognitive behavior therapy is particularly effective for adults with this disorder. Behavioral therapy, particularly systemic desensitization, is an effective form of treatment for children with this disorder. It can help a child and parent overcome feeding problems and the dislike and avoidance of certain foods. By changing the texture of foods and the pace and timings of the feedings, individual can and do improve.

Len Sperry, MD, PhD, and
Elizabeth Smith Kelsey, PhD

See also: Anorexia Nervosa; Behavior Therapy; Bulimia Nervosa; Cognitive Behavior Therapy; *Diagnostic and Statistical Manual of Mental Disorders* (DSM); Psychotherapy; Systematic Desensitization

Further Reading

American Psychiatric Association. *Diagnostic and Statistical Manual of Mental Disorders*, 5th ed. Arlington, VA: American Psychiatric Association, 2013.

Lask, Bryan, and Rachel Bryant-Waugh. *Eating Disorders in Childhood and Adolescence*, 3rd ed. New York, NY: Routledge, 2007.

Mash, Eric J., and Russell A. Barkley. *Assessment of Childhood Disorders*, 4th ed. New York, NY: Guilford Press, 2009.

B

Baby Boomers

The term "Baby boomer" is used to describe a person who was born in the post–World War II era (1946–1964) during the time when the annual birth rate increased exponentially. This generation became a countercultural phenomenon in the United States and Europe as it progressed through adolescence and adulthood, having a historical impact and influencing both the civil rights and feminist movements.

Description

The *Oxford English Dictionary* cites the first recorded use of the phrase "baby boomer" in 1970 in an article in *The Washington Post*. The term has since been used commonly to describe this counterculture. According to the U.S. Census Bureau, "baby boom" refers to a 19-year period following World War II that was marked by a noticeable increase in the birth rate. This cultural phenomenon was documented in North America and Europe. In Canada, this group is referred to as "Boomies," and in Great Britain the time period is termed "the bulge." Historians and authors differ regarding time limits for the era as well as the reasoning for this population spike. Some historians attribute the boom to a desire for normalcy and sense of hopefulness about the future following 16 years of depression and war. Attainment of "the American Dream" felt possible. Others argue that the Cold War campaign urged Americans to outnumber communists. The baby boomer generation is made up of two broadly defined cohorts, the leading-edge boomers and the trailing-edge or late boomers. The leading-edge boomers, encompassing more than half of the generation, are individuals born between 1946 and 1955. The trailing-edge or late boomers are individuals who were born between 1956 and 1964. Subsegments of the generation have also been identified and include the following monikers: "golden boomers," "generation Jones," "alpha boomers," "yuppies," "zoomers," and "cuspers."

Approximately 76 million babies were born in the United States alone during the baby boom, comprising 40% of the total population. Such a rapid increase in population requires nations to prepare for the shift. As a result of the baby boom, many industries and corporations grew more profitable, in particular those associated with housing, retail, and technology. Suburban communities also exploded.

Boomers came of age during the 1960s and 1970s, periods of dramatic social change. Conservative and liberal views clashed. Political controversies were at the forefront: opposition to the Vietnam War, the civil rights movement, and the feminist cause. Thus, baby boomers changed the political landscape of the United States to some extent. This generation has been since associated with qualities such as independent thinking, ingenuity, and resistance to tradition.

Impact (Psychological Influence)

The baby boomers were the most successful, active, and well-educated generation up to that time and among the first to grow up genuinely expecting the world to improve with time. Nearly 90% of boomers completed high school, and almost 30% went onto pursue a college degree or higher. By comparison, Generation X, those born between 1965 and 1980, has been nowhere near as populous or prosperous as their parents. In fact, the birth rate among Americans has dropped dramatically from around 25 per 1,000 in 1957 to 14 per 1,000 in 2011.

With the current average life expectancy projected to be age 75 for males and age 80 for females, boomers will continue to be a dominant force in society for years to come. The first baby boomers reached the standard retirement age of 65 in 2011. According to the Pew Research Center, in January 2015, the millennial generation (aged 18 to 34 in 2015) is expected to grow to 75.3 million, overtaking the projected 74.9 million boomers (aged 51 to 69). By 2030, about one in five Americans will be older than 65, and some experts believe that this will place a strain on social welfare systems.

Melissa A. Mariani, PhD

See also: Millennials

Further Reading

Cheung, Eward. *Baby Boomers, Generation X and Social Cycles, Volume 1: North American Long-Waves.* Charlotte, NC: Longwave Press, 2007.

Fry, Richard. "This Year, Millennials Will Overtake Baby Boomers." Pew Research Fact-Tank. January 16, 2015. http://www.pewresearch.org/fact-tank/2015/01/16/this-year-millennials-will-overtake-baby-boomers/.

Gillon, Steve. *Boomer Nation: The Largest and Richest Generation Ever, and How It Changed America.* New York, NY: Free Press, 2004.

Jones, Landon. *Great Expectations: America and the Baby Boom Generation.* New York, NY: Coward, McCann and Geoghegan, 1980.

Bandura, Albert (1925–)

Description

Albert Bandura is a Canadian American psychologist who is best known for his development of social learning theory and the concept of self-efficacy. He is also known for the controversial 1961 Bobo doll experiment. He is ranked as the fourth most eminent psychologist of the 20th century.

Description

Albert Bandura was born in Mundare, Alberta, Canada, on December 4, 1925. He is of Ukrainian and Polish descent. He was the youngest of six children and the only male child. Mundare, Canada, was a remote town of fewer than 500 inhabitants with limited educational resources, and Bandura attended the one and only school. Due to a shortage of teachers and resources, learning was left to the student's own initiative and motivation. This early educational experience was to play a role in the development of Bandura's social learning theory.

After graduating from high school Bandura worked in the Yukon, repairing the Alaska Highway. Bandura found himself working alongside of criminals, draft dodgers, alcoholics, and other socially challenged individuals. Bandura credits this experience with his interest in psychopathology. Bandura enrolled at the University of British Columbia intending to study the biological sciences. After taking a psychology course just to fill a vacant time slot, he decided to pursue the subject for degree. He graduated in three years (1949) and received his first award: the Bolocan Award in psychology, given only to the top student in psychology. Bandura then attended the University of Iowa and in 1952 graduated with his PhD. Also in 1952 Bandura married Virginia Varns. The couple would have two children and were married for 59 years until Virginia's passing in 2011.

Impact (Psychological Influence)

After earning his doctorate degree Bandura was offered a position at Stanford University, where he continues to work to this day. Bandura began to investigate how family patterns lead to aggressive behavior in children. He discovered that children who behaved very aggressively had parents who had hostile and aggressive attitudes. Bandura concluded that children learned to be aggressive by observation and imitation. He called this process "social learning."

Bandura's early study into human behavior led to an experiment referred to as the "Bobo doll experiment." Using an inflatable doll one group of children was shown a film of a woman beating and yelling at the Bobo doll. Another group of children was not shown the film and another group shown a film of nonaggressive behavior toward the doll. After the film was watched, the children were allowed to play in a room that had a Bobo doll in it. The children who viewed the

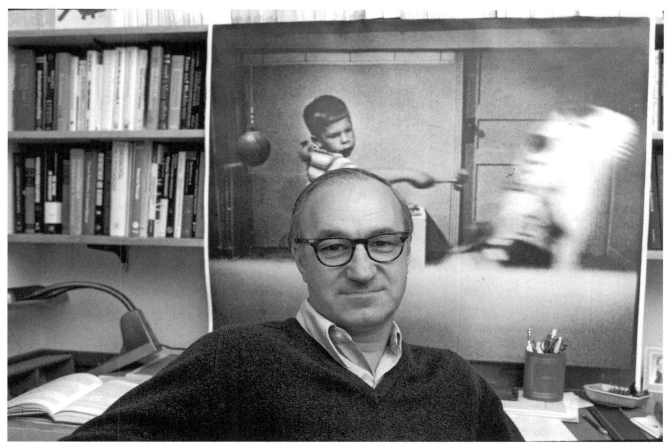

Albert Bandura is a Canadian American psychologist, one of the most influential and distinguished of his time. Best known for his development of social learning theory and the concept of self-efficacy, he's also known for the controversial 1961 Bobo doll experiment, which observed aggressive behavior in children. (Jon Brenneis/Life Magazine/The LIFE Images Collection/ Getty Images)

film of aggressive behavior where much more likely to beat and yell at the doll, imitating the behavior they saw in the film. The other groups did not behave aggressively. The children who beat the Bobo doll did not receive any encouragement or incentives to do so. They did it on their own, simply by observing and then imitating the behavior they saw on the film. At the time most psychologists thought that all behavior had to be reinforced, or rewarded, before it was learned. Bandura's Bobo doll experiment demonstrated that behavior can be learned without being rewarded. This was a very new way of thinking about how people learn, develop, and behave as human beings. Although some people criticized the experiment for training children to act aggressively, the Bobo doll experiments are considered one of the great psychological experiments of the

20th century. In 1977 Bandura's book *Social Learning Theory* was published and had a significant impact on the direction of psychology during the 1980s.

Another significant contribution Bandura has made to the field of psychology is the development of the concept of self-efficacy. "Self-efficacy" refers to a person's attitude about himself or herself and belief in his or her own abilities to complete tasks and reach goals. Bandura demonstrated that people with high self-efficacy are able to accomplish their goals, are not overcome by obstacles, and are able to positively solve problems. People with low self-efficacy give up easily, feel helpless, and are unable to change situations to reach their goals.

Albert Bandura is one of the most influential and distinguished psychologists of the 20th and 21st centuries. He has served on advisory boards, federal agencies, research panels, congressional committees, and commissions of the American Psychological Association. He has received more than 15 honorary university degrees recognizing his contributions to the field of psychology. He has received numerous awards for distinguished scientific contributions to the field of psychology and education. He is also the recipient of the Outstanding Lifetime Contribution to Psychology Award from the American Psychological Association.

Steven R. Vensel, PhD

See also: Social Learning Theory

Further Reading

Bandura, Albert. "Autobiography." In *A History of Psychology in Autobiography (Vol. IX)*, edited by M. Lindzey and W. Runyan. Washington, DC: American Psychological Association, 2006.

Bandura, Albert. "Self-Efficacy: Toward a Unifying Theory of Behavioral Change." *Psychological Review* 84, no. 2 (1977): 191–215.

Haggbloom, Steven, Renee Warnick, Jason E. Warnick, Vinessa K. Jones, Gary L. Yarbrough, Tenea M. Russell, Chris M. Borecky, Reagan McGahhey, John L. Powell III, Jamie Beavers, and Emmanuelle Monte. "The 100 Most Eminent Psychologists of the 20th Century." *Review of General Psychology* 6, no. 2 (2002): 139–152.

Barbiturates

Barbiturates are a class of prescribed drugs that slow the nervous system and are prescribed primarily for sedation, general anesthesia, and treating some types of epilepsy.

Definitions

- **Epilepsy** is a medical condition involving episodes of irregular electrical discharge within the brain that causes impairment or loss of consciousness, followed by convulsions.

- **Benzodiazepines** is a group of central nervous system depressants that are used to relieve anxiety or to induce sleep.

- **Seizure** is a sudden convulsion or uncontrolled discharge of nerve cells that may spread to other cells throughout the brain.

- **General anesthesia** is a drug-induced loss of consciousness and physical sensation.

- **Recreational drugs** refer to the use of a drug with the intention of creating a psychoactive or heightened psychological experience; typically, such use is illegal. These drugs are also called street drugs.

Description

The signature feature of barbiturates is their capacity to effectively depress the central nervous system and produce sedation. In the 1960s and 1970s barbiturates were commonly prescribed to treat anxiety and insomnia. However, because of their abuse potential, the prescription use of barbiturates has declined and the drug has been largely replaced by benzodiazepines. Today, barbiturates are used to sedate patients prior to surgery as well as to produce general anesthesia. They are also used to treat some forms of epilepsy. Barbiturates still in use include Fiorinal (generic name: butalbital) and Seconal (generic name: secobarbital) to treat insomnia and Nembutal (generic name: phenobarbital) to treat seizures.

These drugs are highly addictive and are often abused as recreational drugs. Although still commercially available, barbiturates are no longer routinely recommended for insomnia because of their ability to cause dependence, tolerance, and withdrawal. In general, barbiturates lose their efficacy when they are used to treat insomnia on a daily basis for more than two weeks. These drugs also have significant side effects when taken in large doses and can cause respiratory failure and death.

Precautions and Side Effects

Barbiturate abuse can occur when these drugs are taken for a prolonged period of time or in higher than prescribed doses. Long-term barbiturate use should be avoided unless there is a strong medical need, such as uncontrolled seizures. Women should not use barbiturates during pregnancy unless absolutely necessary. Those addicted to barbiturates while pregnant can give birth to addicted babies who may suffer withdrawal symptoms after birth. Women who are breast-feeding should not take barbiturates because these drugs enter the breast milk and may cause serious side effects in the nursing baby. Children who are hyperactive should not receive phenobarbital or other barbiturates. Some children, paradoxically, become stimulated and hyperactive after receiving barbiturates. Elderly patients must be carefully monitored for confusion, agitation, delirium, and excitement if they take barbiturates. Barbiturates should be avoided in elderly patients who are receiving drugs for other mental disorders such as schizophrenia or depression. While taking barbiturates individuals should not drive, operate heavy equipment, or perform other activities requiring mental alertness.

The most common side effect of barbiturate use is drowsiness. Less common side effects include agitation, anxiety, breathing difficulties, clinical depression, constipation, confusion, dizziness, low blood pressure, nausea, decreased heart rate, nightmares, and vomiting. Rare side effects include fever, headache, anemia, allergic reactions, and liver damage. Overdosing on barbiturates or combining barbiturates with alcohol or other central nervous system depressants can cause unconsciousness and even death. Emergency medical treatment is needed for anyone who shows signs of an overdose or a reaction to combining barbiturates with alcohol or other drugs. Such signs include severe drowsiness, breathing problems, slurred speech, staggering, slow heartbeat, excessive confusion, and severe weakness.

Len Sperry, MD, PhD

See also: Seizures

Further Reading

"Barbiturate Intoxication and Overdose, Systemic." Medline-Plus. http://www.nlm.nih.gov.ezproxy.fau.edu/medlineplus/ency/article/000951.htm.

Henn, Debra, and Deborah de Eugenio, eds. *Barbiturates*. New York, NY: Chelsea House Publishers, 2007.

Preston, John D., John H. O'Neal, and Mary C. Talaga. *Handbook of Clinical Psychopharmacology for Therapists*, 7th ed. Oakland, CA: New Harbinger, 2013.

Beattie, Melody (1948–)

Born in 1948 in St. Paul, Minnesota, Melody Beattie rose to become a widely acclaimed self-help author, particularly among the addiction and recovery circles following the release of her international best seller, *Codependent No More*. The book was published in 1986 and has since sold more than 8 million copies and has been translated into several languages.

Description and History

Codependence is an unhealthy level of emotional or psychological dependence on a loved one whereby one or both individuals in the relationship need the other to feel fulfilled.

Beattie's firsthand knowledge of the difficulty of struggling with addictions began at an early age. After being abandoned by her father, kidnapped at age four, and later sexually abused by a neighbor, she began drinking while still in middle school. She became an alcoholic by the age of 13 and a drug addict by age 18. She started hanging out with a crowd that robbed pharmacies for drugs, and her criminal activity ultimately led her to enter a court-mandated treatment center.

Beattie is considered a beloved self-help author of more than two dozen books and is a household name in addiction and recovery circles. Through her international best seller and writing numerous other books, she has helped millions of followers by sharing her firsthand knowledge of addiction struggles. In addition to surviving abandonment, kidnapping, sexual abuse, and addiction, she has persevered through divorce and the death of a child. For many, her real-life experience gives her credibility and standing to tackle these difficult issues.

Beattie was motivated by her personal struggles of loving someone who suffers from addiction. She has been quoted as saying that there were many books out there about how to help an addict or an alcoholic, but no one was discussing how the addict impacts the lives of the people around him or her.

The concept that she writes about, codependency, is considered an integral part of the relationships among those with addiction or substance abuse issues. Beattie explains that codependent individuals frequently become obsessed with controlling the addict's behavior in an often futile attempt to keep that person from creating chaos and trouble.

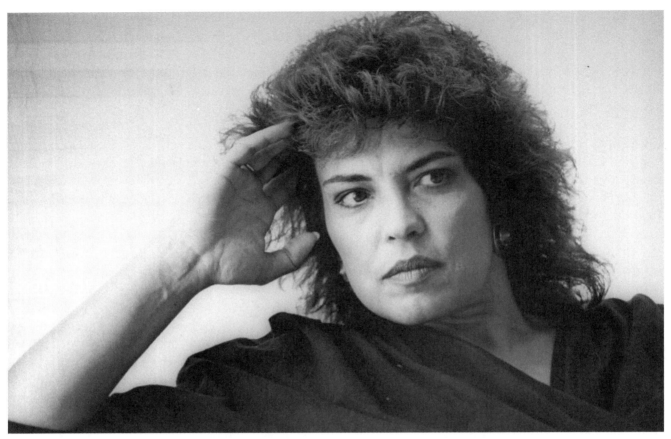

Melody Beattie became a widely acclaimed self-help author, particularly among addiction and recovery circles, following the release of her international bestseller *Codependent No More* in 1986. She has since published several more books. (Michael Mauney/The LIFE Images Collection/Getty Images)

The term "codependence" emerged during the early 1980s and was often used to describe the spouse of an addicted individual. For example, a wife with an alcoholic husband focused her time and resources to making excuses to family and friends, buying alcohol, and keeping the peace within the family. Eventually, all of her activities began to revolve around her husband's drinking. A few of these codependent women founded Al-Anon in 1990, which offers support groups modeled after Alcoholics Anonymous as a way of supporting the needs of family members of alcoholics.

Mindy Parsons, PhD

See also: Addiction Counseling; Peer Groups; Psychoeducation; Psychoeducational Groups; Self-Help Groups

Further Reading

Beattie, Melody. *Codependent No More: How to Stop Controlling Others and Start Caring for Yourself,* 2nd ed. Center City, MN: Hazelden, 1986.

Irvine, Leslie J. Summer. "Codependency and Recovery: Gender, Self, and Emotions in Popular Self-Help." *Symbolic Interaction* 18, no. 2 (1995): 145–163.

Steadman Rice, John. "Discursive Formation, Life Stories, and the Emergence of Co-dependency: 'Power/Knowledge' and the Search for Identity." *The Sociological Quarterly* 33, no. 3 (Autumn 1992): 337–364.

Organizations

Al-Anon: Friends and families of problem drinkers find understanding and support at www.al-anon.org.

Al-Anon Family Group Headquarters, Inc.
1600 Corporate Landing Parkway

Virginia Beach, VA 23454-5617
Telephone: (757) 563-1600
Fax: (757) 563-1655

Co-Dependents Anonymous (known as CoDA) support groups and information for codependents are available at www.coda.org.

CoDA, Fellowship Services Office
PO Box 33577
Phoenix, AZ 85067-3577
Telephone: (602) 277-7991
Toll-free: (888) 444-2359

Beck, Aaron T. (1921–)

American psychiatrist, Aaron T. Beck, is credited as the "father of cognitive therapy" and is known for his extensive research into psychiatric illnesses and for developing various self-report measures to assess anxiety and depression.

Description

Aaron Temkin Beck, was born July 18, 1921, in Providence, Rhode Island, the third son to Russian Jewish immigrants, Elizabeth Temkin and Harry Beck. Two of Beck's siblings died before he was born. His early years were comfortable, growing up in a typical middle-class family and participating in Boy Scouts and athletics. However, at the age of eight he developed a serious staph infection, causing him to be hospitalized and drastically limiting his involvement in sports; he resorted to solitary activities like reading. This experience also resulted in Beck's overwhelming fear of blood, doctors, and hospitals, phobias he would later overcome by training himself to think rationally. Beck proved to be an exemplary student. He attended Brown University majoring in English and Political Science, was a member of the prestigious Phi Beta Kappa Society, served as an editor on *The Brown Daily Herald*, and received several accolades, including the Philo Sherman Bennett Essay Award Francis Wayland Scholarship, the William Gaston Prize for Excellence in Oratory, and the Francis Wayland

Scholarship. He graduated magna cum laude from Brown University in 1942 and continued his education at Yale Medical School, completing his MD in 1946. He did his residency at the Rhode Island Hospital. During his schooling he was trained in the use of medication and psychoanalytic therapy, approaches that he came to believe lacked the ability to empower people to help themselves and take control of their psychological ailments. After graduation, he serviced in the U.S. military as assistant chief of neuropsychiatry at Valley Forge Army Hospital. Aaron married Phyllis in 1950 and the couple went on to have four children. In 1954, he joined the faculty at the University of Pennsylvania, where he later developed his approach

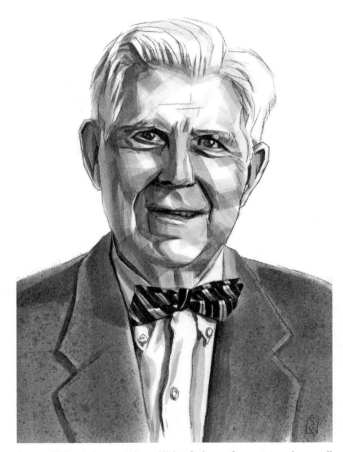

Aaron T. Beck is considered "the father of cognitive therapy" and known for his extensive research into psychiatric illnesses and for developing various self-report measures to assess anxiety and depression. (Jan Rieckhoff/ullstein bild via Getty Images)

while conducting multiple studies on patients suffering from chronic depreson. This approach, which he termed "cognitive therapy" (CT), is a type of talk therapy that employs problem-solving techniques by challenging clients' negative "automatic thoughts" in order to alter faulty thinking, instill hope, and restore a positive outlook on recovery. Cognitive therapy has proven effective in treating a variety of psychological disorders, including anxiety, depression, post-traumatic stress, substance abuse problems, eating disorders, schizophrenia, and suicidal ideation. CT is noted for its solid research support, and is also a cost-effective, time-conscious, and longer-lasting treatment.

Impact (Psychological Influence)

Dr. Beck and his daughter, Dr. Judith Beck, founded the *Beck Institute for Cognitive Behavior Therapy and Research* in Philadelphia in 1994, where he still serves as President Emeritus and his daughter as president. The institute continues to conduct research and provide training and therapy to professionals, educators, and clients from all over the world. He is also director of the *Aaron T. Beck Psychopathology Research Center* at the University of Pennsylvania. Beck has taught at Oxford, Temple, and the University of Medicine and Dentistry of New Jersey, in addition to his long-standing presence at Penn where he presently serves as Professor Emeritus of Psychiatry. He has received honorary degrees from the University of Pennsylvania, Yale University, Brown University, Philadelphia College of Osteopathic Medicine, and Assumption College. A variety of self-report measures to gauge anxiety and depression were developed by Dr. Beck, including the widely used Beck Depression Inventory, as well as the Beck Hopelessness Scale, Beck Scale for Suicidal Ideation, and Beck Anxiety Inventory. Beck has authored or coauthored over 600 professional journal articles and 25 books, some of which include *Cognitive Therapy and the Emotional Disorders, Depression: Causes and Treatment, Cognitive Therapy of Anxiety Disorders: Science and Practice*, and *Anxiety Disorders and Phobias: A Cognitive Perspective*. Dr. Beck's accomplishments are substantial, and he has been the recipient of many awards such as the Heinz Award in the Human Condition, Kennedy

Community Mental Health Award, the Albert Lasker Clinical Medical Research Award, the Anna-Monika Prize, the Adolf Meyer Award, and the Morselli Medal for Lifetime of Research in the Field of Suicide. Cognitive therapy is the most widely used and rigorously studied psychotherapy approach to date. It has profoundly impacted the psychological health of millions of people worldwide so much so that *The American Psychologist* deemed Dr. Aaron T. Beck as "one of the five most influential psychotherapists of all time."

Melissa A. Mariani, PhD

See also: Anxiety Disorders in Adults; Cognitive Therapies; Depression

Further Reading

Beck, Aaron T. *Anxiety Disorders and Phobias: A Cognitive Perspective*. New York, NY: Basic Books, 2005.

Beck, Aaron T. *Cognitive Therapy and the Emotional Disorders*. New York, NY: Meridian, 1976.

Beck, Aaron T., and Brad A. Alford. *Depression: Causes and Treatment*, 2nd ed. Philadelphia, PA: University of Pennsylvania Press, 2009.

Clark, David A., and Aaron T. Beck. *Cognitive Therapy of Anxiety Disorders: Science and Practice*. New York, NY: Guilford Press, 2011.

Weishaar, Marjorie. *Aaron T. Beck* (Key Figures in Counselling and Psychotherapy series). London, UK: Sage, 1993.

Beck Depression Inventory

The Beck Depression Inventory is a widely used clinical measure (questionnaire) of depression.

Definitions

- **Cognitive therapy** is a psychological treatment that focuses on changing cognitive beliefs and thinking patterns to produce behavioral change.

- **Depression** is a mental condition characterized by sadness and loss of interest in life, sleep problems, loss of appetite, loss of concentration, and even thoughts of self-harm.

- **Dysthymic disorder** is a less severe but chronic (ongoing) form of depression.

Description

The Beck Depression Inventory (BDI) is a 21 multiple-choice questionnaire developed to measure the intensity, severity, and depth of depressive symptoms in individuals between the ages of 13 and 80 years. The BDI serves at least two purposes: first, to detect or screen for depression in mental health and primary care settings; and second, to assess and monitor for changes in depressive symptoms. The BDI usually takes between 5 and 10 minutes to complete as part of a psychological or medical examination. The paper and pencil or computer version is either filled out by an individual (self-report) or administered verbally by a trained professional. The BDI also helps measure symptoms related to depression such as fatigue, irritability, guilt, weight loss, and apathy. A shorter form is also available; it is composed of seven questions or items and is used primarily to screen for depression in primary care settings.

Developments and Current Status

The BDI was developed and published in 1961 by Aaron T. Beck, MD (1921–), the founder of cognitive therapy. It was adapted in the 1970s and copyrighted in 1978 (BDI-1A). A more recent version (BDI-II) was developed and published in 1996 by Beck, Robert A. Steer, and Gregory K. Brown. The BDI is divided into two subscales. The affective subscale consists of eight items that measure psychological, or mood, symptoms. These items include negative thoughts involving. pessimism, past failures, guilty feelings, punishment feelings, self-dislike, self-criticalness, suicidal thoughts, and worthlessness. The other subscale focuses on somatic or physical symptoms. It has 13 items, such as loss of energy, agitation, and indecisiveness.

The long form of the BDI is composed of 21 questions, each with four possible responses. Each response is assigned a score ranging from zero to three, indicating the severity of the symptom that the patient has experienced over the past two weeks. The sum of all BDI item scores indicates the severity of depression. The test is scored differently for the general population and for those who have been clinically diagnosed with depression. For the general population, a score of 21 or over represents depression. For those who were clinically diagnosed with depression, BDI-II scores from 0 to 13 represent minimal depressive symptoms, scores of 14 to 19 indicate mild depression, scores of 20 to 28 indicate moderate depression, and scores of 29 to 63 indicate severe depression. The BDI can distinguish between different subtypes of depressive disorders, such as major (severe) depression and dysthymic disorder.

The BDI has been shown to be valid and reliable, with results corresponding to clinician ratings of depression in more than 90% of all cases. Finally, it should be noted that the BDI is one of the most widely used assessment tests by medical and mental health professionals and researchers for measuring depressive symptoms.

Len Sperry, MD, PhD

See also: Cognitive Behavior Therapy; Depression and Depressive Disorders; Persistent Depressive Disorder

Further Reading

Beck, Aaron T., and Brad A. Alford. *Depression: Causes and Treatments*. Philadelphia, PA: University of Pennsylvania Press, 2009.

Clark, David A., and Aaron T. Beck. *Cognitive Therapy of Anxiety Disorders: Science and Practice*. New York, NY: Guilford Press, 2010.

Nezu, Arthur, George F. Ronan, and Elizabeth A. Meadows, eds. *Practitioner's Guide to Empirically Based Measures of Depression*. New York, NY: Springer, 2006.

Pearson Assessments. "Beck Depression Inventory®—II (BDI®—II)." Accessed February 2, 2015. http://www.pearsonassessments.com/HAIWEB/Cultures/en-us/Productdetail.htm?Pid=015-8018-370.

Behavior Therapy

Behavior therapy is a psychotherapy approach that focuses on identifying and changing maladaptive behaviors. It is also referred to as behavioral therapy.

Definitions

- **Behavior modification** is the use of learning principles to increase the frequency of desired behaviors and decrease the frequency of problem behaviors.

- **Behavioral analysis** is a type of assessment that focuses on the observable and quantifiable aspects of behavior and excludes subjective phenomena such as emotions and motives.

- **Dialectical behavior therapy** is a type of cognitive behavior therapy that focuses on learning skills to cope with stress, regulate emotions, and improve relationships.

- **Mindfulness** refers to paying attention in a particular way that is intentional, in the present moment, and nonjudgmental.

- **Reinforcement** is a behavioral modification process in which certain consequences (effects) of behavior increase the probability that the behavior will occur again.

- **Shaping** is a behavioral modification process for reinforcing responses that come sufficiently closer to the desired response.

Description

Behavior therapy (BT) is a treatment approach based on the assumption that behavioral (including emotional) problems are learned responses to the environment and can be unlearned. Traditional BT focuses only on observable behavior and so ignores mental processes. Thus, instead of uncovering and understanding the unconscious processes that underlie maladaptive behavior, behavioral therapists assist clients in directly modifying the maladaptive behavior or developing a new, adaptive behavior. Basic to BT is the antecedent-behavior-consequence model of behavioral analysis, which describes the temporal sequence of a problematic behavior in terms of its "antecedents" (stimulus situation that cues or triggers behavior), "behaviors" (the problematic behavior itself), and "consequences" (the effects or outcomes that follow the behavior). Three types of behavior problems can be identified from this analysis: behavior excesses, deficits, or inappropriateness. Core concepts of BT include respondent and operant conditioning and positive and negative reinforcement.

Various strategies are utilized in traditional BT to promote the desired (new or modified) behavior.

These include shaping the consequences (effects or outcomes) of a behavior so that a desired behavior is reinforced and the undesired ones are extinguished. The desired behavior is then rehearsed (practiced). In addition, therapeutic interventions such as skill training, exposure, response prevention, emotional processing, flooding, systematic desensitization, and homework are used to achieve specific therapeutic outcomes.

Developments and Current Status

BT has evolved over the years. A useful way of understanding this evolution is in terms of its "three waves." The first wave emphasized traditional BT, which focused on replacing problematic behaviors with constructive ones through classical conditioning and reinforcement techniques. Joseph Wolpe (1915–1997) pioneered classical conditioning, particularly systematic desensitization. Traditional BT was a technical, problem-focused, present-centered approach that contrasted with other therapy approaches. The second wave involved the incorporation of the cognitive therapies. These cognitively oriented approaches focused on changing problematic feelings and behaviors by changing the thoughts that cause and perpetuate them. CBT, which was an integration of both behavioral and cognitive techniques, emerged during this phase. The third wave involved the reformulation of conventional CBT approaches. Third-wave approaches were and are more experiential and indirect and utilizes techniques such as mindfulness, dialectics, acceptance, values, and spirituality. Unlike the first and second waves, third-wave approaches emphasize second-order change, that is, basic change in structure and/or function, and are based on contextual assumptions, including the primacy of the therapeutic relationship. Next is a description of CBT followed by descriptions of three common third-wave approaches.

Cognitive Behavior Therapy

Cognitive behavior therapy (CBT) is a psychotherapy approach that addresses maladaptive (faulty) behaviors, emotions, and thoughts with various goal-oriented, explicit systematic interventions. The name refers to behavior therapy, to cognitive therapy, and to therapy based on a combination of basic behavioral and cognitive principles and research. Many therapists working with individuals dealing with anxiety and depression use a combination of cognitive and behavioral therapy. CBT acknowledges that there may be behaviors that cannot be controlled through rational thought. CBT is "problem focused" (undertaken for specific problems) and "action oriented" (therapist tries to assist the client in selecting specific strategies to help address those problems). CBT is thought to be effective for the treatment of a variety of conditions, including mood, anxiety, personality, eating, substance abuse, tic, and psychotic disorders. Many CBT treatment programs for specific disorders have been developed, evaluated for efficacy, and designated as evidence-based treatment. CBT is the most commonly practiced therapy approach in North America.

CBT was developed through an integration of cognitive therapies with behavior modification in the late 1970s. The term "cognitive-behavior modification" was first used by psychologist Donald Meichenbaum (1940–). The cognitive therapies include cognitive therapy, which was developed by Aaron Beck, and rational emotive behavior therapy, which was developed by Albert Ellis. While rooted in rather different theories, these two traditions have been characterized by a constant reference to experimental research to test hypotheses, at both clinical and basic levels. Common features of CBT include its focus on the present, the directive role of the therapist, structuring of the psychotherapy sessions, and on alleviating symptoms.

Dialectic Behavior Therapy

Dialectic behavior therapy (DBT) was developed for the treatment of borderline personality disorder by American psychologist, Marsha Linehan (1943–). More recently, it has been modified and extended for use with other personality disorders as well as Axis I or symptom disorders such as mood disorders, anxiety disorders, eating disorders, and substance disorders. DBT is an outgrowth of BT but is less cognitive than traditional CBT since DBT assumes that cognitions are less important than emotional regulation. Four primary

modes of treatment are noted in DBT: individual therapy; skills training in a group, telephone contact, and therapist consultation.

Cognitive Behavior Analysis System of Psychotherapy

Cognitive behavior analysis system of psychotherapy (CBASP) is a form of CBT that was developed by the American psychologist James P. McCullough (1942–). Basic to this approach is a situational analysis that combines behavioral, cognitive, and interpersonal methods to help clients focus on the consequences of their behavior and to use problem solving for resolving both personal and interpersonal difficulties.

The goal of CBASP is to identify the discrepancy between what clients want to happen (the desired outcome) in a particular situation and what has happened or is actually happening (the actual outcome). Treatment consists of two phases: elicitation and remediation. Elicitation involves a detailed analysis of a specific situation. In remediation, behaviors and thoughts are therapeutically processed so that new behaviors and thoughts will result in their desired outcome.

Mindfulness-Based Cognitive Therapy

Based on the mindfulness teachings of Thich Nhat Hanh (1926–), psychologist Jon Kabat-Zinn (1944–) developed what he called mindfulness-based stress reduction in 1979. This method uses mindfulness techniques to reduce stress associated with various medical conditions. Based in part, on this method, psychologist Zindel Segal (1956–), and his colleagues Mark Williams and John Teasdale, developed mindfulness-based cognitive therapy (MBCT). It was first described in their book, *Mindfulness-Based Cognitive Therapy for Depression* in 2002. MBCT is an adjunctive (extra) or standalone form of treatment that emphasizes changing the awareness of, and relation to, thoughts, rather than changing thought content. It offers clients a different way of living with and experiencing emotional pain and distress. It fosters a detached attitude toward negative thinking and provides the skills to prevent escalation of negative thinking at times of potential relapse. Clients engage in various formal meditation practices designed to increase moment-by-moment nonjudgmental awareness of physical sensations, thoughts, and feelings. Assigned homework includes practicing these exercises along with exercises designed to integrate application of awareness skills into daily life. Specific prevention strategies derived from traditional CBT methods are incorporated in the later weeks of the program.

Len Sperry, MD, PhD

See also: Cognitive Behavior Therapy; Cognitive Therapies; Dialectical Behavior Therapy; Mindfulness; Mindfulness-Based Psychotherapies

Further Reading

Crane, Rebecca. *Mindfulness-Based Cognitive Therapy.* New York, NY: Routledge, 2009.

Miller, Alec L., Jill H. Rathus, and Marsha Linehan. *Dialectical Behavior Therapy with Suicidal Adolescents.* New York, NY: Guilford Press, 2007.

Segal, Zindel V., J. Mark G. Williams, and John D. Teasdale. *Mindfulness-Based Cognitive Therapy for Depression*, 2nd ed. New York, NY: Guilford Press, 2013.

Sperry, Len. *Cognitive Behavior Therapy of DSM-5 Personality Disorders*, 3rd ed. New York, NY: Routledge, 2016.

Behavior Therapy with Children

Behavior therapy with children uses techniques of behavior modification to replace bad habits with acceptable ones.

Definitions

- **Antecedent** is something that occurs before a behavior and includes places, people, and things involved in the environment.

- **Behavior** is an observable action demonstrated by a human being or an animal caused by either internal or external occurrences.

- **Consequence** is the result or outcome that occurs after a behavior is demonstrated.

- **Reinforcement** is the result of a behavior that will strengthen the likelihood of the behavior to happen again in the future.

Description

The aim of behavior therapy with children is to identify and foster the development of personal coping strategies that can replace negative behaviors. The most effective treatments involve the child, parents, teachers, and therapists. All those involved must be taught by a trained therapist about which behavioral interventions are most effective.

Behavior therapy with children focuses on three key elements, which are the antecedent, behavior, and consequence. In the field it is important to identify what happens right before, the antecedent, and after, the consequence, the behavior. This approach is referred to as the antecedent-behavior-consequence model of intervention. It is commonly used in behavior therapy with children to create effective programs at home, in school, and in the community.

One subtype of behavior therapy commonly used with children is applied behavior analysis (ABA). It is one of the most well-researched and supported types of behavior therapy with children. Its goal is to help teach children a variety of ways of responding to challenges in a more positive way. In order to begin behavior therapy, several observations and assessment of a situation have to occur to help identify the function or the purpose of the behavior. Within ABA there are clearly identified reasons why behavior occurs. Some of these include a child's need for attention, to escape, to gain access, and/or to satisfy a sense or physical response like pain. The goal of this therapy is to identify one or many of these reasons for behavior and replace negative behaviors with more positive ones. This occurs often through positive reinforcement, which helps to increase a desired behavior and decrease problem behavior.

Another subset of behavior therapy is cognitive behavior therapy (CBT), which focuses on helping children to identify and improve their thoughts and behaviors. CBT teaches children and teens how to recognize what might trigger undesirable responses and avoid those circumstances. This approach requires that a child have the ability to identify thoughts and consequences. Therefore, CBT can be most effectively used with older children and with parents who can be actively involved.

In behavior therapy for children, several strategies are used. Modeling, role-playing, rehearsal, and rewards are some of them. As an example, role-playing is used to practice interaction with others around real issues in structured situations. This is one example of how children can learn that positive behaviors work and negative behaviors will not result in the same rewards.

Development

One of the founders of behavior therapy with children is considered to be Dr. B. F. Skinner, who identified some of the basic theories of how we learn. Yet before him Dr. John B. Watson was one of the first clinicians to directly use behavior therapy with children in the 1920s. Dr. Watson studied the effects of behavioral conditioning on helping children with phobias or fears. In 1953, Skinner published his first influential book, *Science and Human Behavior*, which included his view on working with children.

Until the late 1970s, behavior therapy was mostly applied in treatment with severely problematic children. Gradually, the work began to be applied to children with different ranges of cognitive and emotional problems. One great success has been in work with children diagnosed with attention-deficit hyperactivity disorder, where behavior therapy can bring positive changes in social relationships and daily functioning.

Behavior therapy has also been used extensively with children on the autism spectrum with positive results. Many practitioners and researchers specifically refer to ABA therapy as one of the most effective treatments for autism. In all cases, when therapy is extended through training both parents and teachers, its benefits are seen in the entire family constellation as well as broadly in the school environment.

Current Status

Today, the field of behavior therapy, especially in the forms of ABA and CBT, is a major part of the treatment protocols for child and adolescent psychology and psychiatry. Ensuring that the child gets the help appropriate to his or her age and circumstances is important in behavior therapy. The younger the child when treatment begins, the greater the chances of behavior therapy being effective. Behavior therapy is proven to work on its own with several populations and groups of children with certain diagnoses. However, there are still cases where a combination of medication and therapy may help behavior changes occur more effectively.

The focus of behavior therapy should always be on treating the child with respect and positive regard. A current focus in behavior therapy is on positive behavior systems and supports. This has helped to put behavior therapy with children into a better position for its introduction into schools and parenting. Many children with different issues benefit from behavior therapy, and it is considered one of the most helpful and effective treatments for young children with a range of challenges.

Alexandra Cunningham, PhD, and William M. Cunningham, MA

See also: Applied Behavior Analysis; Attention-Deficit Hyperactivity Disorder in Youth; Autism Spectrum Disorders; Cognitive Behavior Therapy; Skinner, B. F. (1904–1990)

Further Reading

Beck, Judith S. *Cognitive Behavior Therapy: Basics and Beyond.* New York, NY: Guilford Press, 2011.

Graziano, Anthony M., ed. *Behavior Therapy with Children II.* Vol. 2. Piscataway, NJ: Transaction Publishers, 2008.

Pierce, W. David, and Carl D. Cheney. *Behavior Analysis and Learning.* New York, NY: Psychology Press, 2013.

Behavioral Activation

Behavioral activation is a brief, structured treatment approach that activates those who are depressed so they can again experience pleasure and satisfaction.

Definitions

- **Behavior therapy** is a psychotherapy approach that focuses on identifying and changing maladaptive behaviors.

- **Cognitive behavior therapy** is psychotherapy approach that focuses on maladaptive (faulty) behaviors, emotions, and thoughts. It is also known as cognitive behavioral therapy.

- **Cognitive therapy** is a type of cognitive behavior therapy that focuses on identifying and changing distorted thinking patterns.

- **Depression** is an emotional state that is characterized by feelings of low self-worth, guilt, and a reduced ability to enjoy life.

- **Positive reinforcement** is a way of increasing the strength of a given response by rewarding it.

Description

Behavioral activation is a brief, behavioral treatment for depression that activates individuals in specific ways so they can again engage in pleasant activities. As a result they begin to reexperience pleasure and satisfaction and their depression lifts. Behavioral activation is based on a behavioral theory of depression. In this theory, as individuals become depressed, they increasingly withdraw from their environment, engage in escape behaviors, and disengage from their routines. Depression typically leads to withdrawal, avoidance, and inactivity. This prevents them from experiencing positive reinforcement that provides satisfaction and the desire to be active and involved. Over time, this avoidance exacerbates depressed mood, as individuals lose opportunities to be positively reinforced through pleasurable experiences and social activity, or experiences of mastery.

Behavioral activation treatment is a set of techniques for helping individuals to overcome this pattern. Therapists help their clients to set weekly goals, to identify possible sources of positive reinforcement, and to schedule and structure their activities. Clients are encouraged to develop a list of activities that they enjoy or need to engage in as part of their normal life. Then, beginning with the easiest activities on the list, the individual agrees to carry them out in a systematic way. This reinstates contact with the naturally occurring positive reinforcement of the given activity, which in turn helps overcome the depressed mood.

Developments and Current Status

In the mid-1970s, Peter M. Lewinsohn (1939–), an American psychologist, described a behavioral theory of depression. He speculated that depression reflects low levels of positive reinforcement and high levels of aversive (negative) control. These were due to problems in the environment or to underdeveloped coping skills. Accordingly, he developed a treatment to increase pleasant activities for depressed individuals. As they engaged in an increasing number of pleasant activities, their rate of positive reinforcement began to increase. As activation increased, their symptoms of depression decreased. Unfortunately, his theory and approach was overshadowed in the 1980s and 1990s by the development of Aaron T. Beck's (1921–), cognitive therapy (CT) approach for understanding and treating depression. CT and cognitive behavior therapy (CBT) became known as the most effective treatments for depression. However, in 1996, psychologist Neil S. Jacobson (1949–1999) reported research on the effectiveness of CBT for depression. It showed no differences in treatment outcome between CBT and behavioral activation. A subsequent study showed that behavioral activation was as effective as antidepressant medications for mild to moderate depression. These and subsequent studies have led more therapists to use behavioral activation. Behavioral activation is utilized as either a standalone treatment or an adjunctive (additional) treatment combined with CT, CBT, or other approaches.

Len Sperry, MD, PhD

See also: Behavior Therapy; Cognitive Behavior Therapy; Cognitive Therapies; Depression

Further Reading

Addis, Michael E., and Christopher R. Martell. *Overcoming Depression One Step at a Time: The New Behavioral Activation Approach to Getting Your Life Back*. Oakland, CA: New Harbinger, 2004.

Lewinsohn, Peter M., Mary Ann Youngren, and Antonette M. Zeiss. *Control Your Depression*. New York, NY: Fireside, 1992.

Martell, Christopher R., Michael E. Addis, and Neil S. Jacobson. *Depression in Context: Strategies for Guided Action*. New York, NY: W.W. Norton, 2001.

Martell, Christopher R., Sona Dimidjian, and Ruth Herman-Dunn. *Behavioral Activation for Depression: A Clinician's Guide*. New York, NY: Guilford Press, 2010.

Behavioral Assessment

Behavioral assessment is a form of assessing an individual's behaviors in a specific problem situation.

Definitions

- **Assessment** is the measurement, observation, and systematic evaluation of an individual's thoughts, feelings, and behavior in the actual problem situation.

- **Traits** are patterns of behavior, thought, and emotion, which are stable over time, differ across individuals, and influence behavior.

Description

Behavioral assessment is an approach to assessment that focuses on overt behaviors and the identification of its antecedents (triggers) and consequences (effects) in a problematic situation. The purpose of this assessment is to devise a behavioral plan to correct the problem situation. Correctly identifying the antecedents and consequences points to the function or "why" of the behavior. Behavioral assessment involves observing or otherwise measuring an individual's actual behavior in the specific settings where the individual experiences a behavioral difficulty. Once the behavior is defined and measured, careful consideration is given to factors that may be reinforcing and maintaining the behavior. Specific measures are selected based on the behavior and its context in order to analyze the target behavior prior to, during, and after. This information is used in developing a detailed plan containing strategies for changing or replacing the behavior.

Behavioral assessment typically involves one or more behavioral interviews and observations, and includes direct observation and indirect methods. Direct observation focuses on a specific behavior: frequency (how often a behavior occurs), magnitude (how intense it is), and duration (how long it lasts). Direct observation often includes "anecdotal recording," which involves recording a pattern of behavior using an antecedent-behavior-consequence format. In doing an anecdotal observation, the observer records all behaviors observed, and what was observed to occur before and after the behaviors. For example, if a child is observed to slam the door to his or her bedroom, the observer should record "slammed bedroom door shut" rather than "child frustrated." Then the observations are arranged into a chart which specifies behaviors, antecedents (what happened prior to the behavior), and consequences (what happened as a result of the behavior). Also tracked are the times at which behaviors were observed. Indirect methods include checklists and rating scales. Examples of checklists and rating scales used with children include the Revised Behavior Problem Checklist, the Behavioral Assessment System for Children, and the Behavior Evaluation Scale.

Developments and Current Status

Behavioral assessment evolved from the field of behavior therapy as an alternative to traditional assessment approaches. Traditional assessment approaches were based on the trait model where inferred traits were used to explain and predict behavior of individuals across various contexts and situations. This model had limited utility for behavior therapists and researchers who viewed personality as the total of an individual's habit patterns and behavior. They valued observable phenomena and verifiability of observations and subsequently developed behavioral assessment.

There are two broad categories of behavioral assessment generally: clinical behavioral assessment and functional behavioral assessment (FBA). Clinical behavioral assessment is conducted for problem behaviors exhibited in home, school, work, or other settings, to provide a clear intervention plan for therapists, case managers, family members, or others who work with the individual being evaluated. FBA is an approach used with children who demonstrate chronic behavior problems. It focuses on patterns of behavior and the identification of their purpose or their function. For example, the function might be to avoid something, to get something, or to make something happen. The function is inferred from the carefully observed and analyzed sequence of behavior. FBAs are conducted by a school system when students with disabilities or suspected of having a disability are demonstrating inappropriate behaviors. By federal law, school districts are required to perform FBAs as part of the Individuals with Disabilities Education Act.

Len Sperry, MD, PhD

See also: Diagnosis

Further Reading

Bellack, Allan, and Michael Hersen. *Behavioral Assessment: A Practical Guide*, 4th ed. Needham Height, MA: Allyn & Bacon, 1998.

Cipani, Ennio, and Keven M. Schock. *Functional Behavioral Assessment, Diagnosis, and Treatment: A Complete System for Education and Mental Health Settings*, 2nd ed. New York, NY: Springer, 2011.

Wolpe, Joseph. *The Practice of Behavior Therapy*. New York, NY: Pergamon Press, 1973.

Behavioral Health

Behavioral health is a health-care specialty that focuses on behavior and its effect on mental and physical well-being. It is sometimes referred to as mental health.

Definitions

- **Behavioral health care** is the continuum of health-care services for individuals who suffer from, or are at risk of, mental, behavioral, or addictive disorders.

- **Behavioral medicine** is the interdisciplinary health-care specialty, which integrates knowledge and techniques from behavioral and biomedical science and applies this knowledge and techniques to the diagnosis, treatment, rehabilitation, and prevention of medical conditions.

- **Health Maintenance Organization** is an organization that provides or manages health-care delivery to control costs (managed care).

- **Managed care** is a system of health care that controls costs by placing limits on physicians' fees and by restricting access to certain medical procedures and providers.

- **Medical cost offset** is the cost savings that occurs when the use of medical services decreases as a result of mental or behavioral health interventions.

- **Psychotherapy** is a psychological method for achieving desired changes in thinking, feeling, and behavior. It is also called therapeutic counseling.

Description

Behavioral health is specialty area of health care that addresses the influence and effect of behavior on mental and physical well-being. Over the past decade, the term "behavioral health" is gradually replacing the term "mental health." "Behavioral health" is a broad term that encompasses mental health, psychiatric, marriage and family counseling, and addiction treatment. It includes services provided by psychologists, counselors, psychiatrists, social workers, neurologists, and physicians.

Behavioral health promotes a philosophy of health that emphasizes individual responsibility in the application of behavioral and biomedical science, knowledge, and techniques to the maintenance of health and the prevention of illness and dysfunction with self-initiated, health-enhancing activities. These activities include healthy eating, exercising, no smoking, positive attitude, and limited use of alcohol. Behavioral health is a specialty area of behavioral medicine.

Developments and Current Status

Psychologist Joseph D. Matarazzo (1925–) first defined the health-care specialty of behavioral health in 1979. He distinguished it from the field of behavioral medicine, which was formally introduced in 1978 by the newly formed Society of Behavioral Medicine. Since then, much of the vision, training, clinical practice, and research on behavioral health and medical offset originated with psychologist Nicholas Cummings (1924–). Cummings is considered by many the father of behavioral health-care practice.

Given the changes already noted, it appears that behavioral health practice will become a dominant force in health care. To the extent that behavioral health practice becomes the norm, the practice of psychotherapy and psychological treatments within an integrated health-care setting will be notably different. Shorter and more focused psychological and psychotherapeutic interventions will replace the traditional 50-minute psychotherapy hour. As reimbursement shifts to favor integrated health care, increasing numbers of psychotherapists will work in primary care settings, with smaller numbers in clinics, agencies, or private practice.

Len Sperry, MD, PhD

See also: Behavioral Medicine; Integrative Health; Psychotherapy

Further Reading

Cummings, Nicholas A., and Janet Cummings. *Refocused Psychotherapy as the First Line Intervention in Behavioral Health.* New York, NY: Routledge, 2013.

Hunter, Christopher L., Jeffrey L. Goodie, Mark S. Oordt, and Anne C. Dobmeyer. *Integrated Behavioral Health in Primary Care: Step-by-Step Guidance for Assessment and Intervention.* Washington, DC: American Psychological Association, 2009.

Sperry, Len. *Behavioral Health: Integrating Individual and Family Interventions in the Treatment of Medical Conditions.* New York, NY: Routledge, 2014.

Behavioral Medicine

Behavioral medicine is the interdisciplinary approach to understanding, preventing, diagnosing, and treating medical conditions with behavioral aspects.

Definitions

- **Behavioral** describes the way someone responds to his or her environment. It is also referred to as psychological.

- **Biomedical** is the involvement of biological, medical, and physical sciences.

- **Biopsychosocial** refers to biological, psychological, and social factors.

- **Cochrane Reviews** are evidence-based reviews of health care and health policy research that addresses prevention, treatment, and rehabilitation.

- **Interdisciplinary** is the integration of two or more scientific or educational areas of knowledge.

- **Rheumatic heart disease** is a heart condition caused by rheumatic fever, which is triggered by a preventable infection. The disease is more prevalent in impoverished countries and communities.

Description

Behavioral medicine is the field of medicine that integrates behavioral and biomedical scientific knowledge. It focuses on the role that behavioral factors play in the cause, treatment, and prevention of medical conditions. It also promotes the communication of theory and research, and its application, among the professional fields, particularly medicine and psychology.

The term "behavioral medicine" was first used in 1973 in the title of the book *Biofeedback: Behavioral Medicine* by psychiatrist Lee Birk (1936–2009). It was also used in the names of two organizations, Center for Behavioral Medicine and Study of Behavioral Medicine. The first definition of behavioral medicine was established in 1976 when psychologists Gary E. Schwartz (1944–) and Stephen Weiss held a conference at Yale University for a diverse group of behavioral and biomedical professionals. Together these scientists developed an interdisciplinary definition for the new field of behavioral medicine. They arrived at this definition: "Behavioral medicine is the field concerned with the development and integration of behavioral and biomedical science knowledge and techniques relevant to health and illness and the application of this knowledge and these techniques to prevention, diagnosis, treatment, and rehabilitation. Psychosis, neurosis and substance abuse are included only insofar as they contribute to physical disorders as an end point" (Schwartz and Weiss, 1977, 3). This definition focuses on health as well as illness. Schwartz and Weiss believed the integration of behavioral science and medicine would result in greater knowledge with broader application.

Two examples in which behavioral medicine is used to study and treat physical illness are high blood pressure (hypertension) and rheumatic heart disease.

Behavioral medicine research incorporates the impact of biological, psychological, behavioral, social, environmental, and cultural influences on the occurrence, pattern, treatment, and management of these diseases. Behavioral medicine does not include research on mental illness (i.e., psychosis and neurosis), substance abuse, mental retardation, and social welfare issues (see the previous paragraph).

The advent of behavioral medicine promoted the development of interdisciplinary scientific journals that offer a central venue for behavioral and biomedical researchers to publish scientific findings. It also promoted the development of interdisciplinary organizations that united researchers, practitioners, and educators from different fields. The National Institutes of Health created the Office of Behavioral and Social Sciences Research to coordinate research between the behavioral and social sciences. Finally, the Cochrane Collaboration acknowledged behavioral medicine as an evidence-based field and has included it in the resource database of the Cochrane Reviews.

As far back as 1936, researchers have made the argument that psychosocial factors impact physical health and illness (Suls and Davidson, 2010), namely that psychological stress affects the cardiovascular, respiratory, muscular, metabolic, immune, and central nervous systems. Continuous psychological stress on these systems results in physical changes, which can negatively impact a person's health.

The significance of psychological influences on physical illness and the effects of physical illness on psychological factors illustrate the reciprocal relationship between the mind and body. Behavioral medicine research has several implications for mental health practitioners. First, psychological factors such as anxiety, fear, stress, and self-efficacy impact physical health and behavior. Second an integrative approach from a biopsychosocial perspective is necessary to comprehensively assess, diagnose, and treat individuals. Third, socioeconomic status, race, and ethnicity impact health outcomes and must also be considered during assessment, diagnosis, and treatment.

Len Sperry, MD, PhD, and Christina Ladd, PhD

See also: Biopsychosocial Model; Biopsychosocial Therapy; Integrative Health

Further Reading

Keefe, Francis J. "Behavioral Medicine: A Voyage to the Future." *Annuals of Behavioral Medicine* 41, no. 2 (2011): 141–151.

Schwartz, Gary E., and Stephen M. Weiss. "Behavioral Medicine Revisited: An Amended Definition." *Journal of Behavioral Medicine* 1, no. 3 (1978): 249–251.

Schwartz, Gary E., and Stephen M. Weiss. "Yale Conference on Behavioral Medicine: A Proposed Definition and Statement of Goals." *Journal of Behavioral Medicine* 1, no. 1 (1977): 3–12.

Suls, Jerry M., and Karina W. Davidson. *Handbook of Health Psychology and Behavioral Medicine.* New York, NY: Guilford Press, 2010.

Bender Gestalt Test

The Bender Gestalt Test is a widely used assessment tool for measuring cognitive abilities and assessing brain dysfunction. It is also known as the Bender Visual-Motor Gestalt Test.

Definitions

- **Alzheimer's disease** is a degenerative medical condition that adversely affects the brain and causes dementia within the later years of life.

- **Attention-deficit hyperactivity disorder** is a condition involving hyperactivity in children, characterized by an inability to concentrate and inappropriate or impulsive behaviors.

- **Autism** is a neurological condition that usually begins before the age of three years and develops with respect to disorders involving speech and language, interpretation of the world, social interactions and the formation of relationships, and reaction to stimuli. Repetitive behaviors are often seen within the condition.

- **Visuomotor** refers to visual and motor processes.

Description

The Bender Gestalt Test (BGT), also called the Bender Visual Motor Gestalt Test, is a psychological assessment tool used to evaluate visual-motor functioning and visual perception skills in children and adults. The test requires fine motor skills, the ability to discriminate between varying elements of visual stimuli, the capacity to integrate visual skills with motor skills, and the ability to shift attention from the original design to what is being drawn. The test-taker is instructed to reproduce (copy) simple figures (geometric designs) on a blank piece of paper as well as he or she can. Usually it takes from 7 to 10 minutes to complete. Scores are based on accuracy of the resultant figures and other such relevant factors. The BGT can identify possible organic brain damage and the degree of maturation of the nervous system. It is used to evaluate visual-motor maturity and integration skills, style of responding, reaction to frustration, ability to correct mistakes, planning and organizational skills, and motivation. It is also used within inpatient psychiatric units to differentiate between serious mental disorders and brain impairment.

Developments and Current Status

The BGT was developed by Lauretta Bender, MD (1897–1987), an American child psychiatrist. Bender published the monograph *A Visual Motor Gestalt and Its Clinical Use* in 1935. The original test contains nine geometric figures drawn in black. These figures are presented to the test-taker one at a time, who is asked to copy the unique figure onto a blank sheet of paper with the card still in sight. They are allowed to erase but cannot use rulers or other aids.

The second edition of the Bender Visual-Motor Gestalt Test (Bender-Gestalt II) was published in 2003. It contains 16 figures and has a new recall procedure for visual-motor (visuomotor) memory that provides a more comprehensive assessment of these skills. It also includes supplemental tests of simple motor and perceptual ability to aid in identifying motor-visual deficits. Furthermore, new norms are provided for copy and recall procedures. The main test takes between 5 and 10 minutes to administer, with an additional 5 minutes to complete each of the supplemental visual and motor tests.

The Bender-Gestalt II is used to assess the maturation of visuomotor perceptions of children and adults from age 3 to 85 years. It is useful in assessing various neuropsychological psychological conditions such as Alzheimer's disease, attention-deficit hyperactivity disorder, autism, giftedness, and intellectual and learning disabilities. It is also useful in identifying cognitive decline in older adults. Overall, the Bender-Gestalt II remains a popular psychological test because it is simple to use, is brief to administer, and has proven effective for a wide range of ages.

Len Sperry, MD, PhD

See also: Alzheimer's Disease; Attention-Deficit Hyperactivity Disorder; Autism

Further Reading

Brannigan, Gary G., and Scott L. Decker. *Bender Visual-Motor Gestalt Test*. Itasca, IL: Riverside Publishing, 2003.

Koppitz, Elizabeth M. *The Bender Gestalt Test for Young Children*. Vol. 2. New York, NY: Grune and Stratton, 1975.

Benzodiazepines

Benzodiazepines are a class of drugs that slow the nervous system functioning and are prescribed to relieve nervousness and tension, to induce sleep, and to treat other symptoms. They are highly addictive.

Definition

- **Antianxiety medications** are prescribed drugs that relieve anxiety symptoms. They are also called anxiolytics or tranquilizers.

Description

Benzodiazepines are a class of antianxiety medications that work by slowing the central nervous system functioning. Although anxiety is a normal response to stressful situations, some have elevated levels of anxiety that interfere with daily living. Benzodiazepines help reduce anxious feelings and also relieve other troubling symptoms of anxiety, such as increased heart rate, difficulty breathing, irritability, nausea, and faintness. Other uses of benzodiazepines are for muscle spasms, epilepsy and other seizure disorders, phobias, panic disorder, withdrawal from alcohol, and sleeping problems. However, this medicine should not be used every day for sleep problems that last more than a few days. If used this way, the drug loses its effectiveness within a few weeks. The class of antianxiety drugs known as benzodiazepines includes Xanax, Librium, Valium, and Ativan. The antianxiety effect of this class of medications is experienced shortly after they are taken, typically within 15–60 minutes, depending on the specific medication.

Precautions and Side Effects

Some benzodiazepines increase the likelihood of birth defects, and their use during pregnancy can cause dependency and withdrawal symptoms in the infant. Because benzodiazepines may pass into breast milk, women who are breast-feeding should not use this class of medications without checking with their physicians. Benzodiazepines have considerable addictive potential, and long-term use of benzodiazepines may result in dependence and tolerance, so it is important that their use be monitored by the prescribing practitioner.

The most common side effects are dizziness, light-headedness, drowsiness, clumsiness, unsteadiness, and slurred speech. These problems commonly resolve as the body adjusts to the medication. They do not require medical treatment unless they persist or interfere with normal activities. More serious, but less common side effects include behavior changes, confusion, depression, difficulty concentrating, hallucinations, involuntary movements of the body, memory problems, seizures, or yellow skin or eyes. Medical attention should be sought if these appear. Those who have taken benzodiazepines for a prolonged period or at high doses may notice side effects for several weeks after they stop taking the drug. They should check with their physicians if the following symptoms occur: irritability, nervousness, or sleep problems.

Benzodiazepines interact with other central nervous system drugs and alcohol to further slow central nervous system functioning. These drugs include antihistamines, allergy medicine, cold medicine, muscle relaxants, seizure medications, sleep aids, and some pain relievers. They may also increase the effects of anesthetics, including those used for dental procedures. The combined effects of benzodiazepines and alcohol can result in unconsciousness or even death. Warning signs of this interaction include slurred speech or confusion, severe drowsiness, staggering, and profound weakness.

Len Sperry, MD, PhD

See also: Antianxiety Medications; Ativan (Lorazepam); Valium (Diazepam); Xanax (Alprazolam)

Further Reading

Doble, Adam, Ian Martin, and David J. Nutt. *Calming the Brain: Benzodiazepines and Related Drugs from Laboratory to Clinic.* London, UK: Informa Healthcare, 2003.

Erickson, Carlton K. *Addiction Essentials: The Go-to Guide for Clinicians and Patients.* New York, NY: W.W. Norton, 2011.

Toufexis, Donna. *Anti-anxiety Drugs.* New York, NY: Chelsea House Publishers, 2006.

Bereavement

Bereavement is an individual's emotional reaction to the loss (death) of a loved one.

Definitions

- **Bereavement counseling** is a type of counseling that assists individuals in coping with grief following the death of a loved one or any major life transition that results in grief. It is also called grief counseling.

- **Complicated grief** is the type of grief that is unresolved after an extended period of time and does not follow the typical progression that occurs in common grief reactions.

- **Derealization** is a perceptual reaction in which an individual becomes convinced that life or others are not real.

- **DSM-5** is the abbreviation for the *Diagnostic and Statistical Manual of Mental Disorders, Fifth Edition*, which is the handbook mental health professionals use to diagnose mental disorders.

- **Five stages of grief** are the stages that individuals often experience after the death of a loved one or even after a non-death-related loss. The stages are denial, anger, bargaining, depression, and acceptance.

- **Grief** is a healthy emotional reaction to the loss of another person.

- **V-code** is a DSM-5 designation for a mental condition that is not a disease or injury but results in symptoms or distress that may require some form of intervention.

Description

Bereavement is an emotional response that can be triggered by news of another person's death. Bereavement can vary greatly from person to person, and grief also has a cultural influence. Typical reactions that occur during bereavement are sadness, difficulty concentrating, anger, guilt, temporary decline in daily functioning, derealization, isolation, and frequent crying. The DSM-5 identifies bereavement as a V-code. Resolution of bereavement-related symptoms occurs over a few months, but when symptoms persist, it is called complicated grief.

Bereavement reactions can also occur after a non-death type of loss, for example, a divorce, the loss of functioning of one's legs, or acute illness of a loved one. In 1969, psychiatrist Elisabeth Kübler-Ross (1926–2004) identified the "five stages of grief" in her book *On Death and Dying*. The stages are denial, anger, bargaining, depression, and acceptance. Her research examined the emotional reactions of patient facing terminal cancer or other illnesses, and she described the five stages based on her observations of her patients' experience of grief. Sometimes, individuals do not experience the stages in a linear fashion. Some switch between several stages multiple times, while others may not experience anger or bargaining at all.

Treatment

Bereavement counseling is helpful in dealing with bereavement when symptoms are sufficient to disrupt daily activities. This type of counseling aims to assist individuals in moving from bereavement symptoms to resolution or acceptance of the loss. It assists clients in processing their emotions and other reactions to the loss.

Jon Sperry, PhD, and Len Sperry, MD, PhD

See also: Bereavement Counseling; Grief; Grief Counseling; Kübler-Ross, Elisabeth (1926–2004)

Further Reading

American Psychiatric Association. *Diagnostic and Statistical Manual of Mental Disorders*, 5th ed. Arlington, VA: American Psychiatric Association Press, 2013.

Kübler-Ross, Elisabeth. *On Death and Dying*. New York, NY: Routledge, 1969.

Worden, J. William. *Grief Counseling and Grief Therapy*, 3rd ed. New York, NY: Springer, 2002.

Bereavement Counseling

Bereavement counseling is a type of counseling that assists individuals in coping with grief following the death of a loved one or any major life transition that results in grief. It is also called grief counseling.

Definitions

- **Bereavement** is an individual's emotional reaction to the loss (death) of a loved one.

- **Complicated grief** is the type of grief that is unresolved after an extended period of time and does not follow the typical progression that occurs in common grief reactions.

- **Derealization** is a perceptual reaction in which an individual becomes convinced that life or others are not real.

- **DSM-5** is the abbreviation for the *Diagnostic and Statistical Manual of Mental Disorders, Fifth Edition*, which is the handbook mental health professionals use to diagnose mental disorders.

- **The five stages of grief** are the stages that individuals often experience after the death of a loved one or even after a non-death-related loss. The stages are denial, anger, bargaining, depression, and acceptance.

- **Grief** is a healthy emotional reaction to the loss of another person.

- **V-code** is a DSM-5 designation for a mental condition that is not a disease or injury but results in symptoms or distress that may require some form of intervention.

Description

Bereavement counseling is used with clients who have lost a person or animal due to death. It is often used when a person experiences grief-related behaviors or thoughts that are extremely distressing and are impacting his or her daily functioning. This type of counseling aims to assist individuals in moving from bereavement through resolution or acceptance of the loss. This process is typically done through counseling, by assisting the client in processing his or her emotions and other reactions to the loss. Some common grief presentations that are treated in bereavement counseling include sadness, difficulty concentrating, anger, guilt, temporary decline in daily functioning, derealization, isolation, and frequent crying. Resolution of bereavement-related symptoms typically occurs over a matter of a few months, but when symptoms persist, it is called complicated grief. Complicated grief can occur due to trauma, if the client has a personality disorder, or if the client lacks some of the coping skills or resources to manage grief. Typically bereavement counseling is done in a brief therapy setting, while complicated grief is often done in a long-term setting.

The DSM-5 only lists bereavement as a "condition for further study." Bereavement symptoms may mimic different depressive disorders, but they often pass within a few months and do not meet full criteria for a depressive disorder. When an individual experiences severe and enduring depressive symptoms during bereavement, he or she will be a likely candidate for bereavement counseling. In addition, individuals with a predisposition to depression are vulnerable to experiencing significant challenges with bereavement or major episodes of depression.

Bereavement counseling assists clients through the different stages of grief. One model that explains the grief process was created by psychiatrist Elisabeth Kübler-Ross (1926–2004). She identified the "five stages of grief" in her book *On Death and Dying*. The five stages are denial, anger, bargaining, depression, and acceptance. Her research examined the emotional reactions of clients facing terminal cancer or other illnesses. It is important to note that the individuals do not experience the stages in a linear fashion, as some individuals will switch between several stages multiple times, while others may not experience anger or bargaining at all. In bereavement counseling, the counselor will seek to assess the client's coping skills and symptoms, while aiming to work with the client in moving toward the acceptance stage of grief and at least improved daily functioning. Some clients may grieve for several months, while others may grieve for over a year. Others may grieve for many years with very little improvement.

Bereavement counseling may also be used when a client is aware that he or she or a loved one will likely experience death due to a terminal illness or severe injury. This type of grief is called anticipatory grief, which occurs when a client experiences grief before a loved one dies. Clients may seek counseling services shortly after news of a loved one's terminal illness and likely probability of death as a result.

Jon Sperry, PhD, and Len Sperry, MD, PhD

See also: Bereavement; Kübler-Ross, Elisabeth (1926–2004)

Further Reading

American Psychiatric Association. *Diagnostic and Statistical Manual of Mental Disorders*, 5th ed. Arlington, VA: American Psychiatric Association Press, 2013.
Kübler-Ross, Elisabeth. *On Death and Dying*. New York, NY: Routledge, 1969.
Worden, J. William. *Grief Counseling and Grief Therapy*, 3rd ed. New York, NY: Springer, 2002.

Best Practices

Best practices are methods that have consistently shown results superior to those achieved with other means and that are used as benchmarks.

Definitions

- **Accountability** is the expectation or requirement to conduct evaluations and report performance information.

- **Benchmark** is a standard by which a product or clinical activity can be measured or evaluated.

- **Evidence-based practice** is a form of practice that is based on the integration of the best research evidence with clinical expertise and client values.

- **Health Maintenance Organization** is an organization that provides or arranges managed care.

- **Managed care** is a system of health care that controls costs by placing limits on physicians' fees and by restricting access to certain medical procedures and providers.

- **Practice** is a method or process used to accomplish a goal or objective.

Description

Best practices are methods, procedures, or processes that have been proven to be superior to other methods, procedures, or processes. Benchmarking is a means of comparing various methods and is essential in creating new best practices. Best practices come about when better ways of doing things are discovered. Regular use of best practices leads to consistent outcomes. Best practices improve the quality of a process, and consistency is improved through their use. While the term "best practices" begins in business settings, it is increasingly common in health and mental health settings.

Development and Current Status

The development of best practices in health and mental health care has its roots in managed care. In 1973, the U.S. Congress mandated changes in health care that led to the creation and adoption of best practices. The goal of best practices in business is to increase process efficiency and profit margins. In contrast, the goal of best practices in health and mental health care is to improve clinical outcomes and reduce costs.

Several changes in mental health and psychological services in the United States have occurred in the past two decades. Many of these changes are the result of the increasing expectation for accountability. Increasingly, medical and psychological practice has become more accountable and evidence based. In 2001, the Institute of Medicine defined evidence-based practice (EBP) in medicine as the integration of best research evidence with clinical expertise and patient values. In 2005, the American Psychological Association modified that definition by including client characteristics, culture, and preferences.

It should be noted that EBP is broader than the concept of best practices because it explicitly considers research evidence, client values, and clinician expertise, that is, utilizing clinical skills and past experience to rapidly identify the client's health status, diagnosis, risks and benefits, and personal values and expectations. The current status of best practice is directly related to EBP.

Len Sperry, MD, PhD, and Layven Reguero, MEd

See also: Evidence-Based Practice

Further Reading

American Psychological Association. *American Psychological Association Statement Policy Statement on Evidence-Based Practice in Psychology.* Washington, DC, 2005. http://www.apa.org/practice/resources/evidence/index.aspx.

Drisko, Jim, and Melissa Grady. *Evidence-Based Practice in Clinical Social Work.* New York, NY: Springer, 2013.

Norcross, John C., Larry E. Beutler, and Ronald F. Levant, eds. *Evidence-Based Practices in Mental Health.* Washington, DC: American Psychological Association, 2006.

Beyond Freedom and Dignity (Book)

Beyond Freedom and Dignity is a book written by Dr. B. F. Skinner that highlights his ideas about human behavior and the process of changing human behavior.

Description

Beyond Freedom and Dignity is the name of a book written by American psychologist B.F. Skinner and was first published in 1971. The book challenges the concept of dignity, which Skinner refers to as free will and moral individuality. Instead of the traditional idea that based human choice and development on morality, he took a different approach. He used scientific methods to modify behavior for the purpose of building a happier and better-organized society.

Expanding on the ideas of John B. Watson, Skinner's research led him to believe that human beings are not independent of their physical, social, and cultural environment. He argued that human free will is both false and misleading. This is because Skinner demonstrated that human behavior could be manipulated through both negative and positive reinforcements. In the book he hopes to teach people that we are fooled if we think humans have freedom and free will. This teaching was based on the fact that he proved how actions are both predictable and controllable. Through scientific research he claimed that behavior is based on rewards or punishments.

Perhaps helped by a negative reaction to the freedom movement of the late 1960s, Skinner's ideas presented in *Beyond Freedom and Dignity* struck a chord with many people. This included psychologists, who believed that environment and genetics were important because they molded human decision making. The widespread popularity of the ideas Skinner wrote about in this book helped reinforce a behaviorist approach. This happened within the field of psychology but also in the fields of education and business. The importance of both positive and negative environments in shaping how decisions are made contradicted the concept of free will.

Current Status and Impact (Psychological Influence)

The central insight of behaviorism is the awareness that our activities and choices are heavily influenced by social and environmental factors. This includes things that are rewarding and discouraging. *Beyond Freedom and Dignity* helped popularize the concept, and its principles continue to be represented in higher education.

Although many disliked Skinner's approach, his ideas remain central to the way we understand human behavior. He was one of the first people to use applied behavior analysis to understand human development. He placed this in the context of Individual Psychology as it applies to the environment and people collectively. *Beyond Freedom and Dignity* portrayed these concepts and helped society become aware of human behavior and ways to be as productive as possible in changing it.

Alexandra Cunningham, PhD, and
William M. Cunningham, MA

See also: Applied Behavior Analysis; Behavior Therapy with Children; Skinner, B.F. (1904–1990)

Further Reading

Skinner, Burrhus Frederic. *Beyond Freedom and Dignity.* New York, NY: Bantam Books, 1972.
Toates, F. *Burrhus F. Skinner: The Shaper of Behavior.* Hampshire, UK: Palgrave Macmillan, 2009.

Bibliotherapy

Bibliotherapy is an adjunct to psychological treatment, particularly psychotherapy, which incorporates written materials that are read outside of treatment sessions.

Definitions

- **Adjunct** is a form of treatment that, while not required, can be helpful to the treatment process.

- **Agoraphobia** is anxiety about or avoidance of places or situations from which escape may be difficult or help might not be available in the event of having panic symptoms.

- **Cognitive behavioral therapy** is a form of psychotherapy that emphasizes the correction of distorted thinking patterns and change of maladaptive behaviors.

- **Psychoeducation** is a component of many psychological treatments in which patients are provided knowledge about their psychological condition, its causes, and how a particular treatment might reduce their symptoms and/or increase their functioning.

Description

Bibliotherapy is a form of treatment in which structured readings are used as an adjunct to psychological treatments, particularly psychotherapy. These readings, including biographies, workbooks, and short stories, are used to reinforce learning or insights gained in the therapy. They can also provide additional professional resources to foster personal growth and development. Bibliotherapy has been utilized in a variety of treatment settings for various psychological conditions, including eating disorders, depression, bipolar disorders, agoraphobia, alcohol and substance disorders, and stress-related health conditions.

The goal of bibliotherapy is to increase the patient's understanding of his or her condition or problem that requires treatment. The written materials are used to educate the patient about the condition itself and to increase the patient's acceptance of a proposed treatment. Commonly, reading about one's condition outside of the therapy sessions encourages more active participation in the treatment process and fosters personal responsibility for recovery. Many patients are relieved to learn that others have had the same condition or problem and have been able to successfully cope with or recover from it. Therapists who prescribe bibliotherapy often find that it accelerates treatment progress.

Commonly, bibliotherapy is used as an adjunct to conventional psychotherapy approaches. It is commonly used in cognitive behavior therapy in the developing individualized treatment plans and workbooks for specific disorders. For example, patients with eating disorders, especially bulimia nervosa, can benefit from reading educational information appropriate to their stage of recovery, such as books or articles about cultural biases regarding weight, attractiveness, and dieting. Such information can help patients better understand the rationale for their treatment. In this regard, bibliotherapy is similar to psychoeducation.

Developments and Current Status

For many, written material can reinforce their commitment to getting better. Those who lack the time or finances to participate in weekly psychotherapy sessions may often find that bibliotherapy can bridge the gap between less frequently scheduled appointments. For those experiencing agoraphobia or similar psychological conditions that can preclude in-office treatment, bibliotherapy can be most beneficial. Research indicates that it can be highly effective in helping individuals with agoraphobia better understand and cope with their symptoms.

As with any form of treatment, bibliotherapy is effective to the extent to which it actively engages the patient's desire and readiness for change. The use of bibliotherapy in the form of additional information and workbooks can greatly reinforce the patient's commitment to change.

Len Sperry, MD, PhD

See also: Agoraphobia; Cognitive Behavior Therapy; Psychoeducation; Psychotherapy

Further Reading

Joshua, Janice M., and Donna DiMenna. *Read Two Books and Let's Talk Next Week: Using Bibliotherapy in Clinical Practice.* New York, NY: Wiley, 2001.

Kaywell, Joan. *Using Literature to Help Troubled Teenagers Cope with Abuse Issues.* Santa Barbara, CA: Greenwood, 2004.

Shechtman, Zipora. *Treating Child and Adolescent Aggression through Bibliotherapy.* New York, NY: Springer, 2009.

Binge Drinking

Binge drinking is an irregular episode of heavy alcohol consumption.

Definitions

- **Alcohol abuse disorder** is a mental disorder involving a pattern of problematic alcohol use that leads to significant problems for the user.

- **Alcohol intoxication** is the impairment of ability following the ingestion of alcohol.

- **Alcoholism** is a general term for the compulsive and uncontrolled consumption of alcohol to the detriment of the drinker's health, relationships, and social standing.

- **Standard drink** is considered 12 ounces of beer, 5 ounces of wine, or 1.5 ounces of liquor.

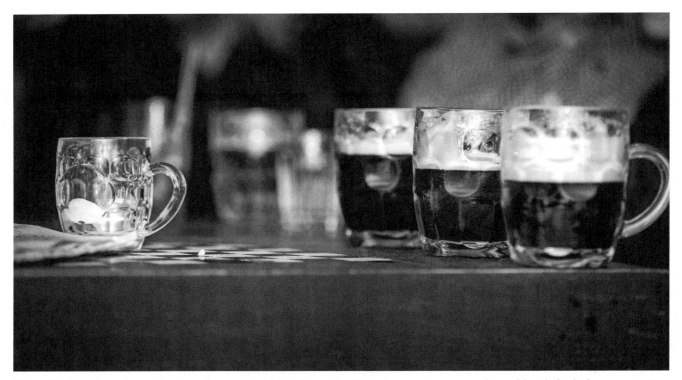

Binge drinking describes episodes of excessive alcohol intoxication where a person reaches a blood alcohol concentration level of 0.08 g/dL. That typically means a person having five alcoholic drinks in two hours for men and four alcoholic drinks within two hours for women, according to the National Institute on Abuse of Alcohol and Alcoholism. (Andreaobzerova/Dreamstime.com)

Description

Binge drinking describes intermittent episodes of excessive drinking that result in alcohol intoxication. The amount of alcohol considered to be excessive in one episode is five standard drinks for men and four for women. Although individuals who binge drink may drink in excess regularly, usually this is not on a daily basis. In contrast, excessive drinking on a daily basis is likely to result in an alcohol abuse disorder or alcoholism.

Binge drinking is most common among young adults, particularly men rather than women. The likelihood of individuals' binge drinking increases if they are college students. This is especially true if they are involved with a fraternity or sorority. It follows that young adults who value "partying" in college also tend to binge drink more than those who do not. A large survey of college students (Courtney and Polich, 2009) found that 44% qualified as binge drinkers. In addition, there is a correlation between those who begin to drink in high school and those who binge drink in early adulthood.

Although this behavior may or may not qualify as alcohol abuse disorder, there are often significant consequences to binge drinking. One of the most likely outcomes is significant impairment of judgment. As a result, binge drinking individuals may act in unusual, harmful, or dangerous ways. For example, drunk driving and unprotected sex may be caused by alcohol intoxication and binge drinking. Furthermore, the consequences of binge drinking are considered to be the leading cause of injury and death in college students in the United States. These are most likely to occur because of car accidents.

Treatment

Binge drinking in itself is not considered a medical condition or mental disorder. Therefore, there is no formal treatment for binge drinking. However, on college campuses prevention programs are commonly used to control this behavior. Another approach is to increase enforcement of the legal drinking age. These programs are generally ineffective.

Jeremy Connelly, MEd, and Len Sperry, MD, PhD

See also: Alcohol Use Disorder

Further Reading

Courtney, K., and J. Polich. "Binge Drinking in Young Adults: Data, Definitions, and Determinants." *Psychological Bulletin* 135 (2009): 142–156.

Miller, William R., and Ricardo F. Muñoz. *Controlling Your Drinking: Tools to Make Moderation Work for You*, 2nd ed. New York, NY: Guilford Press, 2013.

Watson, Stephanie. *Binge Drinking*. Minneapolis, MN: Essential Library/ABDO Publishing, 2011.

Binge Eating Disorder

Binge eating disorder is a mental disorder characterized by binge eating without subsequent purging episodes.

Definitions

- **Addiction** is a persistent, compulsive dependence on a substance or a behavior.

- **Anorexia nervosa** is an eating disorder characterized by refusal to maintain minimal normal body weight along with a fear of weight gain and a distorted body image.

- **Bariatric surgery** is a surgical procedure on the stomach and/or intestines to help those who are extremely obese lose weight. It is also called weight loss surgery.

- **Binge eating** is a pattern of disordered eating consisting of episodes of uncontrolled intake of food.

- **Cognitive behavior therapy** is a form of counseling or psychotherapy that focuses on changing maladaptive (faulty) behaviors, emotions, and thoughts. It is also known as CBT.

- **Eating disorder** is a class of mental disorders that are characterized by difficulties with too much, too little, or unhealthy food intake and may include distorted body image.

- **Obesity** is an excessive accumulation of body fat, usually 20% or more over an individual's ideal body weight.

Description and Diagnosis

Binge eating is central to this disorder, and it involves eating a large quantity of food in a short time. Individuals with binge eating disorder binge regularly for several months. They believe that they cannot control their eating at the time and feel unhappy and upset about it afterward. Binge episodes are experienced as a type of "out-of-body" or "trance-like" experience where the individuals with this disorder experience a loss of control. Individuals with this disorder seem to live from one diet to another and are preoccupied with the need to lose and maintain weight loss. They are often extremely embarrassed by weight gain and are likely to isolate themselves from others.

Binge eating is also central to another eating disorder called bulimia nervosa. But it differs in that those with binge eating disorder do not use purging methods like vomiting or laxatives. Typically, this disorder often leads to obesity. But it also occurs in normal-weight individuals. Obese individuals suffer significantly more medical challenges, such as hypertension (high blood pressure), stroke, heart disease, sleep problems, type 2 diabetes, colon cancer, and breast cancer. Individuals engaging in binge eating often look to diets to help control binge eating.

Binge eating disorder is more prevalent in females but occurs more often in males than do other eating disorders. It is common in individuals who seek treatment for weight loss. Often the client lacks awareness of the psychological or psychiatric components of the disorder. Binge eating is also seen in many seeking bariatric surgery. This disorder usually begins in adolescence and does tend to run in families.

According to the *Diagnostic and Statistical Manual of Mental Disorders, Fifth Edition*, individuals can be diagnosed with this disorder if they exhibit a pattern of consuming excessive amounts of food in a relatively short amount of time (two hours or less) and engage in this bingeing behavior one or more times per week for at least a three-month period of time. A binge is an isolated period of eating in which the individual ingests enormous amounts of food, often at a rapid rate, eating to the point of physical discomfort. While it might be a common experience to witness one or two relatives engaging in binge eating at events like Thanksgiving dinner, the binge eating disorder involves engaging in this type of overeating from 1 to over 14 times per week. Individuals experience the binge as an "out of personal control" experience unrelated to the feeling of hunger. Bingeing often occurs in isolation due to embarrassment regarding the amount of food ingested and is usually accompanied by intense feelings of guilt. Binge eating is diagnosed if the binge occurs without purging and is not an active component of eating disorders like bulimia nervosa or anorexia nervosa. The degree of severity in binge eating ranges from mild with one to three episodes per week to extreme with 14 or more (American Psychiatric Association, 2013).

The cause of this disorder is not well understood. However, it appears to run in families, which may suggest a genetic predisposition to addiction (American Psychiatric Association, 2013). Cultural attitudes about body shape and weight also appear to play a role. Long-term dieting as well as psychological issues appear to increase the risk of this disorder. More specifically, stress, anxiety, and depression can lead to binge eating.

Treatment

The goals for treatment for this disorder are to reduce eating binges, to improve emotional well-being, and, often, to lose weight. Because it typically involves shame, poor self-image, self-disgust, and other negative emotions, counseling is directed at addressing these and other psychological issues. Most commonly, cognitive behavior therapy (CBT), in individual and/or group sessions, is the mainstay of treatment. CBT typically focuses on the situations and issues that trigger binge eating episodes. These include negative feelings about one's body or a depressed mood. If obesity is involved, weight loss counseling is used in addition to CBT. Medication may also play a role in the treatment of this disorder. While no medication is specifically designed to treat binge eating disorder, antidepressants such as Prozac can reduce the urge to binge

and treat associated symptoms like anxiety and depression. When bipolar disorder or a personality disorder is present, treatment is more challenging and may require hospitalization.

Len Sperry, MD, PhD

See also: Anorexia Nervosa; Bulimia Nervosa; Cognitive Behavior Therapy; Prozac (Fluoxetine)

Further Reading

American Psychiatric Association. *Diagnostic and Statistical Manual of Mental Disorders*, 5th ed. Arlington, VA: American Psychiatric Association Press, 2013.

Costin, Carolyn, Gwen Schubert Grabb, and Babette Rothschild. *8 Keys to Recovery from an Eating Disorder: Effective Strategies from Therapeutic Practice and Personal Experience*. New York, NY: W.W. Norton, 2012.

Siegel, Michele, Judith Brisman, and Margot Weinshel. *Surviving an Eating Disorder: Strategies for Family and Friends*, 3rd ed. New York, NY: Harper Perennial, 2009.

Biofeedback

Like any other skill, individuals can learn how to regulate certain unconscious reactions in their bodies. For example, any person—even children—can master how to regulate body temperature with his or her mind. In fact, with proper training, a person can learn how to regulate his or her breathing, muscle tension, heart rate, blood pressure, and even brain waves. To learn these mind–body skills, individuals require the proper instruction and minute-to-minute updates on their bodies' current status. Biofeedback provides this constant stream of information. These streaming updates are critical for a person to understand how his or her body reacts to certain stimuli.

Description

Biofeedback is both the process and device used to train individuals to regulate their own physiologic functions. By giving the individual constant, moment-to-moment updates on specific physiologic functions like heart rate and breathing, this therapy allows him or her to master control over what would otherwise be unconscious bodily reactions.

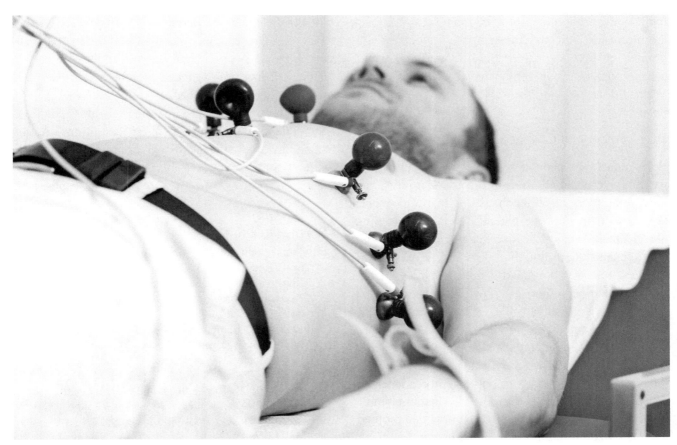

Biofeedback is both the process and device used to train individuals to regulate their own physiologic functions. Biofeedback instruments may include electrodermographs (EDG), capnometers, feedback thermometers, electrocardiographs (ECG), rheoencephalographs (REG), electroencephalograph (EEG) or "neurofeedback," and photoplethysmographs (PPG). (Arne9001/Dreamstime.com)

Biofeedback is a noninvasive therapy that allows a patient to take control of his or her own well-being. It sharpens the mind's hold over various reactions in the body. Through a series of specialized trainings, biofeedback allows an individual to recognize how certain thoughts, situations, or emotions may trigger unhealthy spikes in heart rate, stress levels, blood pressure, or surface temperature.

These biofeedback treatments (or trainings) are focused on the individual. Every patient is different and therefore learns at a different rate and responds to different stimuli. When undergoing biofeedback therapy, a patient is connected to specialized biofeedback equipment that gives the patient constant visual or auditory signals about bodily reactions. In other words,

patients see and hear in real time how their bodies are reacting to various situations.

With this constant stream of information, patients can be trained to manage these reactions. Like physical therapy, patients are encouraged to train and practice at these sessions with a specialized therapist to control these reactions. Through constant repetition, almost anyone can master this type of training, which is why biofeedback is often compared to other trainable skills like learning a language or learning to catch a ball.

One of the most common forms of biofeedback is surface electromyography, which is used to treat many different conditions including chronic pain and joint dysfunction. Other biofeedback instruments include electrodermographs, capnometers, feedback thermometers, electrocardiographs, rheoencephalographs, electroencephalograph or "neurofeedback," and photoplethysmographs, which treat a wide range of conditions.

Development and Current Status

Biofeedback has been extremely effective in helping patients overcome all kinds of disorders, injuries, and conditions. Various biofeedback treatments have been known to help improve patients' memory, sleeping, muscle pain, tension headaches, migraines, anxiety, stress levels, attention-deficit disorder, urinary incontinence, epilepsy, Raynaud's disease, and phantom limb pain, among others.

Studies have shown that biofeedback can assist with learning and other cognitive functions. For example, one study demonstrated how college students used biofeedback to improve their academic performance. Another study showed how a portable biofeedback device allowed a soldier to overcome his insomnia in the middle of a warzone. Other studies show that biofeedback allowed children with various mental handicaps to improve their IQs.

Other studies still show that biofeedback can help adults—and even possibly adolescents—overcome addictions to alcohol, opiates, or other illegal substances. Interestingly, in one study, biofeedback doubled the recovery rate of drug dependence, and it also improved test subjects' ability to process information and focus their attention.

Biofeedback both is noninvasive and poses no known risks to the individual. In fact, biofeedback is often used successfully when other treatments or medications have failed. It's also used on pregnant or nursing women who cannot take other medications.

One drawback to biofeedback is the expense. Biofeedback devices and treatment can be costly. However, as technology is improving, new lower-cost options are becoming available, including some portable biofeedback devices that patients can use at home.

As a modern practice, biofeedback dates back to the mid-20th century. The term "biofeedback" itself was coined in 1969—at the same conference where the Bio-Feedback Research Society first formed. However, some researchers maintain that biofeedback actually began over a century ago in India with certain ancient forms of Yoga and breathing exercises that mimic modern biofeedback.

Today, biofeedback continues to offer solutions for patients with many different conditions. At the same time, biofeedback also gives patients some measure of control over their own health and wellness.

Mindy Parsons, PhD

Further Reading

Dehghani-Arani, Fateme, Reza Rostami, and Hosein Nadali. "Neurofeedback Training for Opiate Addiction: Improvement of Mental Health and Craving." *Applied Psychophysiology Biofeedback* 38 (2013): 133–141, doi:10.1007/s10484-013-9218-5.

Frank, Dana L., Lamees Khorshid, Jerome F. Kiffer, Christine S. Moravec, and Michael G. McKee. "Biofeedback in Medicine: Who, When, Why and How?" *Mental Health in Family Medicine* 7 (2010): 85–91.

Kemper, Kathi J. "Biofeedback and Mental Health." *Alternative and Complementary Therapies* 16, no. 4 (2010), doi:10.1089/act2010.16405.

McKee, Michael G. "Biofeedback: An Overview in the Context of Heart-Brain Medicine." *Cleveland Clinic Journal of Medicine* 75 (2008): 831–834.

McLay, Robert N., and James L. Spira. "Use of a Portable Biofeedback Device to Improve Insomnia in a Combat Zone, a Case Report." *Applied Psychophysiology Biofeedback* 34 (2009): 319–321, doi:10.1007/s10484-009-9104-3.

Organizations

Association of Applied Psychophysiology and Biofeedback
10200 West 44th Avenue, Suite 304
Wheat Ridge, CO 80033
Telephone: (800) 477-8892 or (303) 422-8436
E-mail: info@aapb.org
Website: www.aapb.org

Biofeedback Certification International Alliance
5310 Ward Road, Suite 201
Arvada, CO 80002
Telephone: (720) 502-5829
E-mail: info@bcia.org
Website: www.bcia.org

Biopsychosocial Model

Biopsychosocial model is a way of thinking about health and illness in terms of biological, psychological, and social factors rather than purely in biological terms.

Definitions

- **Biomedical** model of health and disease focuses primarily on biological factors and excludes psychological, environmental, and social influences.

- **Biochemical marker** is any substance in the urine, blood, or other bodily fluids that serves as an indicator of a medical condition.

- **Interdisciplinary** refers to the integration of two or more academic disciplines.

- **Schizophrenia** is a chronic mental disorder that affects behavior, thinking, and emotions, which make distinguishing between real and unreal experiences difficult.

Description

Biopsychosocial model is a way of integrating biological, psychological, and social factors to better understand an individual's experience of disease and illness. This model is used in many fields such as psychiatry, clinical psychology, health psychology, counseling, medicine, nursing, sociology, and clinical social work.

The "biopsychosocial model" was originally developed in 1980 by American psychiatrist George L. Engel (1913–1999), who viewed people as "united, biopsychosocial persons" rather than "biomedical persons" (Dowling, 2005, 2039). Engel promoted the movement from a purely medical model of disease that focuses on biological factors to a biopsychosocial model that incorporates psychological and social factors as well as biological variables. Under the medical model, both physical disease (i.e., diabetes) and mental illness (i.e., schizophrenia) are attributed to the dysfunction of core physical processes. From a biological standpoint, laboratory tests can detect and confirm diabetes or schizophrenia in a person; however, that person may not be experiencing any symptoms and may be completely unaware of any problem. When symptoms begin and how they are physically expressed is influenced by the interaction of psychological, social, and cultural factors *with* biological factors. The severity of a disease is also impacted from a combination of these factors. Psychological and social factors influence when, or even if, a person seeks medical care. Proper medical treatment may manage or eliminate a disease or illness but may not necessarily restore health. In this case, psychological and social influences may be operating as obstacles to the achievement of health. Also affecting the achievement of health is the quality of the patient–doctor relationship and the patient's trust in the physician.

The biomedical model does not take into account variables that aid in the explanation and treatment of mental illness. Engel's biopsychosocial model provides a framework to understand what causes disease and illness, why it appears when it does, the severity of the disease or illness, and how to treat it. It also takes into account the role of the physician and the entire health-care structure. This model helps explain why two people diagnosed with the same disease (measured by biochemical markers) may experience two very different health outcomes. One individual may consider his or her condition to be severe and experience distressing symptoms, while the other may view his or her condition to be mild and experience little symptom distress.

The biopsychosocial model has implications for mental health practitioners and the entire health-care structure. First, it suggests that the treatment of disease and illness necessitates the collaboration of an interdisciplinary team of practitioners from both the medical and mental health fields. Second, the biopsychosocial approach requires practitioners from different fields to understand the interrelationship of physical, psychological, and social factors, and incorporate them throughout the treatment process. This model illustrates that physical and psychological factors may be indirectly affected through health behaviors (e.g., sedentary lifestyle, excessive alcohol use, poor nutrition) and biological factors (e.g., diabetes). Third, practitioners must keep in mind that a purely medical model approach could lead to misdiagnosis. For example, a biochemical measure, such as a blood test, may indicate normal sugar levels in a sick patient or abnormal sugar levels in a healthy patient. Finally, the biopsychosocial model is the basis for behavioral medicine, which is the interdisciplinary approach to understanding, preventing, diagnosing, and treating medical conditions with behavioral aspects. Len Sperry (1943–), a physician and psychologist, has described a treatment approach based on this model called biopsychosocial therapy.

Christina Ladd, PhD, and Len Sperry, MD, PhD

See also: Biopsychosocial Therapy; Health Psychology; Mind–Body; Social Cognitive Theory

Further Reading

Campbell, William H., and Robert M. Rohrbaugh. *The Biopsychosocial Formulation Manual: A Guide for Mental Health Professionals*. New York, NY: Routledge, 2006.

Dowling, Scott A. "George Engel, M.D. (1913–1999)." *American Journal of Psychiatry* 162, no. 11 (2005): 2039.

Engel, George, L. "The Need for a New Medical Model: A Challenge for Biomedicine." *Science* 196 (1977): 129–136.

Sperry, Len. *Psychological Treatment of Chronic Illness: The Biopsychosocial Therapy Approach*. Washington, DC: American Psychological Association, 2006.

Biopsychosocial Therapy

Biopsychosocial therapy is an integrative approach to planning and implementing psychological treatment when biological factors are present along with psychological and sociocultural factors.

Definitions

- **Biopsychosocial perspective** is a way of thinking about health and illness in terms of biological, psychological, and social factors rather than purely in biological terms. It is also referred to as the biopsychosocial model.

- **Psychotherapy** is a psychological method for achieving desired changes in thinking, feeling, and behavior. It is also called therapeutic counseling.

- **Vulnerability** refers to an individual's unique susceptibility to develop a medical or psychological condition or express symptoms based on the individual's genes and psychological history.

Description

Biopsychosocial therapy is an integrative approach to planning and implementing psychological treatment which attends to biological, psychological, and sociocultural factors. Rather than being a "new" treatment or psychotherapy approach, it is a set of strategies for planning and implementing effective treatment interventions within a biopsychosocial (BPS) perspective. It uses basic treatment strategies and treatment tactics to tailor (customize) treatment to the particular needs of clients. Because of its comprehensive and integrative emphasis, biopsychosocial therapy is particularly useful with "difficult," "treatment-resistant" situations or where a medical conation complicates psychiatric (mental) conditions. These include chronic medical conditions like asthma, diabetes, cancer, and chronic fatigue syndrome. It includes depression and anxiety disorders that have not responded to conventional treatment. Also included are comorbid (simultaneous presence) conditions such as substance disorders with an anxiety disorder or heart disease with clinical depression.

Biopsychosocial therapy is based on the BPS perspective. This perspective is an integrative and comprehensive way of thinking about and treating medical and psychological conditions. Since then, it has increasingly influenced the fields of medicine, psychiatry, psychology, social work, and counseling. This perspective emphasizes three sets of vulnerabilities and resources: the biological, the psychological, and the sociocultural domains. In this perspective, stressors, client vulnerabilities and resources, and levels of functioning or impairments are central factors. Four basic premises underlie this perspective. First, a client's problems are best understood in terms of multi-causation involving biological, psychological, and social factors rather than a single etiology. Second, a client's problems are best understood in terms of a client's biological, psychological, and social vulnerabilities. Third, a client's problems are best understood as manifestations of the client's attempts to cope with stressors (biological, psychological, interpersonal, or environmental) given his or her vulnerabilities and resources. Finally, multimodal interventions are used to effect change.

The treatment process includes four phases: engagement, assessment, intervention, and maintenance/

termination. Tailoring treatment to the individual's need is essential at each phase. First, the individual is engaged in the treatment process. Second, an assessment is made of the individual's symptoms and maladaptive pattern. Third, interventions focus on modifying maladaptive patterns and achieving some integration of the chronic illness within the patient's expanded self-conception, such that the illness becomes a part of the self but does not fully define the self. Finally, the focus shifts to maintaining the change and, when appropriate, reducing the individual's reliance on the treatment relationship.

Development and Current Status

The BPS perspective was first proposed by psychiatrist George L. Engel (1913–1999) in a 1977 article in *Science*, where he described the need for a new medical model or perspective. He argued that the biomedical model had proved inadequate in the effective treatment of many patients with medical and psychiatric conditions. Instead, he outlined the BPS model.

Biopsychosocial therapy was formally described and articulated by psychiatrist Len Sperry in 1988 in an article entitled "Biopsychosocial Therapy: An Integrative Approach for Tailoring Treatment." Subsequent articles and books have elaborated this approach and its clinical applications.

The BPS perspective assumes that treatment of medical and mental conditions requires that clinicians (physicians, nurses, psychotherapists) address the biological, psychological, and social influences on a patient's functioning. The reason is that the workings of the body can affect the mind, just as the workings of the mind can affect the body. This means both a direct interaction between mind and body and indirect effects through intermediate factors. A growing body of scientific research indicates that patients' perceptions of health and threat of disease influence the likelihood that they will engage in health-promoting or treatment behaviors. These include taking medication, eating healthy foods, and engaging in physical activity. Research also suggests that when clinicians frame treatment recommendations in a BPS perspective, patients are more likely to better understand and follow such recommendations.

A noticeable shift is under way from a strictly biomedical perspective to a BPS perspective. The trend in U.S. health care is toward integrative care, as mandated by the Affordable Care Act. This focus on integrative services means that clinicians will gather more BPS information from their patients. Integration of professional services through integrated health teams means that patients' psychological and sociocultural needs will be addressed in addition to their biological needs. Members of integrative health teams (nurses, nutritionists, health psychologists, social workers, and professional counselors) will address all three aspects of the BPS perspective. This will allow physicians to focus primarily on biological factors.

Len Sperry, MD, PhD

See also: Biopsychosocial Model; Depression; Psychotherapy

Further Reading

Sperry, Len. "Biopsychosocial Therapy: Essential Strategies and Tactics." In *Brief Therapy with Individuals and Couples*, edited by Jon Carlson and Len Sperry, pp. 535–564. Phoenix, AZ: Zieg, Tucker, and Theisen, Inc., Publishers, 2000.

Sperry, Len. *Psychological Treatment of Chronic Illness: The Biopsychosocial Therapy Approach*. Washington, DC: American Psychological Association, 2006.

Sperry, Len, and Jonathan Sperry. *Case Conceptualization: Mastering This Competency with Ease and Confidence*. New York, NY: Routledge, 2012.

Bipolar Disorder

Bipolar disorder is a mental disorder characterized by a history of manic or hypomanic episodes, usually with one or more major depressive episodes.

Definitions

- **Bipolar and related disorders** are a group of mental disorders characterized by changes in mood and in energy (e.g., being highly irritable and impulsive while not needing sleep). These disorders include bipolar I disorder, bipolar II disorder, and cyclothymic disorder.

- **Cognitive behavior therapy** is a type of psychotherapy that focuses on maladaptive (faulty) behaviors, emotions, and thoughts. It is also called CBT.

- **Cyclothymic disorder** is a mental disorder characterized by alternating cycles of hypomanic and depressive periods with symptoms like those of bipolar disorder and major depressive disorder but of lesser severity.

- **Depression** is a sad mood or emotional state that is characterized by feelings of low self-worth or guilt and a reduced ability to enjoy life. It is not considered a mental disorder unless it significantly disrupts the individual's daily functioning.

- **Depressive disorders** are a group of mental disorders characterized by a sad or irritable mood and cognitive and physical changes that significantly disrupt the individual's daily functioning. These disorders include major depressive disorder, persistent depressive disorder, disruptive mood dysregulation, and premenstrual dysphoric disorder.

- **Depressive phase** is a mental state characterized by sad mood, reduced ability to enjoy life, and decreased energy or activity seen during the course of a bipolar disorder.

- **Hypomania** is a mental state similar to mania but less intense.

- **Major depressive disorder** is a mental disorder characterized by a depressed mood and other symptoms that interfere significantly with an individual's daily functioning. It is also referred to as clinical depression.

- **Mania** is a mental state of expansive, elevated, or irritable mood with increased energy or activity.

- **Manic phase** is a mental state characterized by expansive, elevated, or irritable mood with increased energy or activity seen during the course of a bipolar disorder.

- **SSRI** stands for selective serotonin reuptake inhibitors. They are a class of antidepressant medications that work by blocking the reabsorption of serotonin in nerve cells and raising its level in the brain.

Description and Diagnosis

Bipolar disorder is one of a group of bipolar and related disorders. It is characterized by manic or hypomanic episodes, usually with one or more major depressive episodes that cause clinically significant distress or disrupt everyday functioning. This disorder is often not recognized or is misdiagnosed as major depressive disorder by mental health professionals. Early in its course, bipolar disorder may masquerade as poor school or work performance or as alcohol or drug abuse problem. If left untreated, it tends to worsen and the individual experiences episodes of full-blown mania or depression. Bipolar disorder is a chronic condition. Research indicates that more than half of those diagnosed with this disorder had four or more episodes of mania and depression (Goodwin and Jamison, 1990). The *Diagnostic and Statistical Manual of Mental Disorders, Fifth Edition* (DSM-5), describes two variants of this disorder: bipolar I disorder and bipolar II disorder. Each will be described separately along with its diagnostic features.

Bipolar I disorder. Individuals with this type of bipolar disorder experience periods of mania followed by periods of depression. During the manic phase, they display considerable enthusiasm, hopefulness, confidence, and expansive self-esteem, often to the point of grandiosity. They tend to act impulsively while their thinking is expansive and creative, but distracted. Their enthusiasm contributes to sleeplessness, pressured speech, and increased social participation and to extreme choices that would not be made during non-manic periods. These symptoms reflect the individual's efforts to overcome challenges and create feelings of worth and excitement. While these manic episodes appear to neutralize their underlying discouragement, they create other problems. Largely this is because of their failure to consider the consequences of their actions during these manic periods. This failure later seems to contribute to intensified periods of hopelessness and despair and the inevitable depressive episode that follows.

According to the DSM-5, individuals can be diagnosed with this disorder if they exhibit episodes of persistently elevated, expansive, or irritable mood along with persistently increased goal-directed activity or energy. These episodes last for at least one week and are present most of the day. The mania itself includes elevated self-esteem and grandiosity, decreased need for sleep, increased talkativeness, flight of ideas or sense of racing thoughts, distractibility, and goal-directed behaviors and engagement in activities that have the potential for painful consequences. These symptoms must be significantly distressing and impair the individual's ability to function in important areas of life. Furthermore, these episodes cannot have been caused by substance use or a medical condition or another mental disorder (American Psychiatric Association, 2013).

Bipolar II disorder. The primary difference between bipolar I disorder and bipolar II disorder is the extent of the mania. Bipolar II is characterized by hypomania, which includes less extreme periods of manic features. Why do some individuals exhibit hypomania instead of mania? It may be that those with this bipolar II have a greater awareness of the potential consequences of their actions. This awareness may serve to inhibit the mania. Maybe their ambitions are not as lofty or self-contemptuous as those with a manic episode. It might be that their commitments to family and career serve to limit their mania. Or, the anticipated shame and guilt associated with the failure and disappointment associated with a manic episode serve to retard manic energy.

Unfortunately, there is little research to support these speculations. However, it may be that these are two very different disorders with very different origins. Clinical experience has shown that individuals diagnosed with major depressive disorder who also display hypomanic symptoms are quite different from those with only depressive symptoms. For one, they are likely to have more episodes of severe depressive symptoms, more impaired functioning, and other mental disorders. But even more important, over time these

individuals are more likely to "convert" (meet the criteria) to bipolar I disorder.

According to the DSM-5, individuals can be diagnosed with this disorder if they exhibit one episode of major depression and at least one hypomanic episode. These individuals must never display a full manic episode nor any psychotic feature. For these individuals, the hypomania itself may not significantly contribute to problems in daily functioning. The more significant disruption emerges from the depressed symptoms. These symptoms must be significantly distressing and impair the individual's ability to function in important areas of life. Furthermore, these episodes cannot have been caused by substance use or a medical condition or another mental disorder (American Psychiatric Association, 2013).

The cause of both variants of this disorder is not well understood. However, there is some evidence for genetic and physiological factors as causes or triggers for it (American Psychiatric Association, 2013). Since this disorder runs in families, there appears to be a genetic basis for it. Major depressive disorder, bipolar disorder, and cyclothymic disorder often occur together in families. This occurrence suggests that these mood disorders share similar causes. Levels of the neurotransmitter (brain chemical) called norepinephrine seem to influence bipolar symptoms. Low levels of norepinephrine are associated with depression, while high levels are associated with mania. Imbalanced hormones may be involved in causing or triggering bipolar disorder. An imbalance in hormones may be involved in causing or triggering bipolar disorder. For example, hormone changes related to childbirth may result in bipolar disorder. Environmental factors may also be involved. Stress, significant loss, abuse, or other traumatic experiences may play a role in the development of this disorder. Whether causative or not, stressful life events and alcohol or drug abuse can make the treatment of bipolar disorder more difficult.

Treatment

Effective treatment usually involves psychotherapy and medication for both variants of this disorder.

However, in bipolar II, clinician will be more attentive to the depressed features rather than to the mania, which is a primary focus in the treatment of bipolar I. Psychotherapy, particularly cognitive behavior therapy (CBT), can be quite helpful in increasing emotional regulation. The challenge is to better manage daily life challenges. CBT helps those with this disorder in two ways. The first is to identify unhealthy, negative beliefs and behaviors and replace them with more healthy and positive ones. The second is to identify triggers to both hypomanic and depressive episodes and better cope with upsetting situations. Medication may be helpful in emotional regulation. Medications like Lithium, Depakote, and Tegretol are particularly useful in regulating and stabilizing mood.

Len Sperry, MD, PhD

See also: Cognitive Behavior Therapy; Cyclothymic Disorder; Depression

Further Reading

American Psychiatric Association. *Diagnostic and Statistical Manual of Mental Disorders*, 5th ed. Arlington, VA: American Psychiatric Association Press, 2013.

Duke, Patty, and Gloria Hochman. *Brilliant Madness: Living with Manic Depressive Illness.* New York, NY: Bantam Books, 1997.

Goodwin, Frederick, and Kay Redford Jamison. *Manic-Depressive Illness.* New York, NY: Oxford University Press, 1990.

McManamy, John. *Living Well with Depression and Bipolar Disorder: What Your Doctor Doesn't Tell You . . . That You Need to Know.* New York, NY: William Morrow Paperbacks, 2007.

Miklowitz, David J. *The Bipolar Disorder Survival Guide: What You and Your Family Need to Know*, 2nd ed. New York, NY: The Guilford Press, 2011.

Birth Order

The term "birth order" refers to the rank or position of siblings by their age within a family unit.

Definitions

- **Middle child syndrome** is a phenomenon commonly used to refer to the psychological and emotional results, usually negative, that

a person experiences when wedged between older and younger siblings (typically in a three-child family).

- **Nature versus nurture** refers to the ongoing debate among professionals as to which factors contribute more to differences in personality, intellect, and psychological development, biological/genetic (nature) or environmental/social (nurture) contributors.

- **Sibling rivalry** refers to fighting, resentment, or feelings of animosity felt or displayed among brothers and sisters within a family.

Description

Birth order defines the rank order of brothers and sisters by age within a family. For centuries, theorists and researchers have hypothesized about the impact birth order has on personality, IQ, self-esteem, and overall psychological development. While some evidence suggests that one's position within one's family of origin has a profound effect, there is also research to support the contrary. Factors including parenting style, gender, financial constraints, and health concerns can also influence family dynamics and increase the likelihood of sibling rivalry.

Austrian psychologist Alfred Adler (1870–1937) was the first theorist to propose that birth order could be linked to commonalities among various personality types. Adler, himself a middle child, posited that one's position within a family could have lasting effects on how one perceives situations and progresses through tasks related to work, family, and friends (Adler termed this "lifestyle"). Firstborn children are commonly viewed as reliable, structured, successful, competitive, high achieving, and conscientious. Those who are middle children are often described as flexible, even-tempered, people-pleasers, peacemakers, social, and sometimes rebellious. Lastborn children, also known as youngest children or babies, may be characterized as uncomplicated, fun-loving, pampered, attention seekers, manipulative, and outgoing. Finally, those who grow up as only children are described as mature, diligent, conscientious, leaders, and oftentimes perfectionists. Though these characteristics are widely accepted, exceptions to these can and do exist. Likewise, variations in the traditional family structure can also result in distinctions, including situations that involve divorce, blended families, adoptions, and gap children (siblings who are separated by more than five years).

Current Status and Impact (Psychological Influence)

Research on birth order has been ongoing for decades, suggesting that this remains an area of interest to professionals in the fields of psychology, psychiatry, sociology, medicine, and education. Several of the studies, however, have lacked methodological rigor and adequate sample sizes. Findings, therefore, have been mixed, with some data pointing to the salience of familial rank while other results indicate that birth order does not necessarily leave an indelible mark on one's personality or behavior as was once believed. Family size, which determines birth order, is associated with certain social factors, including ethnicity, education level, and socioeconomic status. Recent evidence has linked birth order and IQ with data reporting that the more older siblings a person has, the lower that person's IQ is. Findings also indicate that birth order influences friendship and spousal choices with selections corresponding to similarities in personality. More rigorous studies are needed on this topic.

Melissa A. Mariani, PhD

See also: Adler, Alfred (1870–1937); Nature versus Nurture

Further Reading

Blair, Linda. *Birth Order: What Your Position in the Family Really Tells about Your Character.* London, UK: Hachette Digital, 2011.

Kluger, Jeffrey. *The Sibling Effect: What the Bonds among Brothers and Sisters Reveal about Us.* New York, NY: Riverhead Books, 2011.

Leman, Kevin. *The Birth Order Book: Why You Are the Way You Are.* Grand Rapids, MI: Revell Books, 2009.

Stewart, Alan E. "Issues in Birth Order Research Methodology: Perspectives from Individual Psychology." *The Journal of Individual Psychology* 68 (2012): 75–106.

Blended Families

Blended families, commonly known as stepfamilies, describe familial structures consisting of children and parents who are not necessarily biologically related to one another.

Definitions

- **Nuclear family**, or elementary family, defines a traditional family unit made up of a mother, a father, and their children.

- **Stepfamily** is another term used to describe a blended family, or a family unit consisting of parents and children who are not biologically related but formed as a result of parental separation, divorce, and possible remarriage.

Description

Blended families, or stepfamilies, are prevalent in today's society, and the traditional nuclear family can no longer be considered the norm. The term "blended" describes family units where the parents and children are not all biologically related but have formed after the ending of a previous relationship. Families that are blended include one or both of the parents whom have children with prior partners that join together through marriage, civil union, or simply by cohabiting. If the couple marries, the parent may be referred to as a "stepmother" or "stepfather" and siblings as "stepsister" or "stepbrother." Stepparents, though they may assume some to all of the responsibilities associated with their new child, have no legal parental rights unless they legally adopt the child(ren). In the United States alone it is estimated that blended families make up approximately 40% of couples with children. Given that over 60% of all marriages now end in divorce, the number of blended families has increased substantially. Statistics further indicate that one-third of all marriages in the United States are remarriages.

Fortunately, a biological connection among family members is not necessary in order to form healthy, caring bonds. However, the transition process involved with blended families can be difficult. If the previous

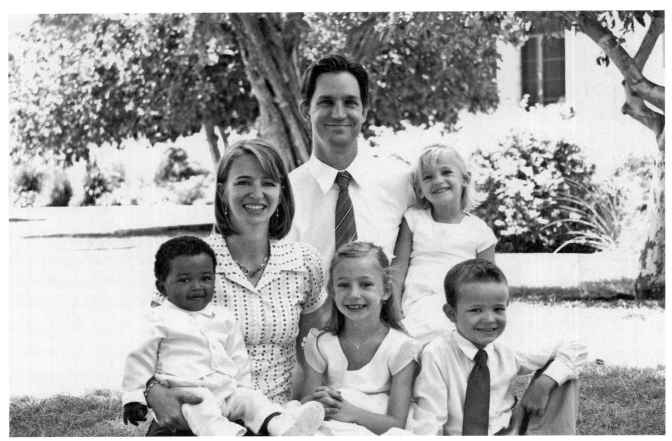

Blended families include those families where one or both parents who have children with other partners join together, whether through marriage, civil unions, or living together. (Ajphotos/Dreamstime.com)

relationship ended negatively, both adults and children may be suffering emotionally, which could place strain on the new unit. Divorce situations can cause angst, particularly if children still have hopes of parents reuniting. Custody disputes can add an additional level of stress. Adjusting to the new family structure, including roles and responsibilities, may take time. Often children resist discipline from their "new" parent, exhibiting overt misbehavior and disrespect. Others internalize pain and engage in destructive patterns that are harder to recognize and address.

Impact (Psychological Influence)

Families today experience more transitions than families of the past. Frequent marriages, quicker divorces, and more short-term cohabiting relationships are common for children and parents. Changes in living arrangements, parenting styles, and familial environments can have a profound impact on child/adolescent well-being. Difficulty accepting the new relationship and adjusting to different home expectations, rules, settings, and schedules can further complicate the process. Loss of familial stability can effect children socially, emotionally, and psychologically. Some may have a hard time maintaining healthy relationships, resulting from lack of trust and support. Research suggests that children from divorced families are at greater risk for delinquency; they display violent behaviors, use alcohol and drugs, and engage in sexual activity at higher rates than youngsters from intact families. Academic achievement also appears to be affected by family structure, with children from intact families performing better in school. Studies indicate that children from broken homes are more prone to hyperactivity, mood swings, anxiety, and depression than their counterparts. However, experts agree that regardless of the familial structure most children thrive in households that are stable, consistent, and caring.

Melissa A. Mariani, PhD

See also: Family Therapy and Family Counseling

Further Reading

Apel, Robert, and Catherine Kaukinen, "On the Relationship between Family Structure and Antisocial Behavior: Parental Cohabitation and Blended Households." *Criminology* 46, no. 1 (2008): 35–70.

Cherlin, Andrew J. *The Marriage-Go-Around: The State of Marriage and the Family in America Today*. New York, NY: Vintage, 2009.

Wisdom, Susan, and Jennifer Green. *Stepcoupling: Creating and Sustaining a Strong Marriage in Today's Blended Family*. New York, NY: Three Rivers Press, 2002.

Body Dysmorphic Disorder

Body dysmorphic disorder is a mental disorder characterized by an excessive preoccupation with an imaginary or minor defect in a part of the body.

Definitions

- **Cognitive behavior therapy** is a form of counseling and psychotherapy that focuses on changing maladaptive (faulty) behaviors, emotions, and thoughts. It is also known as CBT.

- **DSM-5** stands for the *Diagnostic and Statistical Manual of Mental Disorders, Fifth Edition*, which is a diagnostic system used by professionals to identify mental disorders with specific diagnostic criteria.

- **Muscle dysmorphia** is the obsessive belief that one is not muscular enough.

- **Obsessive-compulsive disorder** is a mental disorder characterized by persistent thoughts and compulsive actions, such as cleaning, checking, counting, or hoarding.

Description and Diagnosis

Body dysmorphic disorder is one of the classes of obsessive and compulsive and related disorders in DSM-5. All of these disorders involve some kind of obsessive preoccupation and/or compulsion. Body dysmorphic disorder involves a persistent preoccupation with a part of the body—usually the face, skin, or hair—that is perceived as defective or problematic. Unfortunately for those diagnosed with this disorder, their perceived defect is not recognized by others. Repeated attempts to reduce or eliminate the disorder fail. They also mentally compare their personal appearance to that of others. The extent of the individual's preoccupation causes significant distress or impairment in occupational, social, and other areas of life. There are gender differences in how this disorder presents. Males with it tend to be preoccupied with either genital or muscle dysmorphia. In contrast, females tend to be preoccupied with a wide range of appearance-based concerns.

Typically, those diagnosed with this disorder are ashamed of how they look and embarrassed about the amount of focus that they must put on their appearance. They are convinced that others perceive them as they do themselves and also believe that others are mocking them for these perceived defects. Because of the shame they experience and the belief that others notice their perceived defects, they tend to introverted, quiet, and reserved. They seldom have close, intimate friendships because of their shame, low self-esteem, and related social anxiety. They also may incorrectly and negatively interpret the facial expressions of others, especially in situations where the social cues are vague.

According to the *Diagnostic and Statistical Manual of Mental Disorders, Fifth Edition*, individuals can be diagnosed with this disorder if they exhibit a pattern of fixation and concern about perceived imperfections and flaws in their physical appearance even though these defects go unrecognized or seem minor to others. Some individuals are specifically concerned with having a deficient body build or muscle mass. They also have developed and engaged in repeated patterns in response to their concerns about their appearance.

Such repeated behaviors might include mirror checking, extreme and unnecessary grooming, exercising, or picking at their skin. In addition, individuals will engage in approval-seeking behaviors about their appearance from others. Mental acts of comparing personal appearance to that of others are common. These repeated behavioral and mental acts cause enough distress to impact social, occupational, and other areas of functioning. Preoccupation with appearance cannot be related or attributed to concerns about weight or body fat in persons who have been diagnosed with an eating disorder. Persons with body dysmorphic disorder may differ in their level of insight. In addition, those diagnosed with this disorder may have problems with executive functioning and visual processing (American Psychiatric Association, 2013).

The cause of this disorder is not fully understood. However, it may be genetic in origin and tends to run in families where obsessive-compulsive disorder is diagnosed. It is often associated with childhood abuse and neglect. Individuals may have grown up with limited opportunities to deal with life's demands and may have never "fit in" within the family, the school, or other social settings. As children, they may have developed repetitive patterns of evasion in response to their parent's expectations. Psychologically, individuals are likely to value perfection and believe that appearances are important. They tend to view themselves as defective and unique but unable to be acceptable to others. They tend to view the world as unsafe and that others find them disgusting. Low self-esteem, few social connections, and limited personal responsibility are likely to have predisposed them to be self-absorbed and focused on appearance.

Treatment

The clinical treatment of this disorder is a combination of medications and counseling or psychotherapy. Those with this disorder respond reasonably well to antidepressant medications such as Prozac, Luvox, and Paxil. They tend to require higher dosages of these medications than those who are being treated for depression with these drugs. Cognitive behavior therapy (CBT) is an effective approach to psychotherapy with these individuals. Because the disorder involves inaccurate self-perceptions and beliefs about their appearance, the focus of CBT is to challenge these beliefs. Because of their perfectionism, those who seek cosmetic plastic surgery typically end up feeling the same or worse. For this reason, many plastic surgeons routinely refer those who seek cosmetic surgery for a psychological evaluation prior to surgery.

Len Sperry, MD, PhD

See also: Cognitive Behavior Therapy; Luvox (Fluvoxamine); Obsessive-Compulsive Disorder; Paxil (Paroxetine); Prozac (Fluoxetine)

Further Reading

American Psychiatric Association. *Diagnostic and Statistical Manual of Mental Disorders*, 5th ed. Arlington, VA: American Psychiatric Association Press, 2013.

Nezirogl, Fugen, Sony Khemlani-Patel, and Melanie T. Santos. *Overcoming Body Dysmorphic Disorder: A Cognitive Behavioral Approach to Reclaiming Your Life*. Oakland, CA: New Harbinger Publications, 2013.

Wilhelm, Sabine, Katharine A. Phillips, and Gail Steketee. *Cognitive-Behavioral Therapy for Body Dysmorphic Disorder: A Treatment Manual*. New York, NY: Guilford Press, 2013.

Body Image

The term "body image" is often considered to be the way an individual views his or her body. However, body image also includes how a person thinks and feels about his or her body. Body image is influenced by how a person takes care of his or her body, the absence or presence of medical issues, and reactions from others. Negative thoughts about one's body image can lead to serious challenges, many of which are more common among women, including psychological distress, shame, anxiety, depression, low self-esteem, and even eating disorders.

Definition

Body image is a complex psychological concept that includes a subjective picture of one's own physical appearance that comes both from self-observation and from the reactions of others.

Body image can be negative when compared to unrealistic models for both men (muscular) and women (thin). However, women tend to experience body dissatisfaction more often than men. Body image is influenced from birth. Individuals develop their body image through a combination of their own thoughts and ideas, as well as feedback from their family, friends, culture, and society. While many may not be happy with their body image, there are some who are so unhappy that it may become a component to developing an eating disorder or lead to other mental health challenges, such as anxiety or depression.

Body image is a mental picture that individuals have when they think of what they look like not only to themselves but also to others. However, these thoughts are merely perceptions and may be extremely accurate on one end of the spectrum or completely inaccurate on the other end.

Body image is an important psychological concept because distorted self-views are widespread among American women and those self-views influence an individual's behavior. It is important to note that men are affected by negative body image as well, but it is more readily discussed and recognized in women. Some have taken the position that body image often has a negative connotation to it. There has been an idealized perception of body image that women maintain a thin frame and men have a muscular frame.

Those suffering from a negative body image tend to either avoid their thoughts and emotions regarding their image or take steps toward improving their perceived flaws. At times, this approach can lead to lower self-esteem or disordered eating.

Children and adolescents who report having positive family relationships tend to have higher body image satisfaction. Children and adolescents who sense their parents have negative thoughts about their body image can often hold negative self-views of their bodies. Eating disorders, such as anorexia nervosa or bulimia, have been on the rise since the 1950s. One of the key diagnostic factors is associated with having a negative poor body image, which causes great mental distress. Those working in the field have been calling for the focus to be on wellness and not on weight.

Body image is a constant topic of discussion everywhere from news programs to media. Society especially focuses on the body image of celebrities and is quick to scrutinize when an A-lister gains weight, even during pregnancy. For example, when pop singing sensation Christina Aguilera gained weight and moved from being a tiny starlet to a curvaceous figure, the media and public were quick to criticize her harshly. However, Christina took the platform to encourage people to love their bodies regardless of shape or size.

Dove is a soap company that has been working hard to focus on real beauty and looks to improve women's body image. In its 2013 advertising campaign, the company hired an FBI sketch artist to draw seven women as they described themselves. The artist was not able to see the women and was only able to ask questions having them describe their appearance. Then, strangers were asked to describe these same women to the artist. In each of the sketches, the ones that came from the women's self-descriptions were far less attractive than those that came from a stranger's description. The message was clear for everyone that women are often critical of their appearance and the goal should be to love and find beauty in themselves.

Mindy Parsons, PhD

See also: Anorexia Nervosa; Body Dysmorphic Disorder; Bulimia Nervosa; Eating Disorders; Self-Esteem

Further Reading

De Vignemont, Frederique. "Body Schema and Body Image—Pros and Cons." *Neuropsychologia* 48 (2010): 669–680.

Ganem, Paulina A., Hendrik de Heer, and Osvaldo F. Morera. "Does Body Dissatisfaction Predict Mental Health Outcomes in a Sample of Predominantly Hispanic College Students?" *Personality and Individual Differences* 46 (2009): 555–561.

Gilliland, M. Janice, Michael Windle, Jo Anne Grunbaum, Antronette Yancey, Deanna Hoelscher, Susan R. Tortolero, and Mark A. Schuster. "Body Image and Children's Mental Health Related Behaviors: Results from the Healthy Passages Study." *Journal of Pediatric Psychology* 32 (2006): 30–41.

Hall, Lindsey, and Leigh Cohn. *Bulimia: A Guide to Recovery*. Carlsbad, CA: Gurze Books, 2011.

Body Integrity Identity Disorder

Body integrity identity disorder is a condition characterized by an intense desire to have a healthy body part amputated. It is also known as amputee identity disorder.

Definitions

- **Body dysmorphic disorder** is a mental disorder characterized by an excessive preoccupation with an imaginary or minor defect in a part of the body.

- **DSM-5** stands for the *Diagnostic and Statistical Manual of Mental Disorders, Fifth Edition*, which is a diagnostic system used by professionals to identify mental disorders with specific diagnostic criteria.

- **Gender identity disorder** is a mental disorder characterized by significant dysphoria (discontent) with one's biological sex or the gender roles associated with that sex. It is also called gender dysphoria.

- **Proprioception** is the body's internal sense of its position in space and of the location of body parts in relation to one another.

- **Psychotherapy** is a psychological method for achieving desired changes in thinking, feeling, and behavior. It is also called therapeutic counseling.

Description and Diagnosis

Body integrity identity disorder is a mental disorder characterized by an intense desire, in a nonpsychotic individual, to have one or more body parts (usually limbs) removed by amputation. Usually, body part is healthy, functioning, and not deformed. Individuals with this disorder typically have an idealistic image or view of themselves as amputees and desire to have their body altered to conform to that image. They strongly believe that the body part is foreign or unwanted and will "feel complete" only when it is removed. They may use assistive devices (like crutches) in public in order to appear disabled. Almost always, they feel ashamed, embarrassed, or depressed.

The disorder was proposed for inclusion in DSM-5. But, because it is such a rare condition with very little research, it was not included as a separate disorder. However, it was considered as a possible subtype of body dysmorphic disorder. After serious review,

researchers noted a basic difference between the two disorders. Those with body dysmorphic disorder are excessively concerned about perceived defects in one or more features of their body and want to improve that feature. In contrast, those with body integrity identity disorder want to amputate the defective feature. Actually, this disorder is more similar to gender identity disorder in that the individual believes that a body part is alien to his or her sense of self, similar to the way in which a person with gender identity disorder believes that biological sex is alien to his or her sense of self.

The cause of the disorder is as of yet unknown. It may be that there is damage to the brain involving proprioception. As a result, individuals with this disorder have brains that fail to "recognize" the body parts that they want amputated. Another explanation is that this disorder may be an extension of body alteration methods that are so common today. These include body piercing, breast implants, and other plastic surgery alterations for aesthetic purposes.

Treatment

There is no definitive treatment for this disorder. For some individuals, surgical removal of the body part has been beneficial. However, because such surgery poses significant ethical concerns, it is not the treatment of choice. For others, psychotherapy may be helpful to deal more effectively with other problems in their lives.

Len Sperry, MD, PhD, and Jeremy Connelly, MEd

See also: Body Dysmorphic Disorder; *Diagnostic and Statistical Manual of Mental Disorders* (DSM); Gender Identity Development; Psychotherapy

Further Reading

Furth, Gregg M., and Robert Smith. *Amputee Identity Disorder: Information, Questions, Answers, and Recommendations about Self-Demand Amputation*. Bloomington, IN: AuthorHouse, 2000.

Rowland, David L., and Luca Incrocci. *Handbook of Sexual and Gender Identity Disorders*. Hoboken, NJ: John Wiley and Sons, Inc., 2008.

Stirn, Aglaja, Alexander Thiel, and Silvia Oddo. *Body Integrity Identity Disorder: Psychological, Neurobiological, Ethical and Legal Aspects*. Lengerich, Germany: Pabst Science Publishers, 2009.

Body Piercing

Acts of body piercing and tattooing are the two most common forms of what is known as body modification or body adornment. Although the history of body piercing dates back centuries, today's body piercing often has very different meanings and motivations. In fact, one's self-identity, a desire for beauty, and distinction from others are often the reasons cited for body piercing. However, there have been several studies that show individuals who engage in body piercing have higher incidence rates of sexual abuse, physical injury, and criminal history.

In addition, the body modification population shows tendencies for addictive behavior and often uses the piercings as a way to cope with trauma. Other studies have shown body piercings and tattoos to be strongly related to anger, substance abuse, eating disorders in adolescents, early sexual activity, and self-injury.

Body piercing has become increasingly more widespread in the United States, the United Kingdom, and Europe over the past 20 years. It falls under the category of body modification. This includes procedures that permanently alter a person's body, usually by puncturing the skin to insert a piece of jewelry. Body piercing and tattooing are the two most common forms of body modifications and are practiced by approximately 6.5% and 8.5% of the population, respectively. Piercings are commonly placed in the upper ear, nose, navel, lip, tongue, cheek, and uvula, and are most common among adolescents and young adults.

In history, body piercing was considered a form of cultural expression among a number of civilizations. It has been used to express religious, sexual, and cultural identities. Evidence shows that the Aztecs practiced ear piercing 4,000 years ago. Piercing of the nose has been common among Alaskan natives since the 19th century, tongue piercing was common among Mayan Indians, and genital piercing is mentioned in the *Kama Sutra*, which maintains evidence of penis piercings that included attaching jewelry.

Body piercing became increasingly common during the punk rock movement that began in the late 1970s in Europe. A counterculture was born in an effort to shock and provoke. This practice soon took root in the homosexual and sadomasochist population in the United States and Britain. Shortly thereafter, top music and film celebrities embraced body piercing. Emerging trends in body piercing also include brandings, which is scarring the body by applying heated materials to the skin.

Other forms of body piercing include cuttings, which are cuts in the skin using a sharp knife or blade, as well as implantations of three-dimensional objects placed under the skin to create a sculpture on the surface of the skin. Another form of body piercing is known as pocketing, which is a stapling of the flesh. Stretching or gauging is one form of piercing that is growing in popularity. It involves gradually expanding the ear lobe or any other part of the ear.

Significant medical risks are associated with body piercings. The risks vary in severity from infection and nerve damage to sterility and even death. The most common side effects are bleeding and bacterial and viral infections (e.g., viral hepatitis and HIV), as well as tissue damage and allergies.

Some social scientists believe that individuals who modify their bodies are motivated by rebellion and defiance. They believe that modifications of gauging, piercing, cutting, pocketing, tattoos, and so on, are a way of demonstrating their rejection of conformity to social standards and conventionality.

Mindy Parsons, PhD

See also: Stigma; Tattoos

Further Reading

Chalmers, Claire. "Charting the Existence and Approaches to Management of the Tattooing and Body Piercing Industry—A Historical Overview." *Journal of Infection Prevention* 10, no. 3 (2009): 102–105.

Stirn, Aglaja. "Body Piercing: Medical Consequences and Psychological Motivations." *The Lancet* 361 (2003): 1205–1215.

Stirn, Aglaja, Silvia Oddo, Ludmila Peregrinova, Swetlana Philipp, and Andreas Hinz. "Motivations for Body Piercings and Tattoos—The Role of Sexual Abuse and the Frequency of Body Modifications." *Psychiatry Research* 190 (2011): 359–363.

Body Work Therapies

Knowing the connection between mind and body, physiotherapists and other body work practitioners have developed physical treatments known as body work therapies to help reengage the mind's control over the body and heal or prevent other injuries to the body. A healthy mind has dominion over the body. Likewise, a person with an unhealthy mind or other injuries can lose control over his or her body.

Definition

- **Body work therapy** is a general term that refers to all physical and psychotherapy treatments involving movement or touch to heal the body. These body-based therapies are often designed to unite the body and the mind or heal other injuries in the body.

Description

Often classified as alternative medicine, body work can involve physical techniques, manipulative therapies, massage, and breath work. One goal of this type of therapy is to increase a person's awareness of his or her own body. This therapy can be used to improve posture, heal ongoing stress injuries (as in athletes or dancers), realign the body's structure, increase a person's movement, and even overcome emotional traumas like post-traumatic stress disorder. These body work therapies can take many forms. At times, it can involve deep-tissue work, while the patient lies in a passive state. At times, it can involve applying pressure on hypersensitive spots on the patient's body. At times, it can involve practicing Tai-Chi Chuan (Tai Chi) or other Zen relaxation techniques. At times, it can even involve talk therapy in conjunction with physical treatments.

Since each person is unique, body work therapies focus on addressing the individual. Body work practitioners stress the importance of empathy and intuition when working with new patients to address their specific needs. Examples of popular body work therapies include basic body awareness therapy (BBAT), the Alexander Technique, acupressure, Hellerwork, Shiatsu, Trigger Point Therapy, and Rolfing.

There are a few minor risks involved with body work therapy. For instance, anyone who has recently undergone surgery or suffered a serious injury should not begin body work therapy without first consulting his or her physician. Patients suffering from serious illnesses or infections should wait to start body work therapy. If patients are suffering from post-traumatic stress disorder, body work can trigger violent reactions, flashbacks, anxiety attacks, and feelings of rage. Also, some body work like Rolfing or Hellerwork can cause mild discomfort for new patients.

Development and Current Status

Interestingly, various forms of body work therapy have existed for centuries. One of the oldest forms of body work is Shiatsu, which was discovered in the early 20th century in Japan. However, Shiatsu evolved from an ancient form of Japanese massage that was practiced for centuries known as "Anma." Throughout the 20th and now 21st centuries, new body work practitioners, massage therapists, and physiotherapists have continued to develop new forms of body work therapies to treat all kinds of physical injuries, chronic pain, and emotional trauma. One of the most recent developments has been in using body work to treat mental illness. Scandinavian health services now regularly use a treatment known as BBAT to treat schizophrenia patients. Through various therapy sessions of movement, massage, Tai-Chi, and breathing, schizophrenic patients are often able to overcome or reduce the physical symptoms of schizophrenia like disembodiment, lack of mental awareness, loss of balance, loss of erect posture, or other bodily functions. After this therapy, schizophrenic patients also tended to have higher self-esteem, less anxiety, and an overall feeling that they have more ownership over their bodies.

The body–mind connection is extremely important in this type of therapy. Shiatsu specialists often work with post-traumatic stress disorder victims—including children—to help them overcome their recent emotional traumas. Specifically, Shiatsu has been known to help soldiers who have just returned from combat, children or other individuals who grew up in war zones, trauma victims with missing limbs, abuse victims who suffered from mental or physical abuse, and those who recently experienced a death of a loved one. Body work therapy continues to thrive as a recognized medical practice in both Eastern and Western medicine.

Mindy Parsons, PhD

See also: Psychotherapy

Further Reading

Ferguson, Pamela Ellen, Debra Persinger, and Marianne Steele. "Resolving Dilemmas through Bodywork." *International Journal of Therapeutic Massage and Bodywork* 3, no. 1 (2010): 41–47.

Hedlund, Lena, and Amanda Lundvik Gyllensten. "The Experiences of Basic Body Awareness Therapy in Patients with Schizophrenia." *Journal of Bodywork & Movement Therapies* 14 (2010): 245–254.

McNeill, Warrick, and Jon Gee. "Accessing Intuition in Massage and Bodywork Therapies Using Mindfulness, Knowledge, Empathy and Flow." *Journal of Bodywork & Movement Therapies* 17 (2013): 116–120.

Borderline Personality Disorder

Borderline personality disorder is a mental disorder characterized by a pattern of instability in interpersonal relationships, self-image, affects, self-harm, and a high degree of impulsivity.

Definitions

- **Brief psychotic episode** is a period in which an individual experiences psychotic symptoms such as hearing voices (hallucinations), paranoid thoughts, depersonalization (feeling unreal), or disorganized speech. The episode is usually triggered by substances, medications, or extreme stress.

- *Diagnostic and Statistical Manual of Mental Disorders* is the handbook mental health professionals use to diagnose mental disorders. The current edition (fifth) is known as DSM-5.

- **Dialectical behavior therapy** is a psychotherapy approach that focuses on coping with stress, regulating emotions, and improving relationships.

- **External locus of control** is the belief that one's life is controlled by forces outside the individual's control.

- **Idealizing** is the exaggeration of positive qualities and the minimization of negative qualities.

- **Mindfulness** is the moment-by-moment awareness of one's thoughts, feelings, sensations, and environment without evaluating or judging them.

- **Personality disorder** is a long-standing pattern of maladaptive (problematic) behavior, thoughts, and emotions that deviates from the accepted norms of an individual's culture.

- **Psychotherapy** is a psychological method for achieving desired changes in thinking, feeling, and behavior. It is also called therapeutic counseling.

- **Splitting** is the inability to synthesize (put together) contradictory qualities, such that the individual views others as either all good or all bad.

Description and Diagnosis

Borderline personality disorder is a personality disorder characterized by a pattern of unpredictability, impulsivity, troubled relationships, anger, mood swings, and self-destructive behavior. Individuals with borderline personalities present with a complex clinical picture, including diverse combinations of anger, anxiety, intense and labile affect, and brief disturbances of consciousness such as depersonalization and dissociation. In addition, their presentation includes chronic loneliness, a sense of emptiness, boredom, volatile interpersonal relations, identity confusion, and impulsive behavior that can include self-injury or self-mutilation. Stress can even precipitate a psychotic episode. Of all the personality disorders, they are more likely to have irregularities of circadian rhythms (physiological cycles), especially of the sleep–wake cycle. As a result, chronic insomnia is a common complaint.

The borderline personality in individuals is identified by the following: behavior style, interpersonal style, thinking style, and feeling style. Their behavioral style is characterized by physically self-damaging acts such as suicide gestures, self-mutilation, or the provocation of fights. They tend to accomplish less in their careers and socially than their intelligence and talents would suggest. Their interpersonal style tends to fluctuate quickly between idealizing and clinging to another individual to devaluing and opposing that individual. They are overly sensitive to rejection and abandonment feelings following even slight stressors. Their relationships tend to develop rather quickly and intensely. They are typically intolerant of being alone. As a result they seek out the company of others in indiscriminate sexual affairs, late-night phone calls, or after-hours emergency room visits with vague medical or psychiatric complaints. Their thinking style is best described as inflexible and impulsive. They reason by analogy from past experiences and have difficulty reasoning logically and learning from past mistakes. Because they have an external locus of control, borderlines usually blame others when things go wrong. By accepting responsibility for their own failings, borderlines believe they would feel even more powerless to change circumstances. They often have difficulty recalling images and feeling states which could make sense of their situation and soothe them in times of turmoil. Their inflexibility and impulsivity are further noted in their tendency toward splitting and an inability to tolerate frustration. Finally, because of difficulty in focusing attention and subsequent loss of relevant data, borderlines also have a diminished capacity to process information. Finally, their feeling style is characterized by marked mood shifts from a normal mood to a depressed mood. In addition, inappropriate and intense anger and rage may easily be triggered. Other feelings can include emptiness, a deep "void," or boredom.

The cause of this disorder is not well understood. However, these individuals tend to have characteristic view of themselves, the world, and others and a basic life strategy. They tend to view themselves defective and needy. They tend to view their world as unpredictable and hurtful. Accordingly, their basic life strategy and pattern is to expect others to take care of them and make them happy. They will not likely commit to anything and will reverse roles and vacillate in their thinking and feelings when under actual or perceived attack.

According to the *Diagnostic and Statistical Manual of Mental Disorders, Fifth Edition*, individuals can be diagnosed with this disorder if they exhibit a pervasive pattern of unstable relationships, emotional reactions, identity, and impulsivity. They engage in frantic efforts to avoid abandonment, whether it is real or imagined. Their interpersonal relationships are intense, unstable, and alternate between the extremes of idealization and devaluation. They have chronic identity issues and an unstable sense of self. Their impulsivity can result in self-damaging actions such as reckless driving or drug use, binge eating, or high-risk sex. These individuals engage in recurrent suicidal threats, gestures, acting out, or self-mutilating behavior. They can exhibit markedly reactive moods, chronic feelings of emptiness, emotional outbursts, and difficulty controlling their anger. They may also experience brief, stress-related paranoid thinking or brief psychotic episodes (American Psychiatric Association, 2013).

Treatment

The clinical treatment of this disorder typically involves psychotherapy and may include medication. Decisions about treatment goals and focus are best based on an assessment of the individuals for overall level of functioning. Higher-functioning borderlines have a greater probability for collaborating in psychotherapeutic treatment than the lower-functioning borderlines. Higher-functioning individuals with this disorder may be responsive to traditional psychotherapy that is focused on insight and solving problems of daily living. With lower-functioning individuals, treatment goals may be more limited. The focus of treatment is more likely to be on managing crises and achieving and maintaining more stable functioning. Dialectical behavior therapy (DBT) is one of the most effective treatment approaches with borderlines, particular with lower-functioning individuals. DBT incorporates four treatment components: individual therapy, skills training in a group, telephone contact, and therapist consultation. The rationale for the group component is that the intense interpersonal relationship that forms between the therapist and the client serves as the trigger for the client acting-out. Such acting-out is effectively reduced in a group format. Just as important, skills like emotion regulation and mindfulness are learned in this treatment format. Medication can also be used with this disorder. It is aimed at target symptoms such as impulsivity, insomnia, depression, or anxiety. Such medications include antidepressants, antianxiety, and antipsychotic drugs.

Len Sperry, MD, PhD

See also: Dialectical Behavior Therapy; Personality Disorders; Psychotherapy

Further Reading

American Psychiatric Association. *Diagnostic and Statistical Manual of Mental Disorders*, 5th ed. Arlington, VA: American Psychiatric Association, 2013.

Chapman, Alex L. *The Borderline Personality Disorder Survival Guide: Everything You Need to Know about Living with BPD*. Oakland, CA: New Harbinger Publications, 2008.

Dobbert, Duane L. *Understanding Personality Disorders: An Introduction*. Lanham, MD: Rowman and Littlefield Publishers, 2011.

Kreger, Randi. *The Essential Family Guide to Borderline Personality Disorder: New Tools and Techniques to Stop Walking on Eggshells*. Center City, MN: Hazelden Publishing, 2009.

Sperry, Len. *Handbook of Diagnosis and Treatment of the DSM-5 Personality Disorders*, 3rd ed. New York, NY: Routledge, 2016.

Van Dijk, Sheri. *DBT Made Simple: A Step-by-Step Guide to Dialectical Behavior Therapy*. Oakland, CA: New Harbinger Publications, 2013.

Bowen Family Systems Theory

Bowen family systems theory was developed in the 1950s by Dr. Murray Bowen (1913–1990), a psychiatrist and professor who is considered a pioneer in family therapy. The foundation of his systems theory is the belief that a family is best understood as an interconnected emotional unit and thus any therapeutic intervention needs to address the complex interactions among various family members in the context of the entire family system.

This approach to family counseling is strongly grounded in theory and has provided a majority of the mainstream language utilized when exploring and discussing family systems and family therapy. Bowen introduced the majority of mainstream language in regard to family systems therapy, including ordinal birth position, genograms, and differentiation of self.

Murray Bowen was born in 1913 and was the oldest of five children. He earned his MD from the University of Tennessee Medical School in 1937 and interned at Bellevue Hospital in New York City. His psychiatric training began in 1946 in Kansas. Bowen was also part of a five-year research project through the National Institutes of Mental Health. His research focused on parents and family members of schizophrenic children who had been hospitalized for extended periods of time.

Bowen believed that his efficacy as a therapist was directly linked to his understanding of natural systems theory, something he used as a guide for working with both families and individual patients. He held strongly to the science of human behavior, asserting that there was a difference between what a person was and what he or she felt, imagined, or said. Although there were critics, many agree that family systems theory is among the most fully developed, theoretically grounded views of the family.

Bowen also adopted the idea of family constellation to look at sibling position. This looks at the fixed and ordinal birth positions. Bowen believed that using the ordinal approach he could identify the role the children would play in the emotional aspect of the family life.

In order to help assess these patterns, Bowen was the first therapist to use a genogram. This tool provides a map or diagram of multiple generations and the relationships among the members. This allows for a way of organizing the important information about the family expanding at least three generations. This tool allows for understanding from both the therapist and the family members who now have a visualization of their relationships and patterns. The genogram includes names of family members and dates of birth, marriage, divorce, and death as well as cultural and ethnic origins, religious affiliation, socioeconomic status, and type of relationships.

Bowen also utilized process questions to encourage clients to consider the roles they play in relating with members of their family. He encouraged participants to speak directly to him as opposed to each other during the session. The questions were circular as the focus of change is in relation to others who are viewed as having an effect on functioning. Bowen also encouraged the use of I-positions, which are clear statements of personal opinion and belief that do not have emotional connections. This allows for members to communicate in a more rational manner.

Bowen therapists are concerned with changing individuals within the context of a system. Problems are viewed as stemming from relationship patterns in the family of origin. Therefore, the family of origin must be understood and patterns and relationships addressed.

Bowen therapists are central contributors to the American Association for Marriage and Family Therapy as well as to several current key academic journals such as *The Journal of Marital and Family Therapy*. This theory is actively taught and explored in graduate programs to future clinicians. Bowen's concept of a genogram has been adapted by several other theorists and actively used by many in the family therapy field.

Mindy Parsons, PhD

See also: Family Life Cycle; Family of Origin; Family Therapy and Family Counseling; Genograms; Identity and Identity Formation

Further Reading

Bitter, James R. *Theory and Practice of Family Therapy and Counseling*. Belmont, CA: Brooks/Cole, 2009.
Bowen, Murray. "The Use of Family Theory in Clinical Practice." *Comprehensive Psychiatry* 7 (1966): 345–374.
McGoldrick, Monica, Randy Gerson, and Sueli Petry. *Genograms: Assessment and Intervention*, 3rd ed. New York, NY: W.W. Norton, 2008.
Sperry, Len, Jon Carlson, and Paul R. Peluso. *Couples Therapy: Integrating Theory and Technique*, 2nd ed. Denver: Love Publishing Company, 2006.

Organizations

American Association for Marriage and Family Therapy
112 South Alfred Street
Alexandria, VA 22314–3061
Telephone: (703) 838–9808
Website: www.aamft.org

American Counseling Association

5999 Stevenson Ave.
Alexandria, VA 22304
Telephone: (800) 347-6647
Fax: (703) 823-0252
E-mail: info@aca.org
Website: http://www.counseling.org

The Bowen Center
4400 MacArthur Blvd. NW #103
Washington, DC 20007
Telephone: (202) 965-4400
Fax: (202) 965-1765
E-mail: info@thebowencenter.org
Website: www.thebowencenter.org

Brain

The brain is the organ at the center of the nervous system that controls all other organs and bodily functions.

Definitions

- **Autonomic** means involuntary or unconscious.

- **Central nervous system** is one of the two parts of the nervous system that contains the brain and the spinal cord.

- **Genes** are deoxyribonucleic acid or blueprints that create molecules called proteins. Genes determine heredity.

- **Glial cells** are cells in the central nervous system that provide support for surrounding neurons. Glial cells do not send electrical signals.

- **Homoeostasis** is the tendency of a system to regulate internal processes and maintain a stable and constant condition.

- **Magnetic resonance imaging** is a medical diagnostic test that uses magnetic fields to produce detailed images of the brain and internal organs. It is also referred to as MRI.

- **Nervous system** is the body's control system that is responsible for all voluntary and involuntary actions. It regulates chemical processes and responds to internal and external stimuli. It is made up of the central nervous system and the peripheral nervous system.

- **Neurons** are brain cells that process and send information throughout the body via electrical signals.

- **Neurotransmitters** are chemicals in the brain that send messages across synapses from one neuron to another neuron.

- **Peripheral nervous system** is one of the two parts of the nervous system that connects the central nervous system to the organs, muscles, blood vessels, and glands.

- **Psychotherapy** is a psychological method for achieving desired changes in thinking, feeling, and behavior. It is also called therapy and therapeutic counseling.

Description

The brain is the three-pound organ that controls everything an individual or animal does. It controls all conscious and unconscious processes. It initiates muscle activity and releases chemicals that allow a person or animal to quickly respond to environmental stimuli. In combination with the spinal cord and surrounding nerves, it makes up the central nervous system. The brain is considered in terms of two hemispheres. The right hemisphere is associated with abstract and creative functions and is responsible for induction, or reasoning from specific to general. The left hemisphere is associated with linear and rational functions and is responsible for deduction, or reasoning from general to specific. The brain is composed of three parts: the forebrain, the midbrain, and the hindbrain. The forebrain regulates sensory and information processing, instinctual functions, and voluntary functions. The midbrain regulates vision, hearing, motor control, temperature, sleep, and arousal. The hindbrain is the stem that connects the brain to the spinal cord. It regulates autonomic functions such as heart rate and breathing. It also helps maintain balance, provide movement coordination, and manage sensory information. One of the most important functions of the brain is homeostasis or the regulation of internal chemical processes to maintain a constant balance. The hypothalamus, located at the bottom of the forebrain, is primarily responsible for basic biological functions and homeostasis.

The brain regulates an individual's basic survival instincts and is the motivator that activates behavior to seek food, water, and shelter. It works on a reward-punishment system. When a behavior results in a positive consequence, the reward system produces chemical changes in the brain that cause that behavior to be repeated in similar situations. In contrast, when a behavior results in a negative consequence, the punishment system produces chemical changes in the brain that cause that behavior to be repressed or extinguished. The reward mechanism in the brain plays a significant role in drug and alcohol addiction.

The brain makes it possible for humans and other animals to learn from experiences and modify their behavior. In turn, modified behavior influences brain processes. Santiago Ramón y Cajal (1852–1934), a Spanish neuroscientist, claimed that when learning occurs, there are chemical changes that take place between neurons in the brain. It wasn't until 1971 that physical evidence was found by Terje Lomo (1930–) to support Cajal's claims.

The brain an individual is born with contains the majority of cells it will ever have. What determines brain growth after birth is how much or how little the connections between the brain cells develop. Genes produce proteins that work to connect brain cells. Although the genetics of a brain cannot be altered, the biochemical process within these proteins can. The brain contains two primary groups of cells, neurons and glial cells, which transmit signals to communicate between cells. The points of communication are called synapses. Neurotransmitters are released at synapses. Neurons work together to form a circuit. Circuits work together to form specialized brain systems. Different brain systems regulate functions such as language, perception, or decision making. Environmental influences have the capacity to activate or deactivate the chemical process between cells and impact brain development. Scientific research has shown that growth and development of the brain depends on both genes and experiences.

The debate on the relationship between the brain and mind was started by Rene Descartes (1596–1650) when he made the statement, "I think, therefore I am." The neural activity in the brain is necessary for language, cognitions, emotions, and overall existence of the mind. Researchers indicate that the mind is a complex function of the brain and when the brain is impaired, so is the mind. Similarly, problems with the mind (mental illness) can impair the brain's functioning. For example, depressive illnesses are disorders of the brain. Research studies using magnetic resonance imaging have shown that brains of depressed individuals appear different from individuals without depression. The brain functions that regulate mood, thoughts, behavior, the sleep–wake cycle, and appetite are affected by changes in serotonin levels. Antidepressant medication boosts neurotransmitter levels and assists in restoring homeostasis (balance). Medication in combination with psychotherapy usually results in the better outcome for many depressed individuals.

Christina Ladd, PhD, and Len Sperry, MD, PhD

See also: Depression; Split Brain

Further Reading

Ashwell, Ken, and Richard Restak. *The Brain Book: Development, Function, Disorder, Health.* Ontario, Canada: Firefly Books, 2012.

Greenfield, Susan A. *The Human Brain.* London, UK: Weidenfeld & Nicolson, 1997.

Shelton, C. D. *Brain Plasticity: Rethinking How the Brain Works.* Huntington Beach, CA: Choice PH, 2013.

Brain Imaging

Brain imaging is a set of medical diagnostic techniques for directly or indirectly imaging the structure and function of the brain. It is also known as neuroimaging.

Definitions

- **Brain electrical activity mapping** (BEAM) is a quantitative version of the electroencephalogram (EEG) test, which produces a colored schematic map of the head.

- **Computed tomography** (CT) is a medical diagnostic test in which computer-processed X-rays produce tomographs (cross-sectional images) of body areas.

- **Electroencephalography** is a medical diagnostic test that records electrical activity on the scalp to evaluate various brain functions and psychological disorders.

- **Magnetic resonance imaging** (MRI) is a diagnostic imaging device that uses electromagnetic radiation and a strong magnetic field to produce images of soft tissues.

- **Positron emission tomography** (PET) is a diagnostic imaging technique that uses radioactive substances to produce three-dimensional colored images within the body.

- **Single-photon emission computed tomography** (SPECT) is a diagnostic imaging device that uses gamma rays to produces images of the body.

Description

Brain imaging is a set of medical diagnostic techniques that are useful in providing images (pictures) of the brain used in detecting injury or disease. These images directly or indirectly identify the brain structures and functioning. There are six common types of brain imaging techniques currently in use. They are the EEG, computerized axial tomography (CT), the single-photon emission computed tomography (SPECT), positron emission tomography (PET), magnetic resonance imaging (MRI), and its related functional MRI scan (fMRI).

The first actual neuroimaging technique was the EEG. It was the first effort to measure brain physiology. By taping tiny metal electrodes on the top and sides of a patient's head, the EEG measures neuron-generated evoked potentials (electrical currents) on the surface of the brain. These EEG-generated potentials are valuable in that they measure the functionality of sensory and neuromuscular pathways. Thus, this type of neuroimaging is most commonly used to diagnose epilepsy and sleep disorders. A quantitative version of the EEG,

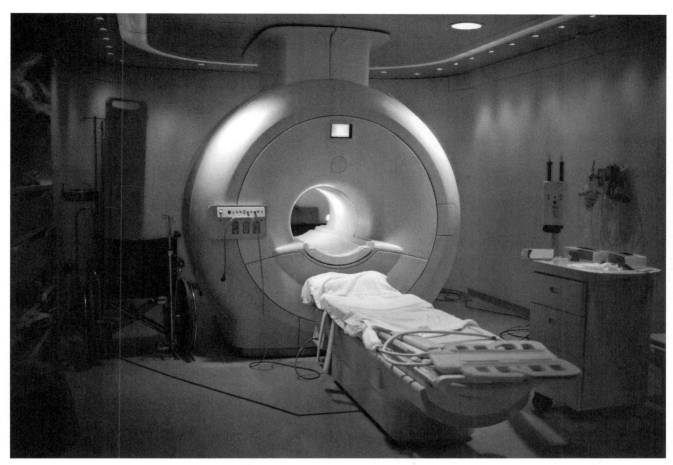

Brain imaging is a set of medical diagnostic techniques that are useful in providing pictures of the brain and used in detecting injury or disease. Magnetic resonance imaging (MRI) is often used for neuroimaging. (Melissa Connors/Dreamstime.com)

called brain electrical activity mapping (BEAM), produces a brain map with electrical potentials identified with colors. This brain map is particularly useful in the diagnosis of Alzheimer's disease and mild closed-head injuries.

Computerized axial tomography scan (CT scan) involves X-rays that move in a small circular arc and penetrate the patient's head. The different intensities of the X-rays measure the location of and variant density of brain tissue and are used by a computer to construct a composite picture of the brain. This type of neuroimaging can be used to identify blockages, clots, and bleeding in the brain. These pathological changes are visually represented on a computer screen. While the CT is effective in displaying brain anatomy, it cannot measure brain functioning. However, the SPECT is an extension of CT scanning that can assess functioning.

SPECT uses radioactive materials injected through a vein to generate high-resolution images. The SPECT scanner monitors the tracer's movement through body tissues. The rate of its radioactive decay allows the clinician to obtain three-dimensional images of blood flow in the heart or electrical activity in different areas of the brain. It can also scan for tumors or bone disease.

Positron emission tomography was the first neuroimaging device to create three-dimensional localization of brain function. PET requires patients to ingest (drink) or be injected with a radioactive substance. This substance emits positrons from which a computer image is generated as with CT scans. Tumors, lesions, and psychiatric abnormalities are visualized. In psychiatric conditions, PRT can identify metabolic activity in the brain. Low levels suggest conditions like depression, while high levels suggest conditions such as schizophrenia.

Magnetic resonance imaging scan is the most popular type of neuroimaging. Because it uses magnetic fields rather than X-rays, it is safer than a CT scan. By placing electromagnets around a patient's head, the MRI works by generating a visual representation of the brain's functioning. MRI is used to identify tumors, tissue degeneration, and blood clots. Like the CT scan, MRI scan provide only anatomical but not physiological information. However, the fMRI scan can provide such physiological or functional information. It is able to measure rapidly changing physiology and generate three-dimensional images of the brain. More specifically, it can measure blood and oxygen flow.

Developments and Current Status

Starting in 1850, clinicians and researchers used invasive techniques to examine the brain. Cutting open a living patient's skull to identify specific brain anatomy and functioning was the only available technique in the pre-neuroimaging era. The obvious advantage of all the neuroimaging techniques that were to emerge in the 20th century was that clinicians and researchers had a noninvasive view of the brain's anatomy and physiology while the patient remained conscious. In the 1920s the ventricles (cavities or open spaces) of the brain and spinal cord were first visualized with X-rays, as were normal and abnormal blood vessels in and around the brain. It was in the early 1970s that CT scanning became available for diagnostic and research purposes. In the early 1980s, SPECT and PET of the brain were introduced. In the late 1980s, the BEAM emerged. It was derived from the EEG. Except for the CT scan, these other imagining techniques were primarily used for research purposes. About the same time, MRI was developed. About 1990 fMRI became available. However, it was not until the early 2000s that brain imaging for clinical purposes became feasible.

Len Sperry, MD, PhD

See also: Computed Tomography (CT); Electroencephalogram (Brain Electrical Activity Mapping);

Magnetic Resonance Imaging (MRI); Positron Emission Tomography (PET); Single-Photon Emission Computed Tomography (SPECT)

Further Reading

Eisenberg, Ronald, and Alexander Margulis. *A Patient's Guide to Medical Imaging.* New York, NY: Oxford University Press, 2011.

Kastler, Bruno. *Understanding MRI*, 2nd ed. Berlin: Springer, 2008.

Levine, Harry III. *Medical Imaging.* Santa Barbara, CA: ABC-CLIO, 2010.

Breakfast Club, The (Movie)

The Breakfast Club (1985) was the second successful movie by writer and director John Hughes about the important, coming-of-age issues that face most teens in high school. The film is known for its accurate and believable dialogue and its realistic depiction of the problems that teenagers face.

Description

In this film, five teenagers are alienated not only from the adult world of their parents and teachers but also from each other because they come from different cliques or social groups in the school which makes them feel like they have nothing in common. All that ends on a long Saturday when the five end up being forced to spend an all-day detention together. The group starts with only a vague knowledge of one another which leads them to rely on stereotypes (classifications of other people by overly simplified conceptions, opinions, or images). Gradually, however, as the day wears on, the five t students open up to one another. The characters include John Bender, acted by Judd Nelson, who plays the "criminal"; Andrew Clark, played by Emilio Estevez, who is the "athlete"; Brian Johnson, played by Anthony Michael Hall, the "brain"; Allison Reynolds, played by Ally Sheedy, who is the "basket case"; and Claire Standish, played by Molly Ringwald, who is the "princess."

These five must remain together in the high school library for a period of 8 hours and 54 minutes: from

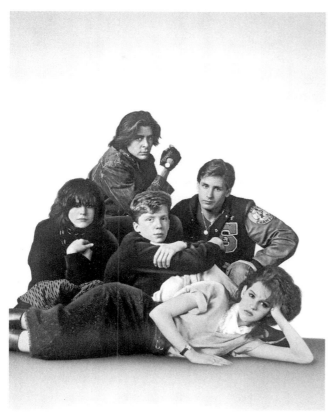

Although released thirty years ago, *The Breakfast Club* (1985), a film by writer-director John Hughes, still speaks to teenagers today. The movie shows teenagers who are alienated not only from the adult world of parents and teachers but also from each other because they come from different school cliques or social groups, making them feel that they have nothing in common. Left to right are Ally Sheedy, Judd Nelson (top), Anthony Michael Hall, Emilio Estevez, and front, Molly Ringwald. (Universal Pictures/Photofest)

exactly 7:06 a.m. to 4:00 p.m. They are instructed to write a 1,000-word essay, in which each student must write about who he or she thinks he or she is. Bender, who rejects authority, disregards the assignment and stirs up the other students.

The students spend the day fighting, talking, smoking marijuana, and dancing. Gradually they open up to each other and reveal their deepest personal secrets. They all discover that they have strained relationships with their parents and are afraid of making the same mistakes as the adults around them. As they grow more involved, they begin to fear that once detention is over they will return to their cliques and never speak to each other again.

Toward the end of the day, the other students ask Brian "the brain" to write the essay assigned earlier. But instead of writing about the given topic, Brian writes a letter objecting to the topic, stating that they have already been judged and labeled. Brian signs the essay on behalf of the group, "The Breakfast Club."

The theme that resonated with audiences was the sense of alienation not only from authority figures but between each of them as stereotyped teens. It is only when they realize how alike their struggles are, especially with their parents, that they become close. They discover that they are more alike than they are different.

Impact (Psychological Influence)

Similar to Hughes's earlier film *Sixteen Candles*, *The Breakfast Club* spoke to teenage problems and angst by taking its characters and their struggles seriously. It also directly addressed the cliques and stereotyping that is often typical of the teenage years, especially during high school. One of the main reasons why this film remains so influential and popular is its authenticity in portraying teenage issues, many of which transcend the time period of the movie.

Alexandra Cunningham, PhD, and
William M. Cunningham, MA

See also: Cliques; *Mean Girls* (Movie); *Sixteen Candles* (Movie)

Further Reading

The Breakfast Club. Directed by John Hughes, 1985. USA: Channel Productions, Universal Studios.
Ebert, Roger. 1985. "Breakfast Club Review." Accessed September 12, 2013. http://www.rogerebert.com/reviews/the-breakfast-club-1985.
Orient, Sio. *The Breakfast Club: Receiving Cult Status*. Culturbia: BBC2 Virtual Revolution, 2010.

Brief Dynamic Psychotherapy

Brief dynamic psychotherapy is a psychological treatment approach that focuses on maladaptive interpersonal patterns that are treated by facilitating new experiences.

Definitions

- **Attachment** is the emotional bond between children and caregivers that can provide a secure (healthy) base from which children are able to safely explore their environment and relate to others.

- **Cognitive behavior therapy** is a type of psychotherapy that focuses on maladaptive (problematic) behaviors, emotions, and thoughts. It is also called CBT.

- **Corrective emotional experience** is a treatment strategy in which a therapist provides a more supportive and new relational response as compared to the assumed expectations of the client.

- **Countertransference** is the unconscious redirection of feelings from the therapist to the client.

- **Cyclic maladaptive pattern** is the pattern (manner) in which a person relates to others and how it influences all aspects of an individual's life.

- **Insight** is the awareness that occurs when an individual attains a fuller understanding of self and others.

- **Interpretation** is a guess or hypothesis made by a therapist about the relationship between an individual's behaviors, thoughts, or emotions and his or her unconscious emotions or thoughts.

- **Psychoanalytic theory** is a psychological theory that explains behaviors and perceptions as the result of unconscious, sexual, and biological instincts. It was originally developed by Sigmund Freud.

- **Psychodynamic therapy** is a form of psychotherapy that emphasizes unconscious (outside awareness) conflicts and focuses on an individual's early childhood and dreams.

- **Psychotherapy** is a psychological method for achieving desired changes in thinking, feeling, and behavior. It is also called therapy and therapeutic counseling.

- **Transference** is the unconscious redirection of feelings from the client to the therapist.

Description

Brief dynamic psychotherapy is a shortened form of psychodynamic therapy. The roots of this approach are in Sigmund Freud's (1856–1939) psychoanalytic theory. The healing process that occurs in long-term psychoanalytic therapy typically requires years of therapy, while brief dynamic therapy can occur in a relatively short amount of time. Given the emphasis on cost savings in health care today, individuals are often eligible for only a limited amount of therapy sessions. Psychologist Hans H. Strupp (1921–2006) developed such a time-limited approach which he called brief dynamic psychotherapy. This approach can effect change in a relatively few sessions, usually 20 or less. Of the several brief approaches to psychotherapy used in clinical practice today, time-limited dynamic psychotherapy is a commonly used and research-based approach.

The goal in brief dynamic therapy is to provide individuals with new experiences of themselves and others through corrective emotional experiences provided in session. Other brief dynamic therapy strategies include interpretation, resolving transference, and fostering insight. Further, therapists aim to assist clients in understanding themselves and developing insight into their relationships by exploring unmet needs that are associated with early attachment figures. The brief dynamic therapy model assumes that individuals' maladaptive interpersonal patterns are reenacted in therapy, and the practitioner will be influenced by the client's dynamics. The therapist's countertransference toward the client also provides information about the client's cyclical maladaptive pattern. Countertransference and transference issues are used in this approach to modify preexisting relational, emotional, and behavioral patterns through in-session processing of these dynamics.

Human suffering, such as depression, is conceptualized from this perspective by examining faulty relationship patterns with caregivers, and these faulty patterns are commonly reflected in presenting symptoms and interpersonal distress. The client's cyclical maladaptive pattern is at the heart of conceptualizing an individual's presenting issues. The four relational components to assess are acts of self, expectations of others reactions, acts of others toward the self, and acts of the self toward the self. Acts of self include thoughts, feelings, wishes, motives, perceptions, and behaviors of the client. Expectations of others reactions include how the clients imagine others will react to them in response to their actions. Acts of others toward the self are the actual behaviors of others, as observed or perceived by the client. Finally, acts of the self toward the self are the clients' behaviors toward themselves and also their relationship with themselves.

Developments and Current Status

While Sigmund Freud's psychodynamic theories are a primary influence, more recent proponents of brief dynamic psychotherapy include Jeffrey L. Binder (1943–) and Hanna Levenson (1945–), who prefer the designation brief dynamic therapy. Both were mentored by Hans Strupp. A relatively small number of professional therapists exclusively use psychodynamic therapy in practice today. However, more therapists use elements of psychodynamic therapy to conceptualize their cases but implement cognitive behavior therapy techniques to treat their clients.

Len Sperry, MD, PhD, and Jon Sperry PhD

See also: Cognitive Behavior Therapy; Psychodynamic Psychotherapies; Psychotherapy

Further Reading

Binder, Jeffrey, L. *Key Competencies in Brief Dynamic Psychotherapy*. New York, NY: Guilford Press, 2004.

Levenson, Hanna. *Brief Dynamic Therapy*. Washington, DC: American Psychological Association, 2010.

Levenson, Hanna. *Time-Limited Dynamic Psychotherapy*. New York, NY: Basic Books, 1995.

Strupp, Hans H., and Jeffrey L. Binder. *Psychotherapy in a New Key*. New York, NY: Basic Boos, 1984.

Brief Psychotic Disorder

Brief psychotic disorder is a mental disorder characterized by psychotic symptoms with a sudden onset, short duration, and the full return of functioning. It is usually triggered by extreme stress. This disorder is also referred to as acute, transient, or reactive psychotic disorder.

Definitions

- **Antipsychotic medication drugs** are prescribed drugs that are intended to reduce psychotic symptoms. It is also known as neuroleptics.

- **Catatonia** is disorganized, limited, or complete absence of normal physical behavior.

- **Cognitive behavior therapy** is a type of psychotherapy that focuses on maladaptive (faulty) behaviors, emotions, and thoughts.

- **Delusions** are fixed false beliefs that persist despite contrary evidence.

- **Family therapy** is a type of psychotherapy for families that focuses on improving relationships and understanding between family members.

- **Hallucinations** are false or distorted sensory perceptions that appear to be real perceptions that are generated by the mind rather than by an external stimuli.

- **Psychotic symptoms** are a group of severe symptoms that include hallucinations, delusions, disordered thinking, or disorganized movement.

- **Schizophrenia spectrum and other psychotic disorders** are a group of mental disorders characterized by psychotic features. These disorders include schizophrenia, delusional disorder, and brief psychotic disorder.

- **Substance-induced psychotic disorder** is a mental disorder characterized by hallucinations or delusions caused by the use of or withdrawal from substance like alcohol or cocaine.

Description and Diagnosis

Brief psychotic disorder is one of the schizophrenia and other psychotic disorders. Individuals with this disorder are likely to present with acute psychotic symptoms that have appeared suddenly. It almost always follows an extreme stressor. Emergency hospitalization is common because of their unexpected and extremely abnormal behavior. As with other psychosis, they are likely to experience hallucinations, particularly of the auditory type. Some individuals may present with various forms of catatonia, including stupor, physical rigidity, expressionlessness, or mutism (not speaking). They may also be experiencing delusions or paranoid thoughts. Approximately 9% of those presenting with a first episode of psychosis receive this diagnosis. Women are twice as likely as men to suffer from this disorder. The age of onset varies, but the average age is mid-30s. In addition, this disorder occurs more frequently in developing nations (American Psychiatric Association, 2013).

An important differentiator between brief psychotic disorder and other disorders is that individuals return to pre-onset functioning in a short time. This means that as their symptoms quickly recede, they regain their same level of abilities and functioning. While this disorder shares some psychotic features with substance-induced psychotic disorder, it is different. Brief psychotic disorder is not caused by substance use or withdrawal.

It is critical that a clinician ascertain the exact time frame involved in both onset and duration in order to make an accurate diagnosis. Brief psychotic disorder can last no longer than one month, or the diagnosis is not applicable. Should it last longer, another disorder from the schizophrenia spectrum and other psychotic disorders group should be considered. Usually, a very stressful event precedes the onset of this disorder. Therefore, it is important to not only ascertain if a stressor is related to the onset of the disorder, but it is imperative to assess for stress-related conditions such as post-traumatic stress disorder.

According to the *Diagnostic and Statistical Manual of Mental Disorders, Fifth Edition*, individuals can be diagnosed with this disorder if they exhibit the abrupt onset of symptoms of delusions, hallucinations, disorganized speech, or bizarre behavior and posture. The episode must last at least one day by less than one month with the eventual return to pre-onset level of functioning. Symptoms of this disorder must be distinguished from culturally sanctioned response patterns that may resemble such symptoms. The diagnosis is not given if there is evidence of the direct physiological effects of a medication, a drug of abuse, or a medical condition (American Psychiatric Association, 2013).

The cause of this disorder is not well understood. However, individuals with a family history of bipolar disorder or depression are more likely to develop a psychotic disorder than those who do not. As already noted, extreme stressors often trigger this disorder. Substances, medications, and medical conditions can cause psychotic episodes. In addition to family history and stressors, substances, medications, and medical conditions can cause, complicate, or trigger psychotic disorders. Accordingly, detailed information about such factors should be identified.

Treatment

Depending on the severity of the symptoms, individuals may require hospitalization for the initial days following the onset of the disorder. During this time, a comprehensive assessment is undertaken to identify the causes and triggers of the disorder. The goal of treatment is to reduce symptoms and to return individuals to their previous level of functioning. Both medication and cognitive behavior therapy are common treatment interventions. Various antipsychotic medication such as Haldol, Risperdal, and Zyprexa are commonly used. In addition to treatment aimed at the reduction of symptoms, it is often recommended that individuals participate in psychoeducation (information sessions) programs aimed at helping them understand their condition. Also, family therapy is beneficial for individuals suffering from brief psychotic disorders. This form of therapy allows other family members to gain insight into the condition and understand how they might support the individual who is suffering in the family setting.

Len Sperry, MD, PhD, and Jeremy Connelly, MEd

See also: Delusions; Family Therapy and Family Counseling; Haldol (Haloperidol); Hallucinations; Psychosis; Risperdal (Risperidone); Schizophrenia; Schizophreniform Disorder; Substance-Induced Psychotic Disorders; Zyprexa (Olanzapine)

Further Reading

American Psychiatric Association. *Diagnostic and Statistical Manual of Mental Disorders*, 5th ed. Arlington, VA: American Psychiatric Association, 2013.

Freudenreich, Oliver. *Psychotic Disorders: A Practical Guide*. Baltimore, MD: Lippincott Williams & Wilkins, 2008.

Fujii, Daryl, and Iqbal Ahmed. *The Spectrum of Psychotic Disorders: Neurobiology, Etiology & Pathogenesis*. Cambridge, UK: Cambridge University Press, 2006.

Torrey, E. Fuller. *Surviving Schizophrenia*, 6th ed. New York, NY: Harper Perennial, 2014.

Brief Therapy

Brief therapy is a form of therapy that can increase an individual's functioning in a relatively short amount of time.

Definitions

- **Acceptance and commitment therapy** is a psychological treatment approach that assists individuals to accept what is outside their control and commit to action that enriches their lives. It is also known as ACT.

- **Adlerian therapy** is a psychological treatment approach that uses encouragement to assist individuals to find constructive actions to deal with their problems while developing an enhanced sense of social interest.

- **Behavioral therapy** is a psychological treatment approach that focuses on identifying and changing maladaptive behaviors. It is also referred to as behavioral therapy.

- **Biopsychosocial therapy** is a psychological treatment approach that focuses on clients' biological, psychological, and social dynamics and focus interventions on those areas.

- **Brief dynamic psychotherapy** is a psychological treatment approach that focuses on maladaptive interpersonal patterns and unmet needs, which are treated by facilitating new experiences in therapy.

- **Brief reality therapy** is a psychological treatment approach that emphasizes problem solving in the here and now. It does not focus on mental illness, rather on the ability to choose and create a better future.

- **Cognitive behavior therapy** is a psychological treatment approach that focuses on maladaptive (problematic) behaviors, emotions, and thoughts. It is also called CBT.

- **Cognitive behavior analysis system of psychotherapy** is a psychological approach that focuses on changing thoughts and behaviors by analyzing desired outcomes in contrast to actual outcomes. It is also called CBASP.

- ***Diagnostic and Statistical Manual of Mental Disorders*** is the handbook mental health professionals use to diagnose mental disorders. The current edition (fifth) is known as DSM-5.

- **Psychotherapy** is a psychological method for achieving desired changes in thinking, feeling, and behavior. It is also called therapy and therapeutic counseling.

- **Solution-focused brief therapy** is a psychological treatment approach that focuses on strengths and problem solving, and examines an individual's past ability to cope effectively.

Description

Brief therapies are an assortment of psychotherapy approaches that can effect change in clients in a short amount of time. Some theories have therapeutic processes that can take years to achieve treatment goals, while brief therapy models utilize techniques that influence change rather quickly. Given the limitations of managed care, individuals are often eligible only for a limited amount of therapy sessions. Third-party payers typically expect therapy to be completed in very few sessions and the treatment provided to be effective and long-lasting. As a result of this, brief therapies have become the treatment of choice for many therapists. Brief therapy models are goal oriented and time-limited and focus treatment to address the individual's strengths and abilities. Rather than looking for the cause of the problem, brief therapies work with clients to make changes in their lives and improve their functioning. Brief models seek to effect change with clients in as little as just one session. Various brief models have been articulated in the literature.

Some brief therapies include brief dynamic therapy, cognitive behavior therapy (CBT), biopsychosocial therapy, brief Adlerian therapy, acceptance commitment therapy (ACT), brief reality therapy, cognitive behavior analysis system of psychotherapy (CBASP), and solution-focused brief therapy. CBT and CBASP are psychological treatment approaches that help clients reduce and modify maladaptive behaviors and cognitions, while brief dynamic therapy works with individuals to examine relationship patterns and unmet needs by changing relational patterns toward a more adaptive approach. Brief Adlerian therapy effects change in clients by helping them implement constructive actions and increase their sense of belonging. ACT assists individuals to accept what is outside their control and commit to action that is in accordance with their goals and values. Solution-focused brief therapy focuses on strengths and problem solving, and examines an individual's past exceptions to when the problem was not a problem. While other brief models exist, the examples provided earlier utilize different therapeutic strategies and interventions to assist individuals who are seeking therapy services in a time-limited setting.

Developments and Current Status

Brief therapy models were developed by various theoretical proponents. Brief therapies are considered some of the most clinical useful and efficient therapy modalities. Research and application of brief therapy approaches continue to occur at an increasing rate. It is anticipated that brief therapies will outnumber the longer-term therapies.

Jon Sperry, PhD, and Len Sperry, MD, PhD

See also: Acceptance and Commitment Therapy (ACT); Adlerian therapy; Biopsychosocial Therapy; Brief Dynamic Psychotherapy; Cognitive Behavior Analysis System of Psychotherapy(CBASP); Cognitive Behavior Therapy; Grief Counseling; Motivational Interviewing; Positive Psychology

Further Reading

Beck, Judith. *Cognitive Therapy: Basics and Beyond.* New York, NY: Guilford Press, 1995.

Binder, Jeffrey, and Ephi Betan. *Core Competencies in Brief Dynamic Psychotherapy: Becoming a Highly Effective and Competent Brief Dynamic Psychotherapist.* New York, NY: Routledge, 2013.

Glasser, William. *Reality Therapy: A New Approach to Psychiatry.* New York, NY: Harper & Row, 1965.

Hayes, Steven C., Kirk D. Strosahl, and Kelly G. Wilson. *Acceptance and Commitment Therapy: An Experiential Approach to Behavior Change.* New York, NY: Guilford Press, 2003.

McCullough, James. *Treatment for Chronic Depression: Cognitive Behavioral Analysis System of Psychotherapy (CBASP).* New York, NY: Guilford Press, 1999.

Bulimia Nervosa

Bulimia nervosa is a mental disorder characterized by recurrent binge eating with loss of control over one's eating and compensation for eating.

Definitions

- **Anorexia nervosa** is an eating disorder characterized by refusal to maintain minimal normal body weight along with a fear of weight gain and a distorted body image.

- **Binge eating** is a pattern of disordered eating consisting of episodes of uncontrolled intake of food.

- **Binge eating disorder** is an eating disorder characterized by binge eating without subsequent purging episodes.

- **Cognitive behavior therapy** is a form of counseling or psychotherapy that focuses on changing maladaptive (faulty) behaviors, emotions, and thoughts. It is also known as CBT.

- **Eating disorder** is a class of mental disorders that are characterized by difficulties with too much, too little, or unhealthy food intake, and may include distorted body image.

Description and Diagnosis

Bulimia nervosa is an eating disorder with a characteristic pattern of recurrent binge eating followed by purging. Bulimics overeat because food gives them a feeling of comfort. However, overeating makes them feel out of control. Then, feeling ashamed, guilty, and afraid of gaining weight, they purge. Basically, this disorder represents a loss of control about overeating and the compensatory behavior of purging for the purpose of regaining a sense of control. Individuals with bulimia nervosa tend to be of normal weight and "low calorie" or "careful restrictive" eaters between episodes of bingeing and purging. About 1.0%–1.5% of females have this disorder, which begins in adolescence and remains a pattern through early adulthood. The female-to-male ratio is 10:0 (American Psychiatric Association, 2013).

This disorder must be distinguished from the binge/purge subtype of anorexia nervosa. Both bulimia nervosa and this subtype involve binge eating and purging. However, whereas the anorexic is unable to maintain even minimal weight, the bulimic contains purging sufficiently to maintain body weight that is minimally normal or above normal level (American Psychiatric Association, 2013). Bulimia nervosa can also be distinguished from binge eating disorder, where there is bingeing but no purging.

Purging typically involves self-induced vomiting, fasting, overexercising, or using medicines like laxatives to induce diarrhea and/or excessive bowel movements. The binge/purge experience is often hidden, occurring during the night or when alone, and bulimics become skilled at inducing vomiting and using diuretics and exercise. Purging can lead to serious and even life-threatening medical conditions. These include dental problems like tooth decay, gum disease, and loss of tooth enamel that result from acid in the mouth following vomiting. It can also lead to osteoporosis (bone thinning), kidney damage, and fatal cardiac arrhythmias (abnormal heart rhythms). Laxative dependence is a common complication of this disorder. Dentists and dental hygienists have a key role in identifying bulimia nervosa since they are often the first to recognize the dental damage caused by purging.

According to the *Diagnostic and Statistical Manual of Mental Disorders, Fifth Edition*, individuals can be diagnosed with this disorder if they exhibit a pattern of binge eating followed by methods of purging or compensating to avoid weight gain. It is not the same as the binge/purge pattern in anorexia nervosa. The purging and/or compensation often involves vomiting, the use of laxatives, diets, and/or fasting. In this disorder the individual is preoccupied with thoughts about appearance, shape, and weight. Depending on the number and duration of binge/purge episodes per week, the disorder is given a severity rating of mild, moderate, severe, or extreme. The disorder can range from mild (1–3 episodes of binge/purge per week) to extreme (14 or more episodes per week) based on the frequency and duration of the episodes of bingeing and purging (American Psychiatric Association, 2013).

The causes and course of this disorder are many and complex. Family history, social factors, and personality traits are usually involved. A family history of obesity or an eating disorder is not uncommon. Expectations for thinness, stressful work situations, divorce, relocation, or loss of a loved one may be involved. It is common in social settings or professions that involve a body performance such as sports, acting, and modeling. Preoccupation with external beauty and "looking good" are common among those with this disorder. Personality traits such as perfectionism, worry, or low self-esteem are common. This disorder may begin with efforts to find social acceptance, attention getting, and the need to please others or seek approval. Sometimes few of these factors are involved, and the disorder begins with the use of purging as a short-term strategy for losing weight.

Treatment

Clinical treatment of this disorder typically involves counseling and sometimes medications. Unlike anorexia nervosa, treatment of bulimia nervosa does not usually involve hospitalization. The goal of the treatment is to reduce bingeing and purging and to foster recovery from the disorder. Because individuals with this disorder are often diagnosed with mood disorders or substance disorders, particularly involving alcohol and/or stimulants, these conditions must be treated simultaneously. Counseling usually involves cognitive behavior therapy and nutritional counseling to change certain behavior and thinking patterns. Antidepressant medicines like Prozac may be used to reduce the binge-purging and to treat related depression or anxiety. Treatment of this and related disorders tends to be long term.

Len Sperry, MD, PhD

See also: Anorexia Nervosa; Binge Eating Disorder; Cognitive Behavior Therapy; Prozac (Fluoxetine)

Further Reading

American Psychiatric Association. *Diagnostic and Statistical Manual of Mental Disorders*, 5th ed. Arlington, VA: American Psychiatric Association Press, 2013.

Costin, Carolyn, Gwen Schubert Grabb, and Babette Rothschild. *8 Keys to Recovery from an Eating Disorder: Effective Strategies from Therapeutic Practice and Personal Experience*. New York, NY: W.W. Norton, 2012.

Siegel, Michele, Judith Brisman, and Margot Weinshel. *Surviving an Eating Disorder: Strategies for Family and Friends*, 3rd ed. New York, NY: Harper Perennial, 2009.

Bullying and Peer Aggression

Bullying, or peer aggression, involves intentionally harmful, repeated acts of aggression toward a person, typically a peer, with lesser power.

Definitions

- **Bully**, the aggressor, victimizer, or perpetrator of bullying; a person who uses his or her power to intimidate, harass, or harm another person.

- **Bullycide** refers to a suicide where the victim's death has been attributed to the victim having been bullied either in person or online.

- **Bystander** is a person who is present at, observes, or witnesses a particular event or circumstance (such as bullying) but who does not have direct involvement.

- **Cyberbullying** refers to using technology (texting, e-mailing, chat rooms, social media sites, pictures, etc.) to repeatedly and intentionally degrade, threaten, or humiliate another person.

- **Mobbing** is defined as when an individual is bullied by a group of people in any context, including a family, school, social setting, or workplace.

- **Victim** is the person who has suffered or been harmed as a result of being the target of bullying behavior.

Description

Bullying, also referred to as peer aggression, is defined as repeated acts of aggression, abuse, or intimidation that are inflicted directly or indirectly over time by one or more dominant persons. This behavior involves the interaction among three parties: the bully (aggressor), the victim (target), and the bystander (witness). Generally, bullying is committed from peer to peer. When bullying is inflicted by a group rather than by one individual, it is termed "mobbing." Three essential components distinguish bullying from other forms of victimization: (1) *intentional* harm to the victim, (2) *repetition* of the harmful acts over time, and (3) the existence of a *power differential* (physically, chronologically, socially, emotionally, psychologically) between bully and victim. There are various types of bullying, including physical, verbal, relational, and cyberbullying. Physical bullying entails behaviors like hitting, slapping, punching, pushing, kicking, tripping, spitting, and damaging another person's property. Insults, name-calling, slurs, threats, and spreading rumors/gossip are forms of verbal bullying. Relational bullying is described as when one uses one's social influence or popularity to isolate, ignore, exclude, or reject another person. Cyberbullying is a more recent phenomenon whereby aggressors use technological means (texting, pictures, social sites, e-mail, etc.) to bully their victims.

Students in grades 6–10 are most likely to be involved in bullying incidents, though bullying has been observed in children as young as three. There are also notable peaks in bullying behavior during the transition years from elementary to middle school and again from middle to high school, pointing to the value of early intervention. Early reports indicated that boys were more likely to engage in physical types of bullying while girls more readily displayed relational bullying. However, recent trends suggest that both boys and girls are involved in relational types of aggression, with a drastic increase noted in recent times in rates of cyberbullying for both genders. The prevalence of technology in today's society has greatly contributed to increased incidents of cyberbullying. Accessibility to technology and anonymity issues further complicates this problem.

Victims of peer aggression may be targeted for differences in their appearance, race, ethnicity, gender, sexual orientation, personality, reputation, or ability. Experts have sought to establish a pattern of behavior for bullies, though no definitive profile exists. It was once believed that bullies harass and torment due to low self-esteem, but this is now considered a myth. Rather, aggressors are attracted to the attention and sense of power they get from putting others down.

The word "bully" can be traced back to the mid-16th century when it was first used as a term of endearment, likened to the word "sweetheart" or "lover" (Dutch/German origin). It was not until the 17th century that the term began to have more of a negative connotation. Reference to the current meaning of "bully" or "bullying" increased around the 1970s–1980s and became more commonplace in everyday vernacular in the late 1990s and early 2000s. The popular book, *Queen Bees and Wannabees* (2009), written by Rosalind Wiseman, exposed the true realities of bullying and relational aggression in girl world. The continued success of the pop culture film, *Mean Girls* (2004), based on Wiseman's book, further points to society's interest in the bullying phenomenon. Wiseman later went on to publish *Masterminds and Wingmen* (2013), addressing relational bullying from a boy's perspective.

As awareness about bullying has increased, more attention has been placed on approaches, policies, and strategies to prevent and combat it. Several have been attempted, ranging in level of effectiveness from zero-tolerance policies, restorative-justice approaches, education and identification training, and punitive measures. Norwegian psychologist Daniel Olweus is considered the pioneer of bullying research. He was the first to examine the prevalence of this problem among school-aged children back in the 1970s. His findings led him to develop a comprehensive approach for addressing bullying school-wide, the *Olweus Bullying Prevention Program*, which focuses on fostering positive peer relationships and creating safe environments where students can learn and develop. This program remains a popular evidence-based approach used today. Recent research supports the effectiveness of social-emotional learning programs that also work to create an overall positive school climate.

Current Status and Impact (Psychological Influence)

Studies have linked experiences with bullying to a wide range of negative consequences (physical, behavioral, academic, social, emotional, and psychological). Victims commonly report headaches, sleep problems, nightmares, and bed-wetting. They also report fear and anxiety about attending school and other social events. Bystanders indicate similar concerns. Being victimized also results in lower self-esteem and an increased risk of experiencing depression. "Bullycide," a term used to describe suicide resulting from peer aggression, is of further concern, as is homicide. There is evidence to support that several school-shooting cases can be traced back to victimization. Success in school can also be affected by bullying. Researchers have tied victimization to increased tardy, absentee, and dropout rates; poorer grades; and more academic struggles. Bullies also experience distinct consequences. Future involvement in spousal abuse, child abuse, and sexual harassment incidents is also more probable for those identified as bullies. In addition, aggressors exhibit lower frustration tolerance, have quicker tempers, and display more impulsive behaviors, which greatly contribute to struggles in school. Poorer grades; increased absentee and dropout rates; substance abuse problems; and high rates of depression, suicide, and self-injurious behaviors have also been noted.

Estimates suggest that some 30%–40% of youngsters, about one out of every four kids, report some level of involvement with bullying on a regular basis. However, these numbers are thought to be grossly underestimated as bullying often goes unrecognized and unreported. Most incidents occur in unsupervised locations such as playgrounds, bathrooms, and hallways, so the true severity of this problem remains unknown. Secrecy also plays a large role, as many victims are scared to report incidents out of fear of retaliation. Bystanders may also be hesitant to report out of concerns that the bully may turn on them next.

Presently, 49 states have anti-bullying laws (all except Montana). Georgia was the first to pass legislation back in 1999. Legislation varies by state according to reporting procedures and guidelines, requirements, and punishments. Educators, researchers, law enforcement officers, psychologists, counselors, parents, and young people remain interested in investigating and remedying the bullying problem.

Melissa A. Mariani, PhD

See also: Cyberbullying; *Mean Girls* (Movie); Mobbing; Peer Groups

Further Reading

Bauman, Sherrie, Donna Cross, and Jenny Walker, eds. *Principles of Cyberbullying Research: Definition, Methods, and Measures.* New York, NY: Routledge, 2013.

Hinduja, Sameer, and Justin W. Patchin. *School Climate 2.0: Preventing Cyberbullying and Sexting One Classroom at a Time.* Thousand Oaks, CA: Corwin, 2012.

Olweus, Daniel. *Bullying at School: What We Know and What We Can Do.* Malden, MA: Blackwell Publishing Ltd., 1993.

Wiseman, Rosalind. *Masterminds and Wingmen: Helping Our Boys Cope with Schoolyard Power, Locker-Room Tests, Girlfriends, and the New Rules of Boy World.* New York, NY: Random House, 2013.

Wiseman, Rosalind. *Queen Bees and Wannabees: Helping your Daughter Survive Cliques, Gossip, Boyfriends, and the New Realities of Girl World.* New York, NY: Three Rivers Press, 2009.

Bystander Effect

The bystander effect, also known as bystander apathy, is a highly researched social psychological phenomenon that occurs when an individual or individuals, who witness dangerous or harmful situations, stand by without offering assistance to the victim or victims.

Definitions

- **Bystander** is a person who is present at, observes, or witnesses a particular event or circumstance (such as bullying) but who does not have direct involvement.

- **Diffusion of responsibility** suggests that bystanders rationalize their hesitance, reluctance, or lack of intervening on a victim's behalf due to a belief that others present will take responsibility.

Description

When dangerous, harmful events or emergency situations occur and an onlooker or onlookers do nothing to intervene, stop, or assist the victim(s), this is referred to as "the bystander effect." This phenomenon has also been termed "bystander apathy," describing what appears to be relative disregard or lack of empathy for what the victim is experiencing. The probability of intervening also appears to decrease as the number of bystanders present increases. Various aspects of this effect have been researched and identified by social psychologists that help explain why the effect occurs. These variables include situational ambiguity, familiarity with the environment, sense of social responsibility, level of group cohesiveness, and diffusion of responsibility.

Development

Sociologists and psychologists have been researching the bystander effect for decades beginning with the groundbreaking study conducted by Bibb Latané and John Darley in 1968. Their interest was piqued following the publicized brutal rape and murder of "Kitty" Genovese by Winston Moseley on March 13, 1964, in Queens, New York. Though it was determined during trial proceedings that a dozen or so people had witnessed various pieces of the attack, media reports initially indicated much higher numbers (36–38), which resulted in public outrage and increasing concerns regarding bystander responsibility. (It was also later publicized that, during the Genovese attack, one person did call the police and one woman rushed to Genovese's side after the attack.) Latané and Darley proceeded with a series of experiments to investigate bystander behavior. Essentially, these studies consisted of staged events whereby a participant or group of participants were placed in emergency and nonemergency situations and observed to see whether they would intervene as well as how long it would take them to act.

Diffusion of responsibility, or the reluctance of observers to initiate assistance or involve themselves when others are around, was suggested as one possible explanation of the phenomenon. Witnesses often believe that someone else, perhaps an individual more qualified, will step up. Others may prefer not to get involved due to fear or intimidation.

Current Status and Results

Research on the bystander effect suggests that whether onlookers perceive the situation as an emergency or not matters. The more serious a situation is viewed, the faster the bystander reacts. An additional finding shows that when a person is alone, rather than with one or more people, he or she also tends to react more swiftly. Degree of connection to the victim is also a contributing factor. Bystanders with some relationship or tie to the victim are more likely to assist. Several examples of the bystander effect have been recorded throughout history. Recent interest in this phenomenon has focused on youth's hesitance to intervene in bullying situations, with experts recommending school violence-prevention programs that address bystander interventions in order to produce lasting change.

Melissa A. Mariani, PhD

See also: Bullying and Peer Aggression; Cliques; Mobbing; Obedience Studies

Further Reading

Cook, Kevin. *Kitty Genovese: The Murder, the Bystanders, the Crime That Changed America.* New York, NY: W.W. Norton, 2014.

Fisher, Peter, Joachim I. Krueger, Tobias Greitemeyer, Claudia Vogrincic, Andreas Kastenmuller, Dieter Frey, Moritz Heene, Magdalena Wicher, and Martina Kainbacher. "The Bystander-Effect: A Meta-Analytic Review on Bystander Intervention in Dangerous and Non-Dangerous Emergencies." *Psychological Bulletin* 137 (2011): 517.

Latané, Bibb, and John M. Darley. *The Unresponsive Bystander: Why Doesn't He Help?* Englewood Cliffs, NJ: Prentice Hall, 1970.

Polanin, Joshua R., Dorothy L. Espelage, and Therese D. Pigott. "A Meta-Analysis of School-Based Bullying Prevention Programs' Effects on Bystander Intervention Behavior." *School Psychology Review* 41 (2012): 47.

C

CACREP

See Council for Accreditation of Counseling and Related Educational Programs

Caffeine-Related Disorders

Caffeine-related disorders are a group of disorders characterized by excessive consumption of caffeine. The disorders in this group include caffeine intoxication and caffeine withdrawal.

Definitions

- **Addictive** refers to a persistent, compulsive dependence on a substance or a behavior.

- **Antianxiety medications** are prescribed drugs that relieve anxiety symptoms. They are also called anxiolytics and tranquilizers.

- **Caffeine** is a naturally occurring stimulant that is derived from plants, which may be addictive or cause withdrawal symptoms.

- **Caffeine-induced anxiety disorder** is an anxiety disorder characterized by state of panic (intense fear of a known danger) or anxiety (intense worry or an imagined danger) as a result of the consumption of caffeine.

- **Caffeine-induced sleep disorder** is a sleep disorder characterized by disturbed sleep as a result of the consumption of caffeine.

- **Substance-related disorders** are a group of mental disorders that are characterized by the problematic use of substances.

- **Withdrawal symptoms** are the symptoms (nervousness, headaches, insomnia, etc.) that occur when an individual who is addicted to a substance (drugs or alcohol) stops using the substance.

Description and Diagnosis

Caffeine-related disorders represent a group of mental disorders that result from excessive consumption of caffeine. This group is part of the substance-related disorders. The two primary disorders of this category are caffeine intoxication and caffeine withdrawal. Because they differ from this group in the severity of symptoms, caffeine-induced anxiety disorder and caffeine-induced sleep disorder are not included.

Caffeine consumption is common and widespread in many cultures. Typically, it is found in coffee, tea, energy drinks, and soda. But it is also in chocolate, in many over-the-counter medicines, and in weight loss supplements. In the United States, it has been estimated that 85% of the population consume caffeine frequently (American Psychiatric Association, 2013). Consequently, these disorders affect people in significant numbers. It is therefore important that clinicians are able to recognize these disorders as well as rule out other similar disorders and treat accordingly.

Here is a brief description of the two most common disorders.

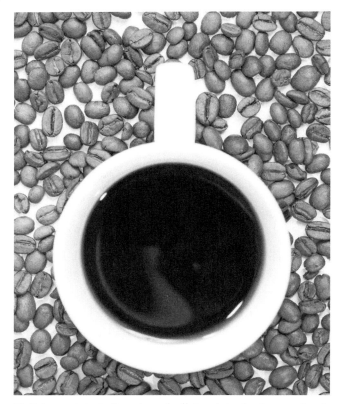

Caffeine related disorders (caffeine intoxication and caffeine withdrawal) represent mental disorders that result from excessive consumption of caffeine, and are part of substance-related disorders. (Richard Nelson/Dreamstime.com)

Caffeine intoxication. Caffeine intoxication is a disorder that results from the consumption of large amounts of caffeine. Individuals diagnosed with this disorder have often consumed 250 mg of caffeine or more, roughly equivalent to 2.5 cups of coffee. To be given this diagnosis individuals must exhibit symptoms that may include agitation, apprehension, excitability, rapid heartbeat, flushed face, frequent urination, and difficulty sleeping. Such symptoms must be distressing to the individual or disrupt daily functioning.

Both children and older adults may be more sensitive to the effects of caffeine than middle-aged adults. It is estimated that 7% of the population may experience many of the earlier-mentioned symptoms every year (American Psychiatric Association, 2013). Treatment of this disorder may include the administration of antianxiety medication to reduce symptoms and laxatives to flush out the caffeine. If the caffeine was ingested recently, activated carbon (a substance that readily absorbs chemicals) may also be administered. Intense symptoms typically last four to six hours and then stop. This means that most individuals will recover fully even without treatment.

Caffeine withdrawal. Caffeine withdrawal is a disorder that results from the abrupt termination of caffeine consumption after having consumed the substance for an extended period of time. Symptoms of this disorder often include migraine (most common), inability to concentrate, moodiness, or symptoms similar to the flu. Typically, symptoms occur within two days following the last ingestion of caffeine. It is estimated that this disorder affects roughly half of those who stop caffeine after extended use (American Psychiatric Association, 2013). One of the most effective ways to reduce caffeine withdrawal symptoms is to provide the individual a small dose of caffeine. Since headaches are the most common withdrawal symptom, individuals may be encouraged to take an over-the-counter headache remedy (like Bayer aspirin) which contains caffeine.

Jeremy Connelly, MEd, and Len Sperry, MD, PhD

See also: Antianxiety Medications

Further Reading

American Psychiatric Association. *Diagnostic and Statistical Manual of Mental Disorders*, 5th ed. Arlington, VA: American Psychiatric Association, 2013.

Garrattini, Silvio. *Caffeine, Coffee and Health.* New York, NY: Raven Press, 1993.

Weinberg, Bennett, and Donnie Bealer. *The World of Caffeine: The Science and Culture of the World's Most Popular Drug.* New York, NY: Routledge, 2001.

Cancer, Psychological Aspects

The psychological aspects of cancer include symptoms of anxiety, depression, and post-traumatic stress, as well as spiritual–existential issues. These may be experienced by the individual with cancer or caregivers.

Definitions

- **Adjustment disorder** is a mental disorder characterized by emotional or behavioral symptoms in response to an identifiable stressor that is significantly distressing or causes impairment.

- **Anxiety** is a negative emotional state characterized by feelings of nervousness, worry, and apprehension about an imagined danger.

- **Chronic disease** is a disease entity which usually does not have a single cause, a specific onset, nor a stable set of symptoms. While cure may be possible, it is unlikely for advanced levels of the disease process. It is also referred to as chronic medical conditions.

- **Depression** is an emotional state characterized by feelings of sadness, low self-esteem, guilt, or reduced ability to enjoy life. It is not considered a mental disorder unless it significantly disrupts one's daily functioning.

- **DSM-5** stands for *the Diagnostic and Statistical Manual of Mental Disorders, Fifth Edition*, which is a diagnostic system used by professionals to identify mental disorders with specific diagnostic criteria.

- **Post-traumatic stress disorder** is a mental disorder characterized by nightmares, irritability, anxiety, emotional numbing, and recurrent flashbacks of a traumatic event that an individual experienced or witnessed. It is also referred to as PTSD.

- **Psychological factors affecting other medical conditions** is a mental disorder characterized by emotional factors that worsen a medical condition.

- **Relapse** is the recurrence of symptoms after a period of improvement or recovery.

Description

While some may consider cancer only a medical condition, there are many psychological aspects that result from this chronic disease. A cancer diagnosis and cancer treatment can result in significant psychological distress. The extent of distress depends on the type of cancer, time since diagnosis, degree of physical and social impairment, and prognosis. Some individuals may not develop symptoms severe enough to qualify for a diagnosis but may still experience psychological problems. Feelings of anger, guilt, sadness, and fear are common in those living with chronic disease. Others may qualify for a mental health disorder diagnosis. These include adjustment disorders or disorders of depression and anxiety.

Common psychological problems faced by individuals with cancer are anxiety, post-traumatic stress, depression, spiritual–existential issues, and interpersonal (relationship) issues. Individuals with cancer may experience anxiety for a number of reasons. These include fears about the cancer progressing or returning after remission (relapse). They may also be due to financial problems resulting from medical expenses, inability to perform previous duties at work or with family, or fears about dying. Experiencing a life-threatening medical condition is one criterion for a diagnosis of post-traumatic stress disorder according to the DSM-5. Depression may be brought on by the loss of familiar routines in daily life. Hopelessness, low self-esteem, and feelings of vulnerability that are associated with cancer may add to this. Individuals may also experience spiritual and existential issues. These involve loss of faith, conflicts in their relationship with God, and finding meaning in their illness. The psychological aspects of cancer impact family members and caregivers as well. Fears of losing a loved one and the stress associated with caring for an individual with cancer can lead to symptoms. Some individuals may develop mental health disorders like post-traumatic stress disorder themselves. This is particularly true for parents of children with cancer. Such stress can lead to a decline in care and increased distress for the individual with cancer.

The psychological problems associated with cancer can also lead to worsening physical symptoms. The DSM-5 diagnosis, psychological factors affecting other medical conditions, describes this relationship. Stress can cause tumors to grow and spread and increase feelings of helplessness. The relationship between psychological factors and cancer can be positive as well, however. Those who are able to manage stress tend to have better outcomes. Exercise, meditation, social support, and counseling are examples of activities used to cope with the psychological problems associated with cancer.

George Stoupas, MS, and Len Sperry, MD, PhD

See also: Adjustment Disorder; Anxiety; Chronic Illness; Depression; *Diagnostic and Statistical Manual of Mental Disorders* (DSM); Post-Traumatic Stress Disorder (PTSD); Psychological Factors Affecting Other Medical Conditions; Re lapse and Relapse Prevention

Further Reading

Barr, Niki. *Emotional Wellness: The Other Half of Treating Cancer.* Seattle, WA: Orion Wellspring, 2013.

Hopko, Derek, and Carl Lejuez. *A Cancer Patient's Guide to Overcoming Depression and Anxiety: Getting through Treatment and Getting Back to Your Life.* Oakland, CA: New Harbinger Publications, 2007.

Rosenbaum, Elana, and Jon Kabat-Zinn. *Here for Now: Living Well with Cancer through Mindfulness*, 2nd ed. Hardwick, MA: Satya House Publications, 2007.

Cannabis Use Disorder

Cannabis use disorder is a mental disorder characterized by cannabis (marijuana) use, which leads to significant problems for the user.

Definitions

- **Addiction** is a chronic disease of the brain which involves compulsive and uncontrolled pursuit of reward or relief with substance use or other compulsive behaviors.

- **Alcoholism** is a general term for the compulsive and uncontrolled consumption of alcohol to the detriment of the drinker's health, relationships, and social standing.

- **Cognitive behavior therapy** is a type of psychotherapy that focuses on maladaptive (problematic) behaviors, emotions, and thoughts. It is also called CBT.

- **Executive functions** are high-level cognitive abilities such as planning, organizing, reasoning, decision making, and problem solving that influence more basic abilities such as attention, memory, and motor skills.

- **Motivational interviewing** is a counseling strategy for helping individuals to discover and resolve their ambivalence to change. It is also referred to as MI.

- **Narcotics Anonymous** is a self-help and support group for those addicted to drugs to help them learn how to live without the use of mind- and mood-altering chemicals. It is a Twelve-Step Program.

- **Psychoactive** is a drug or substance that has a significant effect on mental processes. There are five groups of psychoactive drugs: opioids, stimulants, depressants, hallucinogens, and cannabis.

- **Substance-related and addictive disorders** are a group of mental disorders that include substance disorders characterized by physiological dependence, drug-seeking behavior, tolerance, and social withdrawal. This group also includes the non-substance disorder of gambling.

- **Twelve-Step Program** is a self-help group whose members attempt recovery from various addictions and compulsions based on a plan called the Twelve Steps.

Description and Diagnosis

Cannabis use disorder is one of the substance-related and addictive disorders. It is characterized by a problematic pattern of cannabis use which leads to significant distress or disrupted daily functioning. Problematic use of marijuana includes short-term physical and mental effects. Physical effects include mild sedation, impaired eye–hand coordination, increased appetite ("munchies"), and enhancement of senses. For example, food tends to taste and smell better and with increased appetite can lead to overeating. Mental effects include confusion, drowsiness, difficulty concentrating, exaggerated mood and personality, short-term memory difficulties, and time distortion. Mental effects can also include distortions of sound and color and possible hallucinations. The effects can be unique to the individual. So, while most users will be relaxed, some will be energized by marijuana use. Some may use it only for a specific purpose, such as to be more

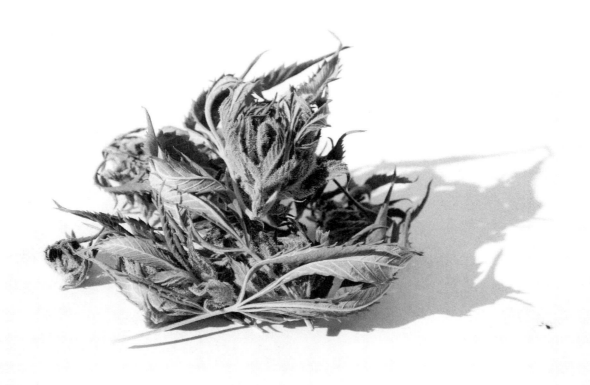

Cannabis use disorder is a substance-related and addictive disorder. It is characterized by a problematic pattern of cannabis (marijuana) use, leading to significant distress or disrupted daily functioning. (Petr Zamecnik/Dreamstime.com)

sociable or to hear music more deeply or differently, while others use it daily. Cannabis is probably the most widely used illicit psychoactive drug in the world. It is used by approximately 5% of adults in the United States, with more males than female users (American Psychiatric Association, 2013).

Long-term effects include respiratory problems, immune system impact, and acute mental effects. Although there is not a direct cancer relationship between long-term marijuana use and cancer such as there is with nicotine use, other respiratory problems include acute and chronic bronchitis and lung tissue damage. Some individuals will experience a great deal of anxiety and paranoia while using marijuana that persists after usage. While not common, cannabis use can precipitate psychosis in those with a predisposition toward it.

According to the *Diagnostic and Statistical Manual of Mental Disorders, Fifth Edition*, individuals can be diagnosed with this disorder if they exhibit a problematic pattern of cannabis use, which leads to significant impairment or distress. This must occur within a 12-month period. This includes taking the substance in larger amounts or for longer than intended. It means wanting to cut down or stop using the substance but not achieving this goal. It involves spending much time getting, using, or recovering from use of the substance. This disorder also involves cravings and urges to use the substance, and continuing to use, even when it causes problems in relationships. It involves failure to meet obligations at home, work, or school because of substance use. It also means reducing or stopping important social, work, or recreational activities because of substance use. This disorder involves repeated substance use even when it is physically dangerous. Despite knowing the risks of the physical and psychological problems that are caused or made worse by the substance, use of it continues. It means tolerance develops (needing more of it to get the desired effect). Finally, it involves withdrawal symptoms, which can be relieved by taking more of the substance (American Psychiatric Association, 2013).

This disorder has many of the same root causes as other substance disorders. The desire for a "high" along with the belief that marijuana is harmless often leads to experimentation during adolescence. However, regular cannabis users typically experience withdrawal symptoms, including stomach pain, aggression, anxiety, and irritability. Many frequent cannabis users are believed to continue using in order to avoid these unpleasant symptoms. Early use of this drug is associated with pervasive cognitive, social, and work-related problems in later life. Long-term use leads to comprised brain activity, particularly cognitive and executive functions (American Psychiatric Association, 2013). Easy availability, higher potency, and lower price for cannabis may all contribute to the increase in cannabis-related disorders.

Treatment

Treatment for this disorder is similar to the treatment of other substance disorders. The goal of treatment is abstinence. Treatment approaches range from inpatient hospitalization and drug rehabilitation centers for detoxification to outpatient programs. Motivational interviewing is useful in identifying reasons to stop using cannabis and to increase motivation and readiness for treatment. Then, cognitive behavior therapy can be used to identify the beliefs, behaviors, and situations that trigger use and cravings. From these clinicians can develop a plan to reduce the likelihood of relapse. Because cannabis addiction is considered a chronic condition, long-term treatment to maintain sobriety and prevent relapse is necessary. This often includes continuing in therapy and/or a Twelve-Step Program like Narcotics Anonymous. For heavy users suffering from withdrawal symptoms, treatment with antianxiety and antidepressant medication may be used.

Len Sperry, MD, PhD

See also: Addiction; Cognitive Behavior Therapy; Motivational Interviewing; Twelve-Step Programs

Further Reading

American Psychiatric Association. *Diagnostic and Statistical Manual of Mental Disorders*, 5th ed. Arlington, VA: American Psychiatric Association, 2013.

Brown, Waln K., and Wendy S. Snyder. *Facts about Marijuana* (*Parent Guides to Childhood Drug Use*), 6th ed. Tallahassee, FL: William Gladden Foundation Press, 2011.

Dodes, Lance. *Breaking Addiction: A 7-Step Handbook for Ending Any Addiction*. New York, NY: Harper Perennial.

Prentiss, Chris. *The Alcoholism and Addiction Cure: A Holistic Approach to Total Recovery*. Malibu, CA: Power Press, 2007.

Capgras Syndrome

Capgras syndrome is a mental disorder characterized by the delusion that someone to whom one is close has been replaced by an imposter. It is also called Capgras delusion.

Definitions

- **Antipsychotic medications** are prescription drugs used to treat psychotic disorders. They are sometimes referred to as antipsychotics or neuroleptics.

- **Cognitive therapy** is a type of cognitive behavior therapy that focuses on identifying and changing automatic thoughts and maladaptive beliefs, including delusional beliefs.

- **Delusional disorder** is a mental disorder characterized by delusions. Previously this disorder was referred to as paranoia or paranoid disorder.

- **Delusions** are fixed false beliefs that persist despite contrary evidence.

- **Dementia** is a group of symptoms including loss of memory, judgment, language, and other intellectual (mental) function caused by the death of neurons (nerve cells) in the brain.

- **DSM-5** stands for the *Diagnostic and Statistical Manual of Mental Disorders, Fifth Edition*, which is a diagnostic system used by professionals to identify mental disorders with specific diagnostic criteria.

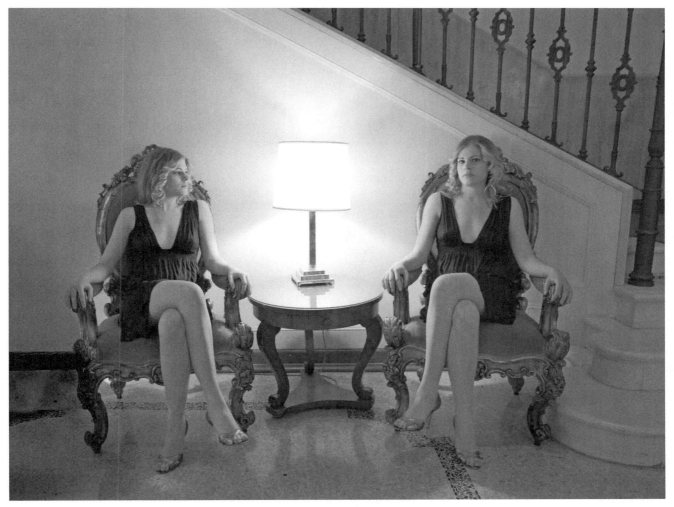

Capgras syndrome is a rare mental disorder characterized by the delusion that someone to whom one is close has been replaced by an imposter. It is also called Capgras delusion. (Bowie15/Dreamstime.com)

- **Schizophrenia** is a chronic mental disorder that affects behavior, thinking, and emotion, which make distinguishing between real and unreal experiences difficult. Symptoms include hallucinations, delusions, thought and communication disturbances, and withdrawal from others.

- **Schizophrenia spectrum and other psychotic disorders** are a group of mental disorders characterized by psychotic features. These disorders include schizophrenia, schizophreniform disorder, schizoaffective disorder, and schizotypal personality disorder, and delusional disorder.

Description

Capgras syndrome is a specific delusion in which an individual believes that one's friend, family member, or spouse has been replaced by an imposter who is identical in appearance. This belief may be of a short duration or chronic. This disorder is named for the French psychiatrist Joseph Capgras (1873–1950), who was the first clinician to recognize and write about the disorder. It is also known as Capgras delusion and delusion misidentification.

The occurrence of Capgras syndrome is unknown but is considered to be rare. This disorder is not a specific diagnosis outlined in the DSM-5. However, it does qualify as a symptom of the schizophrenia spectrum and other psychotic disorders, including delusional disorder and schizophrenia, which it is most commonly associated with. It follows that individuals who experience Capgras syndrome may be diagnosable with one of the previously mentioned disorders.

The specific cause of this disorder is unknown. For individuals who have a primary diagnosis that includes delusional components, the cause is most likely related to the same origin of the primary diagnosis. For those who do not have a delusional disorder, it has been theorized that brain dysfunction caused by illness (e.g., dementia) or brain injury can cause this disorder to manifest. As it pertains to brain injury, it has been suggested that damage to the brain in the areas related to emotional response may be to blame. An individual may see the familiar face of a loved one and be able to recognize it but not experience the emotional response typically associated with that person. Consequently, the individual forms the belief that this person is not the person he or she once knew.

Treatment

Treatment of Capgras syndrome in someone with a primary diagnosis of schizophrenia spectrum and other psychotic disorders is usually the same as the primary diagnosis. Many of the methods employed in these psychotic disorders are effective in treating the characteristic delusion of this syndrome. Specific therapies may include cognitive therapy and antipsychotic medications.

Jeremy Connelly, MEd, and
Len Sperry, MD, PhD

See also: Antipsychotic Medications; Cognitive Therapies; Delusional Disorder; Delusions; Dementia; *Diagnostic and Statistical Manual of Mental Disorders* (DSM); Schizophrenia; Schizophrenia Spectrum and Other Psychotic Disorders

Further Reading

American Psychiatric Association. *Diagnostic and Statistical Manual of Mental Disorders*, 5th ed. Arlington, VA: American Psychiatric Association, 2013.

Freeman, Daniel. *Overcoming Paranoid and Suspicious Thoughts: A Self-Help Guide Using Cognitive Behavioral Techniques.* New York, NY: Basic Books, 2009.

Freudenreich, Oliver. *Psychotic Disorders: A Practical Guide.* Baltimore, MD: Lippincott Williams & Wilkins, 2008.

Fujii, Daryl, and Iqbal Ahmed. *The Spectrum of Psychotic Disorders: Neurobiology, Etiology and Pathogenesis.* Cambridge, UK: Cambridge University Press, 2006.

Kantor, Martin. *Understanding Paranoia: A Guide for Professionals, Families, and Sufferers.* Santa Barbara, CA: Praeger, 2007.

Career Assessment

The purpose of career assessment is to obtain information about a person's interests, abilities, talents, and capacity for growth related to his or her aspirations. In using career assessment tools, a trained practitioner, such as a career counselor or advisor, guides the client toward appropriate placement in hopes of helping the person pursue his or her work-related goals.

Definitions

- **Career counselor,** or vocational counselor, is a counseling professional who has received specialized coursework, training, and certification in career-related guidance in order to provide advisement to persons seeking assistance in this area.

- **Interest inventory** is a type of career assessment that gauges what a person likes or is interested in.

- **Self-assessment (career)** is a self-reporting instrument used to gather information about a person's values, personality, interests, skills, and abilities.

Description

Career assessment describes the process of using tools, tests, questionnaires, and inventories to determine a person's abilities and skills related to work. They are used to identify strengths and weaknesses to help guide possible job choices. Career assessments refer to the specific tests that are used to acquire knowledge about a person's career options. Both quantitative and qualitative information are generated from these tests. Counselors who have been schooled in career or vocational guidance typically conduct them. However, other professionals who have been trained in this type of assessment, including mental health practitioners and educational advisors, may also perform these tests.

There are various types of career assessments, and each uses a different type of criteria to gather information. Interest inventories gauge what one's likes, preferences, or activities one is drawn to. Other tools assess a person's values or what criteria are most important to a person in terms of the person's career. For example, one may value flexibility in work schedule over salary. Aptitude and skills tests seek to determine what a person is best suited for in terms of natural talents or skill sets. Personality inventories place individuals in various type categories and attempt to link these to different careers known to be rewarding for those types.

Development

The foundation for career assessment was laid several decades ago in the early part of the 20th century. A growing need to find proper job placements for soldiers returning from war as well as a new emphasis on math and science preparation in the field of education spawned the career guidance counseling movement. From this came many changes including the development of career assessment tools, such as the Myers–Briggs Type Indicator (MBTI), the Strong-Interest Inventory, and Holland's Codes.

The Myers–Briggs Type Indicator assessment is a psychometric questionnaire that was developed by Katharine Cook Briggs and her daughter Isabel Briggs Myers in 1962. The MBTI measures a person's perceptions of the world and decision-making process. The theoretical basis for the assessment is the principle of typology. Carl Jung was the first psychologist to propose the idea of types back in the 1920s. He theorized that there were four main ways that people experience the world, through sensation, intuition, feeling, or thinking. The MBTI emphasizes the value of personal preferences and how these guide our interests, values, needs, and motivation.

Another career assessment tool is the Holland Codes. Psychologist John Holland developed these codes based on six personality types: Realistic, Investigative, Artistic, Social, Enterprising, and Conventional, each reflective of how a person approaches life. Individuals are categorized based on their top three types. Occupations are also classified and then matches are based on what personality types fit those careers best.

The Strong Interest Inventory (SII), developed by psychologist E. K. Strong, Jr., in 1927, is one of the most popular career assessments. The most recent version (2004) is based on the Holland Codes and is used readily in by career advisors and guidance counselors. The goal of the SII is to determine a person's top interest and use that information to decide on an appropriate career choice.

Current Status and Results

Career assessment tools have been criticized for their lack of validity and reliability. Though these types of tests can be valuable in obtaining useful information, they should be interpreted only by trained professionals and should not be viewed as an end-all determinant. Many of these tools gauge how a person reports feeling, thinking, behaving, or preferring at a given time, which arguably is likely to change over time. However, research trends indicate that a person will change careers at least once in his or her lifetime so career assessments are useful vehicles to guide this process and help a person determine the best suitable job options.

Melissa A. Mariani, PhD

See also: Career Counseling; Career Development

Further Reading

Association for Assessment in Counseling. *A Counselor's Guide to Career Assessment Instruments*. Broken Arrow, OK: National Career Development Association, 2009.

Bolles, Richard N. *What Color Is Your Parachute? 2013: A Practical Manual for Job-Hunters and Career Changers*. New York, NY: Crown Publishing Group, 2013.

Prince, Jeffrey, and Lisa J. Heiser. *Essentials of Career Assessment*. New York, NY: John Wiley & Sons, 2000.

Career Counseling

Career counseling is a collaborative process in which a counselor or advisor works with a person to help identify personal interests, abilities, and goals so the person can make wise career-related decisions.

Definition

- **Career counselor,** or vocational counselor, is a counseling professional who has received specialized coursework, training, and certification in career-related guidance in order to provide advisement to persons seeking assistance in this area.

Description

Career counseling describes a process in which a counselor and counselee form a collaborative relationship focused on identifying and acting on career-related goals. A career counselor employs various techniques that may include individual or group-based discussion, as well as the use of self-assessments, including interest inventories, personality tests, and aptitude tests. By uncovering a person's interests and abilities, the career counselor seeks to expose the counselee to various job possibilities that may be suitable. Goals of a career counseling session may be to bring about self-awareness, identify personal strengths and weaknesses, develop short- and long-term goals, accept responsibility for one's actions, and maintain the proper level of motivation.

Counseling focused on career-related areas can be provided to people of any age and at any stage of their career path. Topics do not have to focus solely on possible job or career changes but may also surround workplace frustrations, decisions about pursuing further education, and/or how to balance personal and professional life. People seeking career counseling services can meet with counselors in a one-on-one setting or in small groups. Though these are the most common settings, career counseling activities may also be presented to larger groups in a classroom or workshop environment. Small group sessions may last anywhere from four to six sessions. An initial or intake career counseling session may entail the use of assessments that will help determine the person's interests, aptitude, and skill sets.

Development (History and Application)

The practice of career counseling has its foundation in career counseling theory. Career counseling theories are different from career theories in that career theories provide possible explanations for how people experience their careers and work environments along with how they make job-related decisions. On the other hand, career counseling theories attempt to provide possible approaches to assist a person along his or her career development path. Several types of career counseling theories exist and can determine the approach, techniques, activities, and assessment tools that a career counselor chooses to employ with a client.

Career counseling services began at the turn of the 20th century with Frank Parsons and the vocational guidance movement. Parsons outlined a career decision-making process whereby people could identify their aptitudes and interests and align them to a fitting career choice. Current theorists, such as John Holland, refer to this concept as "person-environment-fit."

Career counselors typically receive specialized education, training, and/or certification. Most hold a master's level degree in counseling with a specific focus on career assessment, development, theory, and advisement techniques. Professional school counselors, or guidance counselors, obtain coursework and training pertaining to career counseling topics for students in grade prekindergarten through 12th.

Current Status

Career counseling takes place in different settings. Career counseling centers may be free standing or located in educational settings including community colleges and universities. Recent mandates require that career domains be covered in the kindergarten through 12th-grade curriculum. However, how educational systems go about this can vary according to state, district, and school setting. Professional school counselors have been charged with covering career development in their guidance and counseling curriculums. Furthermore, the American School Counselor Association National Model mandates that career standards be incorporated into comprehensive developmental guidance programs. School counseling curriculums may cover career domains in a variety of direct counseling services, including classroom guidance, small group counseling, and individual counseling. Again, the delivery system may also vary according to grade level. For example, high school students may require more individualized career guidance services, so one-on-one advising may occur more often at this level.

Melissa A. Mariani, PhD

See also: Career Assessment; Career Development

Further Reading

Bowers, Judy, and Trish Hatch. *The ASCA National Model: A Framework for School Counseling Programs*, 2nd ed. Alexandria, VA: American Counseling Association, 2005.

Brown, Duane, and Linda Brooks. *Career Counseling Techniques*. Boston, MA: Allyn & Bacon, 1991.

Herr, Edwin L., and Stanley H. Cramer. *Career Guidance and Counseling through the Life Span*, 3rd ed. New York, NY: Longman, 2003.

Osipow, Samuel H., and Louise F. Fitzgerald. *Theories of Career Development*. Boston, MA: Allyn & Bacon, 1996.

Career Development

Career development refers to an ongoing, lifelong process of learning about oneself and developing new skills in relation to work. This process can be influenced by several factors including psychological, educational, physical, economical, and sociological.

Description

Career development refers to how people relate to the world of work and their role in it. This ongoing process involves managing one's career either within an organization or between organizations for the purpose of attaining specific career goals and aspirations. Several factors contribute to the development and success of a career over the lifespan, including personality and trait factors, developmental factors, and systemic factors. These factors have been outlined as the basis of different career development theories.

Career development can be defined within two separate contexts: organizational and personal. When defining the term from an organizational perspective, career development refers to how one manages one's career within an organization or between organizations. It also includes how these organizations structure advancement within the company (i.e., how one progresses in career goals). From a personal perspective, career development is defined as the combination of physical, psychological, sociological, educational, and economic factors that influence the nature and significance of work for a person over his or her lifetime. These factors can also impact one's career patters, decision-making style, sense of self, and personal values.

Prior to the late 1960s, the term "career development" was more commonly referred to as vocational development and its practice as career guidance or vocational guidance. The more recent term, "career development," emerged in the later part of the 20th century and has continued to evolve in the 21st century. Career development derived from the vocational guidance movement. Demographic, economic, and societal changes in the United States during this time urged leaders to respond to growing demands in educational and career domains. Pressure to compete with other nations thus resulted in a need for career guidance and career development practices. The purpose of career development then was to help determine a person's aptitude and ability and properly place the person in a fitting career.

Frank Parsons, the father of the vocational guidance movement, offered a three-step model for counselors to use to guide people through the career development process. He proposed that first, one should have a clear understanding of oneself and one's interests, abilities, talents, and limitations. Second, the person should be educated on what careers are out there that would be a good match for his or her aptitudes, and furthermore, the person should have a working knowledge of the requirements needed in order to be successful in that line of work. With this comes the practical knowledge related to advantages and disadvantages of those career paths. Third, one must have a reasonable ability to incorporate what was learned in the first two steps in order to make the best decision possible.

Current Status and Impact (Psychological Influence)

A person should be introduced to career development early on in life in school if not at home. Though career development has been a focal point of education in elementary and secondary schools since the mid-1900s, specific standards were not outlined in curriculum until much later. The American School Counselor Association's first set of National Standards, developed in 1995, outlined three domain areas that should be the focus of guidance and counseling standards for all students in K-12 settings. These three domains are academic, personal/social, and career development. Career decision making remains an integral part of a student's future success in the world of work.

Melissa A. Mariani, PhD

See also: Career Assessment; Career Counseling

Further Reading

Herr, Edwin L. "Collaboration, Partnership, Policy, and Practice in Career Development." *The Career Development Quarterly* 48 (2000): 293–300.

Osipow, Samuel H., and Louise F. Fitzgerald. *Theories of Career Development*. Boston, MA: Allyn & Bacon, 1996.

Patton, Wendy, and Mary McMahon. *Career Development and Systems Theory: A New Relationship*. Pacific Grove, CA: Brooks/Cole Publishing, 1999.

Sears, Susan. "A Definition of Career Guidance Terms: A National Vocational Guidance Association Perspective." *Vocational Guidance Quarterly* 31 (1982): 137–143.

Caregivers

Caregivers are those who help others who by reason of age, illness, or disability are unable to live self-sufficiently.

Description

A caregiver is a person designated as responsible for the care of someone else who suffers from poor mental health or physical disability or whose health is impaired by sickness or old age. The general term "caregiver" refers to both professional health-care workers and untrained, semiskilled relatives or friends of disabled people. Professional caregivers include graduate school–educated nurses, postsecondary trained assistants, and high school graduates. These professionals also include registered nurses, personal care assistants, or respite care workers. Duties involved in these professional roles range from the provision of medical care to self-help skills and beyond.

Family members, friends, and other relatives of people with disabilities or illnesses also serve as caregivers. Usually these informal caregivers are unpaid and are expected to help the individuals they care for with their daily living activities such as cleaning, cooking, and paying bills. In recent years however, the range of duties has increased to include some traditionally performed only by nursing staff. These duties include administering prescribed medications, dealing as intermediary with doctors and nurses on behalf of the one they care for, and helping the patient with intimate activities such as bathing or dressing, as well as activities such as exercise or physiotherapy. Often caregivers perform these activities over many years and with increasing difficulty as the patient's or relative's condition worsens. Caregivers themselves age and encounter their own physical, psychological, and mental limitations.

Current Status and Impact (Psychological Influence)

In 2009 it was estimated that there were over 60 million people in the United States who were acting as caregivers for others in some capacity. Almost 75% of these people were female and most were between 35 and 59 years of age. With an aging population and limited societal services for individuals who cannot live self-sufficiently, the role of caregiver has become a very common and necessary function in modern society. Caregivers are especially necessary in the beginning stages of debilitating conditions like dementia, Alzheimer's, and Parkinson's. When these patients require assistance mostly to cope with normal daily activities, it is usually relatives or friends who provide the necessary help.

Many nonprofessional caregivers face great challenges in adjusting to their role and its physical and psychological demands. They are often in relationships of familial intimacy with the patients for whom they are responsible. Even though they often say that they find the opportunity to provide care for a loved

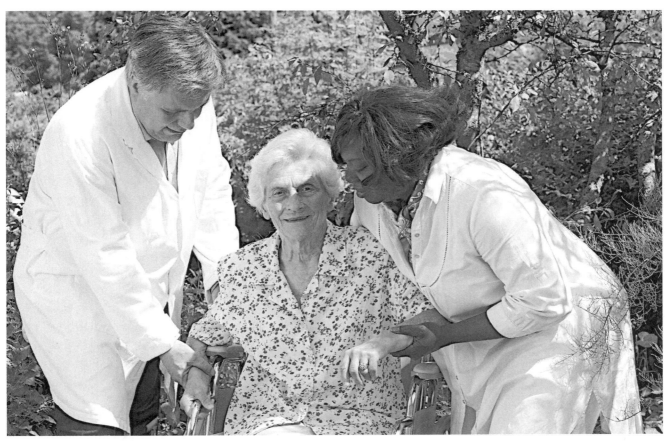

A caregiver is responsible for the care of someone else who suffers from poor mental health or physical disability, or whose health is impaired by sickness or old age. A good caregiver can be crucial to those who suffer from mental health issues. (Jean Paul Chassenet/Dreamstime.com)

one rewarding, it is also true that stress and burnout characterize many caregivers especially after what may be years of continuous responsibility. This condition of exhaustion or discouragement is often referred to as caregiver syndrome.

It is clear that taking care of the caregiver is a challenge for society. Caregivers must have support themselves in order to do their jobs effectively and efficiently. One of the best supports is for the caregiver to get a temporary but regular break from the demands of caregiving for a patient or family member. Psychoeducation and support activities, such as support groups, for caregivers are crucial in the coming years if they are to fulfill their critical duties.

Alexandra Cunningham, PhD, and William M. Cunningham, MA

See also: Psychoeducation; Support Groups

Further Reading

Etters, Lynn, Debbie Goodall, and Barbara E. Harrison. "Caregiver Burden among Dementia Patient Caregivers: A Review of the Literature." *Journal of the American Academy of Nurse Practitioners* 20 (2008): 423–428.

Reinhard, Susan C., Carol Levine, and Sarah Samis. *Home Alone: Family Caregivers Provide Complex Chronic Care.* Washington, DC: AARP Public Policy Institute, 2012.

Sheehy, Gail. *Passages in Caregiving: Turning Chaos into Confidence.* New York, NY: HarperCollins, 2010.

Case Conceptualization

Case conceptualizations provide psychotherapists with an explanation and strategy for planning and focusing treatment interventions to increase the likelihood of achieving treatment goals.

Definitions

- **Diagnostic and Statistical Manual of Mental Disorders (DSM)** is a diagnostic classification framework that characterizes mental disorders with specific diagnostic criteria. It is used by clinicians to diagnose mental disorders. The most current version is DSM-5.

- **Maladaptive pattern** refers to a pattern that is dysfunctional or unhealthy.

- **Pattern** is a description of an individual's characteristic way of perceiving, thinking, and acting.

Description

A case conceptualization is a clinical strategy for obtaining and organizing information about a client, explaining the client's situation and maladaptive pattern, guiding and focusing treatment, anticipating challenges and roadblocks, and preparing for successful termination. While many therapists develop conceptualizations to guide their practice, not all therapists explicitly articulate these conceptualizations because they are not sufficiently confident with this competency. There are a number of internal and external reasons for developing and articulating a case conceptualization. The most important internal reason is that a case conceptualization enables therapists to experience a sense of confidence in their work. This confidence is then communicated to the client, which strengthens the client's trust in the therapist and belief that therapy can and will make a difference.

Developments and Current Status

Since at least 2005, case conceptualizations, previously called case formulations, were a requisite for the effective provision of psychotherapy. There are at least three external reasons for this trend. The first reason is the accountability demand by third-party payers that counselors and therapists justify their treatment with clients. Receiving authorization and payment to treat a client requires documentation of a compelling rationale for treatment. The second reason is the movement toward empirically supported treatment, which emphasizes the use of case conceptualizations. The third reason is that the diagnostic manuals, such as DSM-5,

are largely descriptive and do not provide explanation for causes, precipitants, maintaining factors, or treatment interventions. In contrast, a case conceptualization provides a rationale for all these factors and a link between diagnosis and treatment.

A case conceptualization is essentially a summary statement consisting of four components. The first is a diagnostic formulation that provides a description of the client's presenting situation and its perpetuants or triggering factors. It answers the "What happened?" question and usually includes a DSM-5 diagnosis. The second is a clinical formulation that provides a compelling explanation of the client's presenting symptoms, issues, and maladaptive pattern. It answers the "Why did it happen?" question. The third is the cultural formulation that provides a cultural explanation of the client's presentation and the impact of cultural factors on the client's personality. It answers the "What role does culture play?" question. The fourth is the treatment formulation that provides an explicit blueprint for intervention planning. It answers the "How can it be changed?" questions, contains treatment goals and specific interventions, and anticipates challenges in achieving these goals.

Len Sperry, MD, PhD

See also: Psychotherapy; Psychotherapy Skills and Competency

Further Reading

Eells, Tracy, ed. *Handbook of Psychotherapy Case Formulation*, 2nd ed. New York, NY: Guilford, 2007.

Sperry, Len, and Jonathan Sperry. *Case Conceptualization: Mastering This Competency with Ease and Confidence.* New York, NY: Routledge, 2012.

Case Management

Case management is a collaborative process between a case manager and an individual and his or her family to assess, plan, coordinate, evaluate, and advocate for the individual's health needs.

Definitions

- **Case managers** are health-care professionals who work with individuals and families to plan, coordinate, and monitor the outcomes of health-care services.

- **Evidence-based practice** is a form of practice that is based on the integration of the best research evidence with clinical expertise and client values.

- **Health Maintenance Organization** is an organization that provides or arranges managed care.

- **Managed care** is a system of health care that controls costs by placing limits on physicians' fees and by restricting access to certain medical procedures and providers.

- **Practice** is a method or process used to accomplish a goal or objective.

- **Psychotherapy** is a psychological method for achieving desired changes in thinking, feeling, and behavior. It is also called therapeutic counseling.

Description

Case management has two functions (purposes). The first is to advocate for the client after determining health and mental health needs. The second is to coordinate resources and ensure that the client's needs are satisfied. Case managers are an integral part of case management. Their job is to assess the client's needs to determine the appropriate services to fulfill those needs. They then develop a detailed plan, which includes the services of health-care providers, psychiatrists, psychotherapists, psychological evaluation, substance abuse programs, and life skills counseling. Case manager also works with other agencies and professionals to ensure that clients' needs, including living arrangements, are met.

Case management involves a case-by-case evaluation of clients' need for services. The need is compared to the cost of services and available funding for services. Case management attempts to ethically match appropriate health-care services with client needs. It assists in managing health problems as well as life care planning. First and foremost, the measure of the effectiveness of case management is its advocacy for the client.

While case management and psychotherapy appear to be similar, they are actually quite different. The primary focus of psychotherapy is to develop a therapeutic alliance (relationship) with a client and then work collaboratively to effect a basic change in the client's personality and pattern of functioning. In contrast, while a good working relationship and collaboration with a client are essential for case management to be effective, the goal is not to effect basic changes in the client's personality and pattern of functioning. Rather, it is to coordinate the services of all providers involved with the client, including psychotherapists. It should be noted, however, that occasionally, a psychotherapist may function briefly in the case management role when a client does not have a designated case manager.

Development and Current Status

Case management has its roots in managed care and Health Maintenance Organizations. Managed care was established to increase the efficiency and cost effectiveness of health care. Case management can and does have a critical role in managed care. This is particularly the case when a client has serious, complex, or long-standing health problems that require the coordination of many health providers and services. In this respect, case management has a unique role on the health-care team.

Over the years, case management has become a recognized health-care profession. The Case Management Society of America began in 1990. It was established to assist in defining and promoting the profession of case management. Since 1993, the Commission on Case Manager Certification has awarded the Certified Case Manager designation to professionals who meet certification standards.

Case management systems range in size, bureaucracy, and the number of cases to be managed. Some case management systems are overloaded with clients. The effectiveness of case management is directly related to the amount of time spent with a client. Most frequently, case management is utilized with the elderly, disabled, or chronically ill. Finally, it should be noted that changes to the health-care system in the United States have increasingly impacted the practice of case management.

Len Sperry, MD, PhD, and
Layven Reguero, MEd

See also: Case Manager; Empirically Supported Treatment; Evidence-Based Practice

Further Reading

Kathol, Roger G., Rebecca Perez, and Janice Cohen. *The Integrated Case Management Manual: Assisting Complex Patients Regain Physical and Mental Health.* New York, NY: Springer, 2010.

Powell, Suzanne, and Hussein A. Tahan. *Case Management: A Practical Guide to Success in Managed Care*, 2nd ed. Philadelphia, PA: Lippincott Williams & Wilkins, 2009.

Wong, Daniel F. *Clinical Case Management for People with Mental Illness: A Biopsychosocial Vulnerability-Stress Model.* Binghamton, NY: Haworth Press, 2000.

Case Manager

Case managers are health-care professionals who work together with individuals and families to assess, plan, coordinate, evaluate, and advocate for the individual's health needs.

Definitions

- **Case management** is a collaborative process between a case manager and an individual and his or her family to assess, plan, coordinate, evaluate, and advocate for the individual's health needs.

- **Evidence-based practice** is a form of practice that is based on integration of the best research evidence with clinical experience and client values.

- **Health Maintenance Organization** (HMO) is an organization that provides or arranges managed care.

- **Managed care** is a system of health care that controls costs by placing limits on physicians' fees and by restricting access to certain medical procedures and providers.

- **Practice** is a method or process used to accomplish a goal or objective.

- **Psychotherapy** is a psychological method for achieving desired changes in thinking, feeling, and behavior. It is also called therapeutic counseling.

Description

Case managers have two essential functions (job purposes). The first is to manage advocacy efforts for clients' health and mental health needs. This advocacy occurs after the case manager works to determine what a client's health needs are. The second function includes the coordination of resources necessary to meet those needs. It also includes working with other agencies and professionals to ensure that client needs are thoroughly evaluated, monitored, and treated. Case managers evaluate clients' need for services on a case-by-case basis. They strive to make the most ethical decisions possible regarding matching health services with clients' needs, while considering cost of treatment and available funding. Highly effective case managers successfully advocate and efficiently coordinate services for their clients.

While case managers' and psychotherapists' functions appear to be similar, they are actually quite different. Psychotherapists focus primarily on developing a therapeutic alliance (relationship) with a client and then collaboratively work to effect basic changes in the client's personality and pattern of functioning. In contrast, while effective case managers establish a good working relationship, the purpose of their job is not to effect basic changes in the client's personality and pattern of functioning. Rather, case managers coordinate with all providers of health services required by clients' needs, which often include psychotherapists. However, when a client does not have a case manager, his or her psychotherapist can function briefly in the case management role. Case managers, on the other hand, are not typically trained to function as a psychotherapist.

Development and Current Status

The coordination of health services has evolved throughout the years and has been the responsibility of various health-care professionals. The modern case manager, described earlier, has its roots in managed care and HMOs. Managed care was established to increase the efficiency and cost effectiveness of health care in the 1970s. In 1990, the Case Management Society of America (CMSA) was founded. CMSA assisted in defining and promoting professional case managers. Since 1993, the Commission of Case Manager Certification has awarded the Certified Case Manager designation to professionals who meet certification standards.

Layven Reguero, MEd, and
Len Sperry, MD, PhD

See also: Case Management; Empirically Supported Treatment; Evidence-Based Practice; Managed Care

Further Reading

Longhofer, Jeffrey, Paul M. Kubek and Jerry Floersch. *On Being and Having a Case Manager: A Relational Approach to Recovery in Mental Health.* New York, NY: Columbia University Press, 2010.

Powell, Suzanne K., and Hussein A. Tahan. *CMSA Core Curriculum for Case Management*, 2nd ed. Philadelphia, PA: Lippincott Williams & Wilkins, 2008.

Suber, Robert W., ed. *Clinical Case Management: A Guide to Comprehensive Treatment of Serious Mental Illness.* Thousand Oaks, CA: Sage, 1994.

Catatonic Disorders

Catatonic disorders are mental disorders characterized by catatonia or disturbances in muscle movement often involving rigid body postures.

Definitions

- **Antipsychotic medications** are prescription drugs used to treat psychotic disorders. They are also referred to as neuroleptics or antipsychotics.

- **Bipolar disorder** is a mental disorder characterized by a history of manic episodes (bipolar I disorder), mixed, or hypomanic episodes (bipolar II disorder), usually with one or more major depressive episodes.

- **Catatonia** is a condition of immobility with muscle rigidity or inflexibility and, at times, overactivity and excitability.

- **Delirium** is sudden and severe confusion due to changes in brain function that occur in mental and physical illness.

- **Delusions** are fixed false beliefs that persist despite contrary evidence.

- **Depressive disorders** are a group of mental disorders characterized by a sad or irritable mood and cognitive and physical changes that significantly disrupt the individual's daily routine.

- **DSM-5** stands for the *Diagnostic and Statistical Manual of Mental Disorders, Fifth Edition*, which is a diagnostic system used by professionals to identify mental disorders with specific diagnostic criteria.

- **Electroconvulsive therapy** is a procedure in which electric currents are passed through the brain, intentionally triggering a brief seizure in order to quickly reverse symptoms of certain mental illnesses. It is also referred to as ECT.

- **Hallucinations** are false or distorted sensory perceptions that appear to be real perceptions that are generated by the mind rather than external stimuli.

- **Psychotic disorder** is a severe mental disorder characterized by psychotic features.

- **Psychotic features** are symptoms characteristic of psychotic disorders. They include delusions, hallucinations, and negative symptoms (lack of initiative and diminished emotional expression).

- **Schizophrenia spectrum and other psychotic disorders** are a group of DSM-5 mental disorders characterized by psychotic features. They include schizophrenia, delusional disorder, and catatonic disorders.

- **Specifier** is an extension to a diagnosis that further clarifies the course, severity, or type of features of a disorder or illness.

Description and Diagnosis

Catatonic disorders are classified with the DSM-5 schizophrenia spectrum and other psychotic disorders. Basic to all catatonic disorders is catatonia. It is characterized by a psychomotor (mental processes and physical movement) disturbance that may involve decreased motor activity, dismissiveness during an interview or physical examination, or excessive or strange motor activity. The psychomotor disturbance in an individual may range from being unresponsive to agitated. Motor immobility and dismissiveness may be severe or moderate. Excessive and strange motor behaviors may be simple or complex. The most common presentation is maintaining stiffened and rigid body postures for long periods. In some cases, an individual may alternate between decreased and excessive motor activity. Individuals exhibiting severe stages of catatonia may need supervision from a caretaker to avoid harming themselves or others. Furthermore, catatonia has potential risks, which include exhaustion, malnutrition, extreme fever, and self-harm.

Catatonia is a condition that can occur in several disorders, including neurodevelopmental, psychotic, bipolar, and depressive disorders, and other medical conditions. While catatonia is not a specific disorder in DSM-5, DSM-5 does recognize catatonia associated with other mental disorders (e.g., psychotic disorders, neurodevelopmental disorders, bipolar disorders, depressive disorders, or other mental disorders). There are three types of catatonic disorders in DSM-5. They include catatonia associated with another mental disorder (catatonia specifier), catatonic disorder due to another medical condition, and unspecified catatonia. Following are brief descriptions of each of these disorders.

Catatonia associated with another mental disorder (catatonia specifier). Catatonia associated with another mental disorder (catatonia specifier) may be applied when criteria are met for catatonia during the course of psychotic, neurological, depressive, bipolar, or other mental health disorders. The catatonia specifier is appropriate to use when an individual has characteristics of psychomotor disturbance and involves at least 3 of the 12 diagnostic features indicated in the DSM-5. Some of the diagnostic features include not actively relating to the environment, motionlessness maintained over a long period, resistance to positioning by the examiner, opposition to instructions, and inappropriate posture maintained over a long period. Individuals with this disorder may also exhibit a detailed caricature of normal actions, repetitive movements, agitation, disapproving facial expressions, and mimicking another individual's speech and movements. The majority of catatonia cases involve individuals with bipolar and depressive disorders. However, up to 35% of individuals with catatonia have schizophrenia and are usually diagnosed in inpatient settings (American Psychiatric Association, 2013). Catatonia can occur as a side effect of medications. Before any of the disorders related to the catatonia specifier can be diagnosed, a variety of other medical conditions need to be excluded.

Catatonic disorder due to another medical condition. Catatonic disorder due to another medical condition is the presence of catatonia that is found to be caused by the psychological effects of another medical condition. Catatonia is diagnosed when at least 3 of the 12 clinical features indicated in the DSM-5 are present. The diagnostic features of this disorder are exactly the same as the one's listed earlier in catatonia associated with another mental disorder (catatonia specifier). There must be evidence from a physical examination, an individual's history, or laboratory results that the disturbance is the direct result of another medical condition. This diagnosis is not given if it is better accounted for by another disorder (e.g., depressive episode) or if it takes place solely during the course of a delirium. The disturbance (catatonia) must cause significant impairment and distress in an individual's occupational, social, or other important areas of life. A number of medical conditions may cause catatonia, particularly neurological conditions, such as head trauma, inflammation of the brain, and disease of blood vessels in the brain (American Psychiatric Association, 2013).

Unspecified catatonia. Unspecified catatonia is a category that applies to the appearance of symptoms that are characteristic of catatonia and cause significant impairment or distress in occupational, social, or other important areas of an individual's life. The essential features of the primary mental disorder or other medical condition are not clear. Furthermore, the full criteria for catatonia as indicated in the DSM-5 are not met, and there is not sufficient information to make a more specific diagnosis (American Psychiatric Association, 2013).

Treatment

The clinical treatment of catatonic symptoms involved medication management and electroconvulsive therapy (ECT). Antipsychotics are effective in treating symptoms of catatonia. However, there are concerns with these medications since they can cause or worsen catatonia in some individuals. Still, because they are effective with most individuals with these disorders, they continue to be used. ECT is another form of treatment for catatonia. It involves administering electric shock to the brain, which precipitates a seizure in order to quickly reverse symptoms of catatonia. If an individual does not positively react to medication therapy, ECT has been shown to be the second choice of treatment. ECT has been found to be an effective and safe treatment approach.

Len Sperry, MD, PhD, and
Elizabeth Smith Kelsey, PhD

See also: Benzodiazepines; Bipolar Disorder; Brain; Delirium; Delusions; Depression and Depressive Disorders; *Diagnostic and Statistical Manual of Mental Disorders* (DSM); Electroconvulsive Therapy (ECT); Hallucinations

Further Reading

American Psychiatric Association. *Diagnostic and Statistical Manual of Mental Disorders*, 5th ed. Arlington, VA: American Psychiatric Association, 2013.

Fink, Max, and Michael Alan Taylor. *Catatonia: A Clinician's Guide to Diagnosis and Treatment*. New York, NY: Cambridge University Press, 2006.

Freudenreich, Oliver. *Psychotic Disorders: A Practical Guide (Practical Guides in Psychiatry)*. Philadelphia, PA: Lippincott Williams & Wilkins, 2007.

CBT

See Cognitive Behavior Therapy

Celexa (Citalopram)

Celexa is a prescription antidepressant medication for the treatment of depression and various anxiety disorders. Its generic name is citalopram.

Description

Celexa is one of the selective serotonin reuptake inhibitor (SSRI) antidepressants. Its main use is for the treatment of depression. Other uses include treatment of alcoholism, eating disorders, obsessive-compulsive disorder, panic disorder, post-traumatic stress disorder, premenstrual dysphoric disorder, and social anxiety disorder. Serotonin is a neurotransmitter or brain chemical that carries nerve impulses from one nerve cell to another. It is believed that depression and certain mental disorders are caused by insufficient serotonin in the brain. Like the other SSRI antidepressants, Prozac, Zoloft, and Paxil, Celexa increases the level of brain serotonin. Increased serotonin levels in the brain appear to be beneficial in relieving symptoms associated with depression, anxiety, alcoholism, headaches, and premenstrual tension and mood swings.

Precautions and Side Effects

Individuals who are allergic to other SSRI medications should not be prescribed Celexa. Those with liver problems and those over the age of 65 are best treated with lower doses of the drug. Those with histories of mania, suicide attempts, or seizure disorders should start Celexa with caution and only under close physician supervision. Children and young adults are at higher risk of developing suicidal thoughts and actions. Generally, those under 18 years of age should not take Celexa. Because it interacts with monoamine oxidase inhibitors, like Parnate, an antidepressant, or Buspirone, an antianxiety medication, Celexa should not be used in combination with these medications. Similarly, certain herbal supplements, like Ginkgo and St. John's wort, should not be taken together with Celexa.

Nausea, dry mouth, and insomnia are among the most common side effect of Celexa. Other side effects include anxiety, agitation, headaches, dizziness, restlessness, sedation, tremor, and yawning. Decreased sex drive in women and difficulty ejaculating in men have been reported, while weight gain or loss is not common. In some patients these sexual side effects never resolve. If sexual side effects continue, the dose may be reduced or a switch made to another antidepressant.

Len Sperry, MD, PhD

See also: Antidepressant Medications

Further Reading

Albers, Lawrence J., Rhoda K. Hahn, and Christopher Reist. *Handbook of Psychiatric Drugs*. Laguna Hills, CA: Current Clinical Strategies, 2010.

Baldwin, Robert C. *Depression in Later Life*. New York, NY: Oxford University Press, 2010.

O'Connor, Richard. *Undoing Depression: What Therapy Doesn't Teach You and Medication Can't Give You*, 2ed ed. New York: NY Little, Brown, 2010.

Stahl, Stephen M. *Antidepressants*. New York, NY: Cambridge University Press, 2009.

Certified Addictions Professional (CAP)

Certified Addictions Professional is a credential for individuals who provide treatment services for addictions. It is also known as CAP.

Definitions

- **Addiction** is a chronic disease of the brain that involves compulsive and uncontrolled pursuit of reward or relief with substance use or other compulsive behaviors.

- **Alcoholism** is a general term for the compulsive and uncontrolled consumption of alcohol to the detriment of the drinker's health, relationships, and social standing.

- **Ambivalence** is a human phenomenon that occurs when a client has opposing opinions about behavioral change.

- **Case management** is a process that involves linking clients to community resources that may enhance or promote their well-being or daily functioning.

- **DSM-5** is the abbreviation for the *Diagnostic and Statistical Manual of Mental Disorders, Fifth Edition*, which is the handbook mental health professionals use to diagnose mental disorders.

- **Motivational interviewing** is a counseling approach that is used to assist individuals in considering behavioral change, that is, to stop using alcohol and seek alternative coping strategies.

- **Substance-related and addictive disorders** are a group of DSM-5 mental disorders that include substance disorders characterized by physiological dependence, drug-seeking behavior, tolerance, and social withdrawal. This group also includes the non-substance disorder of gambling.

Description

Certified Addictions Professional (CAP) is a credential that requires training, supervision, and passing a standardized exam. This designation allows clinicians to provide assessment and treatment among individuals living with substance-related and addictive disorders. Individuals with this credential are certified through their state's addictions certification board. This certification requires a minimum of a bachelor's degree and specific education in addictions. Other requirements include supervised work experience with substance abusers and passing a state certification exam. Specific training is required in the following areas: clinical evaluation, case management, counseling, treatment planning, professional documentation, ethical and professional issues, theory and treatment of addictions, client and community education, and application to practice. Training in these content areas can be obtained online or in face-to-face training settings.

Certified Addictions Professionals provide assessment and psychotherapeutic treatment, create treatment plans, and provide case management to individuals living with substance use disorders. Services that CAPs offer include addiction prevention, intervention, and continuing care services. Specific interventions include substance abuse counseling among individuals, couples, families, communities, and group therapy contexts. Substance abuse counseling includes talk therapy interventions such as relapse prevention, learning new coping skills, learning triggers, and cognitive and behavioral replacement strategies. CAPs are trained in working with clients who may be court ordered for treatment or who are not motivated to stop using substances.

Since many clients who enter drug treatment are ambivalent about changing, motivational interviewing is often used. It can assist clients in examining their behaviors and ambivalence in a nonjudgmental and supportive environment. CAPs often utilize this approach to form an alliance with the client but also assist the client in resolving his or her ambivalence about abstaining from substance use and eventually assist him or her in committing to therapy and self-improvement.

Maintenance of the CAP credential requires ongoing continuing education that can be attained from approved providers. Continuing education is required to ensure that clinicians are learning and practicing empirically supported treatments. CAP holders are responsible for obtaining required continuing education through approved or accredited training providers.

The CAP credential is affiliated with the International Certification & Reciprocity Consortium (IC&RC), which monitors the international standards of practice in addiction counseling and other tasks that CAPs engage in. In addition, the IC&RC recognizes the minimum standards to provide reciprocity to professors across state borders. The certification board monitors the code of ethics to ensure quality assurance in the prevention and treatment of individuals living with addictions. Individuals applying for the CAP also take an international exam from the IC&RC.

Jon Sperry, PhD, and Len Sperry, MD, PhD

See also: Addiction; *Diagnostic and Statistical Manual of Mental Disorders* (DSM); Motivational Interviewing; Substance-Related and Addictive Disorders

Further Reading

American Psychiatric Association. *Diagnostic and Statistical Manual of Mental Disorders*, 5th ed. Arlington, VA: American Psychiatric Association, 2013.

Miller, William, and Richardo Muñoz. *Controlling Your Drinking*. New York, NY: Guilford Press, 2005.

Miller, William, and Stephen Rollnick. *Motivational Interviewing: Preparing People for Change*, 2nd ed. New York, NY: Guilford Press, 2002.

Certified Rehabilitation Counselor (CRC)

A Certified Rehabilitation Counselor is a professionally trained therapist who works to help people with various disabilities. It is also known as a CRC.

Definitions

- **Certification** is a formal procedure by which an accredited or authorized person or agency assesses and verifies that a person has the knowledge and skills to perform certain activities.

- **Rehabilitation counseling** is a type of counseling that focuses on helping individuals who have disabilities in order to achieve their career, personal, and independent living goals.

Description

Specific qualifications are required in order to become a Certified Rehabilitation Counselor (CRC). This includes specialized education, training, and field work prior to passing a national exam. Once a person successfully completes these steps, he or she is able to apply to become a CRC. The education and training that CRCs receive focus on understanding the medical and psychosocial aspects of various disabilities.

Those students seeking a master's degree in rehabilitation counseling have undergraduate degrees in rehabilitation services, psychology, sociology, or other human services–related fields. As a master's degree is required at a minimum, rehabilitation counselors are trained at the graduate level. Most earn a master's degree, with a few continuing on to the doctoral level. The Council on Rehabilitation Education accredits programs at universities, but not all programs meet accreditation requirements. This limitation prohibits some graduates from professional certification/licensure.

The primary purpose of rehabilitation counselors is to value a client's rights to be as independent as possible. This includes independent living, promoting advocacy, and empowering the client to be socially included. There are several areas of specialty among rehabilitation counselors. These include specializations in employee assistance, job coaching, substance abuse, life and medical care planning, and mental health counseling. CRCs should also be knowledgeable about assistive technology and devices that can help people overcome obstacles. A CRC is also involved in case management and assessing a client's abilities and strengths to help him or her get jobs.

Current Status and Impact (Psychological Influence)

Although policies vary from state to state, rehabilitation counselors who work in the federal and state systems typically must hold a master's degree in rehabilitation counseling, special education, or a related field, and are required to be certified or be eligible to sit for the certification examination. People accepting employment in government-run vocational rehabilitation programs are required to meet these qualifications by a specific date in order to keep their jobs.

Alexandra Cunningham, PhD

See also: Commission on Rehabilitation Counselor Certification (CRCC); Rehabilitation Counseling; Vocational Counseling

Further Reading

Commission on Rehabilitation Counselor Certification. "Rehabilitation Counseling." Accessed January 15, 2015. www.crccertification.com.

Maki, Dennis R., and Villa M. Tarvydas. *The Professional Practice of Rehabilitation Counseling*. New York, NY: Springer, 2011.

Parker, Randall M., and Jeanne Boland Patterson. *Rehabilitation Counseling: Basics & Beyond*. New York, NY: Pro-ed, 2012.

Chamomile

Chamomile is an herb that has been used to alleviate anxiety and stress, to produce mild sedation, to reduce restlessness and irritability, and to ease depression.

Description

The chamomile flower has been harvested for centuries for various medicinal purposes. Today, various preparations are available. It is commercially available in prepackaged tea bags, in capsule form, as an oil, and as a liquid extract. Chamomile has both internal and external use. It has been used internally for a wide variety of conditions to remove intestinal parasites, to prevent or to reduce inflammation, and to control infection. Chamomile has also been used to relieve intestinal cramping, digestive disorders, menstrual cramps, premenstrual syndrome, headache, and other stress-related disorders. In addition, it is used a sedative, often in the form of tea, to treat anxiety and insomnia. External uses of chamomile include blending its oil with lavender or rose for scenting perfumes, candles, creams, and for other aromatherapy products intended to calm or relax the user's mind and body and reduce anxiety.

Does chamomile actually work? A randomized, double-blind, placebo-controlled study found chamomile extract helped reduce symptoms of mild to moderate generalized anxiety disorder (GAD). Because this is the first controlled clinical trial of chamomile extract for GAD and involved a small sample, additional studies are needed to support its findings. Unlike prescription medications, the U.S. Food and Drug Administration does not evaluate chamomile with regard to its effectiveness, purity, or safety.

Precautions and Side Effects

Generally, chamomile is considered safe. However, it can cause side effects such as allergic reactions in people who are sensitive to ragweed and other substances. Chamomile should not be taken two weeks before or after surgery. Women who are pregnant or could become pregnant should not use chamomile, since its use may increase the risk of miscarriage. Similarly, it should not be used by mothers who are breast-feeding infants. Chamomile can increase the effects of anticoagulant medications and the effects of benzodiazepines. It could also adversely interact with sedatives, antiplatelet drugs, aspirin, and nonsteroidal anti-inflammatory drugs. Individuals prescribed such medications should talk with their doctor before using chamomile. In addition, chamomile can interact with supplements such as ginkgo biloba, garlic, saw palmetto, St. John's wort, and valerian.

Len Sperry, MD, PhD

See also: Ginkgo biloba; St. John's Wort; Valerian

Further Reading

Arrowsmith, Nancy. *Essential Herbal Wisdom: A Complete Exploration of 50 Remarkable Herbs.* Woodbury, MN: Llewellyn, 2009.

Mayo Clinic Book of Alternative Medicine. New York, NY: Time Home Entertainment, 2007.

PDR for Herbal Medicines, 4th ed. Montvale, NJ: Thomson, 2007.

Chicken Soup for the Soul (Book)

Chicken Soup for the Soul is a *New York Times* best-selling book that was first released on June 28, 1993. Since this first publication, 200 variations on the title and translations into 40 different languages have followed. Over 112 million copies have been sold in the United States and Canada alone.

Description

The popular book series, *Chicken Soup for the Soul*, written by Mark Victor Hansen and Jack Canfield, has seen much success grossing over $2 billion to date. The authors both had previous careers as motivational speakers and knew how storytelling could be used to inspire others. For the original book, published in 1993, they gathered 101 of the most powerful stories from ordinary people all over the nation. The book's title came from Canfield's memory of his grandmother and how she always said that her chicken soup could cure any ailment; they applied this same concept to hurts of the soul.

Chicken Soup for the Soul did not gain initial popularity from media attention but rather through simple word of mouth. By September 1994, it was on every major best-seller list in the United States and Canada. It soon received coverage on television shows like *The Oprah Winfrey Show* and *The Today Show* and major sitcoms such as *Friends* and *Everybody Loves Raymond*. In 1995, the book won the prestigious American Booksellers' Book of the Year Award. In 1996, it was honored "Non-Fiction Literacy Award" by the American Family Institute. *Chicken Soup for the Soul* set a record in 1998 when it had seven books from the series on the *New York Times* best-seller list at one time.

Impact (Psychological Influence)

The next two decades saw continued growth for the brand. In 2007, *USA Today* honored *Chicken Soup for the Soul* as one of the five most memorable and affecting books in the last quarter century. In April 2008, the authors sold a large portion of the company to a multimedia group headed by Internet executive, Bill Rouhana, hoping to expand the book's impact further. The newest titles in the series are now distributed through Simon & Schuster, Inc. Over 112 million books have been sold to date, and titles have been translated into more than 40 languages. The *Chicken Soup for the Soul* name is one of the most well known; 88.7% of people recognize it and know what it is (Harris Poll). The company is hoping to expand into other media outlets and is currently working on the development of television shows and Internet sites devoted to providing people with comfort, support, and overall wellness.

Melissa A. Mariani, PhD

See also: Self-Esteem

Further Reading

Canfield, Jack, and Mark Victor Hansen. *Chicken Soup for the Soul.* Deerfield, FL: Backlist, LLC, 1993.

Child Abuse

Child abuse and neglect impacts more children in the United States than all other serious diseases. Every year more than 3 million reports of child abuse that involve more than 6 million children are made in the United States. According to the nonprofit organization Child Help, there is a report of child abuse approximately every 10 seconds, and according to the Centers for Disease Control (CDC), more than four children die every day as a result of abuse.

Description

The Centers for Disease Control defines "child abuse" as the physical, sexual, or emotional maltreatment or neglect of a child or children. It includes any act or series of acts of commission or omission by a parent or caregiver that results in harm, potential for harm, or threat of harm to a child.

Child abuse can occur in multiple different forms of either physical, emotional, or sexual abuse or neglect. Neglect can be physical, educational, emotional, or medical. Physical neglect includes abandonment or lack of supervision as well as failure to provide for the child's safety or physical needs. Educational neglect includes not enrolling the child in school or allowing for frequent truancy. Emotional neglect includes a lack of affection or attention or psychological care for a child's needs. Medical neglect includes delay or withholding medical care, including due to religious beliefs. However, not all states will prosecute in relation to religious beliefs.

Indicators of neglect can include poor hygiene, unsuitable clothing, untreated injury, lack of immunizations, and indicators of prolonged exposure to elements such as extreme heat or cold as well as height and weight significantly below healthy age levels.

Physical abuse is generally the most obvious form of abuse as there can be marks left on the child. This could include everything from punching, beating, burning to shaking of a baby or child. Indicators of physical abuse are recurrent injuries that have either unexplained or inconsistent explanations. The child may be hesitant to show certain parts of his or her body, for instance, not wanting to dress out for physical education classes. The child may also act out aggressively toward others.

Fetal abuse is the result of the parent consuming drugs or alcohol while pregnant. This can result in the child being born addicted. It can also result in premature birth, miscarriage, or developmental delays.

Sexual abuse involves a child in sexual activities. There can be non-touching sexual abuse, which would include an adult exposing himself or herself to the child. Touching sexual abuse would include fondling, making the child touch an adult's sexual organs, or penetration of a child by adult or object. Sexual exploitation includes using the child for prostitution or for pornography. Indicators of sexual abuse include sexually acting out, bruises or bleeding in the genitalia, bed-wetting, excessive bathing, fire setting, aggressive or withdrawn behaviors, or substance abuse. Child sexual abuse is for the benefit of the abuser with lack of regard for the child. Ninety percent of child sexual abuse cases go unreported due to the child being afraid to tell anyone what happened.

Emotional abuse can greatly negatively impact a child's development and self-concept. This is generally the hardest to identify due to lack of physical evidence. This can be done by rejecting the child and humiliating or shaming the child, as well as isolating the child. Indicators of emotional abuse can be seen by the child hiding his or her eyes or avoiding eye contact as well as defensiveness, low self-esteem, regression, difficulty with relationships, depression, or alcohol and drug use.

Children at risk for abuse can come from a family where violence within the intimate partners is present, or are younger than four years. Another risk factor comes from living in communities with high level of violence or in families with great stress, substance abuse, poverty, or chronic illness. However, abuse can happen anywhere. The perpetrator generally has low levels of empathy and low levels of self-esteem.

Current Status and Impact (Psychological Influence)

Each year in the United States more than 3 million reports of child abuse involving over 6 million children are made. Each state in the country has a state-run department that investigates these reports and takes actions to help protect and assist in maintaining and assuring family safety. Regardless of the type of abuse, mental health symptoms such as depression or aggression are common after experiencing a form of abuse.

Research has shown that with a history of sexual abuse in childhood there are a multitude of mental health and behavioral problems in adult life. There is generally a strong link with depressive symptoms as well as post-traumatic stress disorder. Adults with drug and/or alcohol addiction also demonstrate high frequencies of reports of sexual abuse in their childhood. In fact adults with a history of childhood sexual abuse have significantly higher rates of an axis 1 disorder from the *Diagnostic and Statistical Manual of Mental Disorders* (DSM IV-TR).

Child abuse clearly can have long-lasting effects on development of children causing emotional difficulties and aggressive behaviors. There is also strong evidence that children who have been abused or neglected struggle with social relationships and interactions with peers. Children who have been abused or neglected are also at increased risk for juvenile delinquency, substance abuse, and self-destructive behaviors.

Mindy Parsons, PhD

See also: Adverse Childhood Experiences; Child Protective Services; Domestic Violence; Foster Care; Neglect

Further Reading

Briere, John. *Child Abuse Trauma: Theory and Treatment of the Lasting Effects*. Thousand Oaks, CA: Sage, 1992.

Child Help. "National Child Abuse Statistics." Last modified 2014. Accessed February 13, 2015. https://www.childhelp.org/child-abuse-statistics/.

Cutajar, Margaret C., Paul E. Mullen, James R. P. Ogloff, Stuart D. Thomas, David L. Wells, and Josie Spataro. "Psychopathology in a Large Cohort of Sexually Abused Children Followed up to 43 Years." *Child Abuse & Neglect* 34 (2010): 813–822.

Lawson, David M. *Family Violence: Explanations and Evidence-Based Clinical Practice*. Alexandria, VA: American Counseling Association, 2013.

Pelzer, Dave. *A Child Called It: One Child's Courage to Survive*. Deerfield Beach, FL: Health Communications Inc., 1995.

Perez-Fuentes, Gabriela, Mark Olfson, Laura Villegas, Carmen Morcillo, Shuai Wang, and Carlos Blanco. "Prevalence and Correlates of Child Sexual Abuse: A National Study." *Comprehensive Psychiatry* 54 (2013): 16–27.

Troiano, MaryAnn. "Child Abuse." *Nursing Clinics of North America* 46 (2011): 413–422.

Child Onset Fluency Disorder

Child onset fluency disorder is a condition that disrupts a child's speech. It is also called stuttering.

Definitions

- **Fluency** is the ability to speak correctly and easily.

- **Stuttering** is talking with continued involuntary repetition of sounds, especially initial consonants.

Description

Child onset fluency disorder affects how fluently a child speaks and is therefore understood by others. It usually begins at an early age and lasts throughout someone's life to some degree. This condition disrupts the sounds produced from a child and creates a stutter. At some point in time, almost everyone experiences difficulty communicating. In child onset fluency disorder, a child's speech is significantly challenged and creates problems in daily communication.

These problems in daily communication can impact a child's ability to communicate under stressful circumstances. For example, if the home or classroom is a stressful environment, a child will have more disruptions in speech. This can occur commonly when talking on the telephone or in public speaking when speech is relied on heavily for effective communication. For some children their stuttering can occur across environments and situations. This can cause isolation and removal from certain activities that children want to be involved with. Many children with this condition will try to hide their speech problems by using words they can rely on using well or by claiming to forget what they were trying to say or simply my remaining silent.

Child onset fluency disorder usually presents itself around the age of two to four years. In some cases, stuttering will start during later elementary school years but this is rare. It is more common for males to be diagnosed with this condition. Young children who are diagnosed are usually not aware of their speech problems. But children develop, they become aware that they are different from others and notice other people's reactions to their speech.

There are different levels of stuttering that vary across the children who are diagnosed. For some children, speech problems are significant and can persist for days, weeks, and months. Some other children will develop minor speech issues and improve fairly quickly from the first signs of stuttering. Child onset fluency disorder can also improve under certain circumstances and vary daily. This can make it seem like the condition goes away completely and then reappears later. When a child becomes a teenager and later an adult, his or her speech issues tend to stabilize and does not tend to get better or worse with age although under stressful circumstances stuttering tends to worsen.

Causes and Symptoms

The cause of child onset fluency disorder is not known. Research suggests that genetics influences a child's likelihood to be diagnosed with the disorder. When family members inherit stuttering from their family, it directly impacts their ability to speak fluently. But not everyone who is genetically prone to the condition will develop it.

For many people diagnosed with stuttering, stressful life events can often initiate their speech problems. When children are young, their speech issues might be creating more mature sentences. This can occur when a child is attempting to develop from two- or three-word sentences into longer, more complicated statements. Therefore, it may appear that a child does not stutter when he or she uses fewer words and then later speech problems appear. A child who is frustrated by speech is more likely to become physically tense, and this can affect the child's ease of communicating. Other children can make fun of their peers, and this can worsen the symptoms of stuttering. Many diagnosed with this condition experience feelings of anxiety and shame.

Symptoms of the disorder are repeating words or parts of words in addition to lengthening words. Children and adults with the condition might appear to be nervous or out of breath. People with the disorder make a serious effort to complete a word and try not to get stuck on words.

Diagnosis and Prognosis

The accurate diagnosis of child onset fluency disorder should be done by an evaluation by a certified speech-language pathologist (SLP). It might seem easy for others to identify stuttering in some, but not easy in others. SLPs will be able to identify the types of issues that a child presents with and can identify stressors in the environment that impact the speech disorder. Formal assessments, observations, and parent or teacher interviews are typically used during diagnosis and interpreted by the SLP.

After a comprehensive assessment, the results should include when stuttering is most likely to occur. There are specific pieces of information that are important to consider including family history, if the speech problems have occurred for at least six months and if the child is concerned or scared of speaking. When these characteristics are present, a diagnosis of child onset fluency disorder is probably appropriate.

Over half of the children diagnosed between two and four years who stutter will improve and no longer have speech problems. Usually this occurs within a few months of the diagnosis. For others, stuttering will last for years and have periods of supposed improvements with some periods of regression. It is unclear why some children continue stuttering while others do not. Most children who recover from the condition have received speech therapy, but there are some who never receive treatment and also recover. More research needs to be done on this to help determine what helps children become more fluent.

Treatment

Speech-language pathologists (SLPs) are involved in the delivery of speech therapy for children who are diagnosed with stuttering. Many treatment programs are behavioral in nature and focus on teaching the person new skills to improve speech. SLPs who treat these clients use techniques such as monitoring speech pace and relaxation. Learning to control the rate or pace of speech is one of the most effective methods for managing stuttering. This helps people speak more easily and fluidly over time and can create more natural language development and fluency.

Treatment of children during their preschool years is controversial for some SLPs. This is because it is hard to determine whether some children outgrow their issues and many are concerned that treatment could bring damaging awareness to a child who is not able to cope well. In order to prevent this, therapists will recommend a wait-and-see approach in order to give the child time to develop and improve on his or her own. If after a determined period of time therapists, teachers, and parents do not see improvements, individual therapy is warranted.

Parents and other caregivers who are able to interact with children can model fluent speech. Involving the parents and teachers whom the child is exposed to the most has proven helpful in eliminating symptoms in young children. The use of devices and technology has also shown to help children with speech issues. One such way these devices can be used is by recording fluent speech from the child and playing this back to the child.

Support and treatment groups for people with stuttering issues are widely available. These groups are usually self-help in nature and bring together groups of people who face the same problem. People who participate in support groups claim that their experiences in the group give them an opportunity to use techniques they've learned in therapy. They can help each other cope with everyday problems and serve as support. Many of these groups exist in the United States and the world.

Alexandra Cunningham, PhD

See also: Speech-Language Pathology

Further Reading

Guitar, Barry. *Stuttering: An Integrated Approach to Its Nature and Treatment.* Baltimore, MD: Lippincott Williams & Wilkins, 2013.

Yairi, Ehud H., and Carol H. Seery. *Stuttering: Foundations and Clinical Applications.* New York, NY: Pearson, 2014.

Child Protective Services

"Child Protective Services" (CPS) is the name, in many states, of the governmental agency that is responsible for responding to and investigating reports of child abuse and/or neglect. Other states have similar agencies but use other names.

Description

Child Protective Services is a state agency partly funded by the federal government and partly by state and local sources, which handles reports of suspected child abuse or neglect. Each state has its own laws that define abuse and neglect, obligations for reporting, protocol to follow, and penalties for abusers. State agencies receive guidance and structure from the national agency, the Administration for Children and Families, also referred to as the Children's Bureau, which falls under the U.S. Department of Health and Human Services. Depending on the state, the child protective services agency may also be known as the Department of Children and Families, the Department of Children and Family Services, or the Department of Social Services. As the name denotes, the main objectives of this department are to ensure the welfare of minors and provide social services to families. The agency is responsible for a wide range of services, including assisting families with proper care and safety in order to remain together, foster care placement, youth and young adult transition programs out of foster care, and adoption procedures. Personnel work in conjunction with community agencies, tribes, schools, local law enforcement, and the courts.

The law prohibits child maltreatment and Child Protective Services (CPS) may respond to abusive acts by forcefully removing the child from an unsafe home. Any person who suspects child abuse or neglect should promptly report it to CPS. As of August 2012, approximately 18 states and Puerto Rico have issued statutes that require this. Several professionals are classified as "mandatory reporters" including doctors, teachers, and childcare providers, and they are responsible for most of the reports made. Once a report is made, CPS staff may initiate an investigation to determine if the child is at risk and whether the environment is safe for the child to remain in. Initial calls are either "screened out" or "screened in" depending on whether there is sufficient information to warrant an investigation. If a report is screened out, the CPS staff member may refer the reporter to other local agencies or to local law enforcement for help. However, if the report is screened in, then the CPS caseworker must respond to the report in a timely manner, anywhere from a few hours to a few days. This depends on the information provided, including the type of abuse, potential severity of the situation, and the requirements under state law. An investigation will include questioning of the child, the child's parents/guardians, and other people who are in regular contact with the child. If the child is believed to be in imminent danger, then he or she may be removed from the home immediately and placed in the care of a relative or friend or in foster care while court proceedings take place. Depending on the state, additional steps may also be taken to help remediate and support the family in order for them to reconcile. Once the investigation is complete, the CPS caseworker makes one of two findings, either unsubstantiated (unfounded) or substantiated (founded). If unsubstantiated, then the case is filed and essentially dropped; if substantiated, the CPS agency then initiates the authority of the court to determine what actions, if any, are necessary to keep the child safe. The court may then issue order to place the child in the care of another entity, require services be sought, or order that the abuser have no contact with the child. CPS claims that its preferred course of action is to rehabilitate and reunite families; however, this is often not the case. Evidence has also shown that disregard for following proper protocol, delay in the timeliness of responding to reports, and lack of communication between members has contributed to negative perceptions of CPS.

Dating back to 1825, states began enacting laws giving child welfare agencies the authority to remove abused and neglected children from their homes and place them in proper care. In 1874, the first case of child abuse to be prosecuted in the United States, referred to as "the case of Mary Ellen," spurred public outrage and subsequent response from the federal government, including President Roosevelt's public funding of volunteer organizations dedicated to child welfare. The Children's Bureau was established in 1912 by President Taft to coordinate efforts on a national level. The Social Security Act of 1930 outlined further funding toward child maltreatment intervention. C. Henry Kempe referred to "battered child syndrome" in articles published in 1961–1962, raising concerns over the long-lasting effects of abuse. This led to 49 states passing mandatory child abuse reporting laws by the mid-1960s. In 1974, the Child Abuse Prevention and Treatment Act (CAPTA) was passed bringing further national attention to the issue. In addition to providing federal funding toward prevention efforts and treatment, the CAPTA supported research and data collection activities. The CAPTA was recently amended and reauthorized on December 10, 2010. The Adoption Assistance and Child Welfare Act of 1980 (Public Law 96-272), considered the first piece of comprehensive legislation on the problem, promoted state economic incentives for decreasing the length and number of minors placed in foster care. Other similar legislation followed, including the Adoption Assistance Act, the Child Abuse Prevention, Adoption, and Family Services Act of 1988, and the Child Abuse, Domestic Violence, Adoption, and Family Services Act of 1992. All focused on easing the adoption process to promote family permanency for children. In 1997, the Adoption and Safe Families Act was passed, introducing the idea of "concurrent planning" where caseworkers first attempt to reunify families but, in conjunction, work an alternative plan so as not to delay permanency for the child. Current practice is based on this model.

Impact (Psychological Influence)

Child abuse and neglect remains a public concern. According to a 2010 report issued by the National Child Abuse and Neglect Data System, a nationally estimated 754,000 duplicate (repeated victims) and 695,000 unique (first-time reports) number of children were found to be victims of child maltreatment. Based on the unique number of victims, an estimated 78% suffered neglect, 18% were physically abused, 9% were sexually abused, 8% were psychologically abused, and 2% were medically neglected. Recent statistics issued by the U.S. Department of Health and Human Services in 2012 reported that an overwhelming 676,569 children were victims of abuse or neglect (Child Welfare Information Gateway, 2013). Victims of childhood maltreatment suffer from physical, emotional, and psychological distress and are more prone to develop depression, anxiety, and social and behavioral problems. Of further concern are incidents of recidivism, as the cycle of abuse is likely to repeat itself. Prevention efforts should focus on counseling; skill development and remediation; and practical support for victims, perpetrators, and their families.

Melissa A. Mariani, PhD

See also: Child Abuse; Foster Care; Neglect

Further Reading

Child Welfare Information Gateway. *Preventing Child Abuse and Neglect*. Washington, DC: U.S. Department of Health and Human Services, Children's Bureau, 2013.

Fang, Xiangming, Derek S. Brown, Curtis S. Florence, and James A. Mercy. "The Economic Burden of Child

Maltreatment in the United States and Implications for Prevention." *Child Abuse & Neglect* 36, no. 2 (2012): 156–165.

U.S. Department of Health and Human Services. Administration for Children and Families, Administration on Children, Youth and Families, Children's Bureau. *Child Maltreatment 2010.* Last modified 2010. Washington, DC: Government Printing Office. Accessed August 10, 2013. http://www.acf.hhs.gov/programs/cb/research-data-technology/statistics-research/child-maltreatment.

U.S. Department of Health and Human Services. Administration for Children and Families, Administration on Children, Youth and Families, Children's Bureau. *Child Maltreatment 2011.* Last modified 2011. Washington, DC: Government Printing Office. Accessed August 10, 2013. http://www.acf.hhs.gov/sites/default/files/cb/cm11.pdf.

World Health Organization. "Preventing Child Maltreatment: A Guide to Taking Action and Generating Evidence." Last modified 2006. Accessed August 10, 2013. http://whqlibdoc.who.int/publications/2006/9241594365_eng.pdf.

Childhood Disintegrative Disorder

Childhood disintegrative disorder (CDD) is a condition where after healthy development up to the age of approximately 2 but before a child turns 10 years of age, there is loss in many areas of functioning.

Description

Childhood disintegrative disorder, also known as Heller's syndrome, is often considered part of a larger category of developmental disorders. The latest edition of the *Diagnostic and Statistics Manual* places it clearly within the definition of autism spectrum disorder (American Psychiatric Association, 2013). However, unlike others who exhibit autism, those with CDD show severe and abrupt regression following several years of normal development. It is characterized as a more dramatic loss of skills than in other children, and many develop the disorder later than is typical with autism. History and data on this condition is limited, and it may often be misdiagnosed. From the data collected, it seems that the condition occurs in only 2 out of 100,000 children and that most are boys.

Causes and Symptoms

In the absence of brain injury or trauma, science has not determined the characteristic causes for CDD. It is difficult to determine why some children who had previously been on a normal developmental curve begin to lose skills and abilities that they had already acquired. Some research suggests that a combination of genetic issues, including autoimmune factors, and prenatal and environmental stress may explain brain differences for those with CDD. Some scientists have discovered higher-than-normal protein deposits in the brain that can disrupt synaptic transmission.

Symptoms are varied but distinct. In studies at the Yale Child Study Center, it is noted that children with CDD tend to undergo rapid and severe regression. In addition to loss of skills, 70% of these children have episodes of behavior problems before regression. For children between the ages of three and four, some other symptoms of the possible presence of CDD may be increased activity, irritability, or anxiety, which precedes a marked decrease or loss in speaking ability, social skills, and/or motor skills. These motor issues include bladder and/or bowel control problems. Additional symptoms may include difficulty in making the transition from sleep to waking, poor social interactions, tantrums, or withdrawal from peers, as well as poor coordination and awkwardness in walking.

Diagnosis and Prognosis

It is important to note that although some children go through periods of limited regression during normal development, these temporary setbacks are not long lasting. These do not match the severity or lasting impact of the deficits that mark CDD. CDD is characterized by sharp, significant, and often permanent losses of abilities. Although some symptoms may parallel those that occur in autism spectrum disorder and Rett's disorder, clinical analysis will help determine whether the symptoms actually indicate that CDD is the proper diagnosis. In most cases of CDD, the loss of skills reaches a plateau, which unfortunately may last a lifetime. There are some cases when the loss of skills is progressive and leads to early death.

Treatment

There are no medications specific for CDD, although individual symptoms may be addressed with drugs. Therapeutic behavioral interventions are commonly used, such as applied behavior analysis. This treatment is an attempt to slow down the child's deterioration and help stabilize and improve the child's communication, self-help, and social skills.

Alexandra Cunningham, PhD

See also: Autism Spectrum Disorder; Behavior Therapy with Children; Pervasive Developmental Disorders

Further Reading

American Psychiatric Association. *Diagnostic and Statistical Manual of Mental Disorders*, 5th ed. Arlington, VA: American Psychiatric Association, 2013.

Bernstein, Bettina E., Caroly Pataki, and Mary L. Windle. "Childhood Disintegrative Disorder." *Medscape*. Accessed September 9, 2013. http://emedicine.medscape.com/article/916515-overview.

Pelphrey, Kevin, and Alexander Westphal. *In Defense of Childhood Disintegrative Disorder*. New York, NY: Simons Foundation Autism Research Initiative, 2012.

Children's Apperception Test (CAT)

The Children's Apperception Test (CAT) is a projective test used to assess personality traits, maturity level, and overall psychological well-being in children 3 to 10 years of age.

Definitions

- **Apperception** is the process of understanding something through associating it with a previous experience.

- **Projective test** is a type of psychological assessment that seeks to assess a person's true feelings, thoughts, and attitudes based on responses to ambiguous stimuli.

- **Rorschach test**, also known as the "Inkblot Test," was developed by Hermann Rorschach in 1921 and is the most widely used psychological projective assessment. Respondents, ages three and up, are shown a series of inkblot cards and asked a series of questions in order to reveal information about their personality, preferences, and possible internal/external conflicts.

Description

The Children's Apperception Test is a projective personality test for children. Sigmund Freud used the term "projection" to describe how a person may unconsciously project his or her inner feelings onto the external world and vice versa. Projective assessment tools are used to encourage one to openly express what one thinks and feels. General impressions and insights are derived about the person from the answers given. Another commonly used projective assessment is the Rorschach Inkblot test.

The CAT is based on the Thematic Apperception Test (TAT), which was created by psychologist Henry A. Murray for use with people aged 10 years and older. The TAT is comprised of a series of 31 picture cards depicting humans in common social and relational situations. Respondents are asked to develop their own stories based on the scenes on the cards. Answers are believed to reveal underlying themes, emotions, and conflicts about the person's inner world and interpersonal relationships. The CAT follows the same process of assessment as the TAT but is meant to be used with children under the age of ten. The child is presented a series of picture cards and asked to describe what's happening in the situations to the examiner. When this test is used correctly, it is believed to reveal significant aspects of a child's personality. There are three versions of the CAT: the CAT-A (pictures of animals), the CAT-H (pictures of humans), and the CAT-S (pictures of children in typical family situations). Administration of the CAT takes approximately 20 to 45 minutes. However, there is no set time limit. There are no right or wrong answers, and no numerical score are given on the CAT.

Development

The original CAT was developed by psychiatrist Leopold Bellak and psychologist Sonya Sorel Bellak. First published in 1949, it was used to assess personality in children aged 3 to 10. This first version of the CAT, the CAT-A, used animal figures instead of human beings because the authors believed that younger children would identify more easily with pictures of animals. This CAT-A consisted of 10 cards showing animal figures in human social settings. The CAT-H was later developed in 1965 to depict humans. A supplement, the CAT-S, was also added, which included pictures of children in typical family situations. The most recent version of the CAT was published in 1993. Again, the purpose of these tests was to elicit personal identification with what was happening in the picture card scenes.

Current Status and Results

The CAT should be administered only by a trained professional (psychiatrist, psychologist, licensed counselor, social worker, or teacher with specific training in this type of assessment). The results of the CAT alone should never be used to diagnose. Rather, it should be given as part of a larger battery of tests and include an in-depth interview with both the child and his or her parents/guardians. A thorough medical history should also be obtained. This way the assessor has a comprehensive picture of the child's overall psychological functioning.

The Children's Apperception Test is not considered a reliable or valid assessment. There is no clear evidence to support that this test measures what it seeks to or that it measures those constructs consistently from child to child. In addition, because this is a subjective type of assessment based mostly on the opinions and impressions of the examiner, findings are subject to bias and error.

Melissa A. Mariani, PhD

See also: Personality Tests; Rorschach Inkblot Test

Further Reading

Bellak, Leopold, and David M. Abrams. *The Thematic Apperception Test, the Children's Apperception Test, and the Senior Apperception Technique in Clinical Use.* Boston, MA: Allyn & Bacon, 1997.

McCoy, Dorothy. *The Ultimate Guide to Personality Tests.* Inglewood, CA: Champion Press, 2005.

Reynolds, Cecil R., and Randy W. Kamphaus, eds. *Handbook of Psychological and Educational Assessment of*

Children: Personality, Behavior, and Context, 2nd ed. New York, NY: Guilford Press, 2003.

Children's Depression Inventory

The Children's Depression Inventory (CDI) is an assessment that is used to evaluate the symptoms of depression in children and adolescents.

Definition

- **Depression** is an emotional state characterized by feelings of sadness, low self-esteem, guilt, or reduced ability to enjoy life. It is not considered a mental disorder unless it significantly disrupts one's daily functioning.

Description

In its long form the CDI is a list of 27 questions that rates the symptoms of depression in children and teens aged 7 to 17. It measures five different factors. Those are negative mood, self-esteem, interpersonal problems, lack of pleasure, and ineffectiveness. This instrument or tool has a revised version that provides an option for teachers and parents to rate the children they have or are working with.

The CDI is also available in a short, 10-question format. Today, it is highly recommended that the long-form CDI be used, which includes sections for teachers and parents. When CDI results are combined with adult observation and input, they can help provide an accurate description of the child's situation. It helps with early identification of depression and getting treatment to those who need it as quickly as possible.

Development (Purpose and History)

Children can experience mood swings as they develop. But some children suffer from true clinical depression which can be dangerous since self-harm and suicide are possible results. During the 1970s and 1980s childhood depression started to be recognized, and several instruments like the CDI were created.

Maria Kovacs, PhD, was the developer of the CDI. Dr. Kovacs began practicing cognitive therapy in the 1970s as a treatment that was effective for depression, even more so than traditional drugs. For many years Dr. Kovacs worked with Aaron T. Beck, MD, who developed a popular depression inventory instrument, the Beck Depression Inventory (BDI). The BDI was created for adults and based on Dr. Beck's clinical experience with depressed patients. Dr. Kovacs collaborated with him to research and develop the CDI, which was published in 1979.

Current Status and Results

Since it was first published, the CDI has been used in the United States and internationally as a way to identify depression in children and adolescents. The CDI has been validated statistically as a predictor of depressive disorders in children. It is also used to show a distinction between its results for depression and anxiety disorder or conduct disorders.

The CDI does face some criticism as an accurate instrument. One is that it provides too many false negatives, which means that the test shows no depression when depression really exists. Another is that it may identify children who have a general emotional disturbance rather than depression.

Alexandra Cunningham, PhD, and William M.
Cunningham, MA

See also: Depression in Youth

Further Reading

Frick, Paul J., Christopher T. Barry, and Randy W. Kamphaus. *Clinical Assessment of Child and Adolescent Personality and Behavior.* New York, NY: Springer Science + Business Media, 2010.

Jongsma, Arthur E., Jr., and Mark Peterson. *The Child Psychotherapy Treatment Planner.* Hoboken, NJ: John Wiley & Sons, 2014.

Sperry, Len, ed. *Family Assessment: Contemporary and Cutting-Edge Strategies*, 2nd ed. New York, NY: Routledge, 2012.

Chronic Illness

Chronic illness is the subjective experience of a chronic disease.

Definitions

- **Acute disease** is a medical condition with a single cause, a specific onset, and identifiable symptoms which is often treatable with medication or surgery and is usually curable.

- **Chronic disease** is a disease entity that usually does not have a single cause, a specific onset, nor a stable set of symptoms. While cure may be possible, it is unlikely for advanced levels of the disease process. It is also referred to as chronic medical conditions.

- **Disease** is an objective medical condition that can be acute or chronic.

- **Illness** is the subjective experience of a disease.

- **Well-being** is the state of being happy, healthy, prosperous, or successful.

Description

Chronic diseases are medical conditions that are prolonged in duration and do not resolve spontaneously. They are seldom cured completely. Common examples are heart disease, cancer, stroke, diabetes, and arthritis. The Centers for Disease Control and Prevention (CDC) considers chronic diseases to be the most common and costly of all health problems. Nearly 50% of American adults (133 million) live with at least one chronic disease. They account for 70% of all deaths. These diseases account for more than 75% of health-care costs. Chronic medical conditions are three types more common than psychiatric conditions. The reality is that they are preventable. CDC points to four modifiable health behaviors that are responsible for most disability and premature deaths related to chronic diseases. These are tobacco use, inadequate physical activity, poor food choices, and overuse of alcohol. With the average life span now extending in the 80s, the reality is that most individuals can expect to contend with chronic illness in themselves or in the lives of those close to them.

While many use the terms chronic disease and chronic illness interchangeably, they have somewhat different meanings. While disease represents an objective process, illness is a subjective process. As such, chronic illness is experienced differently from individual to individual. Unfortunately, the health-care system has let to offer those with chronic diseases in contrast to those with acute diseases. Largely, this is because medical research and the training of health-care providers has emphasized acute diseases. Furthermore, for treatment to be effective, providers must be sufficiently competent in tailoring treatment that is responsive to multiple factors. These include the individual's unique personality, coping resources, culture, and the type and phase of his or her illness.

There are four main types of chronic diseases. The first is the life-threatening medical conditions such as fast-growing cancers, stroke, and heart attacks. A second type includes the manageable medical conditions such type 2 diabetes, hypertension (high blood pressure), obesity, and chronic sinusitis. While they may become serious, they are seldom life threatening. The third type includes progressively disabling diseases such as Parkinson's disease, lupus, rheumatoid arthritis, and multiple sclerosis. The fourth type includes those that are not life threatening but have a waxing and waning course. Sometimes, but not always, this type can be debilitating. Chronic fatigue syndrome and fibromyalgia are examples.

There are also four phases of chronic illness. These have been described by Patricia Fennell (2003). They are based on her clinical research with several hundred individuals with various types of chronic medical conditions.

Phase One: Crisis. The basic task of this phase is to deal with the immediate symptoms, pain, or traumas associated with this new experience of illness.

Phase Two: Stabilization. The basic task of this phase is to stabilize and restructure life patterns and perceptions.

Phase Three: Resolution. The basic task of this phase is to develop a new self and to seek a personally meaningful philosophy of life and spirituality consistent with it.

Phase Four: Integration. The basic task of this phase is to achieve the highest level of well-being possible despite compromised or failing health status.

It should be noted that not all individuals with a chronic illness proceed through all four phases. In fact, many chronically ill individuals get caught in a recurring loop of cycling between phase one and phase two.

This means that each crisis produces new wounding and destabilization. Such crises are likely to be followed by a brief period of stabilization. But without intervention, a new crises will invariably destabilize the individual again. Only when health providers help these chronically ill individuals to break this recurring cycle can they move to phases three and four.

Len Sperry, MD, PhD

See also: Alcohol Use Disorder; Obesity; Tobacco Use Disorder

Further Reading

Centers for Disease Control (CDC). "Chronic Disease Prevention and Health Promotion." Accessed March 29, 2015. http://www.cdc.gov/chronicdisease/.

Fennell, Patricia. *Managing Chronic Illness Using the Four-Phase Treatment Approach.* Hoboken, NJ: John Wiley & Sons, 2003.

Sperry, Len. *Psychological Treatment of Chronic Illness: The Biopsychosocial Therapy Approach.* Washington, DC: American Psychological Association Books, 2006.

Sperry, Len. *Treating Chronic Medical Conditions: Cognitive Behavioral Strategies and Integrative Protocols.* Washington, DC: American Psychological Association Books, 2009.

Chronic Pain Syndrome

Chronic pain syndrome is a medical condition characterized by the experience of long-standing pain. It is also known as chronic pain.

Definitions

- **Acute pain** is pain that comes on quickly and may be severe but is experienced for a relatively short time (less than six months). It is the opposite of chronic pain.

- **DSM-5** stands for the *Diagnostic and Statistical Manual of Mental Disorders, Fifth Edition*, which is a diagnostic system used by professionals to identify mental disorders with specific diagnostic criteria.

- **Fibromyalgia** is a medical condition characterized by widespread, unexplained pain as well as sensitivity to pressure or touch in specific areas of the body.

- **ICD-10** stands for the *International Statistical Classification and Related Health Problems, 10th edition*. It is published by the World Health Organization and lists all known medical and psychological conditions affecting human beings worldwide.

- **Mindfulness-based stress reduction** is a form of cognitive behavior therapy that utilizes meditation and yoga to change the way an individual perceives and reacts to bodily sensations.

- **Mindfulness practices** are intentional activities that foster living in the present moment and awareness that is nonjudgmental and accepting.

- **Pain** is an unpleasant sensation occurring in varying degrees of severity as a result of injury, disease, or emotional distress.

- **Psychotherapy** is a psychological method for achieving desired changes in thinking, feeling, and behavior. It is also called therapeutic counseling.

- **Rheumatology** is the field of medicine concerned with the painful disorders of the skin, joints, nerves, and bones.

Description and Diagnosis

"Chronic pain syndrome" is a general term and medical condition. In contrast to acute pain, it does not disappear when the underlying cause of pain has been treated or has healed. Chronic pain lasts longer than six months. It is described in the ICD-10 as the experience of ongoing pain that may or may not have a known physiological (related to the body) cause. There is no specific set of symptoms that accurately describes all individuals who suffer from chronic pain syndrome. Symptoms may include dull back pain, severe headaches, and widespread painful sensation of the skin layer. One of the most widely known forms of chronic pain syndrome is fibromyalgia. Although fibromyalgia is considered to be a specific medical diagnosis, the cause is still unknown. Chronic pain syndrome is not described in the DSM-5.

There is no agreement as to what causes chronic pain syndrome. Although this condition is poorly understood,

it is relatively common. Estimates of the occurrence of this disorder exceed 25% of U.S. population.

Treatment

Chronic pain syndrome is treated differently depending on the types of symptoms described by the individual as well as the type of clinician seen. Common treatment may include over-the-counter nonsteroidal anti-inflammatory drugs such as Advil (ibuprofen) or Aleve (naproxen-sodium). Corticosteroid injections and narcotic pain medications may also be prescribed by a physician, often one specializing in rheumatology. Although this condition is considered to be physiological in nature, certain forms of psychotherapy have been shown to be effective in reducing pain. The forms of psychotherapy that are most notable are those that involve mindfulness practice such as mindfulness-based stress reduction. Unfortunately, there are no known treatments considered to be completely curative.

Len Sperry, MD, PhD, and Jeremy Connelly, MEd

See also: *Diagnostic and Statistical Manual of Mental Disorders* (DSM); Fibromyalgia; International Classification of Diseases; Mindfulness; Psychotherapy

Further Reading

American Psychiatric Association. *Diagnostic and Statistical Manual of Mental Disorders*, 5th ed. Arlington, VA: American Psychiatric Association, 2013.

Gardner-Nix, Jackie. *The Mindfulness Solution to Pain: Step-by-Step Techniques for Chronic Pain Management*. Oakland, CA: New Harbinger, 2009.

Kabat-Zinn, Jon. *Full Catastrophe Living: Using the Wisdom of the Body and Mind to Face Stress, Pain, and Illness*. New York, NY: Bantam Dell, 2005.

Turk, Dennis, and Frits Winter. *The Pain Survival Guide: How to Reclaim Your Life*. Washington, DC: American Psychological Association, 2006.

Wallace, Daniel, and Janice Brock Wallace. *Making Sense of Fibromyalgia: New and Updated*. New York, NY: Oxford University Press, 2014.

Circadian Rhythm Sleep–Wake Disorder

Circadian rhythm sleep–wake disorder is a mental disorder that is characterized by irregular patterns of sleep.

Definitions

- **Behavior therapy** is a form of psychotherapy that focuses on identifying and changing maladaptive behaviors.

- **Circadian rhythm** is the approximately 24-hour cycle of physiological and psychological regulation of bodily rhythms such as sleeping and waking. It is commonly referred to as the "internal bodily clock."

- **DSM-5** stands for the *Diagnostic and Statistical Manual of Mental Disorders, Fifth Edition*, which is a diagnostic system used by professionals to identify mental disorders with specific diagnostic criteria.

- **Light therapy** is a medical treatment in which doses of bright light are administered to normalize the body's internal clock and treat depression. It is also called phototherapy.

- **Sleep hygiene** refers to the habits, practices, and nonmedical treatments for insomnia, which improve the quality of sleep.

- **Sleep–wake disorders** are a group of mental disorders that are characterized by various sleeping disturbances including circadian rhythm sleep–wake disorder.

Description and Diagnosis

Circadian rhythm sleep–wake disorder is one of the Sleep–Wake Disorders in DSM-5. It is characterized by a sleep pattern that is out of sync with normal circadian rhythms. Individuals with this disorder have trouble sleeping during the times that others typically sleep. Those with this disorder may not follow the typical circadian rhythms of others, but if allowed to follow their particular patterns, they can experience sufficient and otherwise normal sleep.

To be diagnosed with this disorder, the individual must have recurrent difficulty adapting sleeping patterns to his or her environmental requirements such as job or social demands. In addition, the incongruence of his or her sleeping pattern with these demands must cause sleeplessness, sleepiness, or both. Individuals

may be genetically predisposed to this disorder. Also, atypical light exposure (such as living in northern climates where there is limited daylight) may also be a contributing factor.

DSM-5 identifies five subtypes of circadian rhythm sleep–wake disorder. A brief description of each follows:

Delayed sleep phase type. The delay sleep phase type is characterized by the inability to fall asleep for at least two hours after the preferred sleep time. Individuals with this disorder may also have difficulty waking at the preferred time as a result of a short sleep period. Consequently, individuals may experience sleepiness throughout the day, especially in the morning. Although this disorder affects approximately 17% of the adult population, it is common in adolescence where upward of 7% may experience this type. This diagnosis in adolescence is differentiated from normal sleeping pattern difficulty in that the symptoms typically persist for greater than three months (American Psychiatric Association, 2013). Without treatment, some may experience this disorder intermittently for their entire lives, while for others, symptoms are reduced with age.

Advanced sleep phase type. This type is characterized by earlier than normal sleep–wake times, typically of at least two hours. Also, if an individual delays sleep until the conventional time, he or she will still wake early, thereby causing excessive daytime sleepiness. This type affects approximately 1% of the adult population. Although onset can occur at any age, it is more common in middle-aged and older adults (American Psychiatric Association, 2013). It is important to note that advanced sleep times are common in older adults but are differentiated by adverse symptoms such as daytime sleepiness or shorter than preferred sleep periods.

Irregular sleep–wake type. This type is characterized by fragmented sleep throughout a 24-hour period. An individual with this type does not experience a major sleep period. The individual may experience sleeplessness for long periods of the night and nap excessively during the day. The prevalence of this subtype is not known (American Psychiatric Association, 2013).

Non-24-hour sleep–wake type. This type is characterized by irregular duration of the entire sleep–wake cycle that is out of sync with the normal light–dark 24-hour cycle. Unlike the other types, individuals with this type do not follow a 24-hour pattern of sleeping. They may sleep too much or too little in any given 24-hour period. This type is common in the blind, affecting approximately 50%, but is rare in sighted individuals (American Psychiatric Association, 2013).

Shift work type. This type is characterized by job-related obligation that occur during normal sleeping periods (i.e., at night), thereby causing excessive sleepiness while on the job and sleeplessness while at home. For the diagnosis to apply, both symptoms must be present. Individuals who suffer from this type are more prone to accidents or lowered performance on the job than if they experienced normal, restful sleep. This type is relatively common in night workers, affecting approximately 7.5%. Individuals who are middle aged or older are more prone to this type (American Psychiatric Association, 2013).

Treatment

The treatments for this disorder may include behavior therapy, education on optimal sleep hygiene, and light therapy. The common goal of these therapies is to help the individual in adapting his or her environmental cues to support optimal sleep. Also, individuals may be prescribed sleep aids such as Lunesta or Ambien to help them fall asleep at a conventional or preferred time. Medication may be used as a standalone treatment or in conjunction with therapy.

Len Sperry, MD, PhD

See also: Ambien (Zolpidem); Behavior Therapy; Lunesta; Sleep Disorders

Further Reading

American Psychiatric Association. *Diagnostic and Statistical Manual of Mental Disorders*, 5th ed. Arlington, VA: American Psychiatric Association, 2013.

Choroverty, Sudhansu. *Sleep Disorders Medicine: Basic Science, Technical Considerations, and Clinical Aspects*, 3rd ed. Philadelphia, PA: Saunders, 2009.

Epstein, Lawrence. *The Harvard Medical School Guide to a Good Night's Sleep*. New York, NY: McGraw-Hill, 2007.

Foldvary-Schaefer, Nancy. *The Cleveland Clinic Guide to Sleep Disorders*. New York, NY: Kaplan, 2009.

Perlis, Michael L., Mark Aloia, and Brett Kuhn, eds. *Behavioral Treatments for Sleep Disorders: A Comprehensive Primer of Behavioral Sleep Medicine Interventions*. New York, NY: Academic Press, 2011.

Clinical Health Psychology

Clinical health psychology is a form of psychology that is informed by the biopsychosocial model of health and emphasizes behavioral medicine interventions.

Definitions

- **Behavioral medicine** is an interdisciplinary form of modern medicine that integrates the behavioral, biomedical, and social sciences.

- **Behavioral psychology** is a form of psychology whose aim is to study behavioral adaptation to an environment and its stimuli.

- **Biopsychosocial model** is a way of conceptualizing (thinking about) health and illness in terms of biological, psychological, and social factors rather than purely in biological terms. It is also referred to as the biopsychosocial perspective.

- **Clinical psychology** is a form of psychology that integrates science, theory, and practice to increase the knowledge of the psyche and its function. It is also concerned with predicting, assessing, diagnosing, and alleviating psychological problems and related disability.

- **Cognitive psychology** is a form of psychology whose aim is to study thought and distorted patterns of thinking.

- **Humanistic psychology** is an experiential form of psychology developed from the work of Abraham Maslow and Carl Rogers, which emphasizes a client's capacity for self-actualization and unique positive personal growth.

- **Psychoanalytic psychology** is the form of psychology largely developed by the work of Sigmund Freud, which emphasizes the conflicts and compromises between the unconscious and conscious mind.

- **Psychometric assessment** is the direct or indirect measurement of psychological differences.

- **Psychosomatic model** is a way of conceptualizing (thinking about) certain medical conditions as caused by or resulting from psychological factors.

- **Psychotherapy** is a psychological method for achieving desired changes in thinking, feeling, and behavior. It is also called therapeutic counseling.

Description

Clinical health psychology is a form of clinical psychology that is informed by the biopsychosocial model of health. This contrasts with conventional clinical psychology, which tends to focus on the psychosocial model (psychological and social factors explain health and illness), and conventional medicine, which focuses on the biomedical model (biological factors sufficiently explain health and illness). Clinical health psychology emphasizes the clinical and scientific contributions of behavioral medicine in predicting, assessing, diagnosing, and alleviating psychological problems and related disability. Often the root cause of psychological dysfunction is not isolated to a single contributing factor. Instead, it is usually best explained through the integration of biological, psychological, and social systems contributing factors. For example, behavioral psychology, cognitive psychology, humanistic psychology, psychoanalytic psychology, and biomedical model all have different ways to explain and treat a single psychopathology. It honors the contributions of all applicable biological, psychological, and sociological conceptual models.

Clinical health psychology is a system of psychological subspecialties rather than a separate psychological specialty. As an integrative system, it emphasizes the partnership between psychology and medicine. Such collaborative efforts between clinical health psychologists and other medical and health professionals have markedly contributed to the understanding of psychopathology (dysfunctional thoughts and behavior). These efforts have also furthered the team-based practice of integrative medical and psychotherapeutic interventions. The inclusion of behavioral medicine allows clinical health psychology to expand its focus to include all physiological and psychological factors related to illness. Clinical health psychologists are professionals with a doctoral degree in psychology, specialized training in health, and licensure as a psychologist. They are involved in the treatment of chronic pain, headaches, cessation of cigarette smoking, substance abuse, and management of obesity. Some are also involved in the treatment of heart disease and many other chronic medical conditions. Accordingly, they practice primarily in clinics, hospitals, and other health-care settings.

Development and Current Status

The relationship of the mind and body have been the subject of intense discussion over the centuries. The early Greek philosophers, such as Hippocrates, documented the collaboration between mind, especially with regard to psychology, and body, particularly with regard to medicine. Later influences, including western religion's view of human nature, resulted in a lead to a philosophy of mind–body dualism. Mind–body dualism views illness as either a medical condition caused by biological dysfunction, such as an infection, or a psychological dysfunction caused by trauma or evil spirits. However, in the 19th and 20th centuries, Sigmund Freud (1856–1939) and others developed the foundation for a science of the mind and mind–body interaction. At the same time, Lightner Witmer (1867–1956) established the first psychological clinic at the University of Pennsylvania in 1896. He first used the term "clinical psychology" in 1907 in the journal *The Psychological Clinic*.

Clinical psychology evolved largely from both psychometric assessment and psychoanalytic psychology. The first university programs leading to the doctor of philosophy (PhD) degree were established in 1946 and were accredited by the American Psychological Association (APA). The APA was established in 1892 but did not develop a section devoted to clinical psychology until 1919. This section was revised in 1945 to become APA's Division 12, The Society of Clinical Psychology. Division 12 of the APA is one of the most influential psychological organizations to date. The Veteran's Administration and APA influenced the integration of psychotherapy into graduate training programs in clinical psychology. This integration of scientific research and psychotherapeutic practice in training programs is known as the scientist-practitioner model. It is also known as the "Boulder Model" because Boulder, Colorado, was the location of the professional conference at which the model was accepted by representatives of the profession. It was not until 1973 that the doctor of psychology (PsyD) was accepted by the APA and recognized by the profession. These alternative training programs are known as practitioner-scholar models or the "Vail Model."

Starting in the 1940s, many psychiatrists and clinical psychologists working at the interface of psychology and medicine adopted the psychosomatic model. Franz Alexander (1891–1964), a Hungarian American physician and psychoanalyst, was a main force in advocating for psychosomatic viewpoint. It was largely a psychological explanation that emphasized the power of the mind over the body. For example, duodenal (stomach) ulcers were believed to be caused by frustration and emotional stress. The psychosomatic model began to wane as research determined that there was, in fact, both biological *and* psychological factors involved. Research identified an infection with the *Helicobacter pylori* (*H. pylori*) bacteria along with psychological stress as causative factors in ulcers. Prior to this discovery, the psychiatrist George L. Engel (1913–1999) wrote about the need for a new medical model in a landmark article in *Science* in 1977. Engel proposed the biopsychosocial model, which could integrate the psychosomatic model with the biomedical model.

As the biopsychosocial model has become increasingly accepted in health-care settings, clinical health psychologists have become indispensable team members in behavioral medicine and the health-care system. The cost of health care in the United States has also been a factor in the utilization of clinical health psychologists. Clinical health psychology has made the case that psychologists with specialty training in health psychology and behavioral medicine are invaluable in reducing the financial burden of managing preventable illnesses.

Len Sperry, MD, PhD, and Layven Reguero, MEd

See also: Clinical Psychology; Mind–Body Medicine; Psychosomatic-Psychosomatic Medicine; Somatopsychic

Further Reading

Alexander, Franz. *Psychosomatic Medicine: Its Principles and Applications.* New York, NY: W.W. Norton, 1950.

Belar, Cynthia D., and William W. Deardorff. *Clinical Health Psychology in Medical Settings: A Practitioner's Guidebook*, 2nd ed. Washington, DC: American Psychological Association, 2009.

Boyer, Bret A., and M. Indira Paharia, eEds. *Comprehensive Handbook of Clinical Health Psychology.* Hoboken, NJ: John Wiley & Sons, 2008.

Garchel, Robert J., and Mark S. Oordt. *Clinical Health Psychology and Primary Care: Practical Advice and Clinical Guidance for Successful Collaboration.* Washington, DC: American Psychological Association, 2003.

Clinical Mental Health Counseling

Clinical mental health counseling is a distinct helping profession with national standards for education, training, and clinical practice.

Description

Mental health counselors (MHCs) provide a variety of mental health services including psychotherapy; assessment and diagnosis of mental health disorders; substance abuse treatment; crisis management; treatment planning; psychoeducation, prevention programs; and evidence-based therapies. MHCs provide services in a variety of settings, including agency-based services; substance abuse treatment centers; and hospitals, employee assistance programs, private practice and managed health-care organizations. MHCs provide services to individuals of all ages, families, and couples.

Development

Clinical mental health counseling takes place within a wellness model, meaning the goal of counseling is to help the person move toward higher levels of wellness rather than to cure an illness. Personal and emotional issues are understood from within a human growth and development perspective, which is a holistically focused approach to helping. Prevention is also a key value of clinical mental health professionals. The goal of counseling is to empower and assist clients in solving problems independently. Counseling is considered a collaborative and transitory process through which clients increase their problem-solving skills and self-understanding.

Current Status

Clinical MHCs are highly trained professionals. MHCs earn a master's or doctoral degree from a counselor education or closely related program. Education programs are accredited by the Council for Accreditation of Counseling and Related Educational Programs (CACREP) and range from 48 to 60 semester hours depending on the area of specialization. The core areas of mental health education programs approved by the CACREP include diagnosis and psychopathology, psychotherapy, psychological testing and assessment, professional orientation, research and program evaluation, group counseling, human growth and development, counseling theory, social and cultural foundations, lifestyle and career development, and supervised practicum and internship. Licensure requirements for clinical MHCs are equivalent to two other disciplines (clinical social worker and marriage and family therapist) that require a master's degree for independent practice. A licensed clinical MHC has the following professional qualifications: an earned master's degree in counseling or a closely related mental health discipline, completed a minimum of two-year postgraduate clinical work under the supervision of a licensed or certified mental health professional, and passed a state or national licensure or certification examination.

Clinical MHCs adhere to a rigorous code of ethics and professional practice standards. The American Counselors Association code of ethics consists of eight sectional headings addressing counseling issues: the counseling relationship; confidentiality; professional responsibility; relationship with other professionals; evaluation, assessment, and interpretation; teaching, training, and supervision; research and publications; and resolving ethical issues.

Clinical mental health counseling is a distinct helping profession with a unique focus on wellness, prevention, and empowerment.

Steven R. Vensel, PhD

See also: Mental Health Counselor

Further Reading

American Mental Health Counselors Association. "Standards for the Practice of Clinical Mental Health Counseling." Accessed July 9, 2015. http://www.amhca.org/?page=standardsofpractice.

Clinical Psychology

Clinical psychology is the branch of psychology involved with the assessment and treatment of mental illness, abnormal behavior, and psychiatric conditions.

Definitions

- **Behavioral psychology** is a form of psychology whose aim is to study behavioral adaptation to an environment and its stimuli.

- **Cognitive behavior therapy** is a form of psychotherapy that addresses maladaptive thought distortions that lead to unwanted emotional and behavioral symptoms.

- **Cognitive psychology** is a form of psychology whose aim is to study thought and distorted patterns of thinking.

- **Humanistic psychology** is an experiential form of psychology developed out of the work of Abraham Maslow and Carl Rogers, which emphasizes a client's capacity for self-actualization and unique positive personal growth.

- **Practice** is a method or process used to accomplish a goal or objective.

- **Psychoanalytic psychology** is the form of psychology largely developed by the work of Sigmund Freud, which emphasizes the conflicts and compromises between the unconscious and conscious mind.

- **Psychometric assessment** is the direct or indirect measurement of psychological differences.

- **Psychopathology** is a maladaptive experience of suffering or aspect of a psychological condition incorporating cause, development, structure, and consequences.

- **Psychotherapy** is a psychological method for achieving desired changes in thinking, feeling, and behavior. It is also called therapeutic counseling.

Description

Clinical psychology is the branch of psychology that involves the assessment, diagnosis, and treatment of psychological disorders and behavioral conditions. It integrates knowledge from scientific research and professional practice. The goal of this integration is to enhance the ability to predict, assess, diagnose, and alleviate psychological problems and related dysfunction. Traditionally, there are three major theoretical perspectives in the practice of clinical psychology and psychotherapy. They are the psychoanalytic, cognitive behavioral, and humanistic traditions. More recently, systems theory has been incorporated into many aspects of clinical psychology. Theoretical orientations such as these guide clinical psychologists' research interests or work with clients. Clinical psychology is a system of subspecialties more than it is a single psychological specialty. There is so much diversity in clinical psychology. This leads to the establishment of many sub-specializations within clinical psychology. In addition, the profession undergoes rapid developmental changes as new information is acquired via science and practice. However, clinical psychologists tend to specialize as scientific researchers, clinical practitioners, or some combination of the two. Clinical psychology researchers are primarily interested in empirical study and the publication of novel scientific findings. Research in clinical psychology influences diverse areas of society, including education, medicine, and public policy. Practitioners of clinical psychology utilize the research findings to inform their work with persons suffering from some form of psychopathology. Clinical psychology practice often utilizes psychometric assessment and psychotherapeutic intervention.

Development and Current Status

Lightner Witmer (1867–1956) established the first psychological clinic at the University of Pennsylvania in 1896. Witmer published the term "clinical psychology" in a professional journal he established in 1907, titled *The Psychological Clinic*. Clinical psychology was developed out of psychometric and psychoanalytic forms of psychology. This history is most clearly evidenced by the development and military use of intelligence tests by the United States during World War I. These psychometric assessments, named *Army Alpha* and *Army Beta*, were used to determine how military enlistees would be utilized in the war effort. The United States' Veterans Administration became aware that many veterans returning from the war required treatment related to psychological trauma. After World War II there were increasing numbers of veterans with psychological trauma from "shell shock." As a result, the Veteran's Administration underwrote the development of university doctoral programs in clinical psychology.

The first university programs leading to the doctor of philosophy (PhD) degree were established in 1946 and were accredited by the American Psychological Association (APA). The APA was established in 1892 but did not develop a section devoted to clinical psychology until 1919. This section was revised in 1945 to become APA's Division 12, The Society of Clinical Psychology. Division 12 of the APA is one of the most influential psychological organizations to date. The Veteran's Administration and APA influenced the integration of psychotherapy into graduate training programs in clinical psychology. This integration of scientific research and psychotherapeutic practice in training programs is known as the scientist-practitioner model. It is also known as the "Boulder Model" because Boulder, Colorado, was the location of the professional conference at which the model was accepted by representatives of the profession. It was not until 1793 that the doctor of psychology (PsyD) was accepted by the APA and recognized by the profession.

These alternative training programs are known as practitioner-scholar models or the "Vail Model."

Layven Reguero, MEd, and Len Sperry, MD, PhD

See also: Cognitive Behavior Therapy; Counseling and Counseling Psychology; Psychotherapy

Further Reading

Freeman, Arthur, Stephanie H. Felgoise, and Denise D. Davis. *Clinical Psychology: Integrating Science and Practice.* New York, NY: John Wiley & Sons, 2008.

Trull, Timothy, and Mitchell K. Prinstien. *Clinical Psychology*, 8th ed. Belmont, CA: Cengage Learning, 2012.

Whitbourne, Susan Krauss, and Richard Halgin. *Abnormal Psychology: Clinical Perspectives on Psychological Disorders*, 7th ed. New York. NY: McGraw-Hill, 2013.

Clinical Trial

A clinical trial is a research study for comparing a new medication or treatment with an existing medication or treatment to determine its efficacy and safety. It is also known as clinical research trials.

Definitions

- **Effectiveness** refers to how well a treatment works (produce a beneficial effect) in the clinical practice of medicine.

- **Efficacy** refers to how well a treatment works (produce a beneficial effect) in clinical trials.

- **Food and Drug Administration** is the federal agency responsible for ensuring the safety and effectiveness of all drugs, vaccines, and medical devices.

- **National Institutes of Health** is a federal agency that conducts or supports biomedical research, including sponsoring clinical trials.

- **Placebo** is an inactive form of treatment (often a sugar pill) that has no treatment value.

- **Randomized controlled trial** is a research design in which participants are assigned randomly (by chance) to an experimental treatment or one that receives a comparison treatment or placebo. It is also referred to as randomized clinical trial.

- **Recruiting** is the time frame that a clinical trial has to identify and enroll participants in the trial.

Description

Clinical trials are research studies that utilize medical tests to determine the indications, efficacy, and safety of a new medication or treatment intervention. Such trials involve the monitoring of the various effects on large groups of individuals. They are used to assess the efficacy and effectiveness of a new treatment in comparison with the current standard of care or an existing treatment for a disease or disorder. In the United States, new medical treatments or devices must be approved by the U.S. Food and Drug Administration before they can be released for widespread use. Such approval requires rigorous testing in randomized controlled trials to determine whether it is effective in treating the medical condition. This testing is also used to determine the type and extent of side effects that may result.

Clinical trials are conducted by researchers affiliated with government health agencies such as the National Institutes of Health (NIH), a medical center, medical school, independent researchers, or private industry. Participants are recruited, as either volunteers or paid research subjects. Usually, participants are divided into two or more groups, including a control group that does not receive the experimental treatment, receives a placebo (inactive substance) instead, or receives a conventional treatment for comparison purposes.

For some individuals, clinical trials provide an opportunity for receiving new treatments that are not otherwise available. Those with difficult-to-treat or incurable medical conditions, like AIDS and certain cancers, can participate in clinical trials if standard therapies are not effective.

Developments and Current Status

Clinical trials have a rather long and rich history. About 605 BC what appears to be the first documented clinical trial is recounted in the book of Daniel. In it King Nebuchadnezzar ordered that children of royal blood

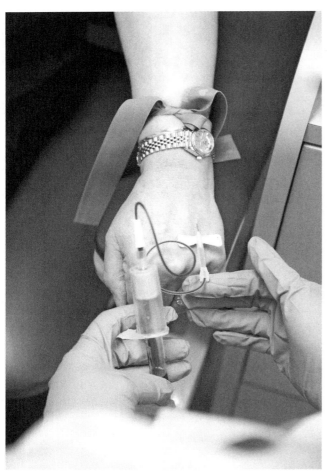

Clinical trials are research studies that use medical tests—often involving blood samples—to determine the indications, usefulness, and safety of a new medication or treatment intervention. Such trials involve the monitoring of the various effects on large groups of individuals. (Jim West/Alamy)

were to eat only meat and wine. Daniel requested an exemption for himself and three other men to eat only bread and water. It wo that the enforced consequences, for example uld be an experiment trial for 10 days in which one group would eat the king's diet and the other group would eat only bread and water. After the trial Daniel and the three children were noticeably healthier. Since this first trial, conducting clinical trials has been greatly refined. In 1747 James Lind conducted the first controlled clinical trial on sailors suffering from scurvy. All sailors were placed on the same diet, but one group was also given cider and vinegar, while the other group was given lemon juice. The group who had the lemon juice supplement recovered from scurvy in just six days.

Placebos were used in clinical trials for the first time in 1863. Since then there have been several refinements in how clinical trials have been designed and run.

There are various types of clinical trials: The most common is treatment trials. These trials test the relative effectiveness of new drugs or treatments or combinations of drugs and treatments. A second type of clinical trial is prevention trials. These trials are used to research ways for preventing a disease in individuals who have not previously had it. They are also used to prevent its return in those who were diagnosed and were then successfully treated. A third type of clinical trial is diagnostic trials. These trials seek to find better ways to diagnose a disorder or illness. A fourth type of clinical trial is screening trials to determine the best way to detect a disease or disorder. A fifth type of clinical trial is the quality-of-life trial. These trials are used to investigate how to increase quality of life (making life easier or more normal) for those diagnosed with a chronic illness.

Clinical trials usually have four phases. Each phase has a different purpose within the trial. Phase I trials involve a small group of participants (20 to 80). It focuses on evaluating the safety and potential side effects of a drug or treatment. It also helps in determining a recommended dosage. In Phase II, the treatment or drug is tested in more participants (100 to 300) to determine its efficacy, effectiveness, and safety. In Phase III, even more participants (1,000 to 3,000) are involved. In this phase the intervention is compared to standard treatments, and further information is collected about its safety and side effects. In Phase IV, post-marketing studies are carried out when the drug or intervention is widely available. The purpose of this phase is to collect additional data on the optimal use of the treatment and to further evaluate its side effects.

The research hospital of the NIH conducts ongoing clinical trials on medical treatments, medications, and therapies for various medical conditions. It continually recruits volunteers in many of these clinical trials. To find out more about medical research studies, various clinical trials, and availability in participating in a clinical trial with NIH, contact the Patient Recruitment and Public Liaison Office at 1-800-411-1222 or visit its website: http://www.cc.nih.gov.ezproxy.fau.edu/participate.shtml.

Len Sperry, MD, PhD

See also: Cancer, Psychological Aspects; HIV/AIDS

Further Reading

Brody, Tom. *Clinical Trials: Study Design, Endpoints and Biomarkers, Drug Safety, and FDA and ICH Guidelines.* New York, NY: Academic Press, 2010.

ClinicalTrials.gov. Accessed October 28, 2014. http://www.clinicaltrials.gov/ct/action/GetStudy.

Friedman, Lawrence M., Curt D. Furberg, and David L. DeMets. *Fundamentals of Clinical Trials*, 4th ed. New York, NY: Springer, 2010.

Norris, Deborah. *Clinical Research Coordinator Handbook*, 4th ed. New York, NY: Plexus Publishing, 2010.

Cliques

Cliques are small groups of friends with shared values, characteristics, and interests, who usually prefer to socialize exclusively with one another.

Definitions

- **Peer groups** are informal associations of people that arise from similarities in age, background, social status, and interests.

- **Peer pressure** describes the positive or negative influence one's peer group, or clique, has on one's attitudes, values, and behaviors.

Description

The term "clique" is derived from the 18th-century Old French term *cliquer*, meaning to "make a noise," and its later derivative, the English term "claque," referring to a group of people hired to applaud or publicly support someone. In the modern sense, the word "clique" describes a small, tight-knit group of people with similar qualities, values, interests, and behaviors. Generally, "cliques" refer to groups of adolescents who hang out primarily with one another. Both males and females form and join cliques. Those who are associated with adolescent cliques generally look, dress, think, and act the same. Some commonly used terms that refer to cliques that may exist in a present-day school include nerds, jocks, preps, Goths, emos, punks, surfers, skaters, gamers, and the "popular" group, or "in crowd." Subgroups have also been identified within these groups (e.g., "band geeks," "football jocks," "Honors kids").

These informal associations of people have positive and negative characteristics, though a prevailing negative connotation of the word "clique" does exist in mainstream culture. On the positive side, cliques can provide a sense of connectedness, belonging, and safety helping members feel important, valued, wanted, and included. In addition, members of cliques often stick up for one another or have one another's back—a quality of particular importance in the adolescent world. On the other hand, cliques can have negative consequences. Cliques, by definition, are exclusionary, so those who are not members may feel judged, undervalued, or rejected. Even those associated with the clique can struggle. Members may experience acting differently when they are in their clique than when they are not with them. Peer pressure is heightened in this type of social environment as well, which can cause the individual to behave in ways that conflict with his or her personal sense of self, values, and feelings. This issue of conformity versus nonconformity is profound in cliques as there is often a set of both spoken and unspoken rules that govern the group's cohesion. Under these circumstances, cliques may engage in bulling behavior—as power and social dominance play a key role in maintaining group dynamics. The book *Queen Bees and Wannabees* articulates this phenomenon from the adolescent girl's perspective. Thus, cliques have established hierarchies both within the group itself and among varying groups within the given setting (i.e., a school), and these levels of power are often made known to members and nonmembers alike.

Impact (Psychological Influence)

Social status among peers and between peer groups has been an area of interest for educators, psychologists, counselors, and sociologists for decades. The peer group one associates with can have an indelible influence on how that person thinks, feels, and acts, essentially affecting the person's overall growth and development. Group association can impact academic performance, behavior, self-esteem, and self-worth, which are critical in determining one's future trajectory and long-term success. Research indicates that an individual's rank in a clique is associated with both the social behaviors the individual uses within the group and the degree of likability by friends and peers. Findings also suggest that, good or bad, the most dominant group members get rewarded. However, there is increasing evidence to support that the range of accepted cliques is on the rise. Furthermore, traditionally deemed "popular" groups no longer have the influence they once had. Though dominant groups may still exist, most young people seek and are often successful in finding a social circle that fits them as individuals. Providing opportunities for youth to engage, including group projects and extracurricular activities, may remedy clique formation and rivalry.

Melissa A. Mariani, PhD

See also: Gangs; *Mean Girls* (Movie); Peer Groups

Further Reading

Closson, Leanna M. "Aggressive and Prosocial Behaviors within Early Adolescent Friendship Cliques: What's Status Got to Do with It?" *Merrill-Palmer Quarterly* 55 (2009): 3. Accessed June 25, 2014. http://digitalcommons.wayne.edu/mpq/vol55/iss4/3.

Gunton, Sharon. *Cliques: Social Issues Firsthand.* Farmington Hills, MA: Greenhaven Press, 2009.

Wiseman, Rosalind. *Queenbees and Wannabees: Helping Your Daughter Survive Cliques, Gossip, Boyfriends, and the New Realities of Girl World.* New York, NY: Random House, 2009.

Clockwork Orange, A (Movie)

A Clockwork Orange is a film directed and released by Stanley Kubrick in 1971, which depicts the isolation and violence among rebellious youth in Britain.

Description

The issue of how society could react to control the growing alienation and violence among young people became a prominent and popular theme, especially because of the social revolutions of the 1960s. Stanley Kubrick's 1971 film *A Clockwork Orange* is an adaptation of Anthony Burgess's 1962 novel of the same name. It employs disturbingly violent images to comment on psychiatry, juvenile delinquency, youth gangs, and other social, political, and economic subjects pertinent to the United Kingdom at that time.

The story depicts the main character, Alex, leading a gang of teenagers who go on the rampage every night, beating, raping, and murdering helpless victims. Eventually Alex is arrested and charged for his crimes. While in jail, he volunteers as a subject for aversion therapy in an effort to shorten his sentence. This kind of therapy is a treatment in which the patient is discouraged from a behavior by being subjected to a punishing stimulus when engaged in that behavior. The aversion therapy itself is violent. When Alex is eventually released from jail because he is cured, he initially hates violence. Eventually the people he meets and interacts with treat him so violently that inevitably he returns to a life of violence and sadism. So while after aversion therapy, Alex behaves for a while as if he were a good member of society, his new behavior does not really result from his own free choice. His goodness is involuntary. In the end he has become the clockwork orange of the title, organic on the outside, mechanical on the inside.

The film's central moral question, as in the book from which the movie was derived, is the definition of goodness. It asks whether it makes sense to use aversion therapy to stop immoral behavior. It is likened to the age-old question of whether a good end can justify evil means. The film raises several interesting questions without resolving them. What is goodness? Is it acceptable to use violent means in an attempt to stop violent behavior? Is aversion therapy effective?

Stanley Kubrick, the director of the movie, described the film in this way: "A social satire dealing with the question of whether behavioral psychology and psychological conditioning are dangerous new weapons for a totalitarian government to use to impose vast controls on its citizens and turn them into little more than robots." He also wrote: "It is a story of the dubious redemption of a teenage delinquent by condition-reflex therapy. It is, at the same time, a running lecture on free-will" (Houston, 1971, 43).

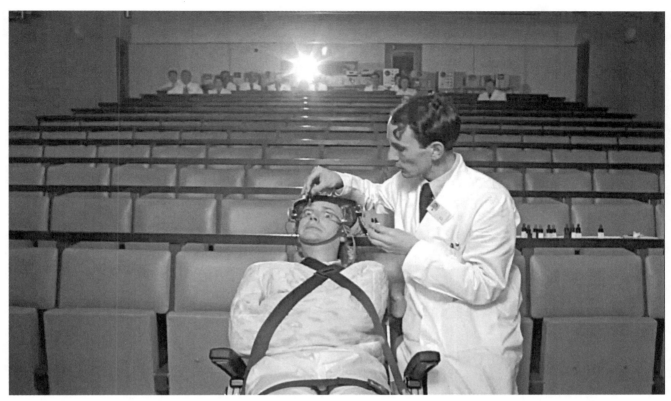

A scene from *A Clockwork Orange*, a classic film from 1971 directed and produced by Stanley Kubrick, shows Alex (Malcolm McDowell), an imprisoned gang leader, being subjected to painful aversion shock therapy in an attempt to reduce his love of physical and sexual violence. (Warner Bros./Photofest)

Impact (Psychological Influence)

The movie is a clear depiction of the dilemma that arises as a result of classical conditioning where the first step is pairing a behavior with a stimulus. In this movie, Alex is conditioned to associate violence with nausea. There is a possible second step, where there is an extinction of the pairing, whether intentional or not, but it is important to know that in the movie it is unintentional. This happens when the person discovers that the enforced consequences, for example, nausea because of drugs not because of violence, are shown to no longer have an effect. Since the change in behavior was artificial, or forced, the subject is then free to resume the original behavior without feeling any further negative consequences. In much less dramatic and dangerous forms, aversion therapy has been tried many times to limit or eliminate habits judged to be negative such as homosexuality and addictions to drugs and alcohol with limited or damaging effect.

Alexandra Cunningham, PhD, and William M. Cunningham, MA

See also: Aversion therapy

Further Reading

Burgess, Anthony. *A Clockwork Orange (Restored Text)*. New York, NY: W.W. Norton & Company, 2012.
A Clockwork Orange. Directed by Stanley Kubrick, 1971. USA: Warner Brothers.
Houston, Penelope. "Kubrick Country." *Saturday Review.* December 25, 1971, 42–44.

Clozaril (Clozapine)

Clozaril is an atypical antipsychotic medication used to alleviate the symptoms and signs of schizophrenia, particularly for those who have not responded to any other antipsychotic drug. Its generic name is clozapine.

Definitions

- **Atypical antipsychotic** is a class of newer-generation antipsychotic medications that are useful in treating schizophrenia and other psychotic disorders.

- **Extrapyramidal symptoms** are side effects caused by certain antipsychotic medications. They include repetitive, involuntary muscle movements, such as lip smacking, and the urge to be moving constantly.

- **Tardive dyskinesia** is a disorder involving involuntary and repetitive body movements that can develop after long-term use of certain antipsychotic medications.

Description

Clozaril is considered an atypical antipsychotic medication that differs from typical antipsychotics in its effectiveness in treating schizophrenia and its profile of side effects. It was the first atypical antipsychotic drug to be developed. Clozaril may reduce the signs and symptoms of schizophrenia in a large proportion of patients with treatment-resistant schizophrenia who have not responded to typical antipsychotics. It is intended for use in those with severe schizophrenia who have not responded to any other antipsychotic drug or who have experienced intolerable side effects. It is estimated that as many as 20%–60% of those with schizophrenia are treatment resistant. Clozaril is believed to work by blocking the neurotransmitters dopamine and serotonin in the limbic system, a region of the brain involved with emotions and motivation.

As an atypical antipsychotic it is to less likely to cause tardive dyskinesia and other extrapyramidal (pertaining to a neural network in the brain) side effects. Tardive dyskinesia involves involuntary movements of the tongue, jaw, mouth, or face or other groups of skeletal muscles. The incidence of tardive dyskinesia increases with increasing age and with increasing dosage. It may also appear after the use of the antipsychotic has stopped. Women are at greater risk than men for developing tardive dyskinesia. There is no known effective treatment for this syndrome, although gradual (but rarely complete) improvement may occur over a long period.

Precautions and Side Effects

Clozaril can cause agranulocytosis, a life-threatening depletion of white blood cells. It can cause epileptic seizures in about 5% of those taking Clozaril. Because seizures are dose related, that is, increasing as the dose of the drug is increased, Clozaril should be discontinued or the dose reduce to stop the seizures. Clozaril should be used in pregnant women only when strictly necessary. Infants born of mothers on Clozaril show extrapyramidal symptoms and symptoms of withdrawal, including agitation, trouble breathing, and difficulty feeding. Clozaril may also be secreted in breast milk, so breast-feeding is not advisable. Clozaril can cause sedation and may interfere with driving and other tasks requiring alertness. The drug may increase the effects of alcohol and sedatives.

Clozaril can cause a number of side effects, including decreases of blood pressure, rapid heart rate, changes in heart rhythm, sedation, increased appetite, excessive salivation, nausea, constipation, abnormal liver tests, elevated blood sugar, blurred vision, dry mouth, nasal congestion, decreased sweating, difficulty urinating, skin rash, weight gain, and fever.

Len Sperry, MD, PhD

See also: Psychosis; Tardive Dyskinesia

Further Reading

Mondimore, Francis Mark. *Bipolar Disorder: A Guide for Patients and Families*, 2nd ed. Baltimore, MD: Johns Hopkins University Press, 2006.

Stahl, Stephen M. *The Prescriber's Guide: Antipsychotics and Mood Stabilizers. Stahl's Essential Psychopharmacology.* Cambridge, UK: Cambridge University Press, 2009.

Torrey, E. Fuller. *Surviving Schizophrenia: A Manual for Families, Patients, and Providers*, 5th ed. New York, NY: Harper Collins, 2006.

Clueless (Movie)

The movie *Clueless*, released in 1995, was a popular teen comedy based loosely on the novel *Emma* directed by Amy Heckerling and starring newcomer Alicia Silverstone.

Description

Clueless is a teen-pop culture film that was released in the United States on July 19, 1995. It was written and directed by Amy Heckerling and produced by Scott Rudin. The comedy is very loosely based on Jane Austen's 1815 novel *Emma*. Alicia Silverstone stars as the lead character, Cher Horowitz. Other actors in the film include Stacey Dash (Dionne Davenport), Paul Rudd (Josh), and Brittany Murphy (Tai Frasier).

The movie is set in Beverly Hills and follows Cher's life as she navigates the social scene in high school. Cher is attractive, popular, wealthy, and fashion-obsessed. Her downfall is that she is also extremely superficial. She lives in a mansion with her father Mel (Dan Hedaya), a powerful litigator in town. Her mother died after suffering complications from a liposuction surgery. Cher is the envy of her peers. Her best friend Dionne is also rich, pretty, and popular. One of the only people to find fault with Cher is her socially conscious ex-stepbrother Josh, who is home visiting on break from college. Cher and Josh verbally spar about one another's shortcomings, though never maliciously. In an effort to prove her selflessness, Cher sets out on several "community service projects." First, Cher decides to play matchmaker to two of her teachers in an attempt to have them soften up on their grading so she can improve her report card. They find happiness and Cher decides that she enjoys helping others, so she moves onto her next project. So she befriends the new, unhip girl at school, Tai, in hopes of turning her popular. This plan backfires when Tai rises to top social status and eventually turns her sights on Josh. It is then that Cher realizes her true feelings for Josh and humbles herself in an effort to win his heart. She allows Tai to be her true self and pursue her feelings for another love interest. In the end, Cher and Josh find love once Cher abandons

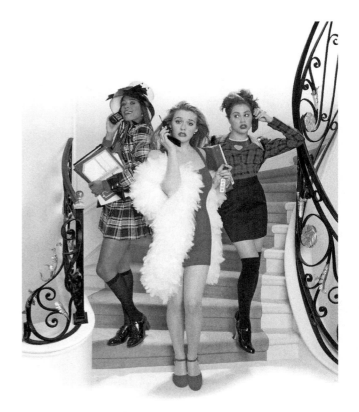

The movie *Clueless*, released in 1995, is a teen comedy based loosely on the Jane Austen novel *Emma*. Directed by Amy Heckerling and starring newcomer Alicia Silverstone, it covers themes of superficiality, kindness, and admitting mistakes. (Paramount Pictures/Photofest)

her selfish ways and begins to appreciate the people in her life.

Impact (Psychological Influence)

Clueless became a surprise sleeper hit when it grossed over $11 million on its opening weekend, finishing no. 2 behind the movie *Apollo 13*. In its box office run it grossed $55 million, the 32nd highest-grossing film of 1995. It catapulted Alicia Silverstone to international star status. Critics have also rated the film favorably. In 2008, *Entertainment Weekly* ranked it 42nd out of 100 "New Classics" released between 1983 and 2008. The magazine also named it the 19th best comedy of the past 25 years. The movie spun off to a television sitcom and a series of books. Much of the pop-culture lingo from the movie is still used by youth today, including phrases like "Whatever," "As-if," and, the movie's title, "Clueless."

Melissa A. Mariani, PhD

See also: Bullying and Peer Aggression; Cliques; Peer Groups

Further Reading

"Clueless, Alicia Silverstone." The Comedy 25: The Funniest Movies of the Past 25 Years." *Entertainment Weekly*. Time. Accessed March 5, 2013.

Clueless. Directed by Amy Heckerling, 1995. USA: Paramount.

"The New Classics: Movies." *Entertainment Weekly*. Time. 2008-06-27. Accessed March 5, 2013.

Coaching

Coaching is a developmental process in which a coach enables an individual to meet his or her goals for improved performance, personal growth, or career enhancement.

Definitions

- **Business coaching** is a form of coaching in which a coach works with an employee (below the level of executive) to enhance the employee's awareness and behavior in order to better achieve the business objectives of both the employee and his or her organization.

- **Executive coaching** is a form of coaching in which a coach works collaboratively with an executive to accomplish specific goals and objectives involving the executive's productivity and well-being. It is short term and focuses on increasing skills and performance or on personal and professional development.

- **Executive consultation** is a form of consultation in which a consultant functions as a sounding board and expert advisor to address a broad range of professional and personal issues of concern to the executive. It is often an ongoing and long-term process.

- **Personal coaching** is a form of coaching in which a coach works to improve the quality of his or her client's life, by offering advice on a broach array of personal and professional matters, including career, health, and personal relationships. It is also known as life coaching.

- **Psychotherapy** is a psychological method for achieving desired changes in thinking, feeling, and behavior. It is also called therapeutic counseling.

Description

When hearing or seeing the word "coaching" many think of sports coaching. In sports, a coach gives directions, instruction, and training of the on-field operations of an athletic team or of individual athletes. Today, many other forms of coaching have developed, in which coaches have different goals and roles than sports coaches. Increasingly, newer forms of coaching are regularly utilized and sought by a broad array of organizations and individuals who are not sports teams nor athletes. A common misconception is that coaching is the same as psychotherapy or therapeutic counseling. In fact they are quite different. The goal of psychotherapy is to assist individuals to recover from emotional or other psychological disorders such as anxiety, depression, or grief. In contrast, the goal of coaching is to assist normal, healthy individuals to achieve personal goals such as clarity on career objectives, increased well-being, or improved work–life balance.

Developments and Current Status

These newer forms of coaching include business coaching, personal coaching, and executive coaching. These forms of coaching focus on one of two objectives. The first is to increase the individual's personal development. The second is to increase the individual's professional performance. It is interesting to note that the original meaning of the word "coaching" is derived from the word "carriage," which in the English language means to convey an individual from where he or she is to where he or she wants to be. The assumption is that focusing on the individual's overall development will lead to increased professional effectiveness and job performance. Those who practice personal coaching, also called life coaching, emphasize this objective. On the other hand, those who view that the purpose of coaching is primarily to improve professional performance enhancement and secondarily personal development are more likely to practice business coaching. If the employee is an executive, it is called executive coaching.

Executive coaching is similar but different from executive consultation. Executive consultation addresses a broader range of professional and personal concern than are typically addressed in executive coaching. Issues in executive consultation can range from complex financial and personnel decisions to delicate personal health issues. Accordingly, it requires a seasoned consultant with an encyclopedic knowledge and broader experience base than is required of executive coaches. The signature characteristic of this form of consultation is that the consultant serves a sounding board and expert advisor who can quickly and effective assess the personal and organizational dynamics influencing the executive's concerns. In executive coaching, the coach also works collaboratively with an executive but with a different focus. The focus of such coaching is on increasing specific skills, performance, or development. It is usually directed at communicating vision and acting strategically, understanding individual and organizational dynamics, building relationships and mobilizing commitment facilitating team performance, or improving specific corporate results. Unless it is part of an ongoing leadership development program, executive coaching tends to be fairly focused and of short duration.

Len Sperry, MD, PhD

See also: Psychotherapy

Further Reading

Kilburg, R. *Executive Coaching: Developing Managerial Wisdom in a World of Chaos.* Washington, DC: American Psychological Association, 2000.

Kilburg, R. *Executive Wisdom: Coaching and the Emergence of Virtuous Leaders.* Washington, DC: American Psychological Association, 2006.

Sperry, L. *Executive Coaching.* New York, NY: Brunner—Routledge, 2004.

Starr, J. *The Coaching Manual: The Definitive Guide to the Process, Principles and Skills of Personal Coaching,* 3rd ed. New York, NY: Prentice-Hall, 2011.

Cobain, Kurt (1967–1994)

Kurt Cobain was the lead singer, guitarist, and songwriter of the pop-culture grunge band, Nirvana. His rise to musical fame in the 1990s is well noted along with his tumultuous relationship with girlfriend and later wife, Courtney Love, and ongoing struggles with drug addiction.

Description

Kurt Donald Cobain was born on February 20, 1967, in Aberdeen, Washington, to his parents, Wendy Elizabeth (Fradenburg) and Donald Leland Cobain, a waitress and automotive mechanic. Kurt had one sibling, younger sister, Kimberly. Cobain's family was filled with artistic and musical influences. His grandmother, Iris Cobain, was a professional artist. Kurt began drawing at an early age and his bedroom was often described as an art studio filled with drawings of his favorite cartoon characters. Musical talent was also present in the family. His Uncle Chuck Fradenburg was in the band The Beachcombers, his Aunt Mari Earle played guitar, and his great-uncle Delbert was an Irish tenor singer who made an appearance in the 1930 film *King of Jazz*. Kurt began singing and playing musical instruments at an early age. His Uncle Chuck gave him his first guitar, a prized gift.

Kurt's parents officially divorced when he was nine years old. This experience had a profound effect as he grew more sullen, withdrawn, and defiant. Though his parents both found new partners, neither household was well received by Kurt. He did not get the level of attention he was used to in his father's, and his mother was involved in a domestic violence situation. After seeking therapy for Kurt, his parents were advised that a single-family environment would be most beneficial, so on June 28, 1979, Cobain's mother granted full custody to his father.

Cobain spent his high school years back and forth between his parents and other family members. His behavior problems continued as well. He dropped out

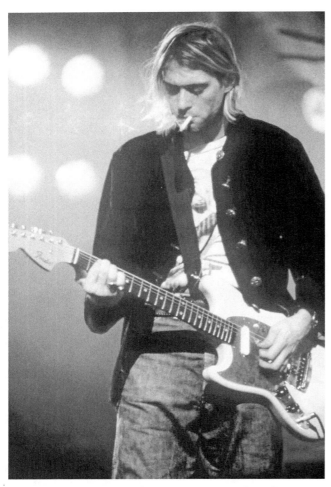

Kurt Cobain, a brilliant American musician best known as the lead singer, guitarist, and primary songwriter of the rock band Nirvana. Cobain struggled with depression and addiction for a number of years, and at the age of 27 ended his life with a shotgun. (AP Photo)

of Aberdeen High School just two weeks shy of graduation after realizing he did not have adequate credits to graduate. His time was then spent at odd jobs, oftentimes unemployed, and following favored punk bands from concert to concert. A few years later he persuaded a fellow devotee, Krist Novoselic, to partner up with him to form the beginnings of Nirvana. The band struggled initially with its first album *Bleach*, trying out a few different drummers and finally settling on Dave Grohl, with whom they found their greatest success. In 1991, their major label debut album, *Nevermind*, was released.

The lead single, "Smells Like Teen Spirit" from that album, was the platform the band needed to catapult into mainstream, rising to the top of the alternative rock/grunge movement. Since the debut of *Nevermind* (1991), Nirvana has sold over 25 million albums in the United States and over 50 million worldwide. Despite this success, Cobain was always uncomfortable with the spotlight and felt misinterpreted by the media. The band released its third album, *In Utero*, in 1993.

Though his professional life was on the rise, Cobain's personal life remained tumultuous. On January 12, 1990, in a Portland nightclub, Kurt Cobain met Courtney Love, the head of the rock band Hole. The two began dating and found common ground in their drug addictions. After dating a short while, Courtney revealed that she was pregnant and the couple subsequently married on Waikiki Beach in Hawaii on February 24, 1992. The couple's daughter, Frances Bean Cobain, was born on August 18, 1992. Tabloid reports then surfaced speculating about Courtney's drug use during her pregnancy. A judge ordered the couple to give up custody and leave Frances in the care of Courtney's sister Jamie. After months of legal battles and conceding to regular drug testing and visits from a social worker, Courtney and Kurt were eventually granted back full custody.

Though Cobain suffered from bouts of depression and drug abuse throughout his life, it was his addiction to heroine that eventually led him to his first stint in rehab in 1992. His recovery did not last long and he ended up overdosing in 1993. He overdosed again in early March 1994, though this incident has been noted as his first suicide attempt. On March 25, 1994, Love staged an intervention and Cobain agreed to enter rehab again but walked out after only 2 days. He returned to his home in Seattle though reports from family and close friends cannot account for his whereabouts during those few days. On April 8, 1994, Cobain's body was discovered at his home in Lake Washington. The coroner's report indicated he suffered one gunshot wound to the head and traces of heroin and diazepam were in his system. A suicide note was also found.

Impact (Psychological Influence)

Cobain's posthumous album "Nirvana: MTV Unplugged" earned him and his band a 1995 Grammy Award. In 2003, *Rolling Stone* magazine named Cobain the 12th greatest guitarist of all time. Dying at the age of 27, he is considered a member of the "27 Club," a group of prominent musicians who all died at the age of 27. Other members include Jimi Hendrix, Janis Joplin, Jim Morrison, and Amy Winehouse. Kurt Cobain is remembered as one of the most iconic alternative rock musicians of contemporary time. Fascination with his life and the struggles he faced continue, as does the popularity that his musical and artistic talents created.

Melissa A. Mariani, PhD

See also: Love, Courtney (1964–)

Further Reading

Azerrad, Michael. *Come as You Are: The Story of Nirvana.* New York, NY: Doubleday, 1994.

Cross, Charles. *Heavier Than Heaven: A Biography of Kurt Cobain.* New York, NY: Hyperion, 2001.

Cocaine

Cocaine is a stimulant drug that is extracted from the leaves of the coca plant. It produces feelings of euphoria and is highly addictive.

Definition

- **Stimulant** is a drug that increases brain activity and produces a sense of alertness, euphoria, endurance and productivity, or suppress appetite. Examples are cocaine, amphetamines, and Ritalin.

Description

Cocaine is one of the oldest-known psychoactive drugs. Extracted from coca leaves, cocaine was used by the Incas and others in the Andean region of South America for thousands of years as a stimulant. It was also used to depress appetite and to treat high-altitude sickness. It is a substance that can be processed into many forms for use as an illegal drug of abuse. In its most common form, cocaine is a whitish crystalline powder, which is known by such street names as "coke," "blow," "C," "flake," "snow," and "toot." It is most commonly inhaled or snorted. It may also be dissolved in water and injected. Cocaine produces feelings of euphoria or intense happiness. It also produces hypervigilance, increased sensitivity, irritability or anger, impaired judgment, and anxiety. Because it is highly addictive, the Federal Drug Administration classifies cocaine as a Schedule II drug, which means it has restricted medical usage. For example, a licensed physician can use it as a local anesthetic for certain eye and ear problems and in some kinds of surgery.

Crack is a form of cocaine that can be smoked and produces an immediate, more intense, and more short-lived high than the powder form. Crack comes in chunks, which are off-white in color, and called "rocks." Besides their standalone use, both cocaine and crack are often mixed with other substances. Cocaine may be mixed with methcathinone to create a "wildcat." Cigars may be hollowed out and filled with a mixture of crack and marijuana. Either cocaine or crack used in conjunction with heroin is called a "speedball." Cocaine used together with alcohol represents the most common fatal two-drug combination.

Cocaine Abuse

The patterns of cocaine abuse in the United States have changed much over the past 30 years. In the annual study, cocaine use among high school seniors was found to have declined from 13.1% in 1985 to 3.1% in 1992. The rate of cocaine use began to rise again and peaked at 5.5% in 1997 (Leshner, 2010). However, use among all ages declined over the same time period, which was attributed in part to education about the risks of cocaine abuse. The incidence of new crack cocaine users has also decreased. A 1997 study by the National Institute on Drug Abuse indicates that among outpatients who abuse substances, 55% abuse cocaine. The lifetime rate of cocaine abuse was reported as 0.2%. More recently, the National Survey on Drug Use and Health reports that in 2009, 4.8 million Americans aged 12 and older had abused cocaine in any form. It also found that adults 18 to 25 years of age had a higher rate of cocaine use than any other age group.

Cocaine abuse affects both genders and various populations across the United States. Males are up to two times more likely to abuse cocaine than females. Cocaine began as a drug of the upper classes in the 1970s, but since then the socioeconomic status of cocaine users has shifted. Cocaine is more likely to be abused by the economically disadvantaged because it is easy for them to get and it is inexpensive. These factors have led to increased violence as those who are cocaine dependent may become involved in illegal activity, like drug dealing to fund their habit. It has also been associated with higher rates of HIV/AIDS among disadvantaged populations.

Len Sperry, MD, PhD

See also: Addiction; Addictive Personality

Further Reading

Erickson, Carlton K. *Addiction Essentials: The Go-to Guide for Clinicians and Patients.* New York, NY: W.W. Norton, 2011.

Higgins, Stephen T., and Katz, Jonathan, L., eds. *Cocaine Abuse: Behavior, Pharmacology, and Clinical Applications.* New York, NY: Academic Press, 2012.

Leshner, Alan. "Cocaine Abuse and Addiction." National Institute on Drug Abuse Research Report Series. NIH Publication Number 99-4342. Washington, DC: U.S. Government Printing Offices, 1999, revised September 2010.

Sabbag, Robert. *Snowblind: A Brief Career in the Cocaine Trade.* New York, NY: Canongate Books, 2002.

Codependency

Codependency is a psychological concept referring to an excessive dependency on others and the thinking, feeling, and behavioral patterns that affect a person's ability to experience healthy relationships.

Description

Codependency is a concept that originally developed in the field of substance abuse recovery. The prefix "co" is Latin for "together." Originally codependency described how family members enable a substance abuser's addictive behaviors (alcohol or drugs use). Enabling is a dysfunctional behavior that is intended to help the substance abuser but actually reinforces the dependency. Enabling behaviors include taking the blame or making excuses for the substance abuser's addiction. For example, the codependent wife of an alcoholic calls the husband's workplace telling the employer that her husband is "sick" and can't come in to work when in fact he is hung-over and shouldn't drive or operate machinery. She believes she is helping him by protecting his employment and reputation, and her financial security, but in fact this enables his alcoholism. Her "helping him" shields him from the consequences of his behaviors and keeps him from being accountable or taking responsibility for his substance abuse. Thus, she is "co" dependent, or with him, in his alcoholism even though she does not drink.

Codependency is not a specific diagnosable mental health condition but it is a term that is used in a variety of situations. The definition of codependency has broadened since it was first identified in the field of addictions. In the fields of counseling and psychology, codependency has come to describe a person's overdependence on and control of another person to feel good about himself or herself. It has been described as "relationship addiction" in which the relationship is more important than the individual. Individuals who are codependent have an underdeveloped sense of self-esteem and only feel good when others are perceived to need them. As a result codependents have poor boundaries; they try to control the relationship by overly caring for the individual. They do more than their fair share of work; they often feel the martyr and have a need for recognition but are embarrassed when they receive it. How they act, feel, and think goes far beyond normal self-sacrifice and caregiving. They feel guilty if they have to assert themselves, fear being rejected, and have difficulty making decisions for fear that others will disapprove of the decision. Codependents believe that others' opinions are of more value than their own. They have difficulty admitting mistakes and go to great lengths to appear right in the eyes of the other, even if that means lying. Codependents are most comfortable when they feel needed. As a result they can be controlling, overly nurturing, or overly compliant depending on the nature of the relationship.

Current Status and Impact (Psychological Influence)

Although codependency is not an officially recognized mental health disorder, it is recognized by most mental health professionals as being a condition that affects a person's ability to have healthy and fulfilling relationships. There is general consensus that codependency develops in childhood as a result of growing up in a dysfunctional family. As such, it is believed that codependent behaviors are learned and can be changed. Individual psychotherapy and couples counseling can be helpful in changing the thoughts, feelings, and behaviors associated with codependency. There are also many books, support groups, website, and online support organizations that address codependency and offer instruction and help to codependents.

Steven R. Vensel, PhD

See also: Addiction Counseling; Beattie, Melody (1948–); Peer Groups; Psychoeducation; Psychoeducational Groups; Self-Help Groups

Further Reading

Beattie, Melody. *Co-dependent No More: How to Stop Controlling Others and Start Caring for Yourself.* New York, NY: Harper & Row, 1987.

Mental Health America. "Codependency." Accessed April 24, 2013. http://www.mentalhealthamerica.net/go/codependency.

Wells, Marolyn, Cheryl Glickauf-Hughes, and Rebecca Jones. "Co-dependency: A Grass Root Construct's Relationship to Parentification, Shame-Proneness, and Self-Esteem American." *Journal of Family Therapy* 27 (1999): 63–71.

Cognitive Behavior Analysis System of Psychotherapy (CBASP)

Cognitive behavior analysis system of psychotherapy is a psychotherapy approach that focuses on identifying and changing hurtful thoughts and behaviors with more helpful ones. It is also referred to as CBASP.

Definitions

- **Behavior therapy** is a psychotherapy approach that focuses on identifying and changing maladaptive (problematic) behaviors.

- **Behavioral analysis** is a type of assessment that focuses on the observable and quantifiable aspects of behavior and excludes subjective phenomena such as emotions and motives.

- **Cognitive therapy** is psychotherapy approach that focuses on identifying and modifying maladaptive (faulty) thoughts.

- **Dialectical behavior therapy** is a type of cognitive behavior therapy that focuses on learning skills to cope with stress, regulate emotions, and improve relationships.

- **Interpersonal psychotherapy** is a psychotherapy approach that focuses on interpersonal relationships and their context and on building interpersonal skills.

- **Psychodynamic psychotherapy** is a psychotherapy approach that assumes dysfunctional behavior is caused by unconscious, internal conflicts and focuses on gaining insight into these conflicts.

- **Psychotherapy** is a psychological method for achieving desired changes in thinking, feeling, and behavior. It is also called therapeutic counseling.

- **Situational analysis** is a type of behavioral analysis in which interpretations (thoughts) and related behaviors in a specific situation are identified.

Description

Cognitive behavior analysis system of psychotherapy (CBASP) is a psychotherapy approach that combines situational analysis with behavioral, cognitive, and interpersonal methods. It works by helping individuals focus on the consequences of their behavior and to use problem solving to resolve personal and interpersonal difficulties. The basic premise of CBASP is that personal and relational problems or symptoms result from a mismatch between what an individual desires or wants and what actually occurs. The focus of therapy is helping clients discover why they did not obtain a desired outcome by evaluating and modifying their limiting or hurtful interpretations (thoughts) and behaviors. In this approach individuals are helped to discover why they did not obtain a desired outcome by evaluating their problematic thoughts and behaviors. They identify the discrepancy between what they want to happen in a particular situation and what has happened or is actually happening.

There are two phases in CBASP treatment: elicitation and remediation. The elicitation phase consists of a detailed situational analysis. This analysis focuses on specific questions: How would you describe the situation? How did you interpret the situation? Specifically, what did you do and what did you say? What did you want to get out of the situation, that is, what was your desired outcome? What was the actual outcome of this situation? And, finally, did you get what you wanted? During the remediation phase, behaviors and interpretations are targeted for change. Then, the individual is helped to select alternative thoughts and behaviors that are more likely to achieve his or her desired outcome. First, each interpretation of the situation is assessed to determine whether it helped or hindered the achievement of the desired outcome. Next, each of the client's behaviors is similarly analyzed to determine whether it helped or hindered in the attainment of the desired outcome.

Developments and Current Status

CBASP is a form of behavior therapy that was developed by the American psychologist James P. McCullough (1942–). It combines methods from behavior therapy, cognitive therapy, interpersonal psychotherapy, and psychodynamic psychotherapy. McCullough sought to find an effective treatment for chronic depression. Since many chronically depressed individuals engage in emotional thinking and do not learn from previous experience, they remain trapped in life. He developed CBASP to help such individuals to move beyond emotional thinking and learn from their experience. Teaching such individuals to learn from their experience and use problem-solving techniques makes it possible for them to become perceptually aware of behavioral consequences. When individuals are able to identify the link between their interpretations and behavior and their consequences, they are then able—often for the first time—to use problem-solving methods to resolve both personal and interpersonal difficulties.

Even though CBASP was initially developed for the treatment of clients with chronic depression, it has extended to mental disorders. These include the various personality disorders, eating disorders, and the anxiety disorder (panic, social anxiety, and general anxiety disorder). It has been said that CBASP can be helpful with nearly all mental disorders except dementia and active psychotic states. It also includes conditions such as anger management, couples issues, parent–child issues, and social skills deficits. It can be used in individual and group formats. CBASP is both a standalone and adjunctive intervention method.

Research has shown that CBASP is a highly effective treatment approach. A national study involving more than 600 chronically depressed individuals showed that CBASP was more effective than either an antidepressant alone or cognitive behavior therapy alone. However, the when CBASP was combined with the antidepressant, 85% achieved an improvement (50% reduction in symptoms) while 42% achieved remission (elimination of all depressive symptoms) (McCullough, 2000).

Len Sperry, MD, PhD

See also: Behavior Therapy; Cognitive Behavior Therapy

Further Reading

Driscoll, Kimberly, Kelly C. Cukrowicz, Maureen Reardon, and Thomas E. Joiner Jr. *Simple Treatment for Complex Problems: A Flexible Cognitive Behavioral Analysis Approach to Psychotherapy.* Mahwah, NJ: Lawrence Erlbaum Associates, 2004.

McCullough, James P. *Skills Training Manual for Diagnosing and Treating Chronic Depression: Cognitive Behavioral Analysis System of Psychotherapy.* New York, NY: Guilford Press, 2001.

McCullough, James P. *Treatment for Chronic Depression: Cognitive Behavioral Analysis System of Psychotherapy.* New York, NY: Guilford Press, 2000.

Cognitive Behavior Therapy

Cognitive behavior therapy is a form of counseling or psychotherapy that focuses on changing maladaptive (faulty) behaviors, emotions, and thoughts. It is also known as CBT and cognitive behavioral therapy.

Definitions

- **Automatic thoughts** are thoughts that spontaneously come to mind when a particular situation occurs.

- **Behavior modification** is the use of learning principles to increase the frequency of desired behaviors and decrease the frequency of problem behaviors.

- **Behavior therapy** is a psychotherapy approach that focuses on identifying and changing maladaptive behaviors.

- **Cognitive restructuring** is a psychotherapy technique for replacing maladaptive thought patterns with constructive thoughts and beliefs.

- **Cognitive therapy** is a type of cognitive behavior therapy that focuses on identifying and changing distorted thinking patterns.

- **Dialectical behavior therapy** is a type of cognitive behavior therapy that focuses on learning skills to cope with stress, regulate emotions, and improve relationships.

- **Psychodynamic therapy** is a psychotherapy approach that assumes dysfunctional behavior is caused by unconscious, internal conflicts and focuses on gaining insight into these conflicts.

- **Rational emotive behavior therapy** is a type of cognitive behavior therapy that focuses on identifying and disputing irrational beliefs.

- **Schema therapy** is a type of cognitive behavior therapy that focuses on identifying and changing maladaptive schemas.

- **Schemas** are core beliefs or assumptions about one's self and the world.

Description

Cognitive behavior therapy (CBT) is a psychotherapy approach that addresses maladaptive (faulty) behaviors, emotions, and thoughts with various cognitive and behavioral interventions. CBT integrates the cognitive restructuring approach of cognitive therapy with the behavioral modification techniques of behavior therapy. The therapist works with the individual to identify thoughts and behaviors that are causing distress, and then to change those thoughts in order to readjust the behavior. Where individuals have schemas which are flawed and require change, CBT can be employed. Unlike other psychotherapy approaches that focus on insight (understanding), such as the psychodynamic psychotherapy, CBT is "problem focused" (focuses on specific problems) and "action oriented" (strategies that focus on changing actions or behaviors). CBT is time-limited, which means treatment is typically completed in 6 to 20 one-hour sessions.

CBT can be used with adults, adolescents, and children. It is thought to be effective for the treatment of a variety of psychological conditions. These include mood disorders, personality disorders, social phobia, obsessive-compulsive disorder, panic disorder, and agoraphobia. CBT has also been found to be effective with eating disorders, substance abuse, post-traumatic stress disorder, chronic pain, and attention-deficit hyperactivity disorder.

There are several approaches to CBT, including cognitive therapy, behavior therapy, schema therapy, and dialectical behavior therapy. While there are differences among these approaches, they all share a number of common characteristics. These are discussed here.

Focus on cognitive and behavioral factors. A basic premise of CBT is that individuals' emotions and behaviors are influenced by their beliefs or thoughts. Because most emotional and behavioral reactions are learned, the goal of therapy is to help individuals unlearn unwanted responses and to learn a new way of responding. The process begins with assessing maladaptive behaviors and thoughts, including automatic thoughts. By assessing, challenging, and modifying maladaptive beliefs and behaviors, individuals are able to gain control over problems previously believed to be insurmountable.

Direct session activity. CBT is a directive approach in which therapists typically direct session activity by setting an agenda, decide, plan what will be discussed prior to the session, and actively direct discussion of specific topics and tasks. Cognitive behavior therapists also endeavor to stimulate and engage individuals in the treatment process and these decisions.

Teach skills. Because CBT is also a psychoeducational approach, cognitive behavior therapists teach individuals skills to help them cope more effectively with problematic situations. Dealing directly with skill deficits and excesses is central to individuals achieving and maintaining treatment gains.

Provide information. Cognitive behavior therapists also discuss the explicit rationale for their treatment and the specific techniques being used. They may provide individuals with detailed information, for example, books or handouts, to orient individuals to the treatment process, to increase their confidence in treatment, and to enhance their ability to cope with problematic situations.

Use homework and between-session activities. Homework and between-session activities are a central feature of CBT. Such activities provide individuals the opportunity to practice skills learned in sessions and transfer gains made in treatment to their everyday life. Such activities can also foster and maintain symptom reduction.

Emphasize present and future experiences. CBT focuses on the impact individuals' present maladaptive thoughts have on their current and future functioning. In addition, skills learned in therapy are designed to promote more effective future functioning.

Developments and Current Status

The term "cognitive behavior therapy" came into usage in the past 40 years or so. It evolved from both the cognitive therapy and behavior therapy traditions in psychotherapy. Behavior therapy in America was pioneered by psychologist Joseph Wolpe

(1915–1997). Cognitively oriented therapies in America were pioneered by psychiatrist Aaron T. Beck (1921–), the developer of cognitive therapy, and by psychologist Albert Ellis (1913–2007), the developer of rational emotive behavior therapy. A useful way of understanding this evolution of CBT is in terms of what has been called the "three waves" of behavior therapy.

First wave. The first wave emphasized traditional behavior therapy, which focused on replacing problematic behaviors with constructive ones through classical conditioning and reinforcement techniques. Joseph Wolpe pioneered classical conditioning, particularly systematic desensitization. Traditional behavior therapy was a technical, problem-focused, present-centered approach that was markedly different than psychoanalysis, individual-centered therapy, and similar approaches of that era that emphasized the therapeutic relationship and the feelings and inner world of the individual.

Second wave. The second wave involved the incorporation of the cognitive therapies which focused on modifying problematic feelings and behaviors by changing the thoughts that cause and perpetuate them. The incorporation of cognitive and behavioral therapies in the 1970s was not initially a cordial or conflict-free union, but today most cognitive therapists incorporate key behavioral interventions while most behavior therapists recognize the role of individuals' beliefs about the consequences of their behaviors The fact that both were problem focused and scientifically based therapies has helped foster this union, resulting in CBT becoming the most commonly practiced treatment method in the United States since the late 1980s.

Third wave. The third wave involved the reformulation of conventional CBT approaches which were based on a modernist paradigm or perspective. In contrast, third wave approaches tend to be more influenced by the postmodern perspective. Accordingly, treatment tends to be more experiential and indirect and utilizes techniques such as mindfulness, dialectics, acceptance, values, and spirituality. Unlike the first and second wave, third wave approaches emphasize second-order change, that is, basic change in structure and/or function, and are based on contextual assumptions, including the primacy of the therapeutic relationship.

Len Sperry, MD, PhD

See also: Behavior Therapy; Cognitive Therapies; Dialectical Behavior Therapy (DBT); Schema-Focused Therapy

Further Reading

Beck, Judith S. *Cognitive Behavior Therapy: Basics and Beyond*, 2nd ed. New York, NY: Guilford Press, 2011.

Craske, Michelle G. *Cognitive-Behavioral Therapy*. Washington, DC: American Psychological Association, 2010.

Sperry, Len. *Cognitive Behavior Therapy of DSM-5 Personality Disorders*, 3rd ed. New York, NY: Routledge, 2016.

Cognitive Behavioral Modification

Cognitive behavioral modification (CBM) is a psychotherapy approach that focuses on identifying dysfunctional self-talk in order to change unwanted behaviors.

Definitions

- **Behavior therapy** is a psychotherapy approach that focuses on identifying and changing maladaptive behaviors. It is also referred to as behavioral therapy.

- **Cognitive behavior therapy** is a form of psychotherapy that focuses on changing faulty behaviors, emotions, and thoughts. It is also known as CBT and cognitive behavioral therapy.

- **Cognitive therapy** is a type of cognitive behavior therapy that focuses on identifying and changing automatic thoughts and maladaptive beliefs.

- **Psychotherapy** is a psychological method for achieving desired changes in thinking, feeling, and behavior. It is also called therapy and therapeutic counseling.

- **Rational emotive therapy** is a form of psychotherapy based on the idea that problems are caused by irrational thoughts, beliefs, and expectations. It was developed by Albert Ellis and is also known as RET. In the 1990s Ellis incorporated the dimension of "behavior" and changed the name to REBT.

- **Self-talk** is one's constant internal conversation which can either be encouraging and motivating or discouraging and self-critical.

Description

Cognitive behavioral modification is a combination of cognitive therapy and behavior therapy techniques for fostering healthy thoughts and behaviors. It focuses on identifying dysfunctional (faulty) self-talk in order to change unwanted behaviors. The assumption is that behavior is the result of one's thoughts and self-talk. The goal of CBM is to teach individuals to observe their own self-talk and behavior and replace it with new, healthier self-talk and behavior.

There are three phases in the CBM process. The first phase involves self-observation. This involves individuals closely listening to their own self-talk and observing their behaviors. Individuals need to be particularly aware of any negative statements they make about themselves as this will likely contribute to symptoms of anxiety and panic. The second phase involves new self-talk. Once an individual recognizes he or she is engaging in negative self-talk, he or she can begin to change it. When an individual catches himself or herself in negative thought patterns, he or she can re-create new positive self-talk. For example, an individual may say "I can't take this exam, and I will fail. I am just not smart enough." A new and healthier self-talk might be: "I know this exam is going to be difficult, but I am going to study and prepare as best as I can." When an individual makes new self-statements, he or she is guided to new behaviors. This leads to better coping skills, and as each small success builds upon another, an individual can make significant gains in his or her recovery. The third phase of CBM involves learning new skills. Each time an individual can identify his or her negative self-talk, modify it, and change his or her behaviors, he or she is learning new skills. When individuals are controlled by negative thoughts, it becomes difficult to control behaviors in unpleasant situations. CBM can help an individual change negative thoughts to positive thoughts, and as a result, the individual will begin to behave and act more effectively.

Psychologist Donald Meichenbaum (1940–) developed CBM in the 1970s. Meichenbaum was greatly influenced by rational emotive therapy. He was one of the first to advocate for combining behavior therapy with cognitive therapy. As a result, he is recognized as one of the founders of cognitive behavior therapy.

Len Sperry, MD, PhD, and
Elizabeth Smith Kelsey, PhD

See also: Behavior Therapy; Cognitive Behavior Therapy; Cognitive Therapies; Psychotherapy; Rational Emotive Behavior Therapy (REBT)

Further Reading

Martin, Garry L., and Joseph Pear. *Behavioral Modification: What It Is and How to Do It*, 7th ed. Upper Saddle River, NJ: Prentice Hall, 2002.

Meichenbaum, Donald. *Cognitive-Behavioral Modification: An Integrative Approach*. New York, NY: Plenum Press, 1977.

Mennuti, Rosemary B., Ray W. Christner, Arthur Freeman, and Judith S. Beck. *Cognitive-Behavioral Interventions in Educational Settings: A Handbook for Practice*. New York, NY: Routledge, 2012.

Cognitive Complexity

Cognitive complexity is an indicator of the degree of complexity (intricacy) or simplicity of an individual's thinking and perceptual skills.

Definitions

- **Cognitive development** is the ability of individuals to think, perceive, and gain an understanding of their world.

- **Cognitive model** refers to how concepts are related. Such models help one to know, understand, or reproduce the idea they represent.

- **Cognitive system** is an interrelated system of beliefs, ideas, assumptions, and knowledge.

- **Concept** is an idea that represents a class of objects or their properties such as "truck" or "green."

- **Construct** is a type of schema which is a cognitive model for understanding meaning.

- **Domain** is a field of personal knowledge.

- **Perceptual skill** is the ability to develop a mental image or awareness of the elements of the environment.

- **Schema** is a cognitive model through which an individual understands or assigns meaning to his or her world. A schema is also referred to as a construct.

Description

Cognitive complexity is described as the level of differentiation and integration in an individual's cognitive system. Differentiation is the number of available constructs in an individual's cognitive system about a particular domain. Integration is the ability to recognize relationships among cognitive constructs (schemas) in a particular domain. The degree of cognitive complexity helps to predict an individual's social and clinical judgment (decisions).

Those who are high in cognitive complexity tend to perceive nuances and subtle differences. Therefore, they are more likely to engage in "both-and" thinking. In contrast, those who are low in cognitive complexity tend not to perceive such nuances and subtle differences. As a result, they are more likely to engage in "black and white" and "either-or" thinking.

Cognitive complexity is also known as a schema, which is an indicator of how individuals structure their world. An individual's level of cognitive complexity relates to an individual's level of cognitive development. The higher the level of an individual's cognitive development, the higher his or her level of cognitive complexity. For example, increasing the growth and thinking process can lead to higher levels of cognitive complexity. Individuals develop constructs as internal ideas of reality of the world around them. These constructs are based on interpretations of an individual's observations and experiences. Complexity of cognition is a result of childhood development and not a personality trait. Parental, familial, and social interactions in early childhood influence the development of the constructs. To the extent that individuals are able to learn from their mistakes and past experiences, their cognitive complexity increases.

Cognitive complexity is particularly important for counselors and therapists. It is often difficult to understand individuals' needs, particularly in counseling, because often times their situations are very complex. An individual's level of cognitive complexity can vary from topic to topic. Given the connection between cognitive complexity and the development of expertise in counseling, programs that train counselors and therapists would do well to integrate cognitive components into their training. Some concrete techniques for integrating cognitive complexity into training curricula include (a) attending to and seeking information about oneself, others, and relationships; (b) organizing and integrating information into conceptual models; and (c) planning, guiding, and evaluating interventions.

Len Sperry, MD, PhD, and
Elizabeth Smith Kelsey, PhD

See also: Schemas and Maladaptive Schemas

Further Reading

Kelly, George. *The Psychology of Personal Constructs.* New York, NY: W.W. Norton, 1955.
Reeves, Wayne, W. *Cognition and Complexity.* Lanham, MD: Scarecrow Press, 1986.
Welfare, Laura, and Diane Borders. "Counselor Cognitions: General and Domain Specific Complexity." *Counselor Education and Supervision* 49, no. 3 (March 2010): 162–178.

Cognitive Deficits

"Cognitive deficit" is a medical term used to describe a variety of brain function impairments.

Description

The word "cognitive" is used to describe any number of mental processes including perception; memory,

judgment, and reasoning. Language and communication are also considered cognitive processes. The term "cognitive deficit" is used to describe a variety of conditions pertaining to problems in a person's mental process. Cognitive deficits include intellectual impairment, speech and communication impairment, memory impairment, and perceptual impairment.

Causes and Symptoms

Cognitive deficits are caused by a number of events and occur in children and adults. Children can be born with cognitive deficits, which can occur as a result of genetic abnormalities, infections, exposure to drugs taken by the mother during pregnancy, and lack of oxygen during birth or in many other ways. Cognitive deficits can occur as a result of acquired brain injuries such as a severe blow to the head, oxygen deprivation from choking or drowning, and brain damage caused by drug use or poisoning. Medical conditions such as strokes or aging-related diseases such as Alzheimer's disease can cause cognitive deficits.

Prognosis

Although there is not a cure for cognitive deficits, they can be treated. Cognitive remediation and cognitive rehabilitation are two types of interventions used to reduce cognitive deficits.

Steven R. Vensel, PhD

See also: Cognitive Remediation; Intellectual Disability

Further Reading

American Psychiatric Association. *Diagnostic and Statistical Manual of Mental Disorders*, 5th ed. Arlington, VA: American Psychiatric Association, 2013.

Cognitive Dissonance

Cognitive dissonance is the emotional discomfort people feel as a result of conflicting beliefs, thoughts, attitudes, and behaviors.

Description

Cognitive dissonance theory is a well-established and highly researched social psychology theory originally proposed by Leon Festinger (1919–1989) in the 1950s. Leon Festinger, one of the top 100 most eminent psychologists of the 20th century, coined the term "cognitive dissonance." He first used the phrase in his 1956 book *When Prophecy Fails*, which looked at what happens in the minds of UFO cult members when their beliefs of a prophecy (a UFO landing and the destruction of the earth) failed to come true. In 1957, Festinger explained cognitive dissonance theory and its importance to social psychology in his book *A Theory of Cognitive Dissonance*. Cognitive dissonance is one of the most highly studied phenomena in the history of psychology.

Cognitive dissonance is the psychological and emotional state produced when someone holds conflicting beliefs, thoughts, attitudes, or values and behaves in ways that are incongruent to those cognitions. The perception of an inconsistency creates a negative internal state of discomfort or dissonance. There are many emotions that may be associated with cognitive dissonance, including anxiety, fear, anger, frustration, and embarrassment.

According to cognitive dissonance theory, people are highly motivated to reduce their cognitive dissonance. Individuals employ several strategies in order to reduce the discomfort. They can modify existing cognitions, that is, change of belief; add new cognitions, that is, add a new belief; or reduce the importance of one of the components of the conflict, that is, change a perception. For example, imagine two separate high school students who aspire to become Olympic athletes. They know that in order to reach their dream they must be dedicated and train several hours each day. Cognitive dissonance would occur when they consider skipping practice for a day at the beach with their friends. They both feel guilty and anxious about missing a day of practice. It is uncomfortable and something must occur in order to reduce the negative feeling. There is a dissonance between their belief of "I want to become an Olympic athlete" and "I want to go to the beach with my friends." One of them thinks "missing one day of training could make the difference between becoming

an Olympian and not making it; besides, I don't really like the beach that much" and that person attends practice. The other athlete thinks "I've been working so hard I deserve a break; missing one day of training can't make that big of a difference," and skips practice. Both were in a state of cognitive dissonance. They were conflicted between their goal of becoming Olympic athletes and going to the beach, a behavior that was in opposition to their goal. One of the students changed her belief by justifying (I deserve a break) and rationalizing (it won't make a difference) the behavior (a day at the beach). The other student reduced the cognitive dissonance by adding a new belief (one day of training could make a difference) and reducing the importance of one of the components (I don't like the beach that much), choosing to attend practice.

Current Status and Impact (Psychological Influence)

A tremendous amount of research has been conducted in examining key components of cognitive dissonance theory in adults and children. The concepts of beliefs, attitudes, and motivational systems; psychological and emotional discomfort; compliance dynamics; use of justification and rationalization; and decision making have been studied.

Cognitive dissonance theory continues to be one of the most studied concepts in psychology. It has been used to examine a multitude of social and psychological problems such as eating disorders, mood and behavior disorders, and substance abuse disorders. It has also been used in studies of relationships, parenting, moral beliefs, racism, prejudice, happiness, attitudes, decision making, motivation, self-perception, and in hundreds of other personal applications. In addition to the social psychology fields, cognitive dissonance research has been conducted in virtually every professional field, including, education, nursing, marketing, economics, finance, law, communication, advertising, and medicine.

Cognitive dissonance theory is a concept that has provided insight into human behavior and functioning. Over the past 60 years studies investigating a wide variety of confusing human behaviors have been conducted. These studies have consistently led to the development of helpful interventions and treatments for a wide variety of problems. Cognitive dissonance theory is sure to continue to offer meaningful insight and understanding into the human condition.

Steven R. Vensel, PhD

See also: Schemas and Maladaptive Schemas

Further Reading

Egan, Louisa, Laurie Santos, and Paul Bloom. "The Origins of Cognitive Dissonance." *Psychological Science* 18, no. 1 (2007): 978–983.

Festinger, Leon. *A Theory of Cognitive Dissonance.* Stanford, CA: Stanford University Press, 1957.

Festinger, Leon, Henry Reicken, and Stanley Schachter. *When Prophecy Fails.* London: Pinter & Martin, 1956.

Haggbloom, Steven, Renee Warnick, Jason E. Warnick, Vinessa K. Jones, Gary L. Yarbrough, Tenea M. Russell, Chris M. Borecky, Reagan McGahhey, John L. Powell III, Jamie Beavers, and Emmanuelle Monte. "The 100 Most Eminent Psychologists of the 20th Century." *Review of General Psychology* 6, no. 2 (2002): 139–152.

Cognitive Problem-Solving Skills Training (CPSST)

Cognitive problem-solving skills training (CPSST) focuses on decreasing inappropriate and disruptive behaviors in children and adolescents by teaching them constructive ways to solve problems.

Description

CPSST was developed to help reduce significant conduct and behavioral problems in children and adolescents at home, at school, and in the social environment. It focuses on helping children and adolescents learn to manage the thoughts and feelings that often provoke or create the problems to begin with. Dysfunctional behaviors include impulsive, disruptive, annoying, and defiant behaviors; aggressive behaviors; and behaviors that infringe upon the rights of others.

The goal of CPSST is to decrease dysfunctional behaviors by increasing an individual's choice in how to respond to social situations. A central precept of CPSST is that children and adolescents are limited in how they interact and respond socially. These limits are often imposed by the family systems of the child. The individual maturity level of the child also imposes limits to his or her response to problems. The early focus is on discovering irrational interpretations and assumptions that lead to dysfunctional behaviors and acting out. For instance, a child who acts out aggressively in a classroom may have wrongly interpreted that someone is laughing at him or her when in fact it is not so.

CPSST consists primarily of individual sessions although group treatment sessions can be utilized. Sessions typically last for 45 to 60 minutes and usually occur weekly but can occur more frequently. CPSST uses a cognitive behavioral approach to managing interpersonal conflict and social relationships. An essential component to early treatment is helping the child or adolescent understand how thoughts, feelings, and behaviors work together to form responses to problems. One of the first goals of CPSST is to address the cognitive aspects of the individual's behavior. How an individual thinks about situations and interprets the actions and behaviors of others is crucial to developing new ways of thinking that lead to new ways of feeling and behaving. Another central aspect of CPSST is helping children gain insight into how they are often a part of the conflict or problem. CPSST then teaches children different skills and techniques in managing thoughts and feelings and in responding appropriately to stressful situations.

CPSST is a collaborative and interactive process between the client and the therapist. Learning new behaviors through modeling and role-playing is key behavioral elements of CPSST. Teaching alternative ways of responding and affirming new skills are also important behavioral components of CPSST. Homework is often assigned in order for the individual to practice the new skills and new ways of thinking. Homework and events during the week are discussed and evaluated in order to reinforce successful problem solving or correct areas of weakness.

Successful CPSST results in children being able to be more flexible in social conflicts and less likely to act impulsively. As CPSST progresses, children become more skilled at generating and implementing alternative solutions to conflicts. Another aspect of successful CPSST is an understanding and anticipation of the social consequences of the child's behaviors on self and others.

Development and Current Status

CPSST continues to be studied and has been found to be effective in changing problem behaviors in children and adolescents. Alan Kazdin, director of Yale Parenting Center, has conducted extensive research into child conduct problems and is the most cited researcher of CPSST. Kazdin's clinical research team has studied child-rearing practices, parenting, and ways in which parenting can be altered to improve child functioning at home, at school, and in the community. The team has also examined child and adolescent treatment practices in use in the mental health professions, the clinical and research bases of these practices, and the implications for mental health services. The result of this extensive research has been the development of the "Kazdin Method" of parenting, which uses a combination of cognitive problem solving and parent training. The Kazdin Method has been examined in controlled studies and found to be effective in reducing conduct problems in children and adolescents aged 2 to 17. It has also been found to be effective across diverse ethnic groups.

Steven R. Vensel, PhD

See also: Cognitive Behavior Therapy

Further Reading

Kazdin, Alan. "Problem-Solving Skills Training and Parent Management Training For Oppositional Defiant Disorder and Conduct Disorder." In *Evidence-Based Psychotherapies for Children and Adolescents*, 2nd ed., edited by J. Weisz and A. Kazdin. New York, NY: Guilford Press, 2010.

Kazdin, Alan, Todd Siegel, and Debra Bass. "Cognitive Problem-Solving Skills Training and Parent Management Training in the Treatment of Antisocial Behavior in Children." *Journal of Consulting and Clinical Psychology* 60, no. 5 (1992): 733–747.

Cognitive Remediation

Cognitive remediation is a type of treatment that assists individuals suffering from psychiatric disorders improve their cognitive skills and increase their social functioning.

Description

Cognitive remediation is a psychological treatment approach focused on the improvement of cognitive deficits and problems in living for individuals suffering from psychiatric disorders such as schizophrenia and attention-deficit hyperactivity disorder. The goal of cognitive remediation is to improve skills most closely tied to living independently, such as holding a job and developing meaningful relationships. Cognitive remediation is used in conjunction with other medical and psychotherapeutic treatments. It has been shown to be effective in the treatment of some psychotic disorders, attention disorders, mood disorders, and eating disorders.

Cognitive remediation and cognitive retraining use similar techniques but have distinct goals. Cognitive retraining focuses on restoring or compensating for cognitive losses after a brain injury. The goal of cognitive remediation is to develop new abilities and skills in individuals suffering from psychiatric disorders.

Development

Cognitive remediation therapy was originally developed at Kings College in London to improve social functioning of patients suffering from psychological and neuropsychological conditions such as schizophrenia. Cognitive remediation uses exercises and tasks to train the brain and improve neuropsychological function. There are two main techniques used to train brain functions. One is to strengthen the deficit function by targeting the specific impairment in order to increase functioning. The second is to target cognitive strengths and develop strategies to compensate for the impaired function. Assisting patients to think more abstractly, increase attention span, organize increasingly complex problems, and develop skills in problem solving and logic are examples of identified treatment goals. Most frequently, the exercises and tasks in cognitive remediation therapy are administered via computer and often take the form of games. Repetition is an important factor in cognitive remediation. Some examples of task used in cognitive remediation therapy include sentence completion exercises; remembering list of numbers, words, or figures; organizing sequences of numbers, letters, or symbols; and other exercises.

Conditions and disorders that have symptoms of attention and concentration issues, memory impairment, and organizational problems include attention-deficit disorders and schizophrenia. Other conditions that have symptoms of cognitive impairment include depression and anorexia. For instance, people suffering from depression often report feeling that their "head is in a cloud" and they are unable to think clearly. Individuals suffering from an eating disorder such as anorexia have very rigid thought patterns when it comes to food.

Current Status

There are numerous studies indicating the effectiveness of cognitive remediation in assisting individuals suffering from a variety of psychological disorders. There are over 100 clinical trials involving more than 2,000 people with schizophrenia indicating cognitive remediation to be effective in improving abilities associated with essential living skills.

In 2010, Til Wykes, professor of clinical psychology and rehabilitation at the Institute of Psychiatry, King's College London, called for greater focus in the research of cognitive remediation therapy. He suggested that all researchers adopt and use no more than 10 standardized measures of performance and categorize study participants into meaningful subgroups, such as age or ways of learning. He also called for researchers to investigate more precisely how cognitive changes are brought about and how significantly they affect a person's life. Further research is currently being conducted investigating the usefulness of this promising technique with other types of conditions in which cognitive impairments are observed.

Steven R. Vensel, PhD

See also: Cognitive Behavior Therapy; Cognitive Deficits; Cognitive Retraining

Further Reading

Elgamal, Safa, Margaret Mckinnon, Karuna Ramakrishnan, Russell Joffe, and Glenda MacQueen. "Successful Computer-Assisted Cognitive Remediation Therapy in Patients with Unipolar Depression: A Proof of Principle Study." *Psychological Medicine* 37, no. 9 (2007): 1229–1238.

Tchanturia, Kate, Helen Davies, Carolina Lopez, Ulrike Schmidt, Janet Treasure, and Til Wykes. "Neuropsychological Task Performance before and after Cognitive Remediation in Anorexia Nervosa: A Pilot Case Series." *Psychological Medicine* 38, no. 9 (2008): 1371–1384.

Wykes, Til. "Cognitive Remediation Therapy in Schizophrenia: Randomized Controlled Trial." *British Journal of Psychiatry* 190 (2007): 421–427.

Wykes, Til. "Cognitive Remediation Therapy Needs Funding." *Nature* 468 (2010): 165–166.

Cognitive Retraining

Cognitive retraining is a form of neuropsychological treatment, which assists brain injury patients restore, or compensate for loss of, cognitive abilities due to a brain injury.

Description

The purpose of cognitive retraining is to assist brain injury patients recover impaired brain functions and improve their quality of life. Cognitive retraining is a rehabilitative technique used by a variety of professionals to improve or restore function to impaired attention, memory, organization, reasoning, understanding, and problem-solving cognitive functions. Assisting brain injury patients improve their awareness of the impact of the injury, accepting their limitations, and adapting to the changes brought about by the injury are important components of cognitive retraining. Developing a sense of well-being within a realistic understanding of the neurobiological changes is an overarching goal of cognitive retraining. Neuropsychologists, counselors, psychologists, psychiatrists, occupational therapists, and speech therapists, among others, can be trained to provide cognitive retraining treatments.

Development

Cognitive retraining is a psychoeducational approach characterized by the therapist's efforts to improve the patient's awareness, acceptance, and realism about his or her injury-related strengths and challenges. Patients are taught to recognize how their neurological strengths and difficulties impact life at home, work, and school and in the environment. There are two categories of cognitive retraining: restorative and compensatory. Restorative retraining helps injured individuals recover functions that have been impaired by injury, stroke, or hypoxia. Compensatory training focuses on assisting patients to cope with and compensate for permanent impairment.

Cognitive retraining begins with a comprehensive neuropsychological assessment of the injured individual. The goal of the assessment is to determine the extent of the injury. It is not uncommon for brain injury patients to be unaware of the extent of their functional impairments, so a complete assessment is essential in planning a course of treatment interventions. The assessment tailors the cognitive retraining to the specific needs of the individual. Studies have indicated that patient buy-in and the ability to "see the big picture" is important to successful outcomes. When patients were able to clearly see the purpose and application of the skills being taught, they were more likely to develop those skills. The relationship between the patient and therapist is also a key factor in positive recovery. A positive working alliance with the therapist, in which there is agreement on therapeutic goals and open and collaborative communication between patient and staff, maximizes treatment potential. Developing a positive working alliance with brain injury patients promotes patient buy-in, fosters positive adaptations, assists in the development of realistic treatment goals, and results in an increase in productivity and quality of life.

Patients receiving cognitive retraining are required to perform a variety of repetitive exercises. Repetition is a key component of cognitive retraining in order for the retrained skill to become automatic. Computers are often used in the cognitive retraining process. Cognitive exercises that target multiple cognitive processes are frequently employed in cognitive retraining. For instance, the "Matching Shapes" exercise addresses functions of memory, motor speed, focused attention, and visual scanning. In the matching shapes exercise, the patient

is shown, at random, one of 15 cards depicting one of four shapes. The patient is required to match the shape on the card by pointing to the correct shape on a picture, which contains 13 different shapes. The patient's score is the time required to match all 15 shapes correctly. Another example of a cognitive exercise is the "block design" exercise which targets attention/concentration skills, motor dexterity, visual scanning, and visual spatial perception. In the block design exercise, the patient is shown 1 of 10 different drawings of colored squares in differing arrangements. The patient is required to construct a matching structure using colored blocks. The patient is scored by cumulative total time it takes to complete 10 structures.

Cognitive retraining is an important therapeutic strategy in the recovery and rehabilitation process for individuals suffering from brain injuries. Whether from stoke, injury, or accident, across all ages, cognitive retraining assists individuals in the development of skills needed to live productive, hopeful, and meaningful lives.

Steven R. Vensel, PhD

See also: Cognitive Deficits; Cognitive Remediation

Further Reading

Klonoff, Pamela S., Karen C. Olson, Melanie C. Talley, Kristi L. Husk, Stephen M. Myles, Jo-Ann Gehrels, and Lauren K. Dawson. "The Relationship of Cognitive Retraining to Neurological Patients' Driving Status: The Role of Process Variables and Compensation Training." *Brain Injury* 24, no. 2 (2010): 63–73.

Klonoff, Pamela S., Melanie C. Talley, Lauren K. Dawson, Stephen M. Myles, Lisa M. Watt, Jo-Ann Gehrels, and Steven W. Henderson. "The Relationship of Cognitive Retraining to Neurological Patients' Work and School." *Brain Injury* 21, no. 11 (2007): 1097–1107.

Cognitive Therapies

Cognitive therapies are a group of psychotherapies that emphasize distorted cognitions and treatment that aims at correcting them. Rational emotive behavior therapy, cognitive therapy, and schema therapy are three common cognitive therapies.

Definitions

- **Automatic thoughts** are thoughts that spontaneously come to mind when a particular situation occurs.

- **Cognitive restructuring** is psychotherapy technique for replacing maladaptive thought patterns with constructive thoughts and beliefs.

- **Cognitive revolution** refers to the shift from a focus on a purely behavioral approach to an acceptance of the role of cognitions as necessary for a fuller understanding of human behavior.

- **Cognitive therapy** is a type of cognitive behavior therapy that focuses on identifying and changing automatic thoughts and maladaptive beliefs.

- **Irrational beliefs** are distorted and/or self-defeating beliefs that are firmly held despite contradictory evidence. It is also known as maladaptive beliefs.

- **Psychoanalysis and the psychoanalytic therapies** are a group of psychotherapy approaches that assumes dysfunctional behavior is caused by unconscious, internal conflicts and focuses on gaining insight into these conflicts.

- **Rational emotive behavior therapy** is a type of cognitive behavior therapy that focuses on identifying and disputing irrational beliefs.

- **Schema therapy** is a type of cognitive behavior therapy that focuses on identifying and changing maladaptive (problematic) schemas.

- **Schemas** are core beliefs or assumptions about one's self and the world.

Description

Cognitive therapies are a group of psychotherapy approaches for which psychological symptoms and conditions are understood to be caused by distorted thinking or thought processes and which can be corrected by changing them. They differ in theory and practice from the psychoanalytic therapies and the behavioral therapies. Three cognitive therapy approaches include rational emotive behavior therapy (REBT), cognitive therapy (CT), and schema therapy (ST). The cognitive therapies view emotional difficulties as rooted in the clients' irrational beliefs—REBT, automatic thoughts and maladaptive beliefs—CT, or maladaptive schemas—ST. Cognitive therapists foster change in clients by assisting them to be more aware of their irrational or maladaptive thoughts and beliefs and their problematic impact, and to replace these problematic thoughts with more adaptive ones. A variety of interventions are utilized in the cognitive therapies, particularly cognitive restructuring which is a broad method, including disputation, guided discovery, Socratic questioning, examining the evidence, reattribution, and cognitive rehearsal.

Developments and Current Status

The cognitive therapies arose as a response to the perceived shortcomings of the psychodynamic therapies and of behavioral therapy. Some of the pioneers in the development of the cognitive therapies had psychoanalytic training. These included psychologist Albert Ellis (1913–2007), the developer of REBT, and psychiatrist Aaron T. Beck (1921–), the developer of CT. Others had training in behavior therapy and other approaches, like psychologist Jeffrey Young (1950–), the developer of ST. The "cognitive revolution" of the 1970s was a turning point in the rapid evolution, acceptance, and legitimacy of the cognitive therapies. Historical precursors of the cognitive therapies have been identified in various ancient philosophical traditions, particularly Stoicism. For example, both Ellis and Beck cite the influence of the Stoic philosophers. One of these, Epictetus, said: "Men are disturbed not by things, but by the view which they take of them." More recent influences on the cognitive therapies include Alfred Adler (1870–1937), who said: "I am convinced that a person's behavior springs from his ideas." Adler developed Individual Psychology in which the cognitive dimension is a central component.

Rational Emotive Behavior Therapy

In 1953, Ellis broke with psychoanalysis and began calling himself a rational therapist. Thereafter, he referred to his approach as rational therapy. His book *How to Live with a Neurotic* published in 1960 elaborated his new method. As he began to emphasize that emotions followed from thoughts, the approach was renamed rational emotive therapy. Later, as cognitive behavior therapy was becoming the dominant therapeutic approach, he renamed his approach rational emotive behavior therapy to reflect its utilization of behavioral methods.

REBT employs the ABCD framework, where "A" is the activating event, "B" is the individual's belief about the event, "C" is the cognitive, emotional, or behavioral consequences of one's beliefs, and "D" is disputation of the irrational belief. In this approach, personal and relational problems as well as symptoms are viewed as resulting from self-defeating thought processes. These thought processes include self- and other-deprecation, catastrophizing, overgeneralizing, and personalizing. The goal of REBT is to change irrational beliefs and self-defeating thought processes into rational beliefs and adaptive thought processes. The focus of treatment is to identify and change the irrational beliefs that underlie disturbed feelings and self-defeating behavior through various cognitive restructuring methods, particularly disputation.

Cognitive Therapy

Like Ellis, Beck also broke with the psychoanalysis in the 1960s. Beck's approach was first articulated in his book *Depression: Clinical, Experimental, and Theoretical Aspects* published in 1967. Soon after, his approach was criticized by behavioral therapists who denied that there was a cognitive cause for mental conditions. Fortunately, as a result of the "cognitive revolution," soon behavior therapy techniques and CT techniques became joined together, giving rise to cognitive behavior therapy. However, even though CT had typically included some behavioral methods, Beck and his associates sought to maintain and establish its integrity as a distinct, clearly standardized therapy.

Theoretically, CT emphasizes the role of cognitive processing in emotion and behavior. It views personality as shaped by central values or superordinate schemas. Psychological distress is influenced by a number of factors, including biochemical predispositions, different learning history, and cognition reaction style. However, presenting problems and symptoms are understood to result from faulty beliefs and/or maladaptive schemas. The focus of treatment is to become aware of limiting automatic thoughts and confront faulty beliefs with contradictory evidence and develop more adaptive beliefs.

Instead of listing specific maladaptive beliefs like Ellis, Beck emphasized that individuals operate from automatic thoughts and core schemas. For example, a woman comes to therapy who is depressed about failing to meet a deadline at her job. Her view of self or self-schema is "I'm worthless and can never do anything right." Strongly believing, this schema tends to activate automatic thoughts like "Things never work our" and "I'm going to get fired." These beliefs further worsen her mood. This is intensified if she reacts by avoiding activities that served to confirm her belief that she is worthless. In therapy, the therapist and client would work together to change this and related automatic beliefs. This is done by addressing the way she thinks and behaves in response to similar situations and by developing more flexible ways to think and respond.

Schema Therapy

Schema therapy is a derivation of CT. Young originally developed it primarily for personality-disordered clients who failed to respond adequately to CT. It was formalized in Young's 1990 book *Cognitive Therapy for Personality Disorders: A Schema-Focused Approach*. Schema therapy is a broad, integrative model that shares some commonalities with object relations therapy, experiential therapy, dialectical behavior therapy, and interpersonal therapy as well as CT and other forms of cognitive behavior therapy. Despite these similarities, ST differs from these approaches with regard to the nature of the therapy relationship, the general style and stance of the therapist, and the degree of therapist activity and directiveness.

Basic to ST are early maladaptive schemas which emerge from aversive childhood experiences such as abuse, neglect, and trauma in early life and lead to maladaptive or unhealthy life patterns. The basic goals of

ST are the following: to identify early maladaptive schemas, to validate the client's unmet emotional needs, to change maladaptive schemas to more functional ones, to promote more functional life patterns and coping styles, and to provide an environment for learning adaptive skills. ST requires considerable training and experience to practice it appropriately and effectively.

Len Sperry, MD, PhD

See also: Cognitive Behavior Therapy; Psychoanalysis; Schema-Focused Behavior Therapy

Further Reading

Adler, A. *The Individual Psychology of Alfred Adler.* Edited by H. Ansbacher and R. Ansbacher. New York, NY: Harper & Row, 1956.

Clark, David A., and Aaron T. Beck, *Cognitive Therapy of Anxiety Disorders: Science and Practice.* New York, NY: Guilford Press, 2010.

Ellis, Albert, and Catharine MacLaren. *Rational Emotive Behavior Therapy: A Therapist's Guide*, 2nd ed. Atascadero, CA: Impact Publishers, 2005.

Young, Jeffrey E., Janet S. Klosko, and Marjorie E. Weishaar. *Schema Therapy: A Practitioner's Guide.* New York, NY: Guilford Press, 2003.

College Counseling

College counseling centers offer a range of services to parents and students about higher education application, admission, and successful completion.

Definitions

- **College advising** is the process of providing students with the information they need to decide on what postsecondary options are right for them, including application, admittance requirements, coursework progression, and financial aid options.

- **College advisor** is a professional who offers parents and students with information about preparing for college readiness and future success.

- **College readiness counseling** is a type of counseling provided individually, in small groups, or in classroom settings to students prior to postsecondary entrance in an effort to boost preparedness and eventual completion.

- **Professional school counselors** are counseling practitioners employed in various educational settings who collaborate with parents and teachers to help students develop across academic, social, and career domains.

Description

"College counseling" refers to the process of providing parents and students with information about application, entrance, coursework, and financial aid for college. College counseling can be provided in various settings and can differ in terms of size, set up, and level of service.

In the high school setting, college counseling may be provided by a guidance counselor or professional school counselor to students on an individual, small group, or classroom basis. Professional school counselors have a master's degree and hold specialized certification or licensure. These professionals are skilled in the practice of guidance and counseling students.

College counseling can also be provided to students at the postsecondary level. College counselors have credentials similar to professional school counselors. However, college advisors, sometimes confused with "college counselors," do not necessarily have backgrounds in counseling. Advisors, rather, have specialized knowledge about the institution or program they service. Many faculty members serve as advisors in higher education settings.

College counseling is an ongoing process. The goal is not reached at admittance into college but continues as the student succeeds throughout his or her college experience and ends ultimately on completion. Students beginning their postsecondary careers need college counselors to provide them with recommendations about how to navigate college successfully. This may include guidance about choosing an appropriate major, outlining a program of study, and providing information about support services.

Development

College counseling practice first appeared in the early 1900s when it was noted that students were struggling to navigate higher education without proper guidance. At this time faculty members and university presidents were providing these types of services. After 1945, veterans returning from war were in particular need of assistance. This spawned an increase in postsecondary educational and vocational counseling, and expansion in the field continued through the 1970s. During the 1990s and on into the early 21st century, college counseling centers became stable fixtures on campuses.

Current Status

In 1991, the American College Counseling Association (ACCA), a division of the American Counseling Association, was established. The mission of the ACCA is to support counselors working in higher education so they can foster student success. The organization serves professionals from various disciplines working in college counseling centers, community colleges, and university settings. Most college counseling centers follow the ethical guidelines, standards, and practices outlined by the ACCA. Though challenges and obstacles related to the practice of college counseling continue to arise, the field itself continues to grow due to the high value placed on obtaining a postsecondary degree.

Melissa A. Mariani, PhD

See also: Counseling and Counseling Psychology; Guidance Counselor

Further Reading

Davis, Deborah C. "The American College Counseling Association: A Historical View." *Journal of College Counseling* 1 (1998): 7–9. doi:10.1002/j.2161-1882.1998.tb00119.x.

Davis, Deborah C., and Keren M. Humphrey. *College Counseling: Issues and Strategies for a New Millennium.* Alexandria, VA: American Counseling Association, 2000.

National Association for College Admission Counseling. *Fundamentals of College Admission Counseling: A Textbook for Graduate Students and Practicing Counselors*, 3rd ed. Arlington, VA: National Association for College Admission Counseling, 2012.

Columbine Shooting

The Columbine shooting is the school rampage shooting that took the lives of 12 students and 1 teacher and injured 24 others.

Definitions

- **Biopsychosocial** is the integration of biological, psychological (thoughts, feelings, and behaviors), and social (environmental and cultural) factors to understand and explain human behavior.

- **School rampage shooting** refers to the act of a student or former student attacking a school with a gun with the initial intent to shoot a specific target but injures or kills at least one other person. It is differentiated from other forms of schools violence and from workplace violence.

- **Sociocultural** refers to the combination of social and cultural factors.

Description

The Columbine shooting is the rampage shooting committed by two seniors at Columbine High School in Columbine, Colorado. On April 20, 1999, these students executed a complex attack on the school that involved guns, bombs, and explosive devices. The perpetrators, Eric Harris (1981–1999) and Dylan Klebold (1981–1999), also took their own lives at the end of their terror attack. In 1996, Harris created a private website where he posted a blog on gaming. Eventually the blog became a place for the troubled teenager to post his negative feelings toward society and instructions on how to make bombs and explosives. The two high school seniors wrote in their personal journals that they wanted to replicate the Oklahoma City Bombing. The bombing of the Alfred P. Murrah Federal Building occurred on April 19, 1995, and killed 168 people

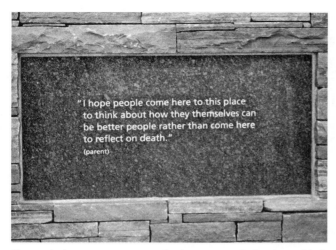

One of the many memorial plaques at Columbine High School in Littleton, Colorado, reflecting on the aftermath of the school rampage shooting that took the lives of 12 students and 1 teacher and injured 24 others. (Bruce Cotler/Globe Photos/ZUMAPRESS.com/Alamy)

and injured at least 680 people. Since their intention was to kill as many people as possible, they placed bombs and explosives in the school cafeteria during the busiest lunch period. However, the cafeteria bombs failed to detonate. Then, Harris and Klebold began randomly shooting people in their path until they entered the library where students and staff were hiding. Here they proceeded to shoot more people until law enforcement officials arrived. At that point, they took their own lives by shooting themselves.

The Columbine shootings have cultural significance. First, the amount of news media coverage it received was only second to the O. J. Simpson murder trial (during the 1990s). Second, at that time, it was the most violent act against a school that killed the most people. Third, the two students used the Internet to create websites to post violent acts committed, bomb-building instructions, hit lists, death threats, and videos. Fourth, after the shootings, many schools installed security measures and adopted a zero tolerance policy toward threats of violence. Finally, the Columbine shootings prompted other individuals who felt victimized, bullied, or somehow marginalized to copy Harris and Klebold's rampage shootings. Harris and Klebold posted their strategies on the Internet and provided others with

specific plans on how to carry out an attack. These postings inspired others to imitate the Columbine shooting and seek revenge on people who they felt wronged them. Furthermore, many subsequent shooters attempted to exceed the death toll of the Columbine shooting.

A sociocultural perspective is taken to understand and make sense of school shootings. The factors considered to have influenced the behavior of Harris and Klebold include bullying, mental illness, video game violence, social climate, Goth subculture, and music. To date, the primary underlying issue for these young men is believed to have been their pain and anger associated with the loss of a place among their peers, in the school community, and in society. An interdisciplinary team effort and a biopsychosocial perspective are both necessary to understand and explain the causes of violence. This team effort includes teachers, school administrators, policy makers, parents, and health-care workers.

Christina Ladd, PhD, and Len Sperry, MD, PhD

See also: Bullying and Peer Aggression; Mass Shootings

Further Reading

Cullen, D. *Columbine*. New York, NY: Twelve Hachette Book Group, 2009.

Larkin, Ralph W. *Comprehending Columbine*. Philadelphia, PA: Temple University Press, 2007.

Stuart, Henry. "School Violence beyond Columbine: A Complex Problem in Need of an Interdisciplinary Analysis." *American Behavioral Scientist* 52 (2009): 1246–1265.

Combined Treatment

Combined treatment is the combination of psychotherapy and medication to treat mental conditions.

Definitions

- **Biopsychosocial** refers to biological, psychological, and social factors and their interaction.

- **Pharmacological** means it relates to pharmacology or the scientific study of drug reactions.

- **Pharmacology** is the study of drugs, how they react, and their use in medicine.

- **Psychopharmacology** is the study of psychotropic drugs and their chemical interactions with the brain.

- **Psychosocial** refers to psychological and social factors and their interaction.

- **Psychotherapy** is a psychological method for achieving desired changes in thinking, feeling, and behavior. It is also called therapy and therapeutic counseling.

Description

Combined treatment is the use of psychological treatment with pharmacological treatment. The objective of combined treatment is to improve an individual's social functioning, quality of life, and treatment outcome. The combination of psychotherapy and medication results in better treatment outcomes for the individual than medication alone. Usually, two clinicians, such as a psychotherapist and a psychiatrist, work collaboratively to develop and implement treatment.

Combined treatment may work better in the prevention and delay of illness onset than either psychotherapy or medication treatment only. Psychotherapy may increase medication compliance and medication compliance may enhance client focus and engagement in the treatment process. Combined treatment is necessary when one type of treatment, either psychotherapy alone or medication alone, is insufficient to decrease or alleviate symptoms.

The term "combined treatment" was originally used by psychiatrist Gerald Klerman (1928–1992) in 1991 in the book entitled *Integrating Pharmacotherapy and Psychotherapy*. Klerman asserted that combined treatment is more efficacious than either medication or psychotherapy alone because it (1) helps to achieve illness remission faster, (2) improves the probability that treatment will commence, (3) decreases or eliminates the probability of relapse, (4) simultaneously treats the client's problems while aiding in the reduction of stress among family members, (5) increases medication compliance, (6) develops and/or improves psychosocial skills, and (7) speeds up the psychotherapy process (Beitman and Klerman, 1991, 3–19). Psychotherapy in combination with medication is better than medication

alone for the treatment of depression, bipolar disorder, schizophrenia, attention-deficit hyperactivity disorder, bulimia, sleep disorders, and post-traumatic stress disorder.

The appropriate combination of treatments is determined from a biopsychosocial approach. An individual's genetic attributes and predispositions, psychological factors, and sociocultural context are considered in the choice of medication and treatment modality (i.e., individual, family, and/or group therapy). From a biopsychosocial perspective, a diagnostic map must be constructed to understand and explain the individual's problems. Then, measurable treatment goals must be identified and assessed throughout the psychotherapy process. Medication, if prescribed, must be monitored and adjusted as necessary. Health practitioners must work collaboratively to determine the sequence and type of combined treatment necessary depending on the diagnosis and its severity. For example, an individual with schizophrenia might receive medication treatment first, followed by individual and family psychotherapy. An individual suffering with psychosis may not be able to take part in any modality of psychotherapy until he or she is properly medicated and psychotic symptoms are managed. Conversely, for individuals with personality disorders, it may be better to begin the combined treatment process with psychotherapy and then include medication to treat symptoms of depression, anxiety, hallucinations, and delusions. Which type of treatment comes first is based on a thorough assessment, professional clinical judgment, and the type and severity of the problem at hand. In addition, clients collaborate with the practitioner in deciding which treatment should be administered and when.

Len Sperry, MD, PhD, and Christina Ladd, PhD

See also: Multimodal Therapy; Psychopharmacology; Psychotherapy

Further Reading
Beitman, B. D., and Klerman, G. L. *Integrating Pharmacotherapy and Psychotherapy*. Washington, DC: American Psychiatric Press, 1991.

Riba, M., and R. Balon, eds. *Pharmacotherapy & Psychotherapy: Collaborative Treatment*. Washington, DC: American Psychiatric Press, 1999.

Sammons, Morgan T., and Norman B. Schmidt. *Combined Treatments for Mental Disorders: A Guide to Psychological Interventions*. Washington, DC: American Psychological Association, 2001.

Commission on Rehabilitation Counselor Certification (CRCC)

The Commission on Rehabilitation Counselor Certification (CRCC) is a not-for-profit organization that sets the standard for quality rehabilitation counseling services through a certification program.

Definitions

- **Certification** is a formal procedure by which an accredited or authorized person or agency assesses and verifies that a person has the knowledge and skills to perform certain activities.

- **Rehabilitation counseling** is a type of counseling that focuses on helping individuals who have disabilities in order to achieve their career, personal, and independent living goals.

Description

The Commission on Rehabilitation Counselor Certification ensures that rehabilitation professionals are accountable for the work they do. Rehabilitation counselors work with people with disabilities to provide vocational services. The skills and training required to do this work vary and can be intensive. The work of these counselors may include interviewing and analyzing a client's disability level to help him or her obtain work and medical and social services. The counselor works to determine what kind of work is appropriate, given the level of disability. When the disabilities are of a catastrophic nature, the rehabilitation counselor may be involved in the full range of life planning for the client.

Development

As the field of rehabilitation counseling grew, it became important to ensure that the counselors had adequate education and skills. The CRCC was founded by two other rehabilitation organizations as a not-for-profit organization established to set standards of quality rehabilitation counseling services. It does this through a standardized certification process for rehab counselors as well as by serving as a lobbying group for the rights of people with disabilities.

The need to ensure quality counselors was reinforced by the passing of the Americans with Disabilities Act in 1990. The CRCC has continued to identify guidelines for conduct and ethical behavior. This is necessary because the field of rehabilitation counseling has grown exponentially in recent years.

Inevitably many ethical questions and issues arise in the course of rehabilitation counseling. Rehabilitation counselors have available training in a Code of Professional Ethics for Rehabilitation Counselors in addition to decision-making models to help them resolve ethical dilemmas. CRCC has also been a lobbying group to ensure the support of rehabilitation efforts and standards of practice.

Impact (Psychological Influence)

Rehabilitation counseling was identified as one of the fastest-growing health professions in the United States in 2011. The CRCC has become the world's largest rehabilitation counseling organization, with over 16,000 professionals currently certified. Since its start the CRCC has certified over 35,000 rehabilitation counselors.

CRCC standards are always in need of review and updating. This includes revising the tests for certification in order to reflect current understanding and best practices of the rehabilitation counselor role and functions. One of the roles of the CRCC is to receive, review, and act on ethical complaints and violations. In the 13 years between 1993 and 2006, 113 complaints were reviewed, of which only 36 resulted in action.

There will continue to be a significant role for CRCC in the rehabilitation field. Among many other challenges is an increasingly diverse patient population. This requires changes in laws and guidelines in health care and insurance that are important for people with disabilities. It is also important for the CRCC to be involved in addressing the many ethical challenges for rehabilitation counselors and provide ways to make sure they are providing the best care for their clients.

Alexandra Cunningham, PhD

See also: American Rehabilitation Counseling Association (ARCA); Rehabilitation Counseling

Further Reading

Chan, Fong, Malachy Bishop, Julie Chronister, Eun-Jeong Lee, and Chung-Yi Chiu. *Certified Rehabilitation Counselor Examination Preparation: A Concise Guide to the Rehabilitation Counselor Test.* New York, NY: Springer, 2011.

Weed, Roger O., and Debra E. Berens, eds. *Life-Care Planning and Case Management Handbook.* London, UK: CRC Press, 2010.

Common Factors in Psychotherapy

Common factors in psychotherapy are basic elements that do not depend on a specific theory or psychotherapy approach.

Definitions

- **Behavior therapy** is a form of psychotherapy that focuses on identifying and changing maladaptive behaviors.

- **Dodo Bird Verdict** is the claim that all psychotherapies are equally effective regardless of their components.

- **Psychoanalysis** is a theory of human behavior and a form of therapy based on psychoanalytic theory. In psychoanalysis, clients are encouraged to talk freely about personal experiences, particularly their early childhood and dreams. It was initially developed by Sigmund Freud.

- **Psychotherapy** is a psychological method for achieving desired changes in thinking, feeling, and behavior. It is also called therapeutic counseling.

Description

Common factors in psychotherapy are basic elements that do not depend on a specific theory or treatment. Throughout history, the followers of different theories have attempted to prove that their theory was superior to others. They argued that their theory led to better outcomes in therapy. For example, those who practice psychoanalysis believed that exploring the past and unconscious drives is necessary for clients to change. Those who practice behavior therapy, however, did not consider these things important and instead focused on behaviors in the present. Currently, there are over 250 different therapeutic approaches. Research has attempted to show which of them is more effective than the others to settle this debate. However, no clear consensus has been reached.

Several factors are common in most psychotherapy approaches. Many of these factors influence the outcomes of psychotherapy. In 1936, psychologist Saul Rosenzweig (1907–2004) published the first paper outlining common factors in psychotherapy. He concluded that all types of therapy could be effective if therapists had these factors. This was also referred to as the Dodo Bird Verdict in reference to a character's quote in Alice in Wonderland ("Everybody has won and all must have prizes"). Rosenzweig's factors included the therapist's personality and theoretical consistency. Psychologist Carl Rogers (1902–1987) later described the "necessary and sufficient" conditions of therapeutic change in 1957. These were empathy, respect, and genuineness. Rogers argued that therapy was effective simply if these elements were present (sufficient). Psychiatrist Jerome Frank (1909–2005) examined many different types of healing practices ranging from traditional psychotherapy to religion. He found four features shared by all effective therapies. These were a confiding relationship with a therapist, a healing setting, a clear explanation for symptoms and the solution, and a collaborative process or ritual to restore the patient's health.

More recent research has continued the investigation into common factors. Psychologist Michael Lambert (1944–) and others reviewed therapeutic outcomes studies. They found that certain factors were responsible for change across different theories and diagnoses and were not connected to a specific theory. They are client variables, the therapeutic relationship, placebo effects, and technique. "Client variables" refer to the qualities that clients themselves possess and bring to therapy. These include such factors as motivation for change, social support, and inner strengths. This is sometimes referred to as "extratherapeutic" change because it is separate from the therapy. According to Lambert's analysis, client variables account for 40% of therapy outcome. The therapeutic relationship factor included variables like empathy, respect, and genuineness previously identified by others. This factor takes place between the therapist and the client, also called the therapeutic alliance. Lambert found that this accounted for 30% of the therapy outcome. Placebo effects refer to clients' degree of hope and expectations for change. Those who believe that positive change will happen are more likely to meet this expectation. Placebo effects account for 15% of therapy outcome according to Lambert. The final common factor is technique. This encompasses features unique to specific theories, such as interpretations or feedback. According to this analysis, 70% of the outcome in therapy is decided by client variables and the therapeutic relationship alone (Lambert, 1992). In other words, therapy will be successful if a client is motivated for change and the therapist has established a strong bond. This formula excludes the specific techniques and theories many thought to be important. Common factors research has led to the development of integrative therapy approaches.

Len Sperry, MD, PhD, and George Stoupas, MS

See also: Behavior Therapy; Dodo Bird Verdict; Psychotherapy; Rogers, Carl R. (1902–1987)

Further Reading

Lambert, Michael J. "Implications for Psychotherapy Outcome Research for Eclectic Psychotherapy." In *Handbook of Eclectic Psychotherapy*, edited by J. C. Norcross, pp. 436–462. New York, NY: Brunner/Mazel, 1992.

Rosenzweig, Saul. "Some Implicit Common Factors in Diverse Methods of Psychotherapy." *American Journal of Orthopsychiatry* 6, no. 3 (1936): 412–415.

Wampold, Bruce, and Zac Imel. *The Great Psychotherapy Debate: Models, Methods, and Findings*. Mahwah, NJ: Lawrence Erlbaum Associates, Inc., 2001.

Community Mental Health

"Community mental health" refers to the delivery of community-based mental health and addictions services to at-risk and underserved populations suffering from mental health conditions and substance use disorders.

Description

The U.S. Department of Health and Human Services (DHHS) is the government agency that provides funding and resources for essential services to underserved populations suffering from mental health conditions and substance use disorders. The Substance Abuse and Mental Health Services Administration (SAMHSA) is an operating division of the DHHS and is tasked with improving the quality and availability of substance abuse prevention, addiction treatment, and mental health services. SAMHSA provides grants and funding to states for substance abuse and mental health services and programs. A major goal of SAMHSA is to improve access and reduce barrier to programs and services for individuals who suffer from, or are at risk for, substance use disorders or mental health disorders.

Development

President John F. Kennedy signed the Community Mental Health Act (CMHA) into law in 1963. The CMHA made a significant impact on the delivery of mental health services and led to the establishment of comprehensive community mental health centers throughout the United States. Prior to the enactment of the CMHA people suffering from chronic mental health conditions were frequently "warehoused" in psychiatric hospitals and institutions. These individuals received little, if any, effective treatment, suffered from poor living conditions with little freedom, and could remain in these institutions for years with little hope of reentering their communities as productive citizens. With advances in psychotropic medications and the development of new approaches to psychotherapy, community-based care became a viable solution to the warehousing of those suffering from chronic mental health disorders.

As treatment of mental illness became more diverse and comprehensive, it became evident that those suffering from addictions also needed services. The combination of mental health interventions and interventions directed at recovery from addiction disorders became known as "behavioral health care." The provision of comprehensive mental health and addiction services is the goal of community-based behavioral health organizations.

Current Status

Community mental health organizations offer a wide variety of support and services to people with mental illnesses and substance use disorders. Examples of services to communities include 24-hour crisis response and suicide preventing training; community reentry support to released prisoners; educational support to organizations in new mental health and addictions therapies; provision and funding of community-based substance use treatment centers; school-based substance intervention educational programs; domestic violence prevention; child and elder abuse prevention and recovery training; and school and gang violence interventions and programs.

According to the National Council for Behavioral Health (National Council), there are approximately 8 million adults and children in the United States living with mental illness and substance use conditions who have severely limited or no access to behavioral health services. The National Council is an example of how the DHHS and SAMHSA provide help to the citizens of the United States. The National Council, funded by DHHS and SAMHSA, represents over 2,000-member organizations that employ over 750,000 people providing care to at-risk individuals and families. The National Council advocates for policies to ensure that people with mental health and addictions disorders have access to comprehensive, high-quality care in order to provide the opportunity for recovery and full participation in community life. The National Council coordinates the Mental Health First Aid (MHFA) program, a national mental health initiative.

In response to gun violence, President Obama called for Mental Health First Aid training across the United States. MHFA is a public education program that teaches community members how to recognize and respond to signs of mental illness and substance use disorders before they become a crisis. MHFA has both youth and adult courses. MHFA consists of eight hours of instruction that introduces participants to the risks factors and warning signs of mental health concerns and links them to local mental health resources, national organizations, support groups and professionals, and online tools. MHFA promotes early detection of specific illnesses such as anxiety, depression, bipolar disorder, psychosis, eating disorder, and addictions. MHFA training is provided to any concerned citizen or group. The National Council seeks to make Youth Mental Health First Aid available in every one of the 4,197 colleges and 13,809 school districts in the United States.

Steven R. Vensel, PhD

See also: Behavioral Health; Mental Health Laws; Substance Abuse and Mental Health Services Administration (SAMHSA)

Further Reading

Department of Health and Human Services. "About Us." Accessed December 23, 2013. http://www.hhs.gov/about/.

National Council for Behavioral Health. "Mental Health First Aid." Accessed December 23, 2013. http://www.thenationalcouncil.org/about/mental-health-first-aid/.

National Council for Behavioral Health. "Mission and Leadership." Accessed December 23, 2013. http://www.thenationalcouncil.org/about/national-mental-health-association/.

Ritter, Lois A., and Shirley Manly Lampkin. *Community Mental Health.* Sudbury, MA: Jones & Bartlett, 2012.

Substance Abuse and Mental Health Services Administration. "About Us." Accessed December 23, 2013. http://beta.samhsa.gov/about-us.

Community Reinforcement Approach (CRA)

Community reinforcement approach is a treatment that rearranges an individual's life so that abstinence and sobriety are more rewarding than substance use. It is also called CRA.

Definitions

- **Abstinence** is the choice not to engage in certain behaviors or give in to desires such as alcohol or drug use.

- **Aversion therapy** uses principles from behavioral psychology to help reduce or eliminate unwanted behaviors.

- **Confrontational counseling** is an intervention used by counselors to promote wellness in an individual by promoting insight, reducing resistance, promoting open communication, and increasing conformity between an individual's goals and behaviors.

- **Family therapy** is a type of psychotherapy approach that is used to help family members resolve conflicts and improve their communication skills.

- **Group therapy** is a type of psychotherapy approach in which a small group of individuals meet regularly with a therapist.

- **Motivational interviewing** is a counseling strategy for helping individuals to discover and resolve their ambivalence to change.

- **Positive reinforcement** is the addition of a reinforcer (reward) following a desired behavior that increases the likelihood that the behavior will reoccur.

- **Recovery** is a series of steps individuals take to improve their wellness and health, while living a self-directed (responsible) life and striving to reach their highest potential.

- **Sobriety** is the condition of complete abstinence from all mind-altering substances as well as increased mental, physical, and spiritual health.

- **Social support system** is feedback and a sense of belonging provided by friends and peers.

- **Substance use disorder** is a mental disorder in which one or more mind-altering substances lead to clinically significant distress or impairment in an individual.

Description

Community reinforcement approach (CRA) is a substance treatment approach for individuals with substance use disorders. It provides individuals with incentives to stop using by eliminating positive reinforcement for using substances and enhancing positive reinforcement for sobriety. The basic premise is that positive reinforcement has a powerful role in encouraging and discouraging substance use. CRA was developed in the early 1970s by psychologist Nathan Azrin (1930–2013). Azrin stressed the interaction between an individual's behavior and his or her environment, particularly the positive reinforcement of an individual's social support system or community. He believed CRA could help individuals decrease their addiction and better enjoy life. CRA uses recreational, social, vocational, and familial reinforcers to help individuals in the recovery process.

CRA integrates several treatment elements into its program. It helps build motivation to stop drinking and using drugs. It assists in analyzing substance abuse patterns and increasing positive reinforcement for an individual to stop using. It involves learning new coping behaviors and involving friends and family members in the recovery process. These elements can be modified to an individual's needs in order to achieve the best treatment outcome. In addition, CRA has been successfully integrated with other treatment approaches. Some of these approaches include motivational interviewing, family therapy, group therapy, aversion therapies, and confrontational counseling. The goal of these various approaches is skills training and improving communication and problem solving.

However, what is unique about CRA is its emphasis on community reinforcement and social support. Individuals with substance use problems, therapists, and friends and family all work together to increase abstinence and sobriety. Having a healthy social support system is a key part of this approach. CRA can be as effective as or more effective than traditional approaches.

Len Sperry, MD, PhD, and Elizabeth Smith Kelsey, PhD

See also: Aversion Therapy; Family Therapy and Family Counseling; Group Therapy; Motivational Interviewing

Further Reading

Meyers, Robert J., and William Miller. *A Community Reinforcement Approach to Addiction Treatment.* New York, NY: Cambridge University Press, 2006.

Meyers, Robert J., and J. E. Smith. *Clinical Guide to Alcohol Treatment: The Community Reinforcement Approach.* New York, NY: Guilford Press, 1995.

Miller, William R., and S. Rollnick. *Motivational Interviewing: Preparing People to Change Addictive Behavior.* New York, NY: Guilford Press, 1991.

Comorbidity

Comorbidity is the presence of an additional mental disorder or medical condition that occurs alongside a mental disorder. It is also referred to as co-occurring illness and dual diagnosis.

Definitions

- **Differential diagnosis** refers to the presentation of symptoms that appear to meet the criteria of multiple diagnoses and the process of ruling out diagnostic alternatives.

- **Dual diagnosis** is the presence of a mental disorder and an addiction to alcohol or drugs.

- **Pathology** is an experience of suffering or aspect of a disease incorporating cause, development, structure, and consequences.

- **Personality disorder** is a type of mental disorders characterized by deeply ingrained maladaptive (problematic) patterns of thinking and acting.

- **Predisposing factors** refer to all the possible factors that account for and explain the client's characteristic way of perceiving, thinking, and responding.

Description

Comorbidity is the occurrence of one or more mental or medical disorders (conditions) along with a primary mental disorder. Usually, these co-occurring pathologies have similar structure, development, or cause. For example, depression is a common comorbidity following a myocardial infarction (heart attack). However, in medicine "comorbidity" can indicate the simultaneous existence of two or more medical conditions that have different causes, structures, or development. This can lead to confusion about the nature of the multiple diagnoses. For treatment purposes, the interrelationship among the multiple conditions must be taken into account. The reason is that individuals with a diagnosed mental disorder have an increased risk of other diagnoses.

Several factors foster comorbidity. These include genetic predisposition, family history, environment, and a history of trauma. It is also possible that different unrelated predisposing factors are operative, leading to different unrelated diagnoses. Finally, it is often the case that the symptoms associated with one mental disorder operate as the predisposing factors of one or more other disorders or physical illnesses. Such differing factors that foster comorbidity may exist in isolation or coexist within the same individual. In brief, comorbidity is having more than one diagnosis at any given time.

Mental health professionals also use the term "comorbidity" when referring to the coexistence of multiple symptoms. This is especially true when a single diagnosis will not account for all client symptoms. The personality of the client is also a factor in comorbidity. Personality traits and coping styles influence the risks associated with developing comorbid mental health disorders. Personality disorder also has a tendency to coexist. It is not uncommon for a client diagnosed with a personality disorder to have features of another personality disorder. In fact, more than half of individuals with personality disorders will be diagnosed with a comorbid personality disorder. Mood disorders and anxiety disorders also have a high rate of comorbidity. The substance disorders often have comorbid mental disorders and/or physical illnesses. The term "dual diagnosis" is especially common when indicating the coexistence of substance-related disorders and other mental disorders. For example, depression is common in individuals with alcohol dependence.

Current research indicates inconsistent use of the term "comorbidity." The primary importance is for the clinician to account for all of the client's problems. It is possible to exclude some of the client's problems if the clinician focuses on only one diagnosis. In this case, comorbidity is related to the term "differential diagnosis." Where the determination of differential diagnosis or process of diagnostic elimination cannot be fully made, the possibility of comorbidity increases.

Development and Current Status

Alvin Feinstein (1925–2001) introduced the term "comorbidity" to medicine in 1970. In the 1990s, researchers identified two major types of comorbidity. "Homotypic comorbidity" refers to the coexistence of two or more diagnoses of the same diagnostic category. "Heterotypic comorbidity" refers to the coexistence of two or more diagnoses of different diagnostic categories. As researchers began to investigate comorbidity, questions arose as to the nature of the relationship between or among coexisting pathologies. A theory of a direct causal relationship was proposed, such that the presence of one disorder causes the presence of another disorder or illness. Another theory of the relationship between comorbid disorders that developed is the theory of the indirect causal relationship. The indirect causal relationship indicates that the presence of one diagnosis increases the likelihood of a second diagnosis. A third theory that developed out of the research on comorbidity is that of common factors. The comorbidity theory of common factors indicates that multiple diagnoses have the same set of predisposing factors.

Len Sperry, MD, PhD, and Layven Reguero, MEd

See also: Depression; Dual Diagnosis; Substance-Related and Addictive Disorders

Further Reading

Daley, Dennis C., and Howard B. Moss. *Dual Disorders: Counseling Clients with Chemical Dependency and Mental Illness*, 3rd ed. Center City, MN: Hazelden Foundation, 2002.

Eaton, William W. *Medical and Psychiatric Comorbidity over the Course of Life*. Arlington, VA: American Psychiatric Publishing, Inc., 2005.

Pagoto, Sherry, ed. *Psychological Co-morbidities of Physical Illness: A Behavioral Medicine Perspective*. New York, NY: Springer, 2011.

Compassion Fatigue

"Compassion fatigue" refers to the emotional strain and stress experienced by a variety of health-care professionals working with victims of traumatic events.

Description

Compassion fatigue, also known as secondary traumatic stress, is a stress condition that some helping professionals experience after working with people who have experienced traumatic events. It is the result of the accumulated emotional and psychological impact of repeated exposure to the traumatic experiences of others. It has been referred to as the "cost of caring" and is experienced by a wide variety of health-care professionals, including counselors, psychologists, social workers, nurses, doctors, emergency room workers, and other care providers. It has also been found to affect clergy, lawyers, firefighters, and other emergency responders. It is estimated that between 16% and 85% of care providers experience compassion fatigue. Compassion fatigue was first recognized in the 1990s and continues to be the focus of research and investigation across professional fields. Charles Figley is recognized for his extensive research and publications concerning compassion fatigue.

Causes and Symptoms

Caregivers who treat trauma victims and listen to repeated stories of tragedy, violence, sorrow, pain, sadness, fear, terror, loss, and death experience compassion fatigue, also referred to as vicarious traumatization. These repeated stories begin to have an affect on the caregiver, and the caregiver experiences what is referred to as secondary traumatic stress.

The effects of compassion fatigue impact helping professionals' emotions, thoughts, and behaviors. They may begin to remember their client's stories during their nonwork hours and may visualize the stories in their mind's eye. Sometimes these images are intrusive and caregivers can't seem to stop thinking about the events even though they did not have the experience themselves. They may experience some of the feelings associated with their client's story. They may become sad or depressed, emotionally detached, anxious, or fearful or experience other feelings their clients or patients experienced. Caregivers may experience physical difficulties such as difficulty sleeping, headaches, or stomach problems. Professionals working with victims of violent crime may become obsessed with fears of their own safety and may avoid places that remind them of the client's experience. Caregivers who work with children may become overprotective of their own children. It is not uncommon for compassion fatigue to result in a change in worldview and beliefs. Caregivers suffering from compassion fatigue may begin to question the meaning of life, question their own religious beliefs, become skeptical, or feel anger toward God.

Diagnosis and Prognosis

Research indicates that certain risk factors exist for the development of compassion fatigue. Exposure is a significant factor. Caregivers who are exposed to traumatic stories on a daily basis are at greater risk of secondary trauma than are those who are exposed less often. It has also been found that those who are more empathic are at greater risk for compassion fatigue. Other risk factors include ability to self-care, coping abilities and stress management, work and peer support, and spirituality.

Compassion fatigue is preventable and treatable. Perhaps the most important strategy to prevent secondary traumatic stress is self-care, which begins with awareness. Professionals who understand compassion fatigue are more likely to recognize the signs of fatigue before they become problematic. Self-care practices such as pursuing enjoyable activities like sports or hobbies, regular exercise, and social activities apart from work are important to a balanced lifestyle that can provide recovery and perspective when working with traumatized clients. It is very important that professionals debrief and talk with other professionals in a supportive role. When compassion fatigue becomes debilitative, psychotherapy has been shown to be effective in the recovery process.

Steven R. Vensel, PhD

See also: Trauma; Trauma Counseling

Further Reading

Figley, Charles. *Compassion Fatigue: Coping with Secondary Traumatic Stress Disorder in Those Who Treat the Traumatized.* New York, NY: Brunner/Mazel, 1995.

Figley, Charles. *Treating Compassion Fatigue.* New York, NY: Brunner-Routledge, 2006.

Competency and Competencies

Within the context of health care, competency is the ability to integrate knowledge, skills, and attitudes to provide high-quality care. Competencies are the specific knowledge, skill, and attitudes by which competency can be evaluated.

Definitions

- **American Counseling Association** is a not-for-profit, professional, and educational organization that is dedicated to the growth and enhancement of the counseling profession. It is also referred to as the ACA.

- **American Psychological Association** is the largest professional organization in the United States and Canada. It publishes the

Publication Manual of the American Psychological Association and is also referred to as the APA.

- **Counseling** refers to professional guidance of an individual by assisting him or her in resolving personal, social, or psychological problems and difficulties.

- **Countertransference** is the redirection of a therapist's feelings toward a client and more generally as a therapist becomes emotionally entangled with a client.

- **Psychotherapy** is a psychological method for achieving desired changes in thinking, feeling, and behavior.

- **Transference** is a phenomenon characterized by unconscious redirection of feelings from one individual to another.

Description

Competency in the field of counseling is the judicious and continuous use of skills, knowledge, emotions, values, clinical reasoning, and reflection in health care. This includes counseling and psychotherapy. The term "competency" was coined by an American psychologist, R. W. White (1904–2001), in 1959. It involves a wide range of professional and personal capacities related to an external standard or requirement. For example, the capacity for analysis, critical thinking, and professional judgment in evaluating a situation and making clinical decisions is based on the competence of a counselor. Because the issues that individuals bring to counseling are often complex, it can be difficult for counselors to effectively treat them. Thus, counselors with a high level of competency are more likely to be effective and successful than those with less competency. It is not surprising that both the American Counseling Association and the American Psychological Association expect competency of its members.

"Competencies" refer to specific knowledge, skill, attitudes, and their integration. Competency can be evaluated in terms of specific competencies. The American psychologist David McClelland (1917–1998) is considered to be the father of the competency movement. There has been a shift in professional training from a core curriculum model to a core competency model of learning (Sperry, 2010). Sperry has identified and described six core competencies in counseling and psychotherapy. These competencies include having a conceptual foundation, relationship building and maintenance, intervention planning, intervention implementation, intervention evaluation and termination, and being culturally and ethically sensitive in practice (Sperry, 2010).

The conceptual foundation provides a conceptual map that will help guide a therapist in determining which clinical data to observe and elicit and how to understand the data. Competent therapy also requires a strong therapeutic relationship between the therapist (counselor) and the client. A strong therapeutic relationship is important because it promotes a bond of trust between the therapist and client and encourages an agreement about the goals for the treatment process. There are two competencies in relationship building. They include establishing a therapeutic alliance and the ability to encourage treatment-promoting behaviors. There are three competencies included in maintaining a therapeutic relationship. One involves being aware of and resolving resistance and having mixed feelings (ambivalence) about something. In addition, being aware of and resolving therapeutic tensions and being aware of and fixing transference and countertransference issues are another aspect to maintaining a therapeutic relationship. Implementation of the intervention process is a part of the core competency model of learning. Therapists who use techniques that focus on intended goals are likely to become proficient in this competency. Intervention planning is a part of the core competency model. It includes accomplishing a comprehensive diagnostic assessment, assigning a DSM-V diagnosis, creating a successful case formulation and treatment plan, and combining a clinical case report. Implementation of an intervention is performed by using modalities and techniques that focus on intended goals that will be helpful in becoming proficient in this competency. Competent counseling requires the capacity for assessing treatment and getting ready for terminating a client. Continually observing a client is vital in order to assess the treatment progress. Lastly, competent therapy insists that the therapist practice in an ethically and culturally sensitive way. Furthermore, cultural competence may help to promote a strong therapeutic alliance.

Len Sperry, MD, PhD, and Elizabeth Smith Kelsey, PhD

See also: American Counseling Association (ACA); American Psychological Association (APA); Counseling and Counseling Psychology; Psychotherapy

Further Reading

Constantine, Madonna G., and Derald Wing Sue. *Strategies for Building Multicultural Competence in Mental Health and Educational Settings.* Hoboken, NJ: John Wiley & Sons, 2005.

Kenkel, Mary Beth, and Roger L. Peterson, eds. *Competency-Based Educational for Professional Psychology.* Washington, DC: American Psychological Association, 2009.

Sperry, L. *Core Competencies in Counseling and Psychotherapy: Becoming a Highly Competent and Effective Therapist.* New York, NY: Routledge, 2010.

Compliance

Compliance is the extent to which an individual follows a prescribed treatment regimen. A related term is "adherence."

Definitions

- **Adherence** involves taking an active role in collaborating with a health provider and treatment regimen.

- **Noncompliance** is the failure, in whole or part, to follow a prescribed treatment regimen.

- **Treatment regimen** is a specified course of treatment for a medical or psychological condition.

Description

"Compliance" is defined as the extent to which an individual's behavior, such as taking medications, keeping scheduled medical appointments, or making lifestyle changes, coincides with his or her prescribed treatment regimen. Patient treatment noncompliance is one of the most vexing challenges facing health-care providers. Noncompliance with medical treatment is very common, ranging from 50% to 75% (Brown and Bussell, 2011). Estimates are that only one-fourth of individuals with hypertension (high blood pressure) are getting medical treatment. Of those, about one-half of those have normal blood pressure readings because only two-thirds use medication as prescribed. In 2006 it was reported that more than 125,000 patients with treatable ailments die each year in the United States because of failure to take their medication properly (American College of Preventive Medicine, 2011). The reality is that most patients find it difficult to take medications as prescribed or make major lifestyle changes consistently over long periods of time.

Compliance and adherence are often used synonymously, but they are different. Compliance literally means complying with (following) the health-care provider's recommended treatment regimen. Compliance implies a paternalistic role for the provider and a passive role for the patient. In contrast, adherence means that the patient is adhering to the treatment regimen. Adherence implies that the patient is empowered to take a reasonable degree of responsibility for his or her own health. It also implies that the patient and provider collaborate to improve the patient's health by integrating the provider's professional opinion with the patient's lifestyle, values, and preferences for care. More specifically, adherence depends not only on patient's acceptance of information about the health condition itself but also on the provider's ability to persuade the patient that the prescribed treatment is worthwhile. It also depends on the individual's perception of the provider's credibility, empathy, interest, and concern.

Developments and Current Status

A medical dictum is particularly relevant to any discussion of compliance. "Drugs don't work in patients who don't take them." So why don't patients comply or adhere? Early research on compliance emphasized the treatment regimen and health provider instructions, and later focused on client perception of his or her illness and expectations of treatment. In the 1990s the focus of adherence research was on the patient–provider relationship and how to improve it. Today, efforts have shifted to increasing the family's influence on compliance.

Len Sperry, MD, PhD

See also: Psychotherapy

Further Reading

American College of Preventive Medicine (ACPM). "Medication Adherence Time Tool: Improving Health Outcomes." Clinical Reference Document. 2011. Accessed March 29, 2015. http://www.acpm.org/?MedAdherTT_ClinRef.

Blackwell, Barry. *Treatment Compliance and the Therapeutic Alliance.* New York, NY: Taylor & Francis, 1998.

Brown, Marie T., and Jennifer K. Bussell. "Medication Adherence: WHO Cares?" *Mayo Clinic Proceedings* 86, no. 4 (April 2011): 304–314. doi:10.4065/mcp.2010.0575.

O'Connor, Patrick. "Improving Medical Adherence." *Archives of Internal Medicine* 166 (2006): 1802–1804.

Sperry, Len. *Treatment of Chronic Medical Conditions: Cognitive-Behavioral Therapy Strategies and Integrative Treatment Protocols.* Washington, DC. American Psychological Association, 2009.

Compulsions

Compulsions are habitual behaviors, practices, or rituals that are impulsively engaged in to defend against perceived threats, to reduce fears or otherwise minimize distress.

Definitions

- **Comorbidity** is the existence of one or more mental disorders or physical illnesses that occur with a primary psychiatric illness. It is also referred to as dual diagnosis.

- **Evidence-based practice** is a form of practice that is based on integration of the best research evidence with clinical experience and client values.

- **Obsessions** are persistent, intrusive, inappropriate, and unwanted thoughts, impulses, or images that result in anxiety or distress.

- **Obsessive-compulsive disorder** is a mental disorder that is distressful to the individual and is characterized by unreasonable obsessions or compulsions that are inappropriately time consuming or cause marked distress or impairment.

- **Obsessive-compulsive personality disorder** is a personality disorder that is defined by a pervasive pattern of preoccupation with control, perfectionism, and meticulousness at the expense of flexibility, openness, and efficiency.

- **Pathology** is an experience of suffering or aspect of a disease incorporating cause, development, structure, and consequences.

- **Practice** is a method or process used to accomplish a goal or objective.

- **Psychotherapy** is a psychological method for achieving desired changes in thinking, feeling, and behavior. It is also called therapeutic counseling.

- **Theoretical integration** is the assimilation of two or more theories of psychotherapy.

Description

Compulsions are habitual behaviors, practices, or rituals that are intended to defend against distress. Obtaining pleasure or gratification is not the primary function of compulsions. A client suffering from compulsivity feels compelled to execute the compulsion. The client feels driven to defend themselves against perceived threats, driven to reduce their anxiety, or driven to minimize their distress. Common compulsive behaviors are hand washing, ordering, checking, hoarding, and requesting or demanding reassurance. Common compulsive mental practices or rituals include praying, counting, and the silent repetition of a word or phrase. Individuals suffering from compulsions are constantly doing and undoing. Compulsions are born out of an individual's desire to avoid the "out-of-control" feeling created by anxieties, perceived threats, and other forms of distress. Compulsions are typically related to an individual's reactive and unwanted emotional response toward an authority that he or she feels forced to be submissive to. The client's reactive emotions are often connected with rebellion, aggression, greed, destructiveness, or disorderliness. Because these emotions are believed by the individual to be unacceptable or dangerous, he or she unwittingly develops compulsions to protect against feeling the reactive emotions. Compulsions are protective psychological defensive mechanisms that prevent unwanted feeling states.

Clients performing defensive compulsions are aware of the fact that their compulsions are excessive or unreasonable. Further, the habitual behavior, practice, or ritual is clearly inappropriate. In fact, compulsions are not at all rationally associated with the perceived threat, anxiety, or distress they are designed to inhibit. Compulsions persist as a result of the tremendous anxiety or distress that is generated through attempts to resist engaging in the compulsion. Clients find relief in yielding to the compulsion and attempt to integrate them into their daily lifestyles. This lifestyle integration may be relatively successful and of little consequence to the individual. In this case compulsions are not pathological. However, it is probable that compulsions will lead to marked distress and require psychotherapy to overcome. Pathological compulsions can be very time consuming and significantly interfere with the client's desired lifestyle. Clients' routines may be interrupted by compulsions. Compulsions may interfere with occupational or academic functioning and impede upon social activities and engagement in meaningful relationships.

Development and Current Status

The *Diagnostic and Statistical Manual of Mental Disorders* published by the American Psychiatric Association has differentiated obsessive-compulsive disorder (OCD) from obsessive-compulsive personality disorder (OCPD) since its third revision (DSM-III). Subsequent editions, including DSM-III-R, DSM-IV, DSM-IV-TR, and DSM-5, maintain the important distinctions between OCD and OCPD. These two distinct mental disorders are rarely comorbid (occurring together). OCD and OCPD are not variations of the same disorder. Compulsions are a feature of OCD but are not of OCPD.

However, the history of term compulsion does not begin with the DSM-III. Medical practitioners in the medieval period utilized the Latin term *compulsio* to talk about compulsions. Many years later, Jean Etienne Dominique Esquirol (1782–1840) opened a clinic for the treatment of involuntary, irresistible, and instinctive activity. In the 1850s French psychiatrists were calling compulsions "insanity with insight" (*folie avec conscience*) and deemed the condition a weakness of willpower. Bénédict Augustin Morel (1809–1873) reclassified OCD from a form of insanity to a disease of the emotions (neurosis). Morel's contribution to OCD laid the groundwork for the modern DSM definition. Freud (1856–1939) also recognized OCD but described it as essentially the same disorder as the OCPD. Needless to say, Freud created unnecessary confusion, which persists even today among some clinicians. Psychological conceptualizations of (ways of thinking about) compulsions evolved from volitional to emotive to intellectual. Until the publication of the DSM-III there was a common belief that pathological personality dynamics caused or triggered compulsions. As noted previously, OCPD was officially distinguished from OCD in 1980.

Len Sperry, MD, PhD, and Layven Reguero, MEd

See also: Evidence-Based Practice; Exposure Therapy; Motivational Interviewing; Self-Efficacy

Further Reading

American Psychiatric Association. *Diagnostic and Statistical Manual of Mental Disorders*, 5th ed. Arlington, VA: American Psychiatric Association, 2013.

Frink, Horace Westlake, and James J. Putnam. *Morbid Fears and Compulsions: Their Psychology and Psychoanalytic Treatment*. Charleston, SC: Nabu Press, 2012.

Hyman, Bruce M., and Cherry Pedrick. *The OCD Workbook: Your Guide to Breaking Free from Obsessive-Compulsive Disorder*, 2nd ed. Oakland, CA: New Harbinger Publications, Inc., 2005.

Nordenfelt, Lennart. *Rationality and Compulsion: Applying Action Theory to Psychiatry*. New York, NY: Oxford University Press, 2007.

Computed Tomography (CT)

Computed tomography (CT) is a medical diagnostic test in which computer-processed X-rays produce tomographs (cross-sectional images) of body areas. It is also referred to as X-ray computed tomography and computed axial tomography (CAT scan).

Definitions

- **Magnetic resonance imaging** is a diagnostic imaging device that uses electromagnetic radiation and a strong magnetic field to produce images of soft tissues.

- **Positron emission tomography** is a diagnostic imaging technique that uses radioactive substances to produce three-dimensional colored images within the body.

Description

Computed tomography (CT scan) is a medical imaging procedure that utilizes computer-processed X-rays to produce tomographic images ("slices") of specific areas of the body. These cross-sectional images are used for diagnostic and therapeutic purposes in various medical disciplines. Digital geometry processing (computer software) is used to generate a three-dimensional image of the inside of an object from a large series of two-dimensional X-ray images.

CT scans are relatively inexpensive compared to magnetic resonance imaging scans and positron emission tomography. CT is a commonly used diagnostic tool that supplements some standard X-ray studies, like the chest X-ray, while it has replaced others. For example, the CT is used to identify tumors, cysts, or infections that may be suspected on a chest X-ray. CT scans of the abdomen are useful in defining body organ anatomy, including visualizing the liver, gallbladder, pancreas, spleen, aorta, kidneys, uterus, and ovaries. Such scans can verify the presence or absence of tumors, infection, abnormal anatomy, or changes caused by trauma.

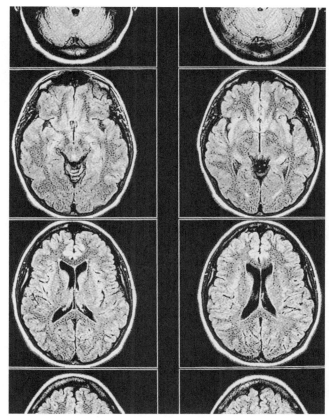

Computed tomography (CT) is a medical diagnostic test in which computer-processed x-rays produce tomographs (cross-sectional images) of body areas, including the brain. (Dave Bredeson/Dreamstime.com)

Developments and Current Status

The CT was invented by Sir Godfrey Hounsfield in England at EMI Central Research Laboratories using X-rays. It was originally known as the "EMI scan" because it was developed at a research branch of EMI. However, EMI is more widely known today for its music and recording business. The first EMI brain scan was done in October, 1971. Soon after, it became known as computed axial tomography and body section röentgenography. Only much later did it become known as the CT scan.

CT produces considerable diagnostic data that can be formatted, through a process known as "windowing," to demonstrate various bodily structures based on their ability to block the X-ray beam. In the past, CT images were represented only in the axial (vertical) or transverse (horizontal) plane. Now, CT images can be represented in various planes, including a volumetric (three-dimensional) representation of body structures.

CT scans have greatly improved the ability of physicians to diagnose many medical conditions earlier in their course and with much less risk than previous diagnostic methods. Further refinements in CT scan technology promise even better picture quality and patient safety. CT scans known as "spiral" or "helical" CT scans are able to provide more rapid and accurate visualization of internal organs. For instance, many trauma centers are using these scans to more rapidly diagnose internal injuries after serious body trauma. High-resolution CT scans are used to accurately assess the lungs for inflammation and scarring. CT angiography is a newer technique that allows noninvasive imaging of the coronary arteries.

Len Sperry, MD, PhD

See also: Magnetic Resonance Imaging (MRI); Positron Emission Tomography (PET)

Further Reading

DeMaio, Daniel N. *Mosby's Exam Review for Computed Tomography*, 2nd ed. St. Louis, MO: Mosby, 2010.

Eisenberg, Ronald, and Alexander Margulis. *A Patient's Guide to Medical Imaging*. New York, NY: Oxford University Press, 2011.

Levine, Harry III. *Medical Imaging*. Santa Barbara, CA: ABC-CLIO, 2010.

Computer-Based Testing

Computers play such an integral role in society that it should come as no surprise that clinicians and psychologists rely heavily on computer-based testing in their evaluation, analysis, and research. In particular, psychologists and researchers alike use computer-based testing programs to standardize testing for personality and actuarial studies. Such computer-based testing also determines an individual's strengths in terms of academics and provides statistical analysis that may lead to indications of a mental health diagnosis.

Definition

- **Computer-based testing** is a form of automated psychological assessment that uses computer software programs to interpret, analyze, and even administer testing procedures. A broader definition of computer-based testing can also include Internet-based assessments, whereby subjects respond through an online medium.

Description

Computer-based testing is not a new phenomenon. Mental health professionals have been using computers for psychological assessment for more than 50 years. Interestingly, computer-based testing as a whole has not changed significantly since the Mayo Clinic released its first computer-based psychological assessment in 1962.

Today, computer-based testing is used in countless psychological studies. Clinicians use this form of testing in nearly every type of personality test. Popular psychological assessments include the Minnesota Multiphasic Personality Inventory-2 (or "MMPI-2"), the MMPI-2-RF, and Wechsler Adult Intelligence Scale.

This type of computer-based testing provides many advantages, including the fact that it's more cost effective than traditional testing methods of paper and pencil. It's also easier to score when a computer evaluates test results. In addition, computer-based testing allows for broad-based statistical analysis of the results once the test is completed. Perhaps, most important, as society becomes more computer literate, clinicians are finding that test subjects prefer to use computer-based testing than the traditional pencil and paper tests.

Studies indicate that test subjects are more open, honest, and forthcoming when answering personality and other questions through a computer-based test compared to a test with paper and pencil. They have also found that test subjects are more likely to respond candidly to sensitive questions in computer-based testing as opposed to traditional, clinician-administered testing methods.

Certain computer-based testing has also evolved to adapt to the individual taking the test. This gives a more precise evaluation of a person's abilities when the computer-based test is tailored to his or her level of knowledge and expertise. While there are many benefits to these computer-based tests, psychologists also warn there are potential disadvantages.

Impact (Psychological Influence)

One of the main issues with these automated tests is their validity. Researchers and psychologists are concerned that such tests may exhibit a certain bias—based on the person administering the test and his or her level of expertise. Another potential disadvantage is the collaboration between the clinician and the computer programmer who designs the test. Some clinicians are concerned that a lack of communication can lead to errors in the programming. However, expert clinicians have called for certain guidelines and standards for computer-based testing to help address these issues. As a whole, clinicians and researchers embrace computer-based testing. By all accounts, this type of testing will be even more critical in the years to come.

Mindy Parsons, PhD

See also: Behavioral Assessment

Further Reading

Greene, Roger L. "Some Considerations for Enhancing Psychological Assessment." *Journal of Personality Assessment* 93, no. 3 (2011): 198–203.

Lichtenberger, Elizabeth O. "Computer Utilization and Clinical Judgment in Psychological Assessment Reports." *Journal of Clinical Psychology* 62, no. 1 (2006), 19–32.

Naus, Mary J., Laura M. Philipp, and Mekhala Samsi. "From Paper to Pixels: A Comparison of Paper and Computer Formats in Psychological Assessment." *Computers in Human Behavior* 25 (2009): 1–7.

Terzis, Vasileios, and Anastasios A. Economides. "Computer Based Assessment: Gender Differences in Perceptions and Acceptance." *Computers in Human Behavior* 27 (2011): 2108–2122.

Conditioned Reflexes: An Investigation of the Physiological Activity of the Cerebral Cortex (Book)

Conditioned Reflexes is a book about how behavior is influenced by the brain. It was written by Ivan Pavlov and discusses his experiments on dogs. It was first published in 1927.

Definitions

- **Behavior therapy** is a form of psychotherapy that focuses on identifying and changing maladaptive behaviors.

- **Classical conditioning** is a process in which a previously neutral stimulus comes to evoke a specific response by being repeatedly paired with another stimulus that evokes the response. In Pavlov's experiments, food was the unconditioned stimulus that produced salivation in the dog—called a reflex or unconditioned response. The bell was the conditioned stimulus, which eventually produced salivation in the absence of food. This salivation was the conditioned response.

- **Conditioning** is a process of changing behavior with a reward or punishment each time an action is performed.

- **Reflex** is the name Pavlov gave to the unconditioned response.

- **Stimulus** is something that triggers a physical or psychological response. The plural is stimuli.

Description

Ivan Pavlov (1849–1936) wrote the book *Conditioned Reflexes: An Investigation of the Physiological Activity of the Cerebral Cortex*. He was a Russian physiologist who studied animals. His research focused on the brain and how it influenced behavior. Pavlov initially believed that animals and humans were simply machines who responded to their environment in predicable ways. His early experiments involved exposing dogs to different stimuli before giving them food and measured the quantity of their saliva. The stimuli ranged from sounds to pictures and touch. When the food was removed, Pavlov found that the dogs still salivated when exposed to the stimulus. They had been conditioned to respond to the stimulus as if it were food. He concluded that the connection between the brain and behavior could be manipulated. This manipulation came to be called classical conditioning. The popular image of Pavlov's dogs drooling to the ringing of a bell comes from ideas introduced in this book.

Pavlov concluded that there are two types of reflexes. *Unconditioned* reflexes happen naturally, such as when a dog sees food and salivates. *Conditioned* reflexes are created through learning, such as when a dog salivates to nonfood stimuli. He discovered that the cerebral cortex (outer part of the brain) was responsible for this. He concluded that nerve pathways within this part of the brain can be changed through learning. It is as if learning "rewires" the brain. Pavlov also found that there were limits to this conditioning. If the brain was given too much to process, it would not change. In addition, new behaviors sometimes wore off over time if they were not reinforced.

Pavlov wrote in this book that all living things respond to their environments through this process of learning in the brain. More advanced organisms like human beings have more complex ways of learning. He viewed humans as different from other animals because they have more conditioned responses than natural ones. Pavlov believed that human civilization was created as a way to manage reflexes. For example, individuals are trained and educated by going to school. They learn about the world around them, how to follow rules, and how to appropriately interact with others. Pavlov also viewed conditioning as changeable. His research had a significant influence on the psychology, in general, and behavior therapy, in particular.

George Stoupas, MS, and Len Sperry, MD, PhD

See also: Behavior Therapy

Further Reading

Pavlov, Ivan. *Conditioned Reflexes: An Investigation of the Physiological Activity of the Cerebral Cortex.* Mineola, NY: Dover Books, 1984.

Todes, Daniel. *Ivan Pavlov: Exploring the Animal Machine.* New York, NY: Oxford University Press, 2000.

Conduct Disorder

Dating back centuries, parents and professionals alike have agonized over how to help children who are seemingly out of control, making conduct disorder among the oldest diagnostic categories currently used by modern-day child psychiatry.

In the early 1900s, one of the pioneers who found success in working with conduct disordered children was August Aichhorn, who left his teaching career at the age of 44 and went to study psychoanalysis under Sigmund Freud. Aichhorn felt that children who had stalled in their development were at risk for later antisocial behavior. He also believed that the cause of these challenges could frequently be traced back to difficulties in the parent–child relationship. Studies suggest that many children diagnosed with conduct disorder later go on to develop antisocial personality disorder.

With support and encouragement from Anna Freud, August Aichhorn is considered among the first to have worked successfully with troubled adolescents. His success came from making modifications to Sigmund Freud's psychoanalytic approach with neurotics. Aichhorn used psychoanalysis in combination with his keen understanding of personality to find positive results in working with juvenile delinquents.

Definition

- **Conduct disorder** is a psychological disorder described in the DSM 5 as having pervasive patterns of behavior that infringe on the rights of others or that violate social norms. These include aggressive, rule breaking, rebellion, and other destructive behaviors. The majority of individuals diagnosed with conduct disorder previously were first diagnosed with oppositional defiant disorder. Conduct disorder is believed to be a precursor to antisocial personality disorder. There are also links to ADHD, substance use, and learning disabilities, which commonly are present in a child or adolescent diagnosed with conduct disorder.

There are two distinct subtypes of conduct disorder, including one with onset in childhood with at least one of the criteria being met before the age of 10 and the second being an onset in adolescence, which requires an absence of any criteria being present before the age of 10. The childhood onset type of conduct disorder includes children who frequently display higher levels of ADHD (attention-deficit hyperactivity disorder) symptoms, family problems, and academic challenges, as well as more aggressive behavior. The adolescent onset type usually has a better long-term prognosis compared to the childhood onset type.

Notably, there seems to be a link between oppositional defiant disorder, conduct disorder, and antisocial personality disorder. Specifically, it has been found that the majority of children who have been diagnosed with conduct disorder were previously diagnosed with oppositional defiant disorder. Moreover, a fair number of individuals who have been diagnosed with conduct disorder later go on to be diagnosed with antisocial personality disorder.

Some of the criteria for conduct disorder include aggression to people and animals (e.g., bullying, fighting, or cruelty to people or animals), destruction of property (e.g., fire setting, damage to property), deceitfulness or theft (e.g., breaking into someone's home or car, or lying), and disregard for rules (staying out late, running away, skipping school). Several risk factors have been identified for conduct disorder, including smoking during pregnancy, low socioeconomic status or poverty, parental misbehavior (drug use, criminal behavior), a poor family environment (unstable, single-parent homes), and exposure to physical or sexual abuse. Treatment of conduct disorder usually requires family therapy, behavior management, and pharmacotherapy.

Mindy Parsons, PhD

See also: American Academy of Child and Adolescent Psychiatry (AACAP); Antisocial Personality Disorder; Attention-Deficit Hyperactivity Disorder; Economic and Financial Stress; Juvenile Offenders; Oppositional Defiant Disorder (ODD); Poverty and Mental Illness

Further Reading

American Psychiatric Association. *Diagnostic and Statistical Manual of Mental Disorders*, 5th ed. Arlington, VA: American Psychiatric Association Press, 2013.

Boden, Joseph M., David M. Fergusson, and John L. Horwood. "Risk Factors for Conduct Disorder and Oppositional Defiant Disorder: Evidence from a New Zealand Birth Cohort." *Journal of the American Academy of Child & Adolescent Psychiatry* 49, no. 11 (2010): 1125–1133.

Burke, Jeffrey, D., Irwin Waldman, and Benjamin B. Lahey. "Predictive Validity of Childhood Oppositional Defiant Disorder and Conduct Disorder: Implications for the DSM-V." *Journal of Abnormal Psychology*. American Psychological Association 119, no. 4 (2010): 739–751.

Conduct Disorder Resource Center at the American Academy of Children and Adolescent Psychiatry (AACAP). http://www.aacap.org/aacap/Families_and_Youth/Resource_Centers/Conduct_Disorder_Resource_Center/Home.aspx.

Gelhorn, Heather L., Joseph T. Sakai, Rumi Kato Price, and Thomas J. Crowley. "DSM-IV Conduct Disorder Criteria as Predictors of Antisocial Personality Disorder." *Comprehensive Psychiatry* 48 (2007): 529–538.

Hill, Jonathan, and Barbara Maughan, eds. *Conduct Disorders in Childhood and Adolescence*. New York, NY: Cambridge University Press, 2001.

Wayward Youth (*Verwahrloste Jugend*) was written by Austrian-born August Aichhorn, who is considered the first expert in dealing with troubled youth and with a forward by Sigmund Freud. Written in 1925, it has been translated into English and is still considered a helpful resource. New York, NY: Viking Press, 1963.

Conflict Resolution

Conflict resolution, sometimes used interchangeably with "dispute resolution," describes a peaceful process or approach that is used to settle disputes, arguments, or conflicts between two opposing parties.

Definitions

- **Compromise** defines when opposing parties move toward one another, finding common ground in order to come to some resolution, understanding, or agreed-upon solution.

- **Conflict management** describes an ongoing process of mediating disputes between two parties where a resolution, though sought after, may not be reached.

- **Mediation** is a process in which one objective party facilitates agreement, understanding, or resolution between two opposing parties.

- **Reconciliation,** a term that often has a religious connotation, describes the act of bringing back together two conflicting parties once agreement has been reached and often after some form of retribution has been made.

Description

Conflict resolution is a process used to facilitate peace or understanding between two or more social entities (individuals, groups, organizations, nations). Win–win solutions in which both sides feel that they have been heard and understood, and that their concerns have been addressed, are sought. Conflict resolution utilizes specific communication skills, including active listening, expression of feelings, empathic responding, open-ended questioning, and problem-solving techniques.

Conflict is an inevitable part of everyday human interaction that can arise from differences in perceptions, feelings, perspectives, interests, or approaches. It is centered in the belief that if one party gets what it wants, then the other party will not be able to do so. When conflict is not dealt with effectively, it can result in feelings of resentment and hurt or damage to relationships. However, when conflict is dealt with in a positive, respectful way, it can alleviate stress, foster acceptance, and even strengthen a relationship. Ownership for resolving conflict is the responsibility of both parties equally. Both need to find common ground, come together, hear one another out, increase understanding, and agree to concede on certain points.

Conflict resolution as a method, though it may vary in language and sequence, has some basic essential components. An initial component required, which can help alleviate tension for those involved, is for each person to recognize, acknowledge, and be able to regulate their emotions. In addition, both parties should have a clear understanding of their own needs. Further progress can be made if the parties are able to effectively communicate their needs to the one another. One must pay attention to what is communicated both verbally and nonverbally. Those involved should remain calm and refrain from attacking one another with either words or actions. Respecting differing backgrounds, perspectives, and views is key. If these components are incorporated, then each person is more likely to be willing to compromise, with the ultimate goal being to find some common ground.

Development

Conflict resolution arose as a defined field of study in the 1950s and 1960s during the Cold War era when fear of nuclear threat was a dominant theme. Scientists began to study conflict and apply similar principles to global problems and national relations, as well as to specific tensions between communities, groups, and individuals. Relations between national superpowers improved during the 1980s and 1990s with the downfall of the Soviet Union. However, tensions between the United States and Middle East have been ongoing since the turn of the century and continue to be of concern. Wars, movements, and threats have all resulted from conflict with varying outcomes. Often conflict between nations, organizations, and groups can result in an increased sense of unity among members of each particular groups. Foundational theorist in the field, Morton Deustch, was the first to define between what he termed "constructive" and "destructive" types of conflict. Other influential writers on the topic, Kenneth Thomas and Ralph Kilman, identified five styles of dealing with conflict during the 1970s: competitive, collaborative, compromising, accommodating, and avoiding. They argued that most people have a preferred conflict resolution style but can learn to respond with differing styles depending on varying situations. Several other models, theories, and approaches have followed with similar terminology, sequences, and themes.

Current Status

The study of conflict resolution is an expanding field both from a scientific perspective and in terms of professional practice. This topic has been studied among countries, government agencies, educational institutions, communities, families, and between individual people. A new area of focus has been on understanding the particular worldviews of each party, remaining multiculturally sensitive and respectful to both. This approach can resolve conflicts more efficiently and effectively.

Melissa A. Mariani, PhD

See also: Coaching

Further Reading

Dana, Daniel, and Roger A. Formisano. *Conflict Resolution.* New York, NY: McGraw Hill, 2001.

Deutsch, Morton, Peter T. Coleman, and Eric Marcus. *The Handbook of Conflict Resolution: Theory and Practice.* Hoboken, NJ: John Wiley & Sons, 2006.

Fisher, Roger, Bruce Patton, and William Ury. *Getting to Yes: Negotiating Agreement Without Giving In.* New York, NY: Penguin Group, 1991.

LeBaron, Michelle, and Venashri Pillay. *Conflict across Cultures: A Unique Experience of Bridging Differences.* Boston, MA: Intercultural Press, 2006.

Rosenberg, Marshall B., and Graham Van Dixhorn. *We Can Work It Out: Resolving Conflicts Peacefully and Powerfully.* Encinitas, CA: Puddledancer Press, 2005.

Conjoint Family Therapy

Conjoint family therapy is a form of psychotherapy developed by Virginia Satir (1916–1988), who is affectionately referred to as the mother of family therapy. Conjoint family therapy uses a comprehensive approach to working with families as a whole system as opposed to working with individuals within the family.

In conjoint family therapy, all family members are seen simultaneously. There must be an alliance between not only the therapist but also within the family unit as well to have a successful outcome. Family members must agree on treatment goals and be willing to work together and confront each other when necessary. Satir believed that oftentimes the presenting issue was not the core problem within a family system but rather the family's way of coping with the underlying problem.

Definition

- **Conjoint family therapy** is a family counseling theory in which a therapist sees a family and addresses the issues and problems raised by the family members as a system rather than addressing the problems being experienced by individual members of the family.

Description

Satir believed that maintaining self-esteem is a primary motivation of individuals and she believed that low self-esteem could lead to significant challenges in interpersonal relationships. Therefore, a family can achieve homeostasis of roles from efforts from each individual to maintain self-esteem. A change in an individual must also incorporate changes from each family member. This is accomplished through conjoint interviews.

In conjoint family therapy, the therapist examines the family rules, roles, and communication. The therapist focuses on group or subgroup actions within the family as opposed to just one individual in the family. Focus on an individual within the family could occur as part of this approach, but it had to be tied back into the context of the family.

Family therapy can be difficult if each member disagrees about what the problem is, what the treatment goals are, or the purpose of therapy. For there to be a successful outcome, each member must be an active participant and invest in the process and each other. The conjoint family therapy model also requires family members to be willing to take risks with each other. To achieve this, therapists must not only be building the therapeutic alliance but also the working alliance between the family members.

It is important that the therapist be in tune with potential ruptures within the family unit and the working alliance as a whole. Ruptures within conjoint family therapy are more complex. They can occur if one family member attempts to force another to participate making that person more likely to resent treatment as a whole. The therapist has to be sure he or she does not show any preferential treatment toward one family member over another. There must be a balance of alliances to work toward successful outcomes.

Development and Current Status

Clinical observation and treatment of the whole family emerged in the 20th century. Interest in the family unit developed from working with individuals and seeing potential connections and impacts. The person who initially sought treatment, or rather the identified patient, was not necessarily the only one affected by problems within the family.

In the mid-1900s there was an emergence of three major forms of family therapy. Conjoint family therapy was the third one, which at the time was growing in popularity. One of the most important contributions of conjoint family therapy was that it led to looking at the family group as a system rather than just a single member of the family who was singled out as the identified patient.

As with any form of therapy, the working alliance is a key component. Virginia Satir played a key role in the development of family therapy and in working within family systems. One of her most well-known books is *Conjoint Family Therapy: A Guide to Theory and Technique*, as well as *Peoplemaking*.

Mindy Parsons, PhD

See also: Family Therapy; Satir, Virginia (1916–1988)

Further Reading

Escudero, Valentin, Emanuelle Boogmans, Gerrit Loots, and Myrna L. Friedlander. "Evidence-Based Case Study Alliance Rupture and Repair in Conjoint Family Therapy: An Exploratory Study." *Psychotherapy* 49 (2012): 26–37.

Fisch, Richard. "Conjoint Family Therapy: A Guide to Theory and Technique." A review of Conjoint Family Therapy: A Guide to Theory and Technique, by Virginia Satir. *The Journal of Nervous and Mental Disease* 148 (1965): 251–261.

Lambert, Jessica E., Alyson H. Skinner, and Micki L. Friedlander. "Problematic Within-Family Alliances in Conjoint Family Therapy: A Close Look at Five Cases." *Journal of Marital and Family Therapy* 38 (2012): 417–428.

Rebner, Isaac. "Conjoint Family Therapy." *Psychotherapy: Theory, Research and Practice* 9 (1972): 62–66.

Satir, Virginia. *Conjoint Family Therapy. Third Edition/Revised and Expanded*. Palo Alto, CA: Science and Behavior Books, 1983.

Conjoint Sexual Therapy

Conjoint sexual therapy is a treatment conducted together for relationship partners, which focuses on aspects of their sexual issues and problems.

Definition

- **Sexual dysfunctions disorders** are a group of mental disorders characterized by significant difficulty in the ability to respond sexually or to experience sexual pleasure. Disorders include delayed ejaculation, female orgasmic disorder, and genito-pelvic pain/penetration disorder.

Description

The term and practice of conjoint sexual therapy came out of the research conducted by Masters and Johnson and published in their 1970 book *Human Sexual Inadequacy*. Conjoint therapy, in general, is behavior-based psychological treatment conducted with individuals together and in the same session. The goal is to help them deal with issues that negatively impact them. Behavior based in this context means that the therapy is not aimed at discovering why the problem exists but rather at dealing with its effects and consequences. For conjoint sexual therapy, sexual exercises and behaviors are often recommended as part of treatment.

In conjoint sexual therapy for sexual partners, the sexual issues or dysfunctions are treated as a separate entity. These include sexual dysfunction disorders such as arousal and orgasmic conditions. The belief is that the sexual problems themselves are the client. This means that issues are seen not as separate problems or individual, his or her, problems. Instead, they are viewed as part of the dynamic of the relationship that both partners share. This is true when the issues may have been problems like erectile dysfunction for the man or painful vaginal experience during intercourse for the woman. In this view, all sexual experiences are shared between partners and they must be worked on in that context for the treatment to be successful.

Development

While there is no question that Masters and Johnson were pioneers in conjoint sexual therapy, the treatment methods and approaches they used were ones that had been available for many years. Techniques described as sensate focus exercises were the basis of their treatment approach. Their aim was to broaden the sexual experience, to reduce anxiety around sexual performance, and to enable couples to enjoy the sexual experience. In all of this they were groundbreaking because they treated men and women as equal in their ability to enter into and enjoy the sexual experience.

Another important researcher in conjoint sexual therapy was Dr. Helen Singer Kaplan. She found that success in an outpatient setting required a slightly different approach. She added psychodynamic therapy and other approaches to increase the likelihood of success for her clients. Both Masters and Johnson and Kaplan were controversial in aspects of their suggestions, which included interventions such as sexual desensitization, masturbation, and sexual surrogates.

Current Status

Although there are many individual success stories from conjoint sexual therapy, it has remained difficult to show consistent experimental results. This makes sense because similar sexual problems may have a variety of physical and psychological causes. It is still a challenge to decide which approach is best for which clients and under what circumstances.

Nevertheless, conjoint sexual therapy remains a treatment of choice for couples who struggle with sexual relationship problems. Most therapists employ a variety of interventions to reduce fear around sexuality, enhance communication and enjoyment, and help people in general to have improved relationships. The aim in current therapeutic approaches is not just to improve sexual functioning but to enhance the partners in their relationship with one another.

Alexandra Cunningham, PhD, and William M. Cunningham, MA

See also: *Everything You Always Wanted to Know about Sex (but Were Afraid to Ask)* (Book and Movie); Female Sexual Interest/Arousal Disorder; Male Hypoactive Sexual Desire Disorder; Sexual Dysfunctions

Further Reading

Kaplan, Helen Singer. *The New Sex Therapy: Active Treatment of Sexual Dysfunctions*. New York, NY: Psychology Press, 1974.

Weeks, Gerald R. *Integrative Sex and Marital Therapy*. New York, NY: Brunner-Routledge, 1987.

Conners Rating Scales

Conners Rating Scales (CRS) are normed behavior rating scales used by mental health professionals to screen and assist in diagnosing attention-deficit hyperactivity disorder (ADHD) in children.

Definitions

- **Attention-deficit hyperactivity disorder (ADHD)**, according to the *Diagnostic and Statistical Manual of Mental Disorders, Fifth Edition* (DSM-5), is a behavioral diagnosis used to describe a combination of problems, including difficulty sustaining attention, hyperactivity, and impulsivity.

- **Rating scales** are semi-objective assessment tools that require individuals completing them to assign a quantitative judgment to their observations of certain behaviors.

Description

Conners Rating Scales are rating forms, completed by parents, teachers, and sometimes self, to determine the presence of behavior issues specifically related to inattention, hyperactivity, and impulsivity. These general screening tools were initially developed to assist in the identification of these types of problems in children; however, they have recently been expanded to use with adults. The most recent version advertises use with ages 6 to 18 (parent and teacher). Psychologist C. Keith Conners published the first of these rating scales in 1964, with follow-up editions in 1989 (Conners Rating Scales-CSR), 1997 (Conners Rating Scales-Revised—CSR-R), and 2008 (Conners 3—C3).

Both long and short versions of the CRS are easy to administer and score. They can be scored by hand or with the accompanying computer software. Number of items vary from version to version, with the most recent, the Conners 3, containing the following: Teacher (long-115; short-39), Parent (long-110; short-43), Self (long-59; short-39). Short version use is recommended for progress monitoring purposes, when one is planning multiple administrations over a period of time. Administration takes approximately 20 minutes for the long version and 10 minutes for the short, but there is no time limit. The Parent and Teacher surveys are written on a fifth-grade reading level and the Self-Report on a third-grade reading level. Both English and Spanish translations are available. The Conners 3 is comprised of six scales: Hyperactivity/Impulsivity, Executive Functioning, Learning Problems, Aggression, Peer Relations, and Family Relations.

The forms are multipaged, carbon copies. Responses circled on the front or back are automatically transferred to a middle section for use by the scorer. The scorer transfers the circled scores into appropriate scales on the middle form and totals each scale at the bottom of the page. After transferring the raw scores to the various scales and totaling them, the total of each scale (A–N) is transferred to another form which represents the findings graphically. The scorer must be careful to transpose the raw scores to the correct age group column within each major scale. Each of these column scores can then be converted to a T-score and then to percentile scores as needed. T-scores above 60 are cause for concern and have interpretive value. Interpretable scores range from a low T-score of 61 (mildly atypical) to above 70 (markedly atypical).

Development

The Conners Rating Scales were initially designed as a comprehensive checklist to identify common behavior problems in children. In the late 1990s, a restandardization of the scales took place, attempting to focus more narrowly on behaviors associated with ADHD. This revision, the CRS-R, was also empirically based and normed on a large, representative sample of North American children. The most recently published version, the Conners 3, includes normative data for 1,200 parents, 1,200 teachers, and 1,000 self-report raters and is matched to the 2000 U.S. Census information on ethnicity/race, gender, and parent education level. Separate norms are provided for males and females in one-year intervals.

Current Status and Results

Debate over the reliability and validity of these assessment tools has been an issue. Therefore, CRS should be used only as part of comprehensive psychoeducational evaluation. They should not be used in isolation to diagnose ADHD symptomatology as there is risk of obtaining false positives (diagnosing when criteria are not present) or false negatives (not diagnosing when the criteria are present). Though theses scales are easy to administer and score, they should be interpreted only by a trained professional. Early versions on the CRS were also criticized for the disparity between results obtained by different ethnic groups, but this has been addressed in the latest revisions.

Melissa A. Mariani, PhD

See also: Attention-Deficit Hyperactivity Disorder

Further Reading

Conners, C. Keith. *Conner's Rating Scales-Revised Technical Manual.* Toronto, Ontario, Canada: Multi-Health Systems Inc., 1997.

Conners, C. Keith. *Conner's 3—SR Technical Manual.* Toronto, Ontario, Canada: Multi-Health Systems Inc., 2008.

Gallant, Stephen, C. Keith Conners, Sara Rzepa, Jenni Pitkanen, Maria-Luisa Marocco, and Gill Sitarenios. *Psychometric Properties of the Conner's*, 3rd ed. Toronto, Ontario, Canada: Mulit-Health Systems Inc., 2008.

Reynolds, Cecil R., and Randy W. Kamphaus. *Handbook of Psychological and Educational Assessment of Children: Personality, Behavior, and Context*, 2nd ed. New York, NY: Guilford Press, 2003.

Contemplative Neuroscience

Contemplative neuroscience is the study of how contemplative practices such as meditation affect the brain and the nervous system.

Definitions

- **Contemplation** is studying or observing something carefully or thinking deeply about it.

- **Contemplative practices** are activities that foster contemplation, such as meditation, reflection, prayer, journaling, and worship.

- **Meditation** is the concentrated focus on a sound, the breath, object, or attention itself to increase awareness of the present moment. Its purpose is to reduce stress, promote relaxation, or increase spiritual growth.

- **Mind–brain relationship** is the interaction of the mind (consciousness) and brain (nerve cells) summed up in the saying "minds are what brains do."

- **Mindfulness** is the moment-by-moment awareness of one's thoughts, feelings, sensations, and environment without evaluating or judging them.

- **Neuroplasticity** is the brain's capacity to restructure itself after training or practice allowing personal growth and development to occur.

- **Neuroscience** is the scientific study of the nervous system, particularly the functioning of the brain.

Description

Contemplative neuroscience is the scientific study of how the brain and nervous system are affected by contemplative practices. Over the past three decades, researchers have discovered how deeply the human brain is influenced by both human experience and the environment. This influence begins early in life and extends throughout the lifespan. This new understanding of the brain's capacity to change and develop, called *neuroplasticity*, provides insight into personal growth transformation (development) that once seemed impossible. This increasing awareness of the brain's plasticity means that the goal of decreasing or eliminating mental and nervous illness may be possible. It also means that mental and emotional health can be greatly increased. Contemplative neuroscience is one method for accomplishing these goals.

Developments and Current Status

Thich Nhat Hanh (1926–), a Zen Buddhist monk and teacher, conducted a retreat on mindfulness in the United States. One of the attendees was the American psychologist Jon Kabat-Zinn (1944–). In 1979, Kabat-Zinn adapted Hanh's teachings on mindfulness into his eight-week Mindfulness-Based Stress Reduction course. This course and its emphasis on mindfulness has since spread throughout North America and to other western countries. At about the same time, the American psychologists Daniel Goleman and Richard Davidson were researching and writing about neuroscience and emotions. In the 1980s, Davidson began a collaboration with the Dalai Lama, Buddhist monk and spiritual leader. As a result, Davidson became increasing involved in practicing and researching meditation. Throughout the next decade of research, he, and several other researchers, extensively studied mindfulness and meditation. Since the early 2000s the terms "contemplative science" and "contemplative neuroscience" emerged, reflecting basic research and applications in clinical and educational settings.

The research on neuroplasticity shows that specific kinds of mental training can influence how the brain functions. More specifically, it shows how emotional and mental well-being can be cultivated through various disciplines, including contemplative practices such as meditation and mindfulness. An individual's emotional set-points can be shifted toward higher levels of well-being. In contrast, conventional psychiatry focuses treatment on reducing symptoms and discomfort with medications, without necessarily addressing the deeper causal issues behind the symptoms and distress. While medication may have a role in treatment of symptoms, it is incapable of teaching the brain new and healthy neurological habits. Contemplative training and meditation, however, can change such habits. Unlike conventional psychiatry, contemplative neuroscience assumes that brain and mind interactions are bidirectional. That means that mind can influence and change the brain, just as the brain can influence and change the mind.

A general goal of contemplative neuroscience is to empower individuals to become the masters of their own minds so they can experience more wholeness, more joy, and more peace. More specifically, loving kindness and compassion can be cultivated and hard-wired (made permanent) in the brain. In short, contemplative neuroscience offers a scientific worldview capable of radically changing what individuals believe is possible for their lives and the lives of future generations.

Len Sperry, MD, PhD

See also: Mindfulness; Mindfulness-Based Psychotherapies

Further Reading

Davidson, Richard J., and Sharon Begley. *The Emotional Life of Your Brain: How Its Unique Patterns Affect the Way You Think, Feel, and Live—and How You Can Change Them.* New York, NY: Penguin, 2012.

Kabat-Zinn, Jon. *Mindfulness for Beginners: Reclaiming the Present Moment—and Your Life.* San Francisco, CA: Harper-Collins, 2012.

Plante, Thomas G., ed. *Contemplative Practices in Action: Spirituality, Meditation, and Health.* Santa Barbara, CA: Praeger Publishing, 2009.

Wallace, B. Alan, and Brian Hodal. *Contemplative Science: Where Buddhism and Neuroscience Converge.* New York, NY: Colombia University Press, 2009.

Conversion Disorder

Conversion disorder is a mental health condition characterized by paralysis, seizures, or other neurologic symptoms that cannot be explained by medical evaluation. It is also known as functional neurological symptom disorder and hysteria.

Definitions

- **Cognitive behavior therapy** is a type of psychotherapy that focuses on maladaptive (faulty) behaviors, emotions, and thoughts.

- **Dissociation** is a detachment from reality. Daydreaming is a non-pathological form of dissociation, while depersonalization (a sense that the self is unreal) is a pathological form of dissociation.

- **Dissociative disorders** are a group of mental disorders characterized by a disturbance of self, memory, awareness, or consciousness which cause disrupted life functioning.

- **DSM-5** stands for the *Diagnostic and Statistical Manual of Mental Disorders, Fifth Edition*, which is a diagnostic system used by professionals to identify mental disorders with specific diagnostic criteria.

- **Malingering** is the practice of intentionally exaggerating or faking physical or psychological symptoms for personal gain. It is also referred to as fictitious illness.

- **Mindfulness practices** are intentional activities that foster living in the present moment and an awareness that is nonjudgmental and accepting.

- **Somatic symptom and related disorders** are a group of DSM-5 mental disorders characterized by prominent somatic symptoms and significant distress and impairment. They include somatic symptom disorder, factitious disorder, and conversion disorder. Previously they were known as somatoform disorders.

- **Somatoform disorders** are a group of mental disorders characterized by physical symptoms that cannot be explained by a medical condition. DSM-5 calls them somatic symptom and related disorders.

- **Stress management** is a set of psychological techniques for increasing the capacity to better cope with psychological stress. It usually includes relaxation methods.

Description and Diagnosis

Conversion disorder is a dissociative disorder that was named to describe a health concern that begins as a psychological stressor or trauma but then "converts" to physical symptoms. Such symptoms appear suddenly and affect individuals' basic senses and movement such as their ability to see, hear, swallow, or walk. While individuals may describe their symptoms in detail, they often show little concern or indifference about symptoms. Historically, this disorder has been referred to as *La Belle Indifference* (American Psychiatric Association, 2013). This indifference can be a useful clue in distinguishing conversion disorder from the medical condition it may mimic. Symptoms can be severe at first. Fortunately for many individuals with this disorder, symptoms tend to improve within a short time.

Conversion disorder is more often diagnosed in women than men. Often these individuals are not psychologically minded (insightful) and they are likely to have an early history of abuse, particularly sexual abuse. The tendency toward dissociation is commonly seen with these individuals. This means they deal with stressors by removing themselves psychologically from these situations as a way of safeguarding themselves. In this way, they pay little or no attention to certain events and so they are less likely to remember or be concerned about them.

According to the *Diagnostic and Statistical Manual of Mental Disorders, Fifth Edition*, individuals can be diagnosed with this disorder if they experience symptoms of voluntary motor function or of sensory function such as weakness or paralysis of a limb or reduced ability to see or hear. What makes these symptoms problematic is that clinical findings cannot explain why these symptoms are occurring, or if there is a neurological disorder present, the symptoms cannot be accounted for by such illness. However, these symptoms contribute to significant disruption in work, relationships, or family life. The symptoms cannot be explained by another medical or mental condition (American Psychiatric Association, 2013).

The cause of this disorder is not well understood, but it appears that it is triggered by a stressful event, a relational conflict, or another mental disorder, such as depression. Individual personality dynamics appear to be involved, particularly feeling avoidance. A careful development history often reveals a pattern of feeling avoidance and confusion of physical sensations with feelings. As children, these individuals seldom experienced empathy or validation of their wishes, thoughts, and feelings. Instead they learned to value logic over feelings. They learned to discount not only their feelings but their bodily sensations as well. As they got older, they may have appeared to others to be healthy on the outside when in fact they were not. For instance, measures of heart rhythms or blood pressure could be clearly abnormal while they appear calm on the outside. In short, because their wishes, thoughts, and feelings were often discouraged or punished, they stopped paying attention to them. These experiences also contribute to a lack of psychological mindedness (insight), which is commonly seen in conversion disorders.

Treatment

For most individuals, symptoms of this disorder resolve (get better) without treatment, often, the reassurance of a health professional that there is no serious medical condition underlying the conversion symptoms. For others, counseling or psychotherapy can be helpful in treating symptoms and preventing their reoccurrence. However, psychotherapy may be necessary if anxiety, depression, or other mental health issues are present. Allowing such individuals to talk about the stressor that triggers their symptoms in a safe environment can be very therapeutic. Cognitive behavior therapy can be particularly helpful in recognizing and distinguishing feelings from somatic (bodily) sensations. Teaching stress management techniques and mindfulness practices can further increase awareness and reduce stress and anxiety.

Len Sperry, MD, PhD

See also: Cognitive Behavior Therapy; Mindfulness; Somatic Symptom Disorder; Stress Management

Further Reading

American Psychiatric Association. *Diagnostic and Statistical Manual of Mental Disorders*, 5th ed. Arlington, VA: American Psychiatric Association, 2013.

Hallett, Mark, C. Robert Cloninger, Stanley Fahn, and Joseph Jankovic. *Psychogenic Movement Disorders: Neurology and Neuropsychiatry*. Baltimore, MD: Lippincott Williams & Wilkins, 2006.

Hallett, Mark, Anthony E. Lang, Joseph Jankovic, and Stanley Fahn. *Psychogenic Movement Disorders and Other Conversion Disorders*. New York, NY: Cambridge University Press, 2012.

Woolfolk, Robert L., and Lesley A. Allen. *Treating Somatization: A Cognitive-Behavioral Approach*. New York, NY: The Guilford Press, 2007.

Coping

Coping is a psychological concept and is defined as the internal mental efforts and the external behavioral efforts a person makes in order to manage and respond to difficult, demanding, and stressful events.

Description

Stress is a part of the human experience and how people cope with stress can influence their lives in significant ways. Stress is defined as the relationship between a person and the environment that is judged by the person as difficult or exceeding his or her ability to experience physical, social, emotional, or psychological well-being.

Richard Lazarus, one of the top 100 most eminent psychologists of the 20th century, was instrumental in developing a theory of stress and coping. Lazarus found that when coping was effective, stress is controlled. When coping is ineffective, stress increases leading to physical and/or emotional difficulties and impaired social functioning. Lazarus used the phrase "cognitive appraisal" to refer to how a person thinks about and evaluates stressful events. There are two cognitive appraisals that take place in a person's mind when faced with stressful events: primary and secondary. Primary appraisals evaluate the impact of an event. Secondary appraisals evaluate what can be done to manage and cope with, or respond to, the event. Each of these appraisals interacts with each other to determine how much stress is experienced. For instance, imagine that there is a major paper due in class on Monday. This paper will have a significant impact on the grade for the course. Also imagine that there is an all-day music festival on Saturday and everyone will be there. How a student spends Saturday, that is his or her behavior, will be determined by his or her primary cognitive appraisal of the importance of the grade (what is at stake) and his or her secondary cognitive appraisal of what he or she needs to do to receive a good grade. One student has already written a complete and thorough draft and only needs to proofread the paper before turning it in. This student attends the festival with little or no stress about the assignment. The student's primary appraisal is that attending the music festival will have no impact on his or her grade. The student's secondary appraisal of what he or she needs to do to receive a good grade (a final proofread that is easily accomplished on Sunday) allows him or her to attend the festival. Another student, however, has put off the assignment and has written very little. The student's primary appraisal is that he or she will fail the class if he or she does not receive a good grade on the assignment. The student is very stressed, that is, the student is anxious and worried about the final grade. The student's secondary appraisal is that if he or she attends the festival, he or she will not have the time to produce a good paper. Another secondary cognitive appraisal is that there will be other music festivals to attend but only one chance to do well on the paper. The student copes with the stress of the assignment by choosing to stay home and work hard on the paper (his or her behavior), which decreases stress (anxiety).

Current Status

Lazarus's theory of stress, appraisal, and coping provided a gold standard model that is widely utilized in many helping techniques, methods, and theories of counseling.

Steven R. Vensel, PhD

See also: Cognitive Behavior Therapy; Cognitive Therapies; Motivation

Further Reading

Haggbloom, Steven, Renee Warnick, Jason E. Warnick, Vinessa K. Jones, Gary L. Yarbrough, Tenea M. Russell, Chris M. Borecky, Reagan McGahhey, John L. Powell III, Jamie Beavers, and Emmanuelle Monte. "The 100 Most Eminent Psychologists of the 20th Century." *Review of General Psychology* 6, no. 2 (2002): 139–152.

Richard Lazarus, and Susan Folkman. *Stress Appraisal, and Coping*. New York, NY: Springer, 1984.

Corrective Emotional Experience

A corrective emotional experience is a novel, positive reexperiencing of a past negative emotional event or pattern.

Definitions

- **Psychodynamic theory** is a broad category of psychological theories that view thoughts, feelings, and behaviors as the result of unconscious process.

- **Psychotherapy** is a psychological method for achieving desired changes in thinking, feeling, and behavior. It is also called therapeutic counseling.

- **Therapeutic alliance** is the moment-to-moment, interactive relationship between an individual and a therapist that should include mutual trust, respect, and collaboration. It is also called a therapeutic relationship.

Description

Corrective emotional experience is a treatment strategy by which an individual experiences a previously negative pattern of thinking, acting, or relating in an unexpected new and healthier way. This change occurs because the individual is better able to tolerate the past negative experience under more favorable circumstances. Such a positive reexperience can contribute significantly to positive outcomes in psychotherapy.

Typically, the event or pattern that is reexperienced is related to the presenting issue or focus of psychotherapy and is facilitated by the therapist. The corrective experience helps the individual to reshape his or her understanding of the "self" (who the individual thinks he or she is) in relationship to others. That is to say that the individual is able to redefine who he or she is by experiencing an interaction with another, in this case a therapist, differently than ever before. It is different from insight, whereby an individual gains a purely intellectual understanding of an issue. Insight alone is not necessarily sufficient for significant growth and healing. This experience may occur during a therapy session, or it can occur outside of therapy as a result of the interactions that took place within the session.

There are two different interpretations of this general term. In the past, this term was most closely associated with psychodynamic theories. Consequently, the original interpretation refers to positive consequences that result from the difference between how a therapist reacts to the individual and how the individual expected the therapist to react. This discrepancy causes the individual to have a new and different interpretation of a relationship with another, thereby causing a corrective emotional experience. Today, the broader term "corrective experience" is used to reflect other perspectives besides psychodynamic theory. This more contemporary interpretation refers to any aspect of the interaction between the individual and therapist that results in the individual having a new and unexpected corrective experience.

There are four types of corrective experiences: emotional, relational, cognitive, and behavioral. Each type represents a differing mechanism of initiating the corrective experience. But all involve an emotional response as the individual learns new ways of responding or experiencing as compared to their previous patterns. An emotional type represents the original understanding of corrective emotional experience whereby the individual experiences a new and different emotional reaction to an unsettled past event. A more specific type is the relational, whereby the individual has a transformational experience as consequence of a new way of interacting with a therapist or another. The cognitive type represents an experience of a new mental process (way of thinking) about a past event. Lastly, the behavioral type represents a new way of acting in response to something or someone.

For a corrective experience to occur, the individual must be engaged in the interaction and must be willing to take risks. It follows that the individual must feel as if the therapeutic environment is safe enough to be sufficiently vulnerable. It is therefore unlikely, if not impossible, that an individual will be able to feel and act in such a way if there is not sufficient trust, respect, and collaboration between the therapist and the individual; this is referred to as the therapeutic alliance or relationship. It is the relationship, not a specific intervention (therapeutic technique), which is of primary importance in creating the opportunity for the corrective experience.

Jeremy Connelly, MEd, and Len Sperry, MD, PhD

See also: Psychodynamic Theory; Psychotherapy; Therapeutic Alliance

Further Reading

Castonguay, Louis, and Clara Hill. *Transformation in Psychotherapy: Corrective Experiences across Cognitive Behavioral, Humanistic, and Psychodynamic Approaches*. Washington, DC: American Psychological Association, 2012.
Sperry, Len, and Jon Carlson. *How Master Therapists Work*. New York, NY: Routledge, 2014.

Council for Accreditation of Counseling and Related Educational Programs (CACREP)

Council for Accreditation of Counseling and Related Educational Programs is the accrediting agency for counseling profession. It is also known as CACREP.

Description

CACREP is a counseling-specific accrediting organization that is recognized by the Council for Higher Education Accreditation. CACREP was created in 1981 by the American Personnel and Guidance Association, which was the predecessor of the American Counseling Association. CACREP was created for the purpose of being the accrediting body for the counseling profession.

More than 30 years ago, leaders in the field of counseling donated their time, expertise, and vision to create an accrediting body that would hold the profession to a higher standard of training and education of graduate students. This includes students at both master's and doctoral levels, although doctoral accreditation came a few years later, but still dates back more than 25 years. It was hoped that by creating these standards of education and training it would, in turn, increase the level of competency of graduating professional counselors entering the field.

Within the U.S. higher education system, accreditation can be achieved in two distinct ways. One is through the university or college and the other is through a specific education program within the university or college. CACREP offers the latter, a specialized accreditation that looks solely at the preparation of graduate students within the counseling profession. However, CACREP has a fairly wide scope of accreditation, including program areas of addiction counseling; career counseling; clinical mental health counseling; marriage, couple, and family counseling; school counseling; student affairs and college counseling; and counselor education and supervision.

The accreditation process can take several years to apply (or reapply) and involves a team of CACREP counselor educators visiting the university to review its programs and ensure that it meets eight core areas of national standards in counseling, including the helping relationship, human growth and development, appraisal, research, professional orientation, social and cultural foundations, and group counseling.

Impact (Psychological Influence)

The most important factor in a counseling program is the proper preparation of students to enter the field as competent professionals who can practice independently. To achieve this, proper gatekeeping policies and procedures must be in place, as well as standards of education and training, since inadequate training can lead to psychological harm to clients, mistrust of the profession, or even ethical misconduct on behalf of the counselor. This is where CACREP standards come in. The current standards being used were updated in

2009. New revisions are being made to these standards, with an update expected in 2016.

According to several studies, the impact of accreditation can be seen in the fact that counselors who receive their training at CACREP-accredited institutions have significantly fewer ethics violations compared to non-CACREP-accredited program graduates. In addition, CACREP program graduates have been found to score higher on their licensure exams, suggesting that they are more knowledgeable in ethics and professional conduct than their non-CACREP-accredited counterparts. Notably, it has also been suggested that CACREP-accredited programs attract and retain higher-caliber students, which could also explain their compliance with ethical codes, higher scores on licensure exams, and holding to higher professional standards. This, in turn, leads to an overall higher level of competency for graduates of CACREP-accredited programs.

Mindy Parsons, PhD

See also: American Counseling Association (ACA)

Further Reading

Adkison-Bradley, Carla. "The Development of the CACREP Doctoral Standards: Counselor Education and Supervision." *Journal of Counseling and Development* 91, no. 1 (2013): 44–49.

Author. *Council for Accreditation of Counseling and Related Educational Programs (CACREP) 2009 Standards.* Alexandria, VA: Author, 2009.

Bobby, Carol L. "The Evolution of Specialties in the CACREP Standards: CACREP's Role in Unifying the Profession." *Journal of Counseling and Development* 91, no. 1 (2013): 35–43.

Even, Trigg A., and Chester R. Robinson. "The Impact of CACREP Accreditation: A Multiway Frequency Analysis of Ethics Violations and Sanctions." *Journal of Counseling and Development* 91, no. 1 (2013): 26–33.

Urofsky, Robert I., Carol L. Bobby, and Martin Ritchie. "CACREP: 30 Years of Quality Assurance in Counselor Education." *Journal of Counseling and Development* 91, no. 1 (2013): 3–5.

Organizations

Council for Accreditation of Counseling and Related Educational Programs (CACREP)
1001 North Fairfax Street, Suite 510
Alexandria, VA 22314
Telephone: (703) 535-5990
Fax: (703) 739-6209
Website: www.cacrep.org

The Council for Rehabilitation Education (CORE), which accredits graduate programs that provide academic preparation for a variety of professional rehabilitation counseling positions.
Council on Rehabilitation Education
1699 E. Woodfield Road, Suite 300
Schaumburg, IL 60173
Website: http://www.core-rehab.org/

Counseling and Counseling Psychology

Counseling and counseling psychology are mental health professions that prevent and treat mental conditions, as well as advocate for optimal human development.

Definitions

- **Behavioral psychology** is a form of psychology whose aim is to study behavioral adaptation to an environment and its stimuli.

- **Biopsychosocial model** is a way of conceptualizing (thinking about) health and illness in terms of biological, psychological, and social factors rather than purely in biological terms. It is also referred to as the biopsychosocial perspective.

- **Clinical health psychology** is the branch of psychology informed by the biopsychosocial model of health and emphasizes behavioral medicine interventions in working with psychological problems and related disability.

- **Clinical psychology** is the branch of psychology that emphasizes the diagnosis and treatment of mental disorders.

- **Cognitive behavior therapy** is a form of psychotherapy that addresses maladaptive thought distortions that lead to unwanted emotional and behavioral symptoms.

- **Cognitive psychology** is a form of psychology whose aim is to study thought and distorted patterns of thinking.

- **Evidence-based treatments** are therapeutic interventions (techniques) that scientific research demonstrates to be effective in facilitating therapeutic change. It is also known as empirically supported treatments.

- **Humanistic psychology** is an experiential form of psychology developed out of the work of Abraham Maslow and Carl Rogers, which emphasizes a client's capacity for self-actualization and unique positive personal growth.

- **Psychiatry** is the branch of medicine and form of psychology that emphasizes the medical management of psychological problems and related disability.

- **Psychoanalytic psychology** is the form of psychology largely developed by the work of Sigmund Freud, which emphasizes the conflicts and compromises between the unconscious and conscious mind.

- **Psychopathology** is a maladaptive experience of suffering or aspect of a psychological condition incorporating cause, development, structure, and consequences.

- **Psychotherapy** is a psychological method for achieving desired changes in thinking, feeling, and behavior. It is also called therapeutic counseling.

Description

Counseling and counseling psychology are two closely related fields within the mental health profession. There are significant similarities and differences between counseling and counseling psychology. The major similarity between counselors and counseling psychologists is that they both primarily practice psychotherapy. The focus of their practice is to treat as well as to prevent psychopathology and related disability. They also help clients resolve hindrances to optimal growth and development. Counselors and counseling psychologists utilize evidence-based psychotherapeutic interventions to reduce the suffering or consequences associated with psychopathology and related disability. Highly effective counselors and counseling psychologists, however, do more than reduce symptoms. For example, they are more likely to focus on solutions rather than on symptom and psychopathology. They may also assist clients in increasing their level of functioning and psychological well-being. In counseling and counseling psychology therapy sessions, the present moment almost always includes an interpersonal interaction between a trained therapist and client(s). The therapeutic relationship is the primary method for remediating the consequences of a client's mental disorder, problem, or complaint.

Counseling and counseling psychology, like clinical psychology and clinical health psychology, are informed by the biopsychosocial perspective of health and illness. Clinical health psychology emphasizes behavioral medicine in working with psychological problems and related disability. Counseling and counseling psychology, in contrast, emphasize psychotherapy or therapeutic counseling. Most counselors and counseling psychologists are integrative and value a team-based approach to mental health. They will refer clients to other mental health specialists, such as psychiatrists, for adjunctive (supportive/secondary) treatment. This holistic approach to mental health enhances the ability to predict, assess, diagnose, and alleviate psychological problems and related dysfunction.

Counseling and counseling psychology share three major traditional theoretical perspectives. These are the psychoanalytic, cognitive behavioral, and humanistic traditions. More recently, systems theory has been incorporated into many aspects of counseling. Theoretical orientations such as these, in addition to client preference, guide psychotherapeutic intervention. Counseling and counseling psychology is a system of subspecialties more than it is a single specialty within the mental health profession. The system of subspecialties continues to be developed and refined as new information is acquired via science and practice. This leads to increasing diversity in ways of conceptualizing (thinking about) client presentations and related psychotherapeutic interventions.

Development and Current Status

The terms "counselor," "psychotherapist," and "therapist" are still used interchangeably. One of the major distinctions between counseling and counseling psychology is the educational requirements necessary to become a counselor versus a counseling psychologist. The term "psychologist" in counseling psychologist has been regulated by law and is limited to use by those who have undergone specialized training. Counseling psychologists have earned a doctor of philosophy (PhD) degree or doctor of psychology (PsyD) degree in psychology and have been licensed in the state(s) in which they intend on practicing. On the other hand, counselors at least earn a master's degree in counseling and have been certified nationally or licensed by the state(s) in which they intend on practicing. These educational requirements are governed by two major professional affiliations. While highly favorable, a degree from an accredited educational program is not required for certification or licensure. The most highly acclaimed educational programs in counseling psychology are accredited by the American Psychological Association (APA). The APA was established in 1892. In 1945, APA established Division 17, the Division of Personnel and Guidance Psychologists. It was renamed the Division of Counseling Psychology in 1951. Division 17 of the APA is not as influential as it once was. For example, counseling psychologists were first utilized to give vocational guidance and advice. Today, vocational guidance is often given by non-licensed career advisors and career coaches, although some counselors and counseling psychologists still practice career counseling. When developing a career in counseling, the most prestigious counseling degrees are governed by the Council for Accreditation of Counseling and Related Educational Programs (CACREP). CACREP was established in 1981. The creation of CACREP occurred only eight years after the PsyD degree was accepted by the APA. The PsyD practitioner-scholar model, otherwise known as the Vail Model, was a departure from the PhD scientist-practitioner model, otherwise known as the Boulder Model. As counseling training programs increasingly deviated from an emphasis on research, a new field of Counselor Education was born. CACREP is gaining much legislative influence and significantly contributing to the development of the counseling profession. This trend may continue because counselors are more cost effective than counseling psychologists. Historically, however, counseling and counseling psychology have shared many similarities. The word "counselor" comes from the Latin word *consulere*, which means to consult, advise, or deliberate. Counselors and counseling psychologists tend to focus on treating clients who are from a "normal" population. In other words, counselors and counseling psychologists make themselves available to work with clients who are without serious or chronic mental illnesses. Counselors and counseling psychologists tend to treat problems of living and concerns related to individual development across the lifespan, including most mental disorders. Chronic and debilitating mental disorders and related disabilities are better treated by clinical psychologists, neuropsychologists, and the medical community.

Len Sperry, MD, PhD, and Layven Reguero, MEd

See also: Clinical Psychology; Mental Health Counselor; Psychiatrist; Psychotherapy

Further Reading

Hill, Clara E. *Helping Skills: Facilitating Exploration, Insight, and Action.* Washington, DC: American Psychological Association, 2009.

Nassar-McMillan, Sylvia C., and Spencer G. Niles. *Developing Your Identity as a Professional Counselor: Standards, Settings, and Specialties.* Belmont, CA: Brooks/Cole, 2010.

Neukrug, Edward S. *A Brief Orientation to Counseling: Professional Identity, History, and Standards.* Belmont, CA: Brooks/Cole, 2013.

Counterdependent Personality Disorder

Counterdependent personality disorder is a mental disorder characterized by denial of dependency on others and an unwillingness to ask for help when in need.

Definitions

- **Avoidant personality disorder** is a mental disorder characterized by a pattern of social withdrawal, feelings of inadequacy, and oversensitivity to negative evaluation.

- **Codependent** is an emotional and behavioral condition that affects an individual's ability to have a healthy relationship because he or she often forms or maintains relationships that are one-sided, emotionally destructive, and often abusive.

- **Depression** is an emotional state characterized by feelings of sadness, guilt, or reduced ability to enjoy life. It is recognized as a mental disorder when it becomes significantly distressing and disrupts daily life.

- **DSM** stands for the *Diagnostic and Statistical Manual of Mental Disorders*, which is the handbook mental health professionals use to diagnose mental disorders. The current edition (fifth) is known as DSM-5.

- **Narcissistic personality disorder** is a mental disorder characterized by a pattern of grandiosity, lack of empathy, and need to be admired by others.

- **Personality disorder** is a long-standing pattern of maladaptive (problematic) behaviors, thoughts, and emotions that deviates from the accepted norms of an individual's culture.

- **PDM** stands for the *Psychodynamic Diagnostic Manual* and is a diagnostic framework that characterizes individuals in terms of their psychodynamics (forces that determine personality).

- **Psychotherapy** is a psychological method for achieving desired changes in thinking, feeling, and behavior. It is also referred to as therapeutic counseling.

Description and Diagnosis

Counterdependent personality disorder is a personality disorder characterized by difficulty being close to others, a strong need to be right all of the time, self-centeredness, resistance in asking for help, and expectations of perfection in self and others. Individuals with this disorder have extreme discomfort when appearing weak or vulnerable and have difficulty relaxing. They are often addicted to several activities (e.g., constantly engaged in work or exercise). They tend to act strong while pushing others away, and exhibit extreme grandiose behaviors, which is a feature of narcissistic personality disorder. They often avoid contact with others (e.g., avoidant personality disorder), particularly out of fear of being crowded, and this can lead to emotional isolation and depression. The counterdependent male may take pride in himself not needing warmth, affection, or support in any relationship. He takes pleasure in being tough and independent. The counterdependent female may take on the attributes of a false self or male persona (image). The independent behavior of the counterdependent individual can act as a powerful lure for a codependent. An individual who is codependent exhibits symptoms of having low self-esteem and poor boundaries (limits), and is a people pleaser and caretaker. As a couple, codependent and counterdependent individuals can often switch roles.

In 1993, Robert Bornstein (1948–) described that there is a continuum from maladaptive dependency (submissiveness) through healthy interdependency (connectedness) to inflexible independence (unconnected detachment). Some individuals at the inflexibility end of the spectrum have powerful dependent longings that they keep out of awareness by denial and reaction formation. Essentially, this develops into having a personality disorder concealed by pseudo-independence. They define themselves in relationships as the individual whom others depend on and take pleasure for being able to take care of themselves. Individuals with this disorder may look skeptically at expressions of need and may regard evidence of emotional vulnerability in themselves or others with contempt. Often, these individuals have some secret of dependency (e.g., addiction to a substance, a partner, an ideology). Some individuals have a tendency toward illness or injury that gives them a justifiable reason to be cared for by others.

According to the *Psychodynamic Diagnostic Manual*, the psychopathic personality disorder is diagnosable by the following criteria. Individuals are possibly more aggressive than openly dependent individuals. They are preoccupied with demonstrating a lack of dependence (e.g., shameful dependence). Individuals exhibit contempt for others and are in denial of weaker emotions, such as sadness, fear, longing, and envy. Their basic belief is that they do not need anyone. Their view of others is that everyone needs and depends on them and requires them in their lives in order to be strong and succeed. Furthermore, these individuals defend themselves through denial (PDM Task Force, 2006).

Treatment

Treatment for individuals with this disorder tends to be challenging. Counterdependent individuals rarely seek psychotherapy in order to avoid the possibility of regression. By eluding psychotherapy, an individual with this disorder can avoid discussing feelings as well as attempting to control the therapist in order to maintain his or her sense of independence. However, if an individual has a partner who is likely feeling a lack of true intimacy, the partner may be forced or given an ultimatum in participating in psychotherapy. While in treatment, individuals with this disorder need assistance in accepting their dependent desires as a natural part of being human before they can develop a healthy balance between separateness and connectedness. Progress in therapy can occur only when the individual can reflect on and mourn his or her early unmet dependency needs and become less defensive (PDM Task Force, 2006).

Len Sperry, MD, PhD, and
Elizabeth Smith Kelsey, PhD

See also: Avoidant Personality Disorder; Depression; *Diagnostic and Statistical Manual of Mental Disorders* (DSM); Narcissistic Personality Disorder; Personality Disorders; *Psychodynamic Diagnostic Manual* (PDM); Psychotherapy

Further Reading

American Psychiatric Association. *Diagnostic and Statistical Manual of Mental Disorders*, 5th ed. Arlington, VA: American Psychiatric Association, 2013.

Bornstein, Robert. *The Dependent Personality Disorder.* New York, NY: The Guilford Press, 1993.

Huprich, Steven K. *Psychodynamic Therapy: Conceptual and Empirical Foundations.* New York, NY: Routledge, 2008.

PDM Task Force. *Psychodynamic Diagnostic Manual (PDM).* Silver Spring, MD: Alliance of Psychoanalytic Organizations, 2006.

Weinhold, Janae B., Barry K. Weinhold, and John Bradshaw. *The Flight from Intimacy: Healing Your Relationship of Counter-dependency—The Other Side of Co-dependency.* Novato, CA: New World Library, 2008.

Counterphobic Personality Disorder

Counterphobic personality disorder is a mental disorder characterized by actively seeking out that which is feared.

Definitions

- **Anxiety** is a negative emotional state characterized by feelings of nervousness, worry, and apprehension about imagined danger.

- **Depression** is an emotional state characterized by feelings of sadness, low self-esteem, guilt, or reduced ability to enjoy life.

- **DSM** stands for the *Diagnostic and Statistical Manual of Mental Disorders*, which is the handbook mental health professionals use to diagnose mental disorders. The current edition (fifth) is known as DSM-5.

- **Obsessive-compulsive disorder** is a mental disorder characterized by unwanted and repeated thoughts and feelings (obsessions), or behaviors that one feels driven to perform (compulsions). It is commonly referred to as OCD.

- **Personality disorder** is a long-standing pattern of maladaptive (problematic) behavior, thoughts, and emotions that deviates from the accepted norms of an individual's culture.

- **PDM** stands for the *Psychodynamic Diagnostic Manual* and is a diagnostic framework that characterizes individuals in terms of their psychodynamics.

- **Psychotherapy** is a psychological method for achieving desired changes in thinking, feeling, and behavior. It is also referred to as therapeutic counseling.

Description and Diagnosis

Counterphobic personality disorder is an uncommon personality disorder. It is characterized by actively seeking out fearful objects and situations. Those with this disorder are attracted to dangerous situations, thrive on taking risks, and have a reputation for intimidating others when exposed to immediate danger. They tend to put themselves in dangerous situations that are so irresistible and forceful that they cannot resist dangerous opportunities to reveal their fearlessness. They may also exhibit magical thinking. For example, they may believe that thinking or wishing for something can cause it to occur. Remarkably, individuals with this disorder have great confidence that they are safe no matter what danger they encounter.

Some children and adolescents appear to have a high threshold for stimulation and the need to deny any fear. Therapists describe these individuals as those who cannot swim yet will jump into the deep end of a swimming pool. Adolescents with this disorder often engage in reckless driving, take drugs on occasion, and engage in high-risk sexual behavior. Younger children with this disorder are often faced with a sense of powerlessness or fear of being lifeless. On the more adaptive (functional) end of the spectrum, children and adolescents become involved in risky activities but in a more controlled way. At the maladaptive (dysfunctional) end of the spectrum, children and adolescents with this disorder tease with the idea of potentially suicidal behavior (PDM Task Force, 2006).

According to the *Psychodynamic Diagnostic Manual*, counterphobic personality disorder is diagnosable by the following criteria. Individuals are preoccupied with safety and danger. Their contributing maturational patterns are unknown. Their main affects or feelings are contempt for others and denial of fear. They view themselves as fearless and able to face anything without fear. They tend to view others as easily frightened and that others admire their courage. Often,

those with this disorder defend themselves through denial, through projection (e.g., making a prediction on known evidence or observations), and by means of defensiveness (PDM Task Force, 2006).

Treatment

Treatment for individuals with this disorder tends to be challenging. Individuals with counterphobic personality disorder rarely seek psychotherapy. However, they may participate in psychotherapy to address symptomatic problems such as depression and obsessive-compulsive disorder. Treatment is also difficult because of their need to deny ordinary anxieties and their tendency to present themselves with a sense of boldness that makes talking with a therapist about any feelings difficult. Therapists may experience anxiety when these individuals talk about their risk-taking behaviors and irritation when they describe their sense of having unlimited power (PDM Task Force, 2006).

Len Sperry, MD, PhD, and
Elizabeth Smith Kelsey, PhD

See also: Anxiety Disorders in Adults; Depression; *Diagnostic and Statistical Manual of Mental Disorders* (DSM); Obsessive-Compulsive Disorder (OCD); Personality Disorders; *Psychodynamic Diagnostic Manual* (PDM); Psychotherapy

Further Reading
American Psychiatric Association. *Diagnostic and Statistical Manual of Mental Disorders*, 5th ed.. Arlington, VA: American Psychiatric Association, 2013.

Millon, Theodore, Carrie M. Millon, Sarah Meagher, Seth Grossman, and Rowena Ramnath. *Personality Disorders in Modern Life*. Hoboken, NJ: John Wiley & Sons, 2006.

PDM Task Force. *Psychodynamic Diagnostic Manual (PDM)*. Silver Spring, MD: Alliance of Psychoanalytic Organizations, 2006.

Couples Therapy

Couples therapy is a form of psychotherapy that focuses on strengthening the relationship bond and resolving conflicts between couples of all types.

Definitions

- **Atheoretical** refers to untested treatments that are not based on theory.

- **Cohabitation** is to live together with someone in a marriage, or marriage like, sexual relationship.

- **Conjoint therapy** takes place when both relationship partners are present in a therapy session.

- **Couples** refer to two people in an established married or unmarried partnership and may include, lesbian, gay, bisexual, transgender, and heterosexual couples.

- **Infidelity** is the act of having a romantic or sexual relationship with someone other than a wife, husband, or committed partner; it is also referred to as cheating, adultery, or having an affair.

- **In-laws** are the people you become related to through marriage, that is, the mother of a wife is referred to as the husband's mother-in-law.

- **LGBT** is an abbreviation for lesbian, gay, bisexual, and transgender couples.

- **Marriage and family therapist** is a protected professional title that designates an individual as meeting the educational standards set forth by the Commission on Accreditation for Marriage and Family Therapy Education.

- **Marriage counseling** is another term for couples counseling.

- **Psychotherapy** is a general term referring to a variety of talking treatments aimed at strengthening mental health, emotional, or relational problems.

- **Theory** refers to a body of knowledge, or set of principles, that explains the phenomenon in question.

Description

Couples therapy (CT) is a form of psychotherapy provided to all types of couples, including lesbian, gay, bisexual, transgender, and heterosexual couples. Historically referred to as "marital" or "marriage" counseling, the term "couples therapy" is increasingly becoming the preferred term. The use of the term "couples" recognizes that many couples cohabitate together while remaining unmarried.

The American Association for Marriage and Family Therapy (AAMFT) is the professional association, which represents over 25,000 marriage and family therapists. The AAMFT also serves as the accrediting organization for graduate training education in marriage and family counseling. Licensure as a marriage and family therapist is regulated by individual states.

Trained therapists provide CT, with most states requiring a graduate mental health degree and state license in order to provide CT. Therapist includes clinical psychologist, mental health counselors, clinical social workers, marriage and family therapist, and pastoral counselors. Couples counseling aims to assist couples strengthen their bond, resolve conflicts, and improve their relationship. CT is usually short term consisting of 12 to 20 sessions. There are a variety of therapeutic approaches and techniques to CT. Couples seek counseling for a variety of reasons, including relationship distress, improve relationship satisfaction, strengthen communication and problem-solving skills, working through issues related to infidelity, sexual difficulties and compatibilities, financial stresses, conflicts, parenting, and in-law issues.

Four phases in the development of CT have been identified, with each phase significantly influencing the expansion of methods and understanding of couples. Phase one (1930 to 1963), the "Atheoretical Marriage Counseling Formation" phase, was the pioneering phase of modern-day CT. Counseling was not based on any theories or scientific understanding of couples. Interventions consisted mostly of advice giving, extoling the virtues of family life, and educating couples on their legal and social obligations.

Phase two (1931–1966), the "Psychoanalytic Experimentation" phase, began to question the effectiveness of a traditional psychoanalytic approach in which partners were seen individually with the hope that as they each progressed through psychoanalysis, their stress would decrease and the relationship would benefit. Psychoanalysis was grounded in the belief that psychological and social dysfunctions were due solely to problems within the individual. Couples who were seen individually rarely, if ever, described a shared event, such as a conflict, in the same way. At the time no theories existed that addressed how to understand multiple perspectives and help multiple people at the same time in a therapy session. This led to conjoint marital therapy in which two individuals are seen at the same time. Conjoint therapy was revolutionary from a psychoanalytic perspective. Phase two was a time of tremendous growth and theoretical development in understanding couples and how to help them. In 1942, the American Association of Marriage Counselors was formed and later renamed as the American Association for Marriage and Family Therapy.

Phase three (1963–1985) is the "Family Therapy Incorporation" stage. Theorists were no longer limited to a psychoanalytic perspective and began to focus on family dynamics. During this time, family therapy became the predominate focus of developing psychotherapies and marital counseling was largely absorbed into the family therapy movement. There was a tremendous increase in the development of theories during this time that focused on understanding the complex interactions and behaviors of families. The years 1975 to 1985 are considered the golden age of family therapy and several groundbreaking theories were developed. Four highly influential clinical family theorists include Don Jackson (Family Rules: Marital Quid Pro Quo), Virginia Satir (Family Therapy: Concepts and Methods), Murray Bowen (Family Systems Theory and Practice), and Jay Haley (Strategic Family Therapy). These, and many other theorists, incorporated ideas into how couples behaved in the family, and toward each other, and what impact the marital relationship had on healthy family functioning.

Phase four (1986–present) is the "Refinement, Extension, Diversification, and Integration" phase. Emerging out of the family therapy movement, CT reasserted its existence in the mid-1980s. Continuing to the present CT theory, research and the development of practical psychotherapies to helping couples have become increasingly refined and integrated with other forms of psychotherapy. For instance, emotion focused couple therapy and behavioral couple therapy are well-established forms of CT first developed in the 1980s and further refined through substantial research support. CT has also been integrated with psychotherapies originally developed as individual therapies such as solution focused therapy.

Couples therapy, in all its forms, has been shown to be effective. Research has consistently established that couples who receive any form of CT are better off after treatment than couples who received no treatment. Although there are numerous types of CT, few studies have examined which models are more effective when compared against each other.

Steven R. Vensel, PhD

See also: Bowen Family Systems Theory; Conjoint Family Therapy; Conjoint Sexual Therapy; Marriage and Family Therapist; Satir, Virginia (1916–1988)

Further Reading

AAMFT. American Association of Marriage and Family Therapy. Accessed March, 27, 2014. http://www .aamft.org/iMIS15/AAMFT/About/About_AAMFT/ Content/About_AAMFT/About_AAMFT.aspx?hke y=a8d047de-5bf7-40cd-9551-d626e2490a25.

Gurman, Alan S. "Couple Therapy Research and Practice of Couple Therapy: Can We Talk?" *Family Process* 50, no. 3 (2011): 280–292.

Gurman, Alan S. "A Framework for the Comparative Study of Couple Therapy: History, Models, and Applications." In *Clinical Handbook of Couple Therapy*, 4th ed., edited by A. S. Gurman, pp. 1–30. New York, NY: Guilford, 2008.

Gurman, Alan S., and Peter Fraenkel. "The History of Couple Therapy: A Millennial Review." *Family Process* 41, no. 2 (2002): 199–260.

Covert Sensitization

Covert sensitization is a therapeutic technique in which an undesirable behavior is associated with an unpleasant image in order to try to control or eliminate the undesirable behavior.

Description

Covert sensitization is used in behavior and cognitive behavior therapy (CBT). By using this technique, the therapist helps the client identify the problem and then uses negative images or experiences to prevent it from happening in the future. The hallmark of covert sensitization is that it happens in the imagination, which makes it covert. Examples of such techniques would be things like vomiting due to overeating or excessive consumption of alcohol in order to reduce addictive behaviors. During treatment, the client is encouraged to imagine the undesirable behavior and then associate it with an unpleasant or disgusting consequence.

The aim in covert sensitization is for the client to move away from his or her present thoughts and behaviors. For example, a client believes what he or she is doing is wrong or undesirable. Then the goal is for the client to shift his or her beliefs about the experience through feeling different unpleasant physical effects. A client who wants to quit smoking may be encouraged to imagine puffing on a cigarette and then associate it with a picture of black and decaying lung tissue. The aversive images are only powerful when they are based on things that the client finds truly negative. This is a form of imaged aversion therapy, and it is based on the idea that behavior is learned and can therefore be changed.

Development

In the 1960s psychologist Joseph Cautela was the first to outline a procedure for covert sensitization. He and his colleague Albert Kearney later published *The Covert Conditioning Handbook* in 1986. This handbook discussed the technique based on research investigations and case studies.

Because it does not require drugs and is relatively simple to implement, covert sensitization has been applied over the years. The technique has been used with many problematic and undesirable behaviors. Among them are alcoholism, smoking, gambling, obesity, and various sexual dysfunctions. Many programs using covert sensitization have had positive clinical results.

Prior to 1974, homosexuality was still identified as a mental illness. During that time covert sensitization was one of the approaches used to try to change or convert sexual orientation. Even though the majority of mental health professionals have changed their stance on this, there are still sexual reorientation or reparation programs that target the homosexual population. Covert sensitization is still used by fundamentalist religious groups, for example, who adhere to the belief that nonheterosexual orientation is a mental illness and continue to use this as a therapeutic technique.

Current Status

Covert sensitization continues to be applied both in therapy and in other fields. This includes people who experience a wide variety of psychosocial problems, from smoking cessation to sexual impulse control, even to drug addiction. One of its appeals is that it avoids the risks involved in drug and pharmacological interventions by using visualization and imagery. Covert sensitization has been used in the treatment of alcoholism, but the results remain controversial.

One critique of covert sensitization is that it does not concern itself with the roots of undesirable behaviors. Many believe that because of this, underlying psychological motivation can persist and therefore real change does not occur. The concern then is that problem thoughts and behaviors can resurface leading to a renewal of problems when and if the aversive imagery loses its power.

Alexandra Cunningham, PhD, and William M. Cunningham, MA

See also: Aversion Therapy; Behavior Therapy; Cognitive Behavior Therapy

Further Reading
Maccio, Elaine M. "Self-Reported Sexual Orientation and Identity before and after Sexual Reorientation Therapy." *Journal of Gay & Lesbian Mental Health* 15, no. 3 (2011): 242–259.
McGrath, Robert J., Georgia F. Cumming, Brenda L. Burchard, and Stephen Zeoli. *Current Practices in Canadian Sexual Abuser Treatment Programs: The Safer Society 2009 Survey*. Canada: Public Safety, 2010.
Witkiewitz, Katie, and G. Alan Marlatt. "Behavioral Therapy across the Spectrum." *Alcohol Research & Health* 33, no. 4 (2011): 313.

Crisis Housing

"Crisis housing" refers to programs that provide short-term housing or residential assistance to people suffering from emergencies or serious mental health issues.

Definition

- **Crisis** is an event, or series of events, in a person's life marked by danger, instability, and chaos that negatively impacts his or her life.

Description

Within the mental health community, crisis housing is a temporary residence or institution for the treatment of people suffering from a recent crisis. Although sometimes referred to as crisis group homes, they differ from therapeutic group homes in their intent, focus, and duration of stay. In many communities, crisis housing has been therapeutically successful. It has also been found to be a cost-effective alternative to expensive psychiatric inpatient hospitalization. The provision of crisis housing has led to a reduction in the number of people who need to be admitted to more traditional clinical settings.

Development

Crisis housing began as a service to help people who were not able to find safe or healthy shelter. Based on emergency situations, crisis housing applies to victims of man-made and natural disasters. But crisis housing has also been important as a response to social, familial, and personal problems for some. It can provide a safe environment for those who are threatened by other people, like abusers, or by their own internal psychological problems, like psychosis.

Beginning in the 1980s, many local communities and governments began to provide crisis housing and case management services as an alternative to psychiatric hospitalization. Crisis housing has taken many forms, from conversion of hotels to refitted private homes. Although not without issues, crisis housing has proved effective in providing space and opportunity for treatment.

One example of a program that uses crisis housing is the Assertive Community Treatment program. This serves as an intervention program that treats people with serious mental illness in a comprehensive, multidisciplinary setting outside of a clinical or hospital setting. The model originated in the late 1970s with the Program of Assertive Community Treatment in Madison, Wisconsin. It grew out of the need to find community-based services as deinstitutionalization, or removal from clinical hospital settings, became the norm. Assertive Community Treatment is often referred to as a hospital without walls.

Current Status

Studies have shown that patients who have the opportunity to live in crisis housing tend to engage in treatment more effectively and have better outcomes. Crisis housing has been publicly supported in many states for patients with mental health issues. This is because it reduces the cost of treatment by avoiding expensive hospital or inpatient programs. Crisis housing can provide clients with the opportunity for a comprehensive approach to treatment.

Alexandra Cunningham, PhD, and
William M. Cunningham, MA

See also: Deinstitutionalization; Hospitalization

Further Reading

DePastino, Todd. *Citizen Hobo: How a Century of Homelessness Shaped America*. Chicago, IL: The University of Chicago Press, 2003.

Honberg, Ron, Sita Diehl, Angela Kimball, Darcy Gruttadaro, and Mike Fitzpatrick. *State Mental Health Cuts: A National Crisis*. A report by NAMI: The National Alliance on Mental Illness, March 2011.

Stone, Michael E. *Shelter Poverty: New Ideas on Housing Affordability*. Philadelphia, PA: Temple University Press, 1993.

Crisis Intervention

Crisis intervention is a fast assessment and response to help people involved in a crisis situation cope and move toward physical and emotional resolution.

Definition

- **Crisis** is an event, or series of events, in a person's life marked by danger, instability, and chaos that negatively impacts his or her life.

Description

Crisis intervention usually occurs when an individual's or group of people's ability to cope has been exhausted or destroyed. Generally, crises usually require outside support where physical, psychological, and social resources are needed to help people overcome intolerable situations. The crisis could be an individual trauma, like suicide, or a natural disaster, like a tornado, or a man-made disaster, such as terrorism. An example of a crisis is the Japanese tsunami of 2011. This natural event caused personal, civic, and regional crises that affected the people directly and the country itself could not address alone. They needed help from others to restore calm and order and even provide both basic and long-term social needs for those in the disaster or crisis zone.

The simplest approach to crisis intervention is the so-called ABC method. A is establishing and maintaining contact, B is identifying the problem clearly, and C is developing coping mechanisms. For health-care professionals the more common situations that demand crisis intervention are based around individual and family issues, horrific events such as death, sexual assault, or other violent crimes. These events shake people so deeply that they are robbed of their usual ability to assess and respond on their own. In this situation crisis intervention is often called crisis counseling and is to be conducted only by those specifically trained to provide this kind of treatment.

Development

There are individual organizations, such as the Red Cross, that have long helped people in disaster situations. The history of crisis intervention as a distinct concept dates back to the 1942 Boston Cocoanut Grove nightclub fire. The fire killed almost 500 people and plunged the community into a traumatic state. Eric Lindemann and Gerald Caplan, known as the fathers of crisis intervention, formed modern crisis intervention based on the response to that experience.

In 1963 federal law mandated the creation of community mental health centers to assist people in crisis. But the early success of these efforts was limited. It was in the late 1970s that the Federal Emergency Management Agency (FEMA) was established by the government. FEMA was created to plan, coordinate, and deliver emergency assistance in cases of widespread social need.

While there are different approaches to crisis intervention, the ACT process created by Albert Roberts, PhD, has been widely used. It has been applied to significant crisis events such as the response to the 9/11 terror attacks. Roberts recommends that those professionals who intervene should take specific steps when intervening to help with a crisis. The first step is to assess the deadly danger or lethality of the situation and the mental state of those involved. The next step is to establish rapport with and get the attention of those impacted by the crisis in order to connect with them. After this it is important to identify the major issues involved and spend time processing and dealing with the feelings of those affected. Next, professionals should apply some immediate emotional coping mechanisms and temporary or partial responses to the event. Once these short-term solutions are put in place, the next step is to develop a long-term action plan, including decisions about when the intervention should end and what will be done to follow up.

Crisis or critical incident debriefing is widely implemented immediately after a disaster. It was used in the crisis event of the mass shooting at a school in Columbine, Colorado, in 1999. Although helpful in the short-term, crisis intervention has been critiqued for being insufficient for long-term problems. This is especially true for those who have symptoms of post-traumatic stress disorder, which may show up only months after a traumatic event occurs.

Current Status

As the world continues to change politically, socially, and environmentally, crises will continue to occur. There is no doubt that crisis intervention skills will continue to be needed on many levels. Although key elements of response by professionals include critical incident debriefing and stabilization, longer-term interventions may also be needed to service those more severely or even chronically affected.

The success of crisis intervention efforts depends on three things. It is important that the intervention be provided in a timely, effective, and well-trained fashion. This should involve not only mental health professionals but police, hot-line operators, clergy, government workers, and more. Crisis prevention and intervention is an important focus for those professionals dealing with people engaging in risky behavior. Often in the workplace, the skills of professionals in human resources are only brought to bear after a traumatic event has occurred.

Alexandra Cunningham, PhD, and William M. Cunningham, MA

See also: Crisis housing

Further Reading

James, Richard K., and Burl E. Gilliland. *Crisis Intervention Strategies*. Independence, KY: Brooks/Cole, 2013.

Roberts, Albert R., ed. *Crisis Intervention Handbook: Assessment, Treatment, and Research*. London, UK: Oxford University Press, 2005.

Cults

"Cults" refer to religious and social fringe groups regarded by the majority culture as engaging in sinister, strange, exploitive, and psychologically harmful beliefs and practices.

Description

The term "cults" has been widely used in popular culture in describing destructive fringe religious and social groups. Religious researchers prefer to use the phrase "new religious movement" (NRM), recognizing that not all NRMs are harmful to their followers. Here "cult" will be used to refer to intense groups, frequently religious but not rooted in a mainstream religion, formed around a controlling and manipulative charismatic leader, which demand unwavering devotion, and pose a physical, psychological, or exploitive danger to their followers.

Impact (Psychological Influence)

Thousands of different cults exist. Destructive cults include apocalyptic groups such as "Heaven's Gate"

in which 38 followers committed mass suicide after the UFO that was to usher in the end of world failed to arrive. Other cults have political, social and religious, motivations, such as the "People's Temple" infamous for the 1978 "Jonestown Massacre" in which over 900 followers committed "revolutionary suicide" by drinking poisoned drink mix at the urging of the Reverend Jim Jones. Although "Flavor Aid" was the actual drink brand used in the poisonings, the phrase "Don't drink the Kool-Aid" became culturally iconic when referring to unquestioned beliefs related to political or religious agendas.

Cult members use a variety of techniques to control and manipulate potential followers. Cults are usually isolated and exert considerable control over communication with the outside world. They use intense indoctrination techniques often referred to by the popular culture as "brain washing" or "mind control." They employ intense and cunning emotional manipulation; use guilt, shame, and fear tactics; subject recruits to emotionally charged meetings and rituals lasting for hours; and use sleep deprivation and other forms of influence to convert recruits. Cults dictate and control how followers should think, act, and feel. These practices are so effective that followers give up all they have and all they are to the cult.

Cults most frequently target young adults for recruitment. This is a stage in life when young adults are seeking their own self and spiritual identity distinct from that of their parents. This leaves them especially vulnerable to charismatic leaders who "have all the answers" and "know the one way." Young adults are emotionally manipulated and made to feel especially understood, accepted, and cared for increasing their vulnerability to recruitment and eventual conversion.

Cults are powerful and destructive social phenomenon, and awareness of their tactics is especially important for young adults. Becoming knowledgeable of the beliefs and practices of any religious group, or NRM, before becoming involved is an essential safeguard of one's spiritual and psychological well-being.

Steven R. Vensel, PhD

See also: Identity and Identity Formation; Spiritual Identity

Further Reading

Bohm, Jonathan, and Laurence Alison. "An Exploratory Study in Methods of Distinguishing Destructive Cults." *Psychology, Crime & Law* 7 (2001): 133–165.

Martin, Walter. *Kingdom of the Cults*. Grand Rapids, MI: Bethany House, 2003.

Walsh, Yvonne. "Deconstructing 'Brainwashing' within Cults as an Aid to Counselling Psychologists." *Counselling Psychology Quarterly* 14, no. 2 (2001): 119–128.

Cultural Competence

Cultural competence is the ability to interact effectively with individuals from other cultures. It is also known as multicultural competence and intercultural competence.

Definitions

- **Cultural competence** is the capacity to recognize, respect, and respond with appropriate words and actions to the needs and concerns of individuals from different ethnicities, social classes, genders, ages, or religions.

- **Cultural encapsulation** is a way of relating to another from one's own biased worldview and perspective.

- **Cultural incompetence** refers to acting from one's culturally encapsulated perspective and failing to consider the other's worldview.

- **Culture** refers to the values, norms, and traditions that affect how individuals of a particular group perceive, think, act, interact, and make judgments about their world.

- **Multicultural counseling** is an approach to counseling clients that is responsive to their cultural beliefs and the effect these beliefs can have on their treatment.

- **Worldview** refers to basic assumptions that individuals and groups have about other people and the world. It defines one's cultural perspective.

Description

Cultural competence is increasingly important in the helping professions of counseling and psychotherapy. It is the capacity to recognize and respond appropriately to the needs and concerns of individuals from other cultures. There are four dimensions of cultural competence: cultural knowledge, cultural awareness, cultural sensitivity, and cultural action. Briefly, cultural knowledge is acquaintance with facts about ethnicity, social class, acculturation, religion, gender, and age. Cultural awareness builds on cultural knowledge. It includes the capacity to recognize a cultural problem or issue in a specific client situation. Cultural sensitivity is an extension of cultural awareness. It also involves the capacity to anticipate likely consequences of a particular cultural problem or issue and to respond empathically. Cultural action follows from cultural sensitivity. It is the capacity to translate cultural sensitivity into action that results in an effective outcome. The higher one's level of culturally competence increases the more likely one will make appropriate decisions and take effective cultural action in a given situation.

Possessing only basic cultural knowledge, awareness, sensitivity and skillful, actions is insufficient to function effectively in a multicultural world. A low level of cultural competence is evident when one demonstrates deficits in these requisite components, is unable to perceive the need to apply them, or is unable to do so. In contrast, a high level of cultural competence is evident when one knows, recognizes, respects, accepts and welcomes, and takes effective and appropriate skillful action with regard to another's culture. In other words, cultural competence requires both sufficiency of its basic components and the proficiency to implement them.

Individuals vary in their capacity for demonstrating cultural competence. In fact, cultural competence has been conceptualized as a continuum ranging from a very low level of cultural competence at one end to a very high level of cultural competence at the other end. For example, a low level of cultural competence is called cultural incompetence. It reflects a lack of or minimal acquaintance and recognition of cultural knowledge and cultural awareness. Because there is a lack of cultural sensitivity, one's cultural decisions and actions are likely to be inappropriate, ineffective, or even harmful or destructive. Individuals are likely to be culturally encapsulated. Besides a failure to understand the worldview and cultural identity of another, it is the failure to incorporate whatever cultural knowledge one might have of the other into interactions with others. In contrast, a high level of cultural competence reflects more cultural knowledge and awareness, and there is no indication of cultural encapsulation.

Developments and Current Status

Awareness of cultural factors in mental health is the basis of what is called the multicultural movement in counseling. In 1962, psychologist Gilbert Wrenn (1902–2001) described the culturally encapsulated counselor and how such counselors negatively impacted culturally different or minority clients. The movement gained momentum with psychologist Stanley Sue's (n.d.) 1977 article in which he indicated that minority clients received unequal and poor mental health services. In 1978 psychologist Derald Wing Sue (n.d.) described the term "worldview" and its influence on counseling. Soon after, the first edition of Derald Sue's book *Counseling the Culturally Different* appeared in 1981. It provided background on several different minority groups and became the model for similar books. Sue's book is now in its sixth edition. It has the distinction of being the most frequently cited publication in multicultural psychology. This book is estimated to be used in nearly 50% of the graduate counseling and psychology courses. In 1992, Darryl Sue and colleagues identified 31 standards of cultural competence arranged in three categories: awareness of one's own worldview, knowledge of the worldviews of culturally different clients, and skills needed to work with such clients. In a recent series of articles and book chapters, psychiatrist and psychologist Len Sperry (1943–) distinguished the four components of cultural competency: cultural knowledge, cultural awareness, cultural sensitivity, and cultural action.

Len Sperry, MD, PhD

See also: Acculturation and Assimilation; Culturally Sensitive Treatment; Culture

Further Reading

Lee, Courtland, ed. *Multicultural Issues in Counseling*, 4th ed. Alexandria, VA: American Counseling Association, 2013.

Paniagua, Freddy A. *Assessing and Treating Cultural Diverse Clients: A Practical Guide*. Thousand Oaks, CA: Sage, 2005.

Sperry, Len. "Cultural Competence: A Primer." *Journal of Individual Psychology* 68 (2012): 310–320.

Sue, Derald W., Patricia Arredondo, and Robert J. Davis. "Multicultural Competencies and Standards: A Call to the Profession." *Journal of Counseling & Development* 70 (1992): 477–486.

Sue, Derald W., and David Sue. *Counseling the Culturally Different: Theory and Practice*, 6th ed. Hoboken, NJ: John Wiley & Sons, 2012.

Culturally Sensitive Treatment

Culturally sensitive treatment is a medical or psychotherapeutic treatment that is sensitive to the client's culture.

Definitions

- **Acculturation** is the degree to which individuals integrate new cultural patterns into their original cultural patterns.

- **Clinician credibility** is the culturally diverse individual's perception that the practitioner is effective and trustworthy based on how the practitioner instills faith, trust, and confidence in the client for the treatment process and outcomes.

- **Cultural identity** is an individual's self-identification and perceived sense of belonging to a particular culture or place of origin.

- **Cultural sensitivity** refers to practitioners' awareness of cultural variables in themselves and in their clients that may affect the professional relationship and treatment process.

- **Culture** refers to the values, norms, and traditions that affect how individuals of a particular group perceive, think, act, interact, and make judgments about their world.

Description

Even though most practitioners believe that culturally sensitive treatments are important in providing effective care to culturally diverse clients, very few practitioners actually provide such treatment. The most common reason for this omission is that few have had formal training and experience with these competencies. Such treatments include cultural intervention, culturally sensitive therapy, and culturally sensitive interventions.

Developments and Current Status

A cultural intervention is an intervention that is useful in effecting a specified change because it is consistent with the individual's belief system regarding healing. Examples include healing circles, healing prayer, exorcism, and involvement of traditional healers from that client's culture.

Culturally sensitive therapy is a psychotherapeutic intervention that directly focuses on the individual's cultural beliefs, customs, and attitudes. Since this therapy utilizes traditional healing methods, such approaches are appealing to certain clients. Examples include "cuento therapy," which focuses on "familismo" and "personalismo" through the use of folk tales ("cuentos"). "Morita therapy" is a therapy used for various disorders ranging from shyness to schizophrenia and is particularly effective in those with lower levels of acculturation.

A culturally sensitive intervention is a psychotherapeutic intervention that has been adapted or modified to be responsive to the cultural characteristics of a particular client. Cognitive behavior therapy is the most common of such intervention because it is structured, educationally focused, and easily modified to be culturally sensitive. For example, disputation and cognitive restructuring are not effective with individuals with lower levels of acculturation. However, culturally sensitive problem solving, skills training, and cognitive replacement interventions are more appropriate and effective.

Len Sperry, MD, PhD

See also: Cognitive Behavior Therapy; Cultural Competence; Culture

Further Reading

Hays, P., and G. Iwanasa, eds. *Culturally Responsive Cognitive-Behavioral Therapy: Assessment, Practice, and Supervision.* Washington, DC: American Psychological Association, 2006.

Paniagua, F. *Assessing and Treating Cultural Diverse Clients: A Practical Guide.* Thousand Oaks, CA: Sage, 2005.

Sperry, L. *Core Competencies in Counseling and Psychotherapy: Becoming a Highly Competent and Effective Therapist.* New York, NY: Routledge, 2010.

Culture

"Culture" refers to the values, norms, and traditions that affect how individuals of a particular group perceive, think, act, interact, and make judgments about their world.

Definitions

- **Acculturation** is the degree to which individuals integrate new cultural patterns into their original cultural patterns.

- **Acculturative stress** is the stress experienced when struggling to adapt to a new culture psychologically and socially and its impact on health status.

- **Clinician credibility** is the culturally diverse individual's perception that the practitioner is effective and trustworthy based on how the practitioner instills faith, trust, and confidence in the client for the treatment process and outcomes.

- **Cultural competence** is the capacity to recognize, respect, and respond with appropriate words and actions to the needs and concerns of individuals from different ethnicities, social classes, genders, ages, or religions.

- **Cultural diversity** is the presence of a number of diverse or different cultures within a society. It is also known as cultural pluralism.

- **Cultural identity** is an individual's self-identification and perceived sense of belonging to a particular culture or place of origin.

- **Cultural sensitivity** is the practitioners' awareness of cultural variables in themselves and in their clients that may affect the professional relationship and treatment process.

- **Culture-bound syndromes** are recurrent, patterned, and problematic behaviors or experiences that are specific to a geographical region or culture.

- *Diagnostic and Statistical Manual of Mental Disorders* is the handbook mental health professionals use to diagnose mental disorders. The current edition (fifth) is known as DSM-5.

- **Indigenous medicine** is a cultural system of practicing medicine that was developed prior to modern medicine and is part of a cultural heritage. It is also known as folk medicine and traditional medicine.

- **Multicultural counseling** is a form of psychotherapy in which the therapist and client (individual, couple, or family) who are of different cultural backgrounds collaborate in a psychotherapeutic relationship.

- **Psychotherapy** is a psychological method for achieving desired changes in thinking, feeling, and behavior. It is also called therapeutic counseling.

Description

Culture is frequently conceptualized (thought about) as a way of categorizing different approaches to living. Cultural differences include heritage, customs, language, values, and beliefs. They also include ethnicities, races, and religious beliefs. Furthermore, cultural differences exist between social classes, gender identities, sexual orientations, and age groups. Artifacts or objects that are distinct to a group of people are also part of culture. For example, particular food, clothing, and housing norms may differ from group to group. These are the various ways in which culture is defined.

Cultural identity is the sense of belonging to a particular cultural group or place of origin. Cultural identity affects one's psychological experience of living. As a result, the mental health professions have integrated cultural sensitivity into their work. Cultural sensitivity is an ethical requirement of the profession. Cultural sensitivity requires basic knowledge and awareness of cultural factors and how they impact individuals. A culturally competent psychotherapist is aware of, knowledgeable about, and sensitive to a range of diverse human behaviors and experiences. This cultural competence is especially relevant to multicultural counseling. In the United States, the therapist and client are often members of different cultural groups. Effective psychotherapy accommodates cultural factors. Cultural factors influence the ways in which a client's presenting problem is expressed and understood. Psychotherapeutic interventions that are culturally sensitive lead to better treatment outcomes. Culturally sensitive psychotherapy includes an assessment of acculturation. Acculturative stress occurs when an immigrant experiences difficulty integrating new cultural patterns with his or her original cultural patterns. In addition, clients from cultures with histories of being oppressed may have difficulty trusting a therapist from cultural groups other than their own.

Development and Current Status

Nearly every cultural group throughout history has practiced the art and science of restoring health. Contemporary mental health practices are informed by this ancient heritage. Practitioners of indigenous medicine are more likely to work on healing physical, psychological, social, or spiritual ailments. In contrast, modern health-care professionals have become increasingly specialized in the practice of medicine. At the end of the 19th century, psychology established itself as a distinct profession. However, cultural considerations in the mental health professions were largely ignored until the middle of the 20th century. At that time the third major mental health reform was under way. The third major mental health reform was called the Community Mental Health Movement. The Community Mental Health Movement was a backlash against institutionalization and led to greater social integration.

Alexander H. Leighton (1908–2007) and Dorothea C. Leighton (1908–1989) were pioneers in culturally sensitive mental health research and practice. Their observations of indigenous healers illuminated similarities and differences between many traditional and modern health-care practices.

One of the major differences between indigenous and mainstream American culture is culture-bound syndromes. Until 1967 they were considered peculiar psychiatric disorders. Today, these syndromes are considered to be illnesses or afflictions that are specific to a given culture. The first culture-bound syndrome identified is amok and is associated with Malaysian culture. *Amok* describes a period of brooding followed by assaultive or murderous behavior. It is usually precipitated by a perceived insult or slight. Often, culture-bound syndromes are believed by the cultural group to be caused by evil spirits. There are many culture-bound syndromes listed in the *Diagnostic and Statistical Manual of Mental Disorders*.

The mental health professions have become increasingly sensitive to the impact of culture on psychotherapy since the 1950s. Culturally sensitive and evidence-based mental health practices have become more common. The surgeon general of the United States reported on the contributions of such research efforts in 2001. However, in the same report the surgeon general noted that major insufficiencies in cultural knowledge still existed. Mental health care for populations of cultural minorities is still not sufficiently evidence based. Modern science allows contemporary multicultural interventions to study the integration of traditional and modern treatments. Evidence-based treatments have been proven to produce therapeutic change in the controlled contexts of scientific research. However, the majority of evidence-based psychotherapy research does not emphasize cultural sensitivity. Counseling research has largely been based on white male middle-class American culture. The results of these scientific studies and resultant treatments might not be generalizable to members of cultural minority groups. Interventions that were invented in one culture may not be applicable across cultural barriers. The increasing diversity in the United States requires that evidence-based treatments be reevaluated for use with various cultural groups. Insensitivity to cultural factors in psychotherapy can lead to misunderstanding, conflict, oppression, and a minimization of positive outcomes. Common cultural differences leading to therapeutic obstacles include social class, gender, and sexual orientation. It is not surprising that dropout rates in psychotherapy are higher for culturally diverse clients than for clients in the cultural majority. Culturally sensitive therapeutic approaches have been developed to better serve the needs of culturally diverse clients.

Len Sperry, MD, PhD, and Layven Reguero, MEd

See also: Cultural Competence; Culturally Sensitive Treatment; Multicultural Counseling

Further Reading

American Psychiatric Association. *Diagnostic and Statistical Manual of Mental Disorders*, 5th ed. Arlington, VA: American Psychiatric Association, 2013.

Leach, Mark M., and Jamie D. Aten, eds. *Culture and the Therapeutic Process: A Guide for Mental Health Professionals*. New York, NY: Routledge, 2010.

Sue, David, and Diane M. Sue. *Foundations of Counseling and Psychotherapy: Evidence-Based Practices for a Diverse Society*. Hoboken, NJ: John Wiley & Sons, 2008.

Sue, Derald W., and David Sue. *Counseling the Culturally Diverse: Theory and Practice*, 6th ed. Hoboken, NJ: John Wiley & Sons, 2012.

Custody and Custody Evaluations

Custody explores the rights of the parent or guardian over children. The primary purpose of an evaluation is to assess the best psychological interest of the child. In separation or divorce, custody evaluations review who has residential or primary care of the child or children as well as identify visitation rights and expectations. Custody evaluations are conducted to help determine which parent or caregiver best meets the child's needs and are generally conducted by a child psychologist appointed by the court or guardian ad litem (GAL).

Description

Custody evaluations have not always been as complicated and challenging as they currently are. Prior to the turn of the 20th century, children were automatically put into the care of their fathers as it was believed the fathers could care for children better financially. However, the industrial revolution brought to light the mother's role in child care. This led to a belief that younger children were better in their mother's care, resulting in a switch toward favoring mothers in custody disputes.

The 1960s to current day has brought attention to focusing on the best interest of the child as opposed to the gender of the parent. The 1970s introduced the Uniform Marriage and Divorce Act, which was adopted by the majority of states. This act focused on the best interest of the child and identified several factors that should be considered. These factors include parental preference regarding custody, the desire of the child, interactions and relationships of the child with the parent as well as siblings and any other person who could be involved in the adjustment of the child, and the mental and physical health of the parents as well as any other relevant factors. However, in the two decades mothers still predominately receive primary custody of the children in custody agreements.

Anyone the child resides with or who is responsible for caring for the child is a part of the child custody evaluation. This includes both natural parents and significant others such as stepparents, live-in partners, grandparents, and live-in help. The process includes interviews and observations, as well as cognitive and personality functioning tests. Information is obtained from school records, medical records, and legal and court records as well as from any relevant party involved. For instance, teachers may be interviewed for their perception of interactions and parental investment.

The purpose of the evaluation is the fitness of the parent. The evaluator and courts are looking at the emotional, financial, and residential stability. Any psychiatric hospitalizations and use of psychotropic medication, as well as the reasons for therapy can all be assessed. Any drug- or alcohol-related problems will also be evaluated. The evaluator will also look at what parents can best support the child academically as well as for needs of daily living. Cooperation both with the other parent and the courts is assessed as well as behavior during meetings. The parent's social skills and judgment are also explored, as well as the interaction between the child and parent and their ability to communicate openly. These factors are all incorporated into the Ackerman-Schoendorf Scales for Parent Evaluation of Custody (ASPECT and ASPECT-SF).

The evaluation is generally completed by a child psychologist and may work in collaboration with an adult psychologist. Ideally it should be a single professional completing the evaluation. The evaluator should have a doctorate in psychology and be licensed in that state. Traditionally both parents would hire an expert to evaluate them separately. Due to the cost and time of this, there has been a shift to court-appointed evaluators who serve both parents. Some states, however, still use the traditional method. It is common now that the evaluator be appointed either by the court or by a GAL. The evaluator works as a team member with the GAL as they are obligated to make recommendations based on best interest of the child.

Current Status

Currently child custody evaluations have a purpose of assessing the best psychological interest of the child as well as the child's well-being. There is a focus on the developing needs of the child as well and the ability of the parent to meet those needs.

Mindy Parsons, PhD

See also: Divorce; Family Therapy and Family Counseling

Further Reading

Ackerman, Marc J. *Clinician's Guide to Child Custody Evaluations*, 2nd ed. New York, NY: John Wiley & Sons, 2001.

Cutting

Cutting is a form of self-injury whereby one makes cuts on his or her body, usually on the arms or legs, without attempting to commit suicide.

Definitions

- **Deliberate self-harm,** or self-inflicted injury, refers to acts of harming oneself with non-suicidal intent.

- **Self-inflicted injury** is a term used to refer to a range of behaviors that encompass self-harm where one deliberately injures oneself but without suicidal intentions.

- **Self-injury,** also referred to as self-harm, is the act of intentionally harming one's own body (by cutting or burning), without the intention of committing suicide.

Description

Cutting is considered a type of deliberate self-harm or self-injury. A person who engages in cutting behavior intends to hurt himself or herself but does not do it with the intention of committing suicide. Rather, this type of self-harm is used as an unhealthy way to cope with emotional pain, anger, or frustration. However, as with any form of self-inflicted injury, there is the possibility of more serious and even fatal consequences.

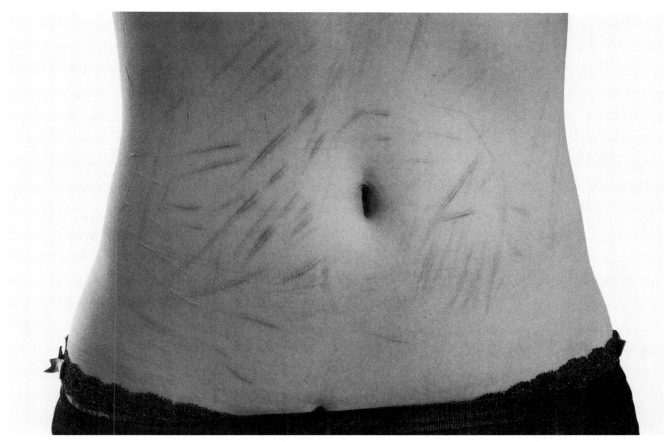

Cutting is a form of self-injury whereby an individual makes cuts on his or her body with sharp objects such as razor blades, usually on the arms or legs. Cutting is not a suicide attempt but is rather a maladaptive coping mechanism for dealing with stress, anxiety, or other negative emotions. (Axel Bueckert/Dreamstime.com)

When a person cuts, he or she usually makes small, shallow incisions, using a razor or other sharp object, on his or her legs or arms. Typically these cuts are made in places that are not readily visible to family or friends. Cutting behavior is associated with an inability to cope and regulate one's impulses. It has been linked to a variety of mental disorders, including depression, anxiety, eating disorders, bipolar disorder, schizophrenia, and borderline personality disorder. Perfectionistic tendencies among some cutters have also been noted. People who self-injure have often experienced some form of abuse, physical, verbal, emotional, and/or sexual.

Cutters report that the act helps them to get rid of negative emotions, release endorphins, and/or gain some sense of control. Though feelings of calm or an easing of tension may result immediately on cutting oneself, this is often replaced later by feelings of guilt or shame. Oftentimes, cutting behaviors are associated with long-term psychological issues such as anxiety and depression. People who cut are also more likely to have experienced some form of abuse, physical, emotional, and/or sexual, in their past. Cutting behavior is a behavioral sign of deeper, underlying problems, and thus, treatment for this type of behavior should be sought out immediately. Consultation with a pediatrician or health-care provider may be the first step. Follow-up treatment may include working on behavior and proper coping skills with a counselor or therapist and/or medication.

Impact (Psychological Influence)

Research estimates that adolescents and young adults, ranging in age from 12 years to early 30s, report cutting behaviors most often. Children as young as nine years have reported cutting. Females are more likely to be cutters than males. Cutting and other forms of self-injurious behavior have been identified across all cultures and socioeconomic statuses. Though the practice of cutting may have existed in secrecy for some time, recent media attention has caused a rise in the number of young people who engage in this form of self-injury. To further complicate the matter, there have been relatively few research studies done on cutting which makes definitive statistics on the subject hard to come by.

Melissa A. Mariani, PhD

See also: Self-Mutilation/Self-Harm

Further Reading

Conners, Robin E. *Self-injury: Psychotherapy with People Who Engage in Self-Inflicted Violence*. Northvale, NJ: Jason Aronson, 2000.

Hollander, Michael. *Helping Teens Who Cut: Understanding and Ending Self-Injury*. New York, NY: Guilford Press, 2008.

Levenkron, Steven. *Cutting: Understanding and Overcoming Self-Mutilation*. London, UK: W.W. Norton, 1998.

Cyberbullying

"Cyberbullying" refers to using electronic technology (cell phones, computers, tablets, gaming devices) to repeatedly and intentionally degrade, threaten, or humiliate another person.

Definitions

- **Bullycide** refers to a suicide where the victim's death has been attributed to his or her having been bullied either in person or online.

- **Bullying** describes deliberate, repeated acts of aggression that are inflicted directly or indirectly over time by one or more dominant persons.

- **Mobbing** defines when an individual is bullied by a group of people in any context, including a family, school, social setting, or workplace.

Description

Using technology and electronic communication as a means to threaten, harm, humiliate, or intimidate another person is known as cyberbullying. Cyberbullying is a distinct type of bullying or peer aggression. Technology devices such as computers, cell phones, tablets, or gaming devices can be used as vehicles for bullying behavior. Those who cyberbully may do so through calling, texting, e-mailing, instant messaging, posting comments, making

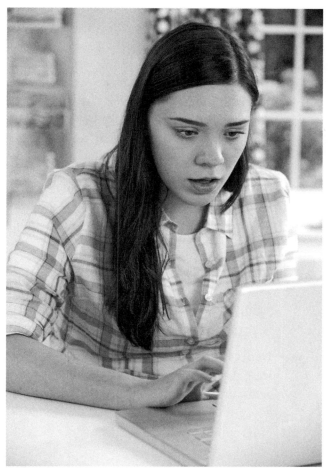

"Cyberbullying" refers to using electronic technology (e.g., cell phones, computers, and tablets) to repeatedly and intentionally degrade, threaten, or humiliate another person. It can have devastating psychological consequences for the victims and may even lead them to commit suicide. (Ian Allenden/Dreamstime.com)

verbal/written threats on social media and gaming sites, or taking pictures and transmitting them electronically. Canadian educator and anti-bullying activist, Bill Belsey, is credited with coining the term "cyberbullying."

Certain characteristics of cyberbullying make it more difficult to identify and report, given that the incidents do not happen in person as is the case with other forms including physical, verbal, or relational bullying. Anonymity is an issue as there is no way to be certain of the true identity of the aggressor. Temporary e-mail accounts, using pseudonames, anonymous postings, or sending messages from another

person's phone or computer can be accomplished nowadays with little trouble. Another characteristic that contributes to the ease of cyberbullying is lack of supervision. While teachers, administrators, and staff can deter bullying from occurring in schools simply by their presence, close monitoring of electronic devices and proper Internet usage during personal time is more complicated. In addition, parents may not be as technologically savvy as their children, making it more difficult for them to adequately supervise their usage. Furthermore, the simplicity of accessing mobile devices, particularly smartphones with Internet capabilities, has made cyberbullying an around-the-clock issue. Homes are no longer safe havens, and aggressors can target their victims anywhere and anytime. The level of impact in terms of the number of people that can be reached through cyberbullying also makes it distinct from other types of bullying. Mobbing, or bullying by a group of people rather than an individual, can be accomplished almost effortlessly through group messages, chat rooms, and social networking sites. These factors also contribute to the lasting impact this type of harassment can have on an individual's emotional and psychological well-being.

Cyberbullying can result in serious consequences. Victims often report higher levels of fear, anxiety, and stress. In addition, those who have been cyberbullied have lower self-esteem, may become socially withdrawn/isolated, and are at greater risk for depression and suicide. The term "bullycide" has been used to refer to suicides where bullying was determined to be a primary contributing factor. Cases such as that of Ryan Halligan (2003), Megan Meier (2006), Pheobe Prince (2010), and Tyler Clementi (2010) brought media attention to the detrimental effects of cyberbullying specifically.

Current Status and Impact (Psychological Influence)

Since the 1990s there has been a rise in reported incidents of cyberbullying as society's reliance on technology has increased. Recent reports indicate that the majority of teens aged 12 to 17, approximately 95%, access the Internet on a regular basis. Smartphones, which have become an increasingly popular vehicle used for social interactions, permit users to go online from any location at any time of the day. Research has found that most parents are concerned with what information their child may access or share online. Given this fact and the relative ease with which cyberbullying occurs, certain measures should be taken to help combat this growing problem. Experts agree that close monitoring can prevent and reduce cyberbullying. They recommend that parents discuss online etiquette and what constitutes appropriate sharing of information with their children and that they educate them about cyberbullying and its consequences as well as what to do if they see this behavior occurring. Parents are also encouraged to require their children to keep computers, tablets, and other devices in a centrally located, open room in the house to deter youngsters from engaging in negative interactions themselves or hiding the inappropriate behaviors of others.

Melissa A. Mariani, PhD

See also: Bullying and Peer Aggression; Peer Groups; Mobbing

Further Reading

"Cyberbullying Statistics." *NOBullying.com: The Movement against Bullying.* Accessed May 23, 2014. http://nobullying.com/cyber-bullying-statistics/.

Hinduja, Sameer, and Justin W. Patchin. *Bullying beyond the Schoolyard: Preventing and Responding to Cyberbullying.* Thousand Oaks, CA: Corwin, 2009.

Kowalski, Robin M., Susan P. Limber, and Patricia W. Agaston. *Cyberbullying: Bullying in the Digital Age.* London, UK: Blackwell Publishing, Ltd., 2012.

Madden, Mary, Amanda Lenhart, Maeve Duggan, Sandra Cortesi, and Urs Gasser. "Teens and Technology 2013." Pew Research Center, March 13, 2013. Accessed May 22, 2014. http://www.pewinternet.org/2013/03/13/teens-and-technology-2013/.

Patchin, Justin W., and Hinduja, Sameer. *Cyberbullying Prevention and Response: Expert Perspectives.* New York, NY: Routledge, 2012.

Cyclothymic Disorder

Cyclothymic disorder is a mental disorder characterized by alternating cycles of hypomanic and depressive symptoms.

Definitions

- **Bipolar and related disorders** are a group of mental disorders characterized by changes in mood and in energy (e.g., being highly irritable and impulsive while not needing sleep). These disorders include bipolar I disorder, bipolar II disorder, and cyclothymic disorder.

- **Bipolar disorders** is a mental disorder characterized by a history of manic episodes (bipolar I disorder), mixed, or hypomanic episodes (bipolar II disorder), usually with one or more major depressive episodes.

- **Cognitive behavior therapy** is a type of psychotherapy that focuses on maladaptive (faulty) behaviors, emotions, and thoughts. It is also called CBT.

- **Depression** is a sad mood or emotional state that is characterized by feelings of low self-worth or guilt and a reduced ability to enjoy life. It is not considered a mental disorder unless it significantly disrupts the individual's daily functioning.

- **Depressive disorders** are a group of mental disorders characterized by a sad or irritable mood and cognitive and physical changes that significantly disrupt the individual's daily functioning. These disorders include major depressive disorder, persistent depressive disorder, disruptive mood dysregulation, and premenstrual dysphoric disorder.

- **Hypomania** is a mental state similar to mania but less intense.

- **Major depressive disorder** is a mental disorder characterized by a depressed mood and other symptoms that interfere significantly with an individual's daily functioning. It is also referred to as clinical depression.

- **Mania** is a mental state of expansive, elevated, or irritable mood with increased energy or activity.

- **SSRI** stands for selective serotonin reuptake inhibitors. They are a class of antidepressant medications that work by blocking the reabsorption of serotonin in nerve cells and raising its level in the brain.

Description and Diagnosis

Cyclothymic disorder is one of a group of depressive disorders. It is characterized by a chronic fluctuating mood with distinct periods of hypomanic symptoms and distinct periods of depressive symptoms. The symptoms are like those of bipolar disorder and major depressive disorder but of lesser severity. Cyclothymic disorder is similar to bipolar II disorder. It is seen in individuals unable to regulate their emotions effectively. They may lack the willingness to think beyond themselves, consider their impact on others, and take the initiative in meeting their responsibilities. This disorder usually begins early in life. It appears to be equally common in men and women although women are more likely to seek treatment for it than men (American Psychiatric Association, 2013).

According to the *Diagnostic and Statistical Manual of Mental Disorders, Fifth Edition*, individuals can be diagnosed with this disorder if they exhibit a pattern of chronic, fluctuating mood disturbance involving numerous periods of hypomanic symptoms and periods of depressive symptoms. These fluctuating depressive and hypomanic symptoms must be distinct from one another and have lasted at least two years. The hypomania and depression is not sufficient to warrant either a bipolar I or II diagnosis, yet sufficient to disrupts one's ability to function efficiently (American Psychiatric Association, 2013).

The cause of this disorder is not well understood. However, there is some evidence for genetic and physiological factors as causes or triggers for it (American Psychiatric Association, 2013). Since this disorder runs in families, there appears to be a genetic basis for it. Major depressive disorder, bipolar disorder, and cyclothymic disorder often occur together in families. This suggests that these mood disorders share similar causes. These individuals also tend to have skill deficits in emotion regulation.

Treatment

Effective treatment of this disorder usually involves psychotherapy and medication. Psychotherapy, particularly cognitive behavior therapy (CBT), can be quite helpful in increasing emotional regulation. The challenge is to better manage daily life challenges. CBT helps those with this disorder in three ways. The first is develop better emotion regulation skills. The second is to identify unhealthy, negative beliefs and behaviors and replace them with more healthy and positive ones. The third is to identify triggers to both hypomanic and depressive episodes and better cope with upsetting situations. Medication may be helpful in emotional regulation. Medications like Lithium, Depakote, and Tegretol are particularly useful in regulating and stabilizing mood.

Len Sperry, MD, PhD

See also: Bipolar Disorder; Cognitive Behavior Therapy; Depakote (Divalproex Sodium); Depression; Lithium; Major Depressive Disorder; Tegretol (Carbamazepine)

Further Reading

American Psychiatric Association. *Diagnostic and Statistical Manual of Mental Disorders*, 5th ed. Arlington, VA: American Psychiatric Association, 2013.

Duke, Patty, and Gloria Hochman. *Brilliant Madness: Living with Manic Depressive Illness*. New York, NY: Bantam Books, 1997.

McManamy, John. *Living Well with Depression and Bipolar Disorder: What Your Doctor Doesn't Tell You . . . That You Need to Know*. New York, NY: William Morrow Paperbacks, 2007.

Miklowitz, David J. *The Bipolar Disorder Survival Guide: What You and Your Family Need to Know*, 2nd ed. New York, NY: The Guilford Press, 2011.

Cymbalta (Duloxetine)

Cymbalta is a prescribed medication used to treat depression and neuropathic pain. Its generic name is duloxetine.

Definitions

- **Antidepressant medications** are prescription drugs that are primarily used to treat depression and depressive disorders. They are known as antidepressants.

- **Neuropathic pain** is pain generated by the nervous system. It is also called neurogenic pain.

- **Selective serotonin norepinephrine reuptake inhibitors (SSNRI)** are medications that act on and increase the levels of serotonin and norepinephrine in the brain that influences mood. They differ from selective serotonin reuptake inhibitors, which act only on serotonin.

- **Serotonin discontinuation syndrome** is a condition caused by abrupt discontinuation of an SNRI resulting in withdrawal symptoms. These include flu-like symptoms, anxiety, agitation, vivid or bizarre dreams, insomnia, nausea, diarrhea, dizziness, headache, numbness and tingling of the extremities. This syndrome can be avoided by dose reduction over time.

- **Serotonin syndrome** is a serious medication reaction resulting from an excess of serotonin in the brain. It occurs when a number of medications that increase serotonin are taken together. Symptoms include high blood pressure, high fever, headache, delirium, shock, and coma.

Description

Cymbalta belongs to a class of antidepressant medications known as selective serotonin norepinephrine reuptake inhibitors (SSNRI). It is used to treat various disorders, including clinical depression, generalized anxiety disorder, and neuropathic pain associated with diabetic peripheral neuropathy and fibromyalgia. SSNRIs specifically act on two chemicals called serotonin and norepinephrine. It is believed that a decrease in serotonin and norepinephrine contributes to depression, anxiety, and pain. SSNRIs work by counteracting this by increasing the actions of both neurotransmitters. An increase of serotonin and norepinephrine in the brain is believed to reduce depressive symptoms, while an increase of both in the spinal cord reduces pain associated with diabetic neuropathy or fibromyalgia. Cymbalta has a high success rate in treating depression and

is often the first SSNRI to be prescribed. Cymbalta can be used alone or in combination with other medications depending on the medical condition and the individual's health history.

Precautions and Side Effects

Antidepressant drugs, including Cymbalta, have been associated with an increased risk of suicidal thoughts and behaviors in children and adults up to age 24. Any patient taking an antidepressant drug should be monitored for changes in behavior and worsening depression. If treatment with Cymbalta is ceased, it should be slowly discontinued to avoid the development of SNRI discontinuation syndrome. Close medical monitoring is needed if Cymbalta is used with those with liver or kidney function impairment, seizure disorder, bleeding disorders, glaucoma, dehydration, and history of alcohol abuse and in patients younger than 25 years of age or those over 60 years. Cymbalta should be used only for a short time and with careful monitoring in those with bipolar disorder as it can induce mania. The safety of Cymbalta use during pregnancy and breast-feeding is unknown, so its use is not recommended.

Because SSNRIs have fewer side effects than SSRIs and tricyclic antidepressants, they tend to be the drug of choice in treating depression. Nevertheless, side effects may still occur. The most common are nausea, headache, dizziness, constipation, sexual dysfunction, diarrhea, sweating, dry mouth, shakiness, loss of appetite, hot flashes, high blood pressure, yawning, anxiety, and insomnia. Rare but serious side effects include mania, worsened depression and suicidality, seizures, serotonin syndrome, SNRI discontinuation syndrome, electrolyte imbalances, urinary retention, skin reactions, abnormal bleeding, liver damage, and glaucoma.

To reduce the likelihood of serotonin syndrome, Cymbalta should not be combined with antipsychotics like Thorazine or Prolixin or herbal supplements such as Yohimbine, ginkgo biloba, and St. John's wort. Drug interactions may occur when alcohol, Haldol, or NSAIDs are taken with Cymbalta. Other medications that can cause drug interactions with Cymbalta include Tagamet, Lithium, Inderal, and anticoagulant medicines. Others include diuretics (water pills), diet pills such as Meridia, caffeine, antibiotics such as Cipro, mood stabilizers such as Lithium, antipsychotics such as Haldol and Clozaril, and antiseizure medications like Dilantin. There is increased risk of internal bleeding when Cymbalta is used with anticoagulant drugs such as aspirin and warfarin, and large doses of the herbal supplements red clover, ginkgo biloba, feverfew, or green tea.

Len Sperry, MD, PhD

See also: Antidepressant Medications; Depression

Further Reading

Baldwin, Robert C. *Depression in Later Life*. New York, NY: Oxford University Press, 2010.

O'Connor, Richard. *Undoing Depression: What Therapy Doesn't Teach You and Medication Can't Give You*, 2nd ed. New York, NY: Little, Brown, 2010.

Stahl, Stephen M. *Antidepressants*. New York, NY: Cambridge University Press, 2009.

Stargrove, Mitchell Bebel, Jonathan Treasure, and Dwight L. McKee. *Herb, Nutrient, and Drug Interactions: Clinical Implications and Therapeutic Strategies*. St. Louis, MO: Mosby, 2007.

Dahmer, Jeffrey (1960–1994)

Jeffrey Dahmer was a sexual predator and serial killer notorious for cannibalizing, that is, eating, many of his victims. He killed 17 males between 1978 and 1991, and was sentenced to 15 consecutive life terms in 1992. On November 28, 1994, he was murdered by a prison inmate.

Description and History

Dahmer was born in Milwaukee, Wisconsin, on May 21, 1960, to Lionel and Joyce Dahmer. His early upbringing was unremarkable until age 6, when he underwent minor surgery to correct a double hernia, and his brother was born. He is said to have become socially withdrawn and less self-confident. After high school, he enrolled in college but dropped out after one-quarter because of drinking and failure to attend class. Then he enlisted in the army but was dishonorably discharged because of his alcoholism. When his army superior berated him and said he would never amount to anything, Dahmer is reported to have said, "Just wait and see, someday everyone will know me."

As an adult, Dahmer appeared to blend in easily in the middle-class neighborhood in which he lived. He was described as a quiet but likeable young man who held a job. At that same time he was a killer and sexual predator who murdered men and boys—most of whom were of African or Asian descent. Dahmer's murders were particularly gruesome because they involving rape, torture, dismemberment, necrophilia, and cannibalism. By the summer of 1991, Dahmer was murdering approximately one person each week and probably would have continued had he not finally been arrested after police searched his apartment.

Impact (Psychological Influence)

The story of Dahmer's arrest and the inventory in his apartment quickly gained national and international attention. Many were shocked to learn that several corpses were stored in acid-filled vats, and materials for an altar of candles and human skulls were found in his closet. Seven skulls were found in the apartment and a human heart was recovered from his freezer. Like many facile psychopaths, Dahmer had managed to avoid detection for years because of his uncanny ability to deceive police, parole personnel, and even mental health professionals with highly plausible stories and explanations.

He would entice victims to his apartment where he would drug them, strangle them, and then engage in various deviant sexual behaviors with the corpse prior to dismembering and eating it, at least parts of it. The key to this deadly sequence was drugging his victims, usually with benzodiazepines like Valium and Ativan or sleep-inducing medications like Ambien. Dahmer would grind the pills and mix them with coffee which he persuaded his victims to drink. The source of these pills were various physicians, including some psychiatrists with extensive training in forensics. He would complain of difficulty with anxiety and sleeplessness and convince these doctors that he really needed these medications. The fact that he had a long history of chronic alcoholism, dating from his high school and army days, should have been a contraindication to prescribing such medications. Nevertheless, he was consistently successful in conning physicians to provide him with the means to kill his next victims.

High-visibility psychopaths and serial killers seem to arise in every generation, but few have been as

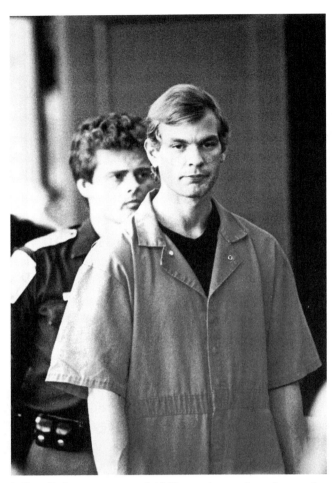

Jeffrey Dahmer was a serial killer and sexual predator who murdered men and boys—most of whom were of African or Asian descent. Dahmer's murders were particularly gruesome because they involved rape, torture, dismemberment, necrophilia, and cannibalism. (AP Photo/Eugene Garcia)

gruesome and evil as to strangle, kill, sexually abuse, and cannibalize their victims like Dahmer. Jeffrey Dahmer appears to have made good on his promise to his army superior that "someday everyone will know about me."

Len Sperry, MD, PhD

See also: Lies and Deceit; Mass Shootings; Psychopathic Personality Disorder; Sexual Predator

Further Reading

Dahmer, Lionel. *A Father's Story*. New York, NY: William Morrow, 1994.
Davis, Donald. *The Jeffrey Dahmer Story: An American Nightmare*. New York, NY: Macmillan, 1991.

Sperry, Len. "Duped, Drugged, and Eaten: Working with the Jeffrey Dahmers of the World." In *Duped: Lies and Deception in Psychotherapy*, edited by Jeffrey Kottler and Jon Carlson. New York, NY: Routledge, 2011.

Dance Therapy

Dance therapy is the psychotherapeutic use of movement to promote emotional, social, cognitive, and physical integration of the individual. It has been shown to be an effective therapeutic treatment by improving the well-being of those with social, physical, and/or psychological challenges.

Description

Dance therapy has been utilized as a healing ritual for thousands of years. Although dance therapy finds its roots among indigenous people, it wasn't formalized into a specific treatment modality until the 20th century. Thus, dance therapy is considered to be a relatively new practice; however, it has already been shown to be a viable treatment for a wide variety of mental and physical challenges.

For example, dance therapy has been studied as a treatment for dementia, depression, alcoholism, heart disease, diabetes, and many more mental and physical ailments—often with statistically significant positive results. It is important to note that there has long been a connection between therapy and dance; however, as a formal discipline, it remains a fairly new approach.

With the growing development of counseling theories and techniques, new ways of treating mental health challenges are being identified. Dance therapy, depending on the theoretical perspective of the therapist, is conducted either individually or in a group format. Regardless of perspective, the participant's dance identity must be considered. Dance therapy has been identified as an alternative medicine by the National Institute of Mental Health as it is an expression of the mind and body. Movement reflects personality and has an advantage over traditional talk therapy since it includes assessment of the nonverbal body movements. Dance therapy is considered to have a positive impact on a person's well-being.

There are two models that tend to be the most commonly utilized by practitioners. The first is Dance/Movement Therapy, which was developed in the United States during the 1940s. This model has been widely accepted by dance therapists in the United States. This model has its roots in modern dance tradition and encourages movement without any form of limitation. Here, the emphasis is on body-self, body weight, knowledge of the body, and creation of a safe space. This therapy is conducted either individually or in a group format.

The other model is Expression Primitive, which originated in France in 1984. This model came from the French Society of Dance Therapy. The view of this model is that dance therapy is ritualistic and present in every aspect of life. Dance is conducted in a group format with the individual following verbal or physical directives given by the therapist.

These two models are distinct from one another, and those in the field tend to choose the model they identify with and often question the effectiveness of the other. One large difference between the two is that The American perspective is that dance occurs under special conditions. The focus of disagreement between the two models is also focused on the differences in the forms of dance.

Current Status

Dance therapy is currently a supported form of alternative medicine by the National Institute of Mental Health. It has also been accepted by the Association for Creativity in Counseling, which is a recognized division of the American Counseling Association. Current research has found support for its effectiveness with specific disorders, such as eating disorders and alcoholism.

Mindy Parsons, PhD

See also: Eating Disorders; Expressive Arts Therapy; Substance-Related and Addictive Disorders

Further Reading

American Dance Therapy Association. "About Dance/Movement Therapy." Last modified 2014. Accessed December 12, 2014. www.adta.org/About_DMT.

Chace, Marian, Susan L. Sandel, Sharon Chaiklin, and Ann Lohn, eds. *Foundations of Dance/Movement Therapy: The Life and Work of Marian Chace.* Columbia, MD: American Dance Therapy Association, 1993.

Kiepe, Marie Sophie, Barbara Stockigt, and Thomas Keil. "Effects of Dance Therapy and Ballroom Dances on Physical and Mental Illnesses: A Systematic Review." *The Arts in Psychotherapy* 39 (2012): 404–411.

Panagiotopoulou, Efthimia. "Dance Therapy Models: An Anthropological Perspective." *American Journal of Dance Therapy* 33 (2011): 91–110.

Organizations

American Dance Therapy Association (ADTA)
10632 Little Patuxent Parkway, Suite 108
Columbia, MD 21044
Telephone: (410) 997-4040
Fax: (410) 997-4048
E-mail: info@adta.org
Website: www.adta.org

The Association for Creativity in Counseling (ACC)
A Division of the American Counseling Association
6101 Stevenson Ave.
Alexandria, VA 22304
Telephone: (800) 347-6647
Fax: (800) 473-2329
E-mail: webmaster@counseling.org
Website: http://www.counseling.org

Darkness Visible: A Memoir of Madness (Book)

Darkness Visible: A Memoir of Madness was written by William Styron (1925–2006) and published in 1990. Although an abridged version of the book was originally published in 1989 in the magazine *Vanity Fair*, the origins can be traced back to a lecture the author gave on affective disorders at the Department of Psychiatry at Johns Hopkins University's School of Medicine. This first-person account of his near-fatal descent into depression is considered one of the most vivid and insightful, even after more than 25 years since it was first published. The title of Styron's book is highly symbolic; it was taken from John Milton's description of hell in *Paradise Lost*.

William Styron was considered among the greatest American writers of his time following the release of his first novel, *Lie Down in Darkness*, published in 1952 when he was just 26 years old. He won a Pulitzer Prize for his second novel, *The Confessions of Nat Turner*, and his 1979 novel *Sophie's Choice* was made into an Academy Award–nominated movie in 1982 and an opera in 2002. However, he may be best known for his 1990 personal memoir of depression, *Darkness Visible: A Memoir of Madness*, which became a national best seller in 1990.

The impact of *Darkness Visible* has yet to wane, even though decades have passed since its original publishing. Although just 85 pages, the clarity of Styron's description of his depressive condition led to the book being embraced by both critics and mental health professionals alike. At the time, the memoir was considered groundbreaking in that it served to greatly increase knowledge about major depressive disorders and the often-accompanying act of suicide. It also helped to decrease the stigma and shame associated with depression that had long been kept silent among its sufferers.

Styron chronicles the rapid onset of his depression and blames the abrupt end to years of alcohol abuse in combination with a prescription of Halcion (triazolam). Although he never attempted suicide, he painfully shares his intense suicidal ideation that kept him bedridden for months and ultimately led to his hospitalization.

One of the most valuable contributions of Styron's memoir is that it was the first book to help break the silence surrounding depression and refuted the idea that depression was suffered mainly by weak-minded individuals, especially those who attempted or completed suicide. However, perhaps the greatest impact of *Darkness Visible* is the message that no matter how severe depression may get, hope and even redemption is possible through perseverance.

Mindy Parsons, PhD

See also: Major Depressive Disorder; Suicide

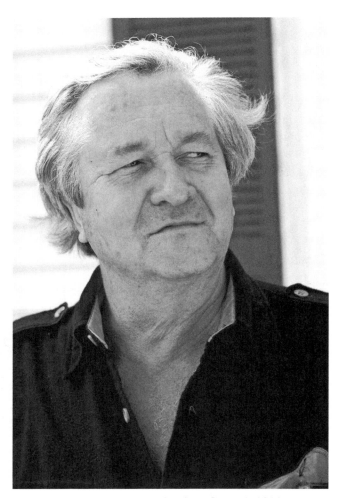

Prominent American author William Styron's 1990 memoir, *Darkness Visible*, chronicled his terrible struggles with depression. (ZUMA Press, Inc./Alamy)

Further Reading

Kosner, Edward. "Writing in Darkness and Light." *The Wall Street Journal*. November 30, 2012. http://online.wsj.com/article/SB100014241278873233532045781295339388550000.html.

Solomon, Andrew. *The Noonday Demon: An Atlas of Depression*. New York: Scribner, 2001.

Styron, Alexandra. *Reading My Father: Growing up with William Styron*. New York: Scribner, 2012. The book chronicles her experience growing up as the daughter of one of the greatest novelists of the 20th century but a man who was also devastated by a deep depression that greatly impacted their family.

Styron, William. "Darkness Visible." *Vanity Fair*. 1989. http://www.vanityfair.com/magazine/archive/1989/12/styron198912.

Styron, William. *Darkness Visible: A Memoir of Madness*. New York: Random House, 1990.

Date Rape

The term "date rape" refers to an act of sexual assault perpetrated by a person with whom the victim has been acquainted with (not a stranger). It is also referred to as "acquaintance rape."

Definitions

- **Consent** is an act of voluntary willingness.

- **Rape** occurs when sexual intercourse (vagina, anus, or mouth) is not consensual, or the perpetrator forces himself on the victim sexually against the victim's will.

- **Sexual assault** is an involuntary sexual act whereby a person is forced to engage in any type of sexual activity (touching, kissing, sexual penetration) against his or her will; it is used in legal terminology to refer to a statutory offense.

Description

"Date rape" refers to an act of nonconsensual sexual intercourse that is committed by a person the victim knows, usually a friend or acquaintance. It is also referred to as "acquaintance rape" or "drug-induced sexual assault." Date rape is distinguished from rape in that the victim knows the attacker socially. The victim may even have been involved in a romantic relationship with the attacker. Both men and women can be victims of date rape. Incidents of date rape oftentimes occur when the victim is under the influence of alcohol or drugs. Rohypnol and gamma-hydroxybutyrate are considered "date rape drugs" and have been linked to these cases of sexual assault. Date rape is a serious crime and is classified as a felony offense. Victims of date rape suffer from physical and emotional abuse.

Impact (Psychological Influence)

Date rape is much more common than incidents of rape perpetrated by a stranger. Estimates suggest that 80%–85% of all reported rapes can be classified as date rape. However, instances of date rape are also underreported

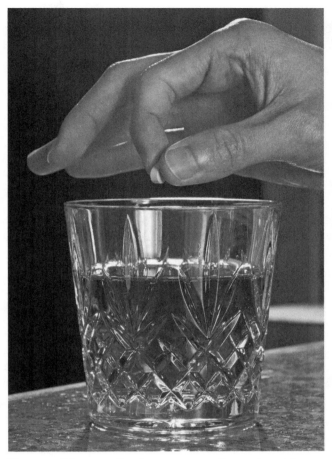

The term "date rape" refers to an act of sexual assault perpetrated by a person with whom the victim is acquainted (rather than a stranger). Incidents of date rape oftentimes occur when the victim is under the influence of alcohol or drugs. All forms of rape can have profound psychological consequences, including depression, anxiety, feelings of shame, and post-traumatic stress disorder (PTSD). (Innovatedcaptures/Dreamstime.com)

as victims may not recognize these acts as a crime. Feelings of guilt over not knowing what happened, perhaps due to drugs or alcohol, are also contributing factors. The United States Bureau of Justice indicated that 38% of reported rapes were perpetrated by a friend or acquaintance, and in 28% of cases, the attacker was considered "an intimate," while in 7% of the cases the attacker was "a relative" (Rape Statistics, 2012).

Melissa A. Mariani, PhD

See also: Sexual Abuse; Sexual Predator

Further Reading

Rape Statistics. U.S. Bureau of Justice, CDC, Koss, Gidycz & Wisniewski College Study, United Nations. 2012.

Söchting, Ingrid, Nichole Fairbrother, and William J. Koch. "Sexual Assault of Women: Prevention Efforts and Risk Factors." *Violence against Women* 10 (2004): 73–93.

USLegal—Date Rape Law & Legal Definition. Accessed April 4, 2013. Definitions.uslegal.com.

Zurbriggen, Eileen L. "Understanding and Preventing Adolescent Dating Violence: The Importance of Developmental, Sociocultural, and Gendered Perspectives." *Psychology of Women Quarterly* 33, no. 1 (2009): 30–33.

Dating and Flirting

Dating is social courting done by two people who each want to see if the other is a possible intimate relationship partner or spouse. Flirting includes verbal and nonverbal communication by one person to another that suggests an interest in a physical or romantic relationship with the other person.

Description

Social rules regarding dating vary according to variables such as country, social class, religion, age, sexual orientation, and gender. Behavior patterns of dating and flirting are generally unwritten and constantly changing. There are considerable differences between social and personal values. Each culture has particular patterns that determine flirting and dating norms. These include choices such as whether the man asks the woman out and where people might meet. Other questions include whether kissing is acceptable on a first date and who should pay for meals or entertainment. Depending on where you live and who you are, the social choices and questions involved are complex.

The term "dating" most commonly refers to a trial period in which two people explore each other. Dating can also refer to the time when people are physically together in public as opposed to the earlier time period in which people are arranging the date, perhaps through corresponding by e-mail or text or phone. Another meaning of the term "dating" is to describe a stage in a person's life when he or she is actively pursuing romantic relationships with different people.

One of the main purposes of dating is for two or more people to evaluate one another's suitability as a possible long-term companion or spouse. Often physical characteristics, personality, financial status, and other aspects are judged and as a result feelings can be hurt and confidence shaken. Dating can be stressful for those involved because of the uncertainty of the future, the desire to be acceptable to the other person, and the possibility of rejection. Dating often lets those involved get a chance to decide where to take the relationship. If the dating experience is positive, two people usually move into a more permanent or committed relationship.

Flirting requires several different skills that involve body language, empathy, and creativity. Flirting can be used either in trying to find someone to date or in trying to get a desired object or outcome in a situation. Research has been conducted on flirting techniques used in bars, malls, and other places where young people go to meet each other. Results of this research indicate that it is not the most physically appealing people who get approached but the ones who send specific signs. These people signal their availability and confidence through basic techniques like eye contact and smiles. Signaling your interest in someone gets you halfway there, whether you're a man or a woman.

Two types of flirting exist and are fairly universal. Smiling and eye contact indicate flirting and are effective in most places and for most people. But an even more effective flirting technique is touch. Research has been done to identify which types of touching are flirting, such as touching the shoulder, waist, forearm, and, most intimately, the face. Flirting can be done to let another person know you're interested in him or her romantically or sexually. It usually occurs before and during the dating process. Touching that is gentle and informal, and that occurs face-to-face or involves hugging, lets someone else know that the person intends to continue pursuing the relationship.

Impact (Psychological Influence)

There are some identifiable differences in the ways that men and women in heterosexual relationships date and flirt. Research suggests that men prefer women who seem to be flexible and admired. Men also tend to date younger women with subordinate jobs such as assistants rather than executive women. Online dating patterns suggest that men are more likely to initiate online exchanges. It also indicates that men are less picky than women and seek younger partners and tend to cast a wider net in the pool of women they choose. The stereotype for heterosexual women is that they seek well-educated men who are usually older and have high-paying jobs. Much of the research suggests that women are the pickier of the genders and that is linked to reproductive decision making.

Alexandra Cunningham, PhD

See also: Self-Esteem; Shyness

Further Reading

Ferrante-Shepis, Maria, and G. Michael Maddock. *Flirting with the Uninterested: Innovating in a "Sold, Not Bought" Category.* Charleston, SC: Advantage, 2012.

Regan, Pamela C. *Close Relationships.* New York, NY: Routledge, 2011.

Regan, Pamela C. *The Mating Game: A Primer on Love, Sex and Marriage.* Thousand Oaks, CA: Sage Publications, 2008.

de Shazer, Steve (1940–2005)

Steve de Shazer was a psychotherapist who, along with his wife Insoo Kim Berg, developed solution-focused brief therapy.

Description

Steve de Shazer (1940–2005) and his wife, Insoo Kim Berg (1934–2007), had both been trained in traditional psychoanalytic or Freudian therapy. They were frustrated because they found that it often didn't work to help clients resolve their issues. In fact they felt it was harmful and led to an endless cycle of investigating the origins of the client's issues. Because of these concerns, de Shazer and Kim Berg developed a new form of therapy called solution-focused.

Solution-focused brief therapy (SFBT) differs from other approaches to the treatment of psychological problems. The couple based SFBT on the concept that although causes of problems may be extremely complex, their solutions do not necessarily need to be. Their therapeutic approach decided to focus on simple, doable solutions. Together de Shazer and Kim Berg founded the Brief Family Therapy Center in Milwaukee, Wisconsin, during the 1980s.

SFBT, as a therapy model, does not put emphasis on the need to examine past problems. The approach focuses on the clients' assessment of how their lives or experiences might be different if they didn't exist at all. From this focus, the therapist builds approaches based on the clients' own strengths and previous successes. SFBT is based on solution building rather than problem solving.

Steve de Shazer and his wife were able to help clients build those solutions from insights and responses to what they called "the Miracle Question." The miracle question was an intervention; it asked the client to think differently by responding to this question: "If you woke up tomorrow and a miracle occurred and the problem had completely disappeared, even though you didn't know why, what small changes would tell you that it had been solved?" By asking their clients to describe how they would know the problem was resolved, and to evaluate how important the symptoms of improvement were, they could work with them to create change.

Impact (Psychological Influence)

SFBT has been widely practiced and accepted in the therapeutic community. Its hallmark is to focus on creating solutions rather than rehashing problems. de Shazer was specifically in charge of researching the approach, which helped solidify SFBT not only as a foundational theory but also as a practice that could be taught to future practitioners. The small, positive changes that are based on the client's perspective make it appealing to both professionals and their clients.

The SFBT approach is criticized for some weaknesses such as not allowing for exploration of family history and patterns as well as the limited applicability to those experiencing chronic or severe disorders. Steve de Shazer and Kim Berg admitted that their approach would not be effective in about 20% of client cases. But it has been adapted for use in a variety of different environments. This includes clinical therapy groups, schools, and hospital nursing staffs. Clinical and research results indicate that SFBT makes a positive difference and Steve de Shazer helped to validate and make this approach known among mental health professionals.

Alexandra Cunningham, PhD, and William M.
Cunningham, MA

See also: Solution-Focused Brief Therapy (SFBT)

Further Reading

de Shazer, Steve, and Yvonne Dolan. *More Than Miracles: The State of the Art of Solution-Focused Brief Therapy.* New York, NY: Taylor & Francis, 2007.

Kelly, Michael S., Johnny S. Kim, and Cynthia Franklin. *Solution Focused Brief Therapy in Schools: A 360 Degree View of Research and Practice.* Cary, NC: Oxford University Press, 2008.

Metcalf, Lisa. *The Miracle Question: Answer It and Change Your Life.* Wales, UK: Crown House Publishing, 2004.

Dead Poets Society (Movie)

Dead Poets Society is a 1989 American-period film directed by Peter Weir and starring Robin Williams.

Description

In the movie *Dead Poets Society*, Robin Williams (1951–2014) portrays an inspiring English teacher at an exclusive Vermont private boys' academy in 1959. *Dead Poets Society* is perhaps best known for several iconic scenes in which Williams's character, John Keating, dramatically and idealistically inspires his students. Central themes include individualism, freethinking, self-empowerment, and living significant, meaningful lives in light of issues of mortality and death.

Set in 1959 the movie follows a class of students at the Welton Academy, a conservative prep school for boys. The story focuses on the impact a new and unconventional English teacher, John Keating, has on their lives. Keating, a former student at Welton, exposes the students to classic poetry in ways that are controversial and unorthodox for the time and setting. For instance, finding the mathematical formula to rate

poetry absurd, Keating has students rip out the introduction of the poetry textbook. In another scene, Keating has students stand on their desks in order to see life from a different perspective. In perhaps the most iconic scene, Keating gathers his students in front of a trophy case with pictures of alumni from years long past. Quoting from a poem by Robert Herrick "Gather ye rosebuds while ye may," Keating tells the boys that the meaning of the poem is about "carpe diem," which means "seize the day." Keating tells his students "Because we are food for worms, lads. Cause believe it or not each and every one of us in this room is one day going to stop breathing, turn cold, and die. Therefore, seize the day, boys. Make your lives extraordinary" (Internet Movie Database, 2013).

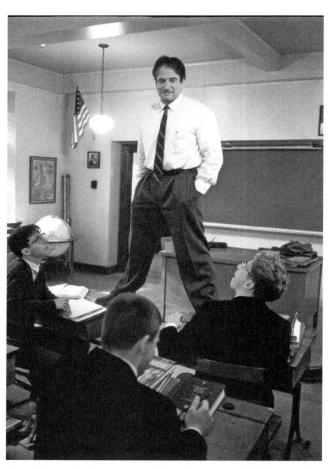

Dead Poets Society portrays an inspiring English teacher (played by Robin Williams) at an exclusive Vermont private boys' academy in 1959. The film has been used to illustrate concepts such as empowerment and individuality. (Buena Vista/Photofest)

The students are both captivated and inspired by Keating's ideals. Keating encourages the students to revive the "Dead Poets Society," which meets secretly in a cave where they may reflect on how to "suck the marrow out of life," pursue their dreams, and find their voice. The movie follows several of the students' personal difficulties, challenges, and triumphs as they are changed by what they are leaning. For one student, Neil, his quest to find his own voice leads him to pursue acting and perform in a local play. This is in defiance of the plans his controlling authoritarian father has for him to become a medical doctor. Neil turns to Keating who encourages Neil to speak with his father to help him understand how he feels. Neil attempts to confront his father but is bullied and threatened with military school. Unable to reason with his father, Neil commits suicide.

An investigation is launched, and Keating is accused of abusing his authority, inciting rebellion, and encouraging Neil to defy his father. After being betrayed by one of the students, Keating is made a scapegoat for Neil's death and is fired. Entering the classroom one last time to retrieve his personal belongings, Keating is honored by the students standing on their desks in defiance of the headmaster.

Impact (Psychological Influence)

Dead Poets Society was well received by the viewing public and maintains an 85% Rotten Tomatoes rating. The film was nominated for four Academy Awards and won for best Original Screenplay (Tom Schulman). It is recognized as one of Robin Williams's best roles and performances.

Dead Poets Society is used as a teaching film in a wide range of topics, including innovative teaching techniques, teacher/student relationships, mentoring, and lessons on empowerment and individualism. More recently, *Dead Poets Society* has been criticized for whether the main character, John Keating, is a positive or negative example for a teacher. Was he inspiring students to love poetry or to love him; to think for themselves or to think like him? The film also called into question the ethical responsibilities teachers have when instructing and mentoring impressionable students. How responsible was Keating in Neil's death?

Dead Poets Society is a highly popular and highly rated American film that explores issues of self-empowerment and meaning in life. The movie remains one of the most popular Robin Williams films and continues to be used in a wide range of educational settings.

Steven R. Vensel, PhD

See also: Self-Identity

Further Reading

Internet Movie Database. 2013. "Dead Poet's Society." Accessed November 3, 2013. http://www.imdb.com/title/tt0097165/.

Roger Ebert. 1986. "Dead Poet's Society." Accessed November 3, 2013. http://www.rogerebert.com/reviews/dead-poets-society-1989.

Rotten Tomatoes. 2013. "Dead Poet's Society." Accessed November 3, 2013. http://www.rottentomatoes.com/m/dead_poets_society/.

Death, Denial of

The denial of death is when someone refuses to accept the concept of mortality for either himself or herself or someone else. Death is something that all living creatures experience at some point in their lives. It is an inevitable part of life that affects everyone. Many struggle to come to terms with the inevitable end of their own life or the loss of another.

Description

Within the United States the discussion of death is often considered a taboo topic of conversation. There are many implications with dealing with grief and loss for the loss or pending loss of a loved one or demise of one's self. Denial of death can occur for those who are terminally ill and seeing the end of their own life coming or for those who are anticipating the loss of a loved one or have already lost that person.

The loss of a loved one can lead a person to experience shock, increase his or her desire to connect with others, or bring on sadness, regret, and other mixed emotions. It is important to note that there are different attitudes toward death among various cultures. These variations can play a role in how an individual deals with death.

Humans have always contemplated the meaning of life and mortality. Regardless of how hard someone tries to ignore the awareness of the loss, symptoms will present through stressors, depressing thoughts, anxieties, or conflicts. Unfortunately, to be focused on the denial or fear of death can prevent people from living fully because so much energy is spent on the denial and avoidance of death. Freud argued that denial and fear of death is universal and a biological inheritance; however, therapists can help clients move past this fear or denial of death by working on acceptance.

Current Status

In the time of grief and loss or when someone is struggling with the acceptance of the end of life, therapists may be called on to assist with the transition. Tragic or unexpected loss can be very difficult for a person to come to terms with, especially the loss of a loved one. In 2012 and 2013, U.S. citizens experienced several large-scale tragedies, the Sandy Hook Elementary school shooting in Newtown, the Colorado movie theater shootings, devastating tornados in Oklahoma, the Boston Marathon bombing, and a plant explosion in Texas, all which cost many their lives. Agencies such as the Red Cross and other disaster reliefs are now including therapists and licensed practitioners as part of the first responders to meet the mental and emotional needs of those dealing with the loss of a loved one.

Mindy Parsons, PhD

See also: Grief; Palliative Care; Psychological Factors Affecting Other Medical Conditions; Terminal Illness, Psychological Factors

Further Reading

Becher, Emily H., Tomoko Ogasawara, and Steven M. Harris. "Death of a Clinician: The Personal, Practical and Clinical Implications of Therapist Mortality." *Contemporary Family Therapy* 34 (2012): 313–321.

Becker, Ernest. *The Denial of Death.* New York, NY: Free Press, 1997.

Meladze, Victor. "Denial of Death: America in Decline." *The Journal of Psychohistory* 39 (2012): 180–202.

Wong, Paul T.P., and Adrian Tomer. "Beyond Terror and Denial: The Positive Psychology of Death Acceptance." *Death Studies* 35 (2011): 99–106.

Defense Mechanisms

Defense mechanisms are unconscious psychological processes by which individuals unknowingly attempt to reduce anxiety or conflict. These can be either healthy or detrimental for the individual.

Definitions

- **Coping strategy** is a conscious process employed by an individual to reduce anxiety or resolve a conflict or problem.

- **DSM-5** stands for the *Diagnostic and Statistical Manual of Mental Disorders, Fifth Edition*, which is a diagnostic system used by professionals to identify mental disorders with specific diagnostic criteria.

- **Psychoanalytic theory** is a psychological theory that explains behaviors and perceptions as the result of unconscious, sexual, and biological instincts. This is the original theory of Sigmund Freud.

- **Unconscious** is an aspect of the mind which operates without awareness and over which one does not have active control. In contrast, the subconscious mind lies just below consciousness (awareness), and it is easily accessible if attention is paid to it.

Description

Defense mechanisms are psychological processes by which an unconscious drive that is incompatible with the world or one's sense of self is resolved. This process can also serve to protect an individual from the experience of fear, anxiety, and guilt. It can occur without the individual being initially aware that it is happening. Defense mechanisms are sometimes confused with coping strategies. The difference is that coping strategies are conscious efforts for dealing with conflicts. In contrast, defense mechanisms are unconscious efforts.

Defense mechanisms date back to the work of Sigmund Freud, the originator of psychoanalytic theory. Originally called "ego defense mechanisms," Freud suggested that drives associated with the id (unconscious and primitive instincts) conflicted with the superego (moral part of self) representing societal rules and ideas of fairness. The reason it was called ego defense mechanism is that he believed the ego was the part of the self that resolved the conflict between the id and the superego. Although his model of ego is no longer used, his work served as the basis of contemporary defense mechanisms.

Defense mechanisms are numerous and unique. Here are descriptions of some of the more common defense mechanism.

- **Denial** is the defense mechanism whereby the consequences, implication, or a disturbing event is blocked or denied, as if they have never happened. For example, an individual who is on the verge of bankruptcy may continue unsustainable spending when it is otherwise obvious that he or she should change spending habits. Individuals may completely deny an obvious fact, or they may also acknowledge that fact but deny the consequences. This is similar to repression except for in repression it is disturbing thoughts, not a physical reality that is denied.

- **Displacement** is the unconscious refocusing of negative feelings or impulses on to a different object, usually one that has less power to retaliate or threaten. For example, an employer, someone who is very difficult to retaliate against, may unfairly reprimand an individual. Instead of responding to the employer, the employee unknowing takes his or her aggression out on the family pet on returning home. This is similar to sublimation, except for in sublimation the transmutation of the impulse of thought is typically more acceptable.

- **Intellectualization** is characterized by unknowingly denying the emotional or meaningful content of thoughts or events. Instead, the individual considers the event in a removed or overly objective manner. That is to say that they deal with the event intellectually and not emotionally. For example, a parent may

be unable to knowingly accept the death of a child and subsequently may act robotic and unemotional toward spouse or others.

- **Projection** is a mechanism in which individuals extend some thought or quality about themselves on to another. For example, an individual may be unconsciously unwilling to accept that he or she has not achieved a high level of success and project this notion on to others. Subsequently, the individual may see or accuse others of being lazy or not achieving their potential.

- **Rationalization** is the most commonplace of defense mechanisms. This is characterized by explaining unacceptable events or thoughts with a logical argument while not acknowledging an apparent truth. For example, a student who receives a poor grade on a test may blame a professor for poor teaching when, in fact, the student did not study sufficiently.

- **Reaction formation** is the mechanism whereby an individual acts in a way contrary or opposite to his or her true sentiments. For example, if a man is attracted to a woman but unconsciously fears rejection, he may act cold and uninterested even if the woman acts as if she may be interested.

- **Regression** is characterized by a reaction to a disturbing event that is indicative of a less mature level of development. For example, an adult may experience significant financial hardship and revert to a childlike dependency on friends or parents.

- **Repression** is characterized by the unconscious blocking of disturbing thoughts from conscious awareness. An individual unknowingly represses difficult or unacceptable thoughts to such an extent that he or she is completely unaware of the disturbing thought having ever taken place. For example, an individual may have been exposed to abuse and acknowledge that it happened but be consciously unaware of any feelings about the event. This is similar to denial, but different in with denial is the event itself that is blocked, not thoughts.

- **Sublimation** is a defense mechanism whereby an individual transfers the energy of a disturbing event or thought and expresses it in a more acceptable form. For example, someone who experienced a great deal of pain in childhood made unknowingly express his or her pain in art of exercise. This mechanism is similar to displacement except for in displacement the energy is transferred in to another object and is not necessarily dealt with in a more acceptable manner.

Defense mechanisms are no longer listed in DSM-5; however, they were listed in the previous DSM-4 as an area to be studied further. Although they are not listed in the current DSM, they are nonetheless useful to a clinician in assessing clients and understanding their behavior.

Len Sperry, MD, PhD, and Jeremy Connelly, MEd

See also: Diagnostic and Statistical Manual of Mental Disorders (DSM)

Further Reading

American Psychiatric Association. *Diagnostic and Statistical Manual of Mental Disorders*, 5th ed. Arlington, VA: American Psychiatric Association, 2013.

Cramer, Phebe. *Protecting the Self: Defense Mechanisms in Action*. New York, NY: The Guilford Press, 2006.

Valliant, George. *Ego Mechanisms of Defense: A Guide for Clinicians and Researchers*. Washington, DC: American Psychiatric Press, 1992.

Deinstitutionalization

Deinstitutionalization is the release of a person with mental or physical disabilities from a hospital, asylum, or other medical institution, usually with the intention of providing treatment, support, or rehabilitation through outpatient community resources.

Description

Until the 1960s, American citizens who were diagnosed with severe mental illnesses, like schizophrenia, were institutionalized in government-run mental hospitals.

These people were deemed to require long-term or permanent professional care and institutions were often called asylums for the insane. Government policy beginning in the 1960s refocused the concept of care for those with severe mental illnesses. In the movement of deinstitutionalization, the government decided to transfer responsibility for mental health care from state government to local care centers that would be funded largely by the federal government.

The deinstitutionalization of mental health care was made possible by several factors. The first was a change in the way society viewed the need and benefit of institutionalizing people with mental health issues. Mental health professionals began to feel that the large-scale institutionalization of people made them more dependent. Many believed that it accustomed patients to being passive recipients of care without encouraging them to change their circumstances or return to the outside world. Overall, people began to develop new attitudes toward those with mental health issues. People began seeing them no longer as patients for life but rather as people with treatable problems. Many believed that their issues could be resolved better within society rather than by removing them from society.

The second factor that promoted this movement was the possibility of controlling thinking and behavior through drug treatment. With patients whose symptoms indicated they were doing well and whose medication was managed, it was deemed that they could once again participate in normal society. And, finally, the last factor that made deinstitutionalization possible was the shift of financial support of these facilities from states to federal budgets. This process began in the United States and soon spread to Europe.

Current Status and Impact (Psychological Influence)

Among most people deinstitutionalization was considered a success in terms of reducing the number of mental health patients in hospitals by 75% between 1955 and 1980. But there have been criticisms of the movement. One is that there is a high cost in terms of the poorer quality of patient care that may be available in community service settings. Some say that hospitalization programs provide better quality care. Another factor that many believe credible is that some patients who would have been cared for in psychiatric institutions are now in prisons. This likely includes people who suffer from paranoid delusions or types of dementia. Those disorders may lead them to refuse help because they either believe that people are trying to hurt them or that they do not need the help. Many people experiencing psychosis break the law and end up in the prison system instead of in medical treatment.

Inpatient hospital treatment does still exist in the United States and internationally. Most of these institutions, however, are privately owned and operated. Several privately run mental institutions provide services to patients who have broken the law but have been deemed mentally unfit and therefore instead of prison sentences they are ordered to seek inpatient hospital treatment. For these patients, their stays can range in time from a few months to decades.

The shift from hospitalization to community-based treatment has resulted in some concerns. From some perspectives, community-based services are not always adequate to the task of meeting the complex needs of all patients. This could lead to a portion of those with mental health issues who are living homeless, jobless, or with limited social connections. Today, many families are forced to provide care that once would have been more widely available from state institutions. Deinstitutionalization by itself is not the simple solution to a difficult and long-term mental health-care problem. But it has given people with mental illness or disabilities the opportunity to have access to the community and gain as much independence as possible.

Alexandra Cunningham, PhD, and
William M. Cunningham, MA

See also: Crisis Housing; Homelessness; Hospitalization

Further Reading

Johnson, Kelley, and Rannveig Traustadottir. *Deinstitutionalization and People with Intellectual Disabilities: In and Out of Institutions.* London, UK: Jessica Kingsley, 2005.

Paulson, George. *Closing the Asylums: Causes and Consequences of the Deinstitutionalization Movement.* Jefferson, NC: McFarland, 2012.

Torrey, Fuller E. *Out of the Shadows: Confronting America's Mental Illness Crisis.* New York, NY: John Wiley & Sons, 1997.

Delayed Ejaculation

Delayed ejaculation is a mental disorder characterized by a male's delay, difficulty, or inability to reach sexual orgasm. It is also referred to as male orgasmic disorder.

Definitions

- **Cognitive behavior therapy** is a type of psychotherapy that focuses on maladaptive (problematic) behaviors, emotions, and thoughts. It is also called CBT.

- **DSM-5** stands for the *Diagnostic and Statistical Manual of Mental Disorders, Fifth Edition*, which is a diagnostic system used by professionals to identify mental disorders with specific diagnostic criteria.

- **Orgasm** is the peak of sexual excitation characterized by extremely pleasurable sensations.

- **Sensate focus exercises** are series of touching *exercises* designed to increase intimacy in a relationship. It is also called sensate focusing.

- **Sexual dysfunctions disorders** are a group of mental disorders characterized by significant difficulty in the ability to respond sexually or to experience sexual pleasure. Disorders include female organismic disorder and delayed ejaculation.

- **Sexual orgasm** is orgasm attained through sexual intercourse instead of self-stimulation or oral stimulation.

- **Systematic desensitization** is a form of cognitive behavior therapy that gradually exposes individuals to their phobia, while remaining calm and relaxed.

Description and Diagnosis

Delayed ejaculation disorder is one of the DSM-5 sexual dysfunction disorders. It is characterized by delay, difficulty, or complete absence of sexual orgasm in males during otherwise normal sexual activity. Some with this disorder indicate that they avoid sex because of it. There is no consensus on what constitutes a delay in ejaculation. For this reason, the male's self-report is the basis for making the diagnosis. Delayed ejaculation is relatively rare, affecting less than 1% of men (American Psychiatric Association, 2013). However, this disorder is more likely to occur after the age of 50.

According to the *Diagnostic and Statistical Manual of Mental Disorders, Fifth Edition*, this diagnosis requires the following criteria to be met. First, the male must experience a delay or absence of sexual orgasm in 75% or more occasions of sexual activity with his partner. This delay must be present for at least six months and cannot be attributable to relationship stress, use of medications, another disorder, or a medical condition. In addition, it must cause the male considerable distress. Some individuals may experience this disorder for their entire lives or may develop symptoms following a period of otherwise normal sexual functioning. Also, symptoms may be present in certain situations or may always be present. The condition is further specified (diagnosed) as mild, moderate, or severe.

The cause of this disorder is not well understood. However, it is believed to be associated with relationship or partner issues, a history of sexual abuse, and stress. Cultural factors, religious issues, and social factors can also cause or complicate the disorder.

Treatment

The goal of treatment is to restore normal sexual functioning. The first step in the treatment of this disorder is to identify and treat any physical cause or mental disorder. Like female orgasmic disorder, this dysfunction may have numerous cultural or social factors that must be considered. Therefore, treatment must be focused not only on the physical aspects of the disorder but also on the individual's beliefs and personal history. Treatment most commonly includes psychotherapy. Typically, this involves cognitive behavior therapy and specifically sensate focus exercises and systematic desensitization. Involving the spouse or sexual partner may be necessary if relational issues are present or sensate focusing is used. It is not uncommon for the partner to believe that he is no longer attracted to her because of his inability to reach climax. This and other concerns can lead to additional complications unless

they are addressed in treatment. Specific medications are sometimes used in the treatment of this disorder.

Len Sperry, MD, PhD, and Jeremy Connelly, MEd

See also: Cognitive Behavior Therapy; *Diagnostic and Statistical Manual of Mental Disorders* (DSM); Female Orgasmic Disorder; Sexual Dysfunctions; Systematic Desensitization

Further Reading

American Psychiatric Association. *Diagnostic and Statistical Manual of Mental Disorders*, 5th ed. Arlington, VA: American Psychiatric Association, 2013.

Berkowitz, Bob, and Susan Yager-Berkowitz. *Why Men Stop Having Sex: Men, the Phenomenon of Sexless Relationships, and What You Can Do about It*. San Francisco, CA: Harper Perennial, 2009.

Rowland, David. *Sexual Dysfunction in Men: Advances in Psychotherapy, Evidence-Based Practice*. Cambridge, MA: Hogrefe Publishing, 2012.

Deliberate Practice

Deliberate practice is the intentional effort to achieve a level of expertise that is just beyond an individual's level of proficiency. It is also known as purposeful practice.

Definitions

- **Deliberate practice** is the intentional effort in striving to attain increased expertise just beyond an individual's level of proficiency.

- **Expertise** is the special knowledge or skills in a particular subject or area learned from experience or training and a high level of proficiency in utilizing that knowledge or skills.

- **Feedback** is information about how well or badly an individual is performing a task and is intended to help the individual perform it better.

- **Practice** is the act of rehearsing or engaging in an activity repeatedly in order to improve performance.

- **Self-reflection** is the process of examining one's own thoughts, feelings, and motivations in order to grow and change.

Description

Expertise is a lifelong process of continued development extending over several years of professional practice. More specifically, it requires years of professional training, professional experience, and challenges to be confronted and overcome on the path to expertise. It also requires an awareness of one's limitations, which motivates the individual to continue learning and developing throughout his or her career. Research suggests that it takes a minimum of 10 years for a high level of expertise to be achieved. This means 10 years of progressively increasing expertise, rather than 1 year of limited expertise that is repeated 10 times. The difference between the two is deliberate practice.

Deliberate practice differs considerably from practice. The key difference is intentional, stretching beyond one's current level of proficiency. Deliberate practice involves setting a stretch goal for performance, using specific interventions to master a specified task, seeking and using feedback, and engaging in self-reflection to optimize performance and increase expertise. In learning new skills, deliberate practice involves engaging in increasingly difficult elements of the skill. Setbacks and frustration are inevitable, and persistence and learning through failure, although unpleasant, are also necessary. Seeking ongoing feedback can greatly enhance deliberate practice. Then, it means using the feedback to alter the course or direction of treatment. Being open to feedback is part of deliberate practice. Finally, deliberate practice is fostered by the use of self-reflection.

Developments and Current Status

In 1980, two researchers, Stuart Dreyfus (n.d.) and Hubert Dreyfus (1929–), proposed that a learner passes through five distinct stages of developing expertise. These two brothers named the stages: novice, competence, proficiency, expertise, and mastery. Since then, the scientific study of expertise has expanded rapidly. Initially, this research focused on athletes, musicians, and chess players. Studies by psychologist K. Anders Ericsson (1948–) found that at least 10,000 hours of deliberate practice spread over at least 10 years was necessary to develop expertise. Now, this research has extended to physicians, psychotherapists, and elementary school students.

Len Sperry, MD, PhD

See also: Evidence-Based Practice; Psychotherapy

Further Reading

Clark, Ruth C. *Building Expertise: Cognitive Methods for Training and Performance Improvement*, 3rd ed. New York, NY: John Wiley & Sons, 2009.

Ericsson, K. Anders, Neil Charness, Paul J. Feltovich, and Robert R. Hoffman, eds. *The Cambridge Handbook of Expertise and Expert Performance*. Cambridge: Cambridge University Press, 2006.

Ronnestad, Michael H., and Thomas M. Skovholt, eds. *The Developing Practitioner: Growth and Stagnation of Therapists and Counselors*. New York, NY: Routledge, 2013.

Sperry, Len, and Jon Carlson. *How Master Therapists Work: Effecting Change from the First to the Last Session and Beyond*. New York, NY: Routledge, 2014.

Delirium

Delirium is a mental disorder characterized by rapid onset of extreme disorientation and confusion.

Definitions

- **Dementia** is the deterioration or loss of mental processes, particularly memory and confusion.

- **DSM-5** stands for the *Diagnostic and Statistical Manual of Mental Disorders, Fifth Edition*, which is a diagnostic system used by professionals to identify mental disorders with specific diagnostic criteria.

- **Neurocognitive disorders** are a group of disorders in DSM-5 that are characterized by a decline from a previous level of neurocognitive (mental) function.

Description and Diagnosis

Delirium is one of the neurocognitive disorders of the DSM-5. It is characterized by severe disorientation and confusion. Individuals who experience delirium appear to be bewildered and are unable to comprehend attempts to communicate. While this condition is most often acute, it can be chronic for some, particularly the elderly. Since the symptoms of delirium and dementia can be similar, it is essential that an accurate diagnosis be made by a trained physician or clinician.

This disorder is relatively rare in the population as a whole, affecting between 1% and 2%. However, over the course of an individual's lifetime it is not unlikely that the individual may experience delirium at some point. With increasing age, the chances of experiencing delirium increase significantly, especially in hospital and nursing facilities. In fact, delirium occurs in 15%–53% of individuals after a surgery and approximately 80% of those in intensive care. In addition, 83% of individuals experience delirium as they are dying (American Psychiatric Association, 2013).

According to the *Diagnostic and Statistical Manual of Mental Disorders, Fifth Edition*, individuals can be diagnosed with this disorder if they experience difficulty in focusing their attention and awareness, and are disoriented. These symptoms must have developed over a short time period and tend to fluctuate in severity. Also, the symptoms must be accompanied by some limitation in memory, coordination, or ability to communicate. Finally, there must be evidence that the disturbance has been caused by a substance, medication, or a medical condition or exposure to a toxic substance (American Psychiatric Association, 2013).

Unlike most mental disorders, the cause of delirium is well understood. It usually results from medical conditions that deprive the brain of oxygen or induce chemical imbalances. Most commonly these are dehydration or infections such as pneumonia, urinary tract infection, and abdominal infections. Other causes include alcohol or drug intoxication or withdrawal, exposure to a poison or toxic substance, and surgery. Some medications, like allergy medications, or combinations of medications can trigger delirium.

Treatment

The primary focus of treatment is to address the underlying cause or causes. Usually this means treating an infection, giving oxygen, or stopping the use of the medication or substance. Treatment then focuses on calming the brain and reducing disorientation using reorientation techniques. These include memory cues such as a calendar and clocks, and making the environment stable, quiet, and well-lighted. In many cases, the condition will resolve without the use of drugs or treatment.

Len Sperry, MD, PhD, and Jeremy Connelly, MEd

See also: Dementia; Alzheimer's Disease

Further Reading

American Psychiatric Association. *Diagnostic and Statistical Manual of Mental Disorders*, 5th ed.. Arlington, VA: American Psychiatric Association, 2013.

Kempler, David. *Neurocognitive Disorders in Aging*. Thousand Oaks, CA: Sage Publications, 2005.

Page, Valerie, and E. Wesley Ely. *Delirium in Critical Care*. New York, NY: Cambridge University Press, 2011.

Delusional Disorder

Delusional disorder is a mental disorder characterized by delusions. Previously this disorder was referred to as paranoia or paranoid disorder.

Definitions

- **Antipsychotics** are prescription medications used to treat psychotic disorders, including schizophrenia, schizoaffective disorder, and psychotic depression.

- **Delusions** are fixed false beliefs that persist despite contrary evidence. The can be bizarre or non-bizarre (could occur in real life, such as being followed or conspired against).

- **Hallucinations** are false or distorted sensory perceptions that appear to be real perceptions that are generated by the mind rather than by an external stimuli.

- **Psychoeducation** is a psychological treatment method that provides individuals with knowledge about the condition as well as advice and skills for reducing their symptoms and improving their functioning.

- **Psychosis (psychotic disorder)** is a mental disorder characterized by a loss of touch with reality and psychotic features.

- **Psychotic features** are characteristics of psychotic disorders: delusions, hallucinations, disorganized thinking and speech, grossly disorganized or abnormal motor behavior, and negative symptoms, for example, lack of initiative and diminished emotional expression.

- **Schizophrenia spectrum and other psychotic disorders** are a group of mental disorders characterized by psychotic features. These disorders include schizophrenia, schizophreniform disorder, schizoaffective disorder, and schizotypal personality disorder, and delusional disorder.

Description and Diagnosis

Delusional disorder is one of the schizophrenic spectrum and other psychotic disorders. It is characterized by non-bizarre delusions, which is the signature feature of this disorder. This diagnosis requires the presence of persistent, non-bizarre delusions, without the other psychotic features characteristic of other schizophrenia disorders. In fact, most with the disorder can be sociable and appear quite normal as long as their delusions are not triggered in conversation. But, when triggered, these individuals are likely to express their strange beliefs. Because their psychosis is limited and contained, these individuals are able to function reasonably well in other areas of their life. That means that professionals like physicians, lawyers, and teachers who are delusional can otherwise function in their jobs and personal lives. However, there are some who become so preoccupied with their delusion that their lives become disrupted.

Several types of delusional disorders can be specified, each of which reflects a dominant delusional theme. These include the *Erotomanic Type*, with the theme that someone of a higher status is in love with the individual. In the *Grandiose Type*, the theme involves inflated power or a special relationship to a deity or famous individual. In the *Jealous Type*, the theme involves the unfaithful of the individual's sexual partner. In the *Persecutory Type*, the theme involves being abused or treated malevolently. In the *Somatic Type*, the theme involves having a physical defect or medical condition. Delusional disorder is a rare disorder and is found in approximately 0.2% of adults. The jealous type is more common in females, while the persecutory type is more common in males (American Psychiatric Association, 2013).

According to the *Diagnostic and Statistical Manual of Mental Disorders, Fifth Edition*, individuals can be diagnosed with this disorder if they exhibit one or more delusions. Such delusions are manifest for at least one month. In addition, there are no positive symptoms of schizophrenia such as hallucinations. If hallucinations are present, they are related to the theme of the delusions. Functioning at work or in relationships is not significantly impaired. Nor is the individual's behavior considered odd, bizarre, or eccentric. If a major depressive episode or a manic episode has occurred concurrently, these episodes have been relatively brief. The symptoms of this disorder must develop during or within one month of intoxication by or withdrawal from the substance. Finally, the disorder cannot be caused by a substance, a medical condition, or another mental disorder (American Psychiatric Association, 2013).

The cause of this disorder is not well understood. However, genetic, biochemical, and environmental factors may play a significant role in its development. There is a strong family link with this disorder and both schizophrenia and schizotypal personality disorders, suggesting a genetic basis (American Psychiatric Association, 2013). Biochemically, those with this disorder may have an imbalance in neurotransmitters (brain chemicals) that accounts for their symptoms. Also, environmental factors such as social isolation, drug abuse, excessive stress, and recent immigration may increase the risk of developing this disorder.

Treatment Considerations

By definition, delusional beliefs are resistant to compelling contrary evidence and rational disputation. Individuals with this disorder are convinced that their delusional beliefs are correct and that there is no need to change them. Accordingly, treatment of this disorder can be extraordinarily difficult. The longer the symptoms have been present, the more refractory they are to simple treatments such as psychoeducation, psychotherapy, or medication. When those with this disorder agree to psychotherapy, it should be initiated in such a way that its benefits outweigh their reluctance to discuss their beliefs. Accordingly, early therapy sessions should emphasize developing a trusting relationship with a neutral and accepting therapist. Cognitive behavior therapy can be useful in changing delusional behavior. Antipsychotic medication can be also effective with this disorder. Such medication can take the "edge" off delusions and facilitate psychotherapy. However, those with this disorder are often resistant to taking medication.

Len Sperry, MD, PhD

See also: Antipsychotic Medication; Cognitive Behavior Therapy; Delusions; Hallucinations; Schizophrenia; Schizotypal Personality Disorder

Further Reading

American Psychiatric Association. *Diagnostic and Statistical Manual of Mental Disorders*, 5th ed. Arlington, VA: American Psychiatric Association, 2013.

Freeman, Daniel. *Overcoming Paranoid and Suspicious Thoughts: A Self-Help Guide Using Cognitive Behavioral Techniques.* New York, NY: Basic Books, 2009.

Kantor, Martin. *Understanding Paranoia: A Guide for Professionals, Families, and Sufferers.* Santa Barbara, CA: Praeger, 2007.

Torrey, E. Fuller. *Surviving Schizophrenia*, 6th ed. New York, NY: Harper Perennial, 2014.

Delusions

Delusions are fixed, false beliefs that persist despite contrary evidence.

Definitions

- **Antipsychotic medications** are prescription medications used to treat psychotic disorders, including schizophrenia, schizoaffective disorder, and delusional disorder.

- **Delusional disorder** is a mental disorder characterized by delusions. Previously this disorder was referred to as paranoia or paranoid disorder.

- **Hallucinations** are false or distorted sensory perceptions that appear to be real perceptions that are generated by the mind rather than by an external stimuli.

- **Paranoia** is an unfounded or exaggerated distrust or suspiciousness of others.

- **Psychosis (psychotic disorder)** is a mental disorder characterized by a loss of touch with reality and psychotic features.

- **Schizophrenia** is a chronic mental disorder that affects behavior, thinking, and emotion which make distinguishing between real and unreal experiences difficult. Symptoms include hallucinations, delusions, thought and communication disturbances, and withdrawal from others.

Description

Delusions are unshakeable false beliefs. They are irrational, defy normal reasoning, and remain firm even in the face of overwhelming proof to the contrary. These beliefs are not accepted by others in the individual's culture or subculture (American Psychiatric Association, 2013). They are psychotic symptoms that are often accompanied by hallucinations or paranoia which act to strengthen the delusions. Delusions must be distinguished from overvalued or unreasonable ideas. With such ideas individuals usually have some doubt about the validity of their ideas. In contrast, delusional individuals are absolutely convinced that their delusions are valid.

Delusions are categorized as either bizarre or non-bizarre. Bizarre delusions are false beliefs that could never occur in real life, such as the belief that president is an alien. Non-bizarre delusions are false beliefs that could occur in real life, such as being followed or conspired against. Delusions can be symptoms of many physical and mental disorders, as well as reactions to some medications. They are most common in schizophrenia and delusional disorder. Delusional disorder is a rare disorder and is found in approximately 0.2% of adults. Jealous delusions are more common in females, while persecutory delusions are more common in males (American Psychiatric Association, 2013). Other common disorders that may involve delusions include depression, bipolar disorder, and some types of alcohol and drug abuse. Many with Alzheimer's disease eventually develop delusions.

There are several types of delusions. The most common are described here.

Persecutory delusions. Individuals with this delusion falsely believe that they are being followed, cheated, drugged, conspired against, spied on, attacked, or obstructed in their pursuit of a goal. This type of delusion can be so broad and complex that it can appear to explain everything that happens to an individual. This is the most common type of delusions.

Jealous delusions. Individuals with this delusion falsely believe that their romantic partner is having an affair. Those with this belief may try to restrict their partner's activities or gather "evidence" and confront the partner about the nonexistent affair. This type of delusion is most likely to be associated with violent behavior. It is the second most common type of delusions.

Erotomanic delusions. Individuals with this delusion falsely believe that a famous individual or someone of higher status is in love with them. Usually, they attempt to contact the other through phone calls, letters, or gifts. Sometimes this delusion leads to stalking or violence against that individual or a perceived romantic rival.

Grandiose delusions. Individuals with this delusion falsely believe that they have special talents, powers, or abilities. They may even believe that they are famous or that they have a special mission in life. For example, they may believe they are a rock star or sent by God to save the world. More often, they believe that they have made a significant contribution for which they have not gotten sufficient recognition.

Somatic delusions. Individuals with this delusion falsely believe that their body is somehow diseased, deformed, or infested. For example, they may believe that their body is infested with parasites. Often this delusion leads to excessive and irrational concerns about their body so that they continually seek medical treatment for their imagined condition.

Delusion of reference. Individuals with this delusion falsely believe that insignificant remarks, events, or objects in their environment have personal meaning for them. They may believe that they are receiving special messages from a newspaper story or a television announcement. Often, the meaning assigned to such messages is negative.

While delusions of reference may be bizarre, most persecutory, somatic, erotomanic, grandiose, and jealous delusions are considered non-bizarre.

While delusions are usually caused by an underlying medical condition, other mental disorders, or drug reaction, the exact cause is unknown. Genetics, neurotransmitter (brain chemicals) abnormalities, and psychological factors may also play a role. Delusions can be caused by drugs such as amphetamines, cocaine, and phencyclidine. Delusions can occur both during use and withdrawal from drugs or alcohol. Some prescription drugs, including stimulants, steroids, and medications for Parkinson's disease, can cause delusions.

Treatment

Individuals with delusions often resist diagnosis and treatment. Because of their firm convictions in their delusions, they believe that there is nothing about them that needs to change. Treatment depends on the underlying cause of the delusions. Antipsychotic medications and psychotherapy, particularly cognitive behavior therapy, are commonly used. The prognosis for delusions depends on the underlying cause. Those caused by schizophrenia usually disappear within a few weeks of starting antipsychotic medication. With appropriate treatment, even those with diagnoses of delusional disorder can experience some relief of symptoms.

Len Sperry, MD, PhD

See also: Antipsychotic Medication; Cognitive Behavior Therapy; Delusional Disorder; Hallucinations; Schizophrenia

Further Reading

American Psychiatric Association. *Diagnostic and Statistical Manual of Mental Disorders*, 5th ed. Arlington, VA: American Psychiatric Association, 2013.

Freeman, Daniel. *Overcoming Paranoid and Suspicious Thoughts: A Self-Help Guide Using Cognitive Behavioral Techniques.* New York, NY: Basic Books, 2009.

Kantor, Martin. *Understanding Paranoia: A Guide for Professionals, Families, and Sufferers.* Santa Barbara, CA: Praeger, 2007.

Dementia

Dementia is the deterioration or loss of mental processes, particularly memory.

Definitions

- **Alzheimer's disease** is a medical and mental disorder that causes dementia, particularly late in life. It is also referred to as Neurocognitive Disorder Due to Alzheimer's Disease.

- **DSM-5** is the abbreviation for the *Diagnostic and Statistical Manual of Mental Disorders, Fifth Edition*, which is the handbook mental health professionals use to diagnose mental disorders.

- **Neurocognitive disorders** are a group of disorders in DSM-5 that are characterized by a decline from a previous level of neurocognitive (mental) function.

Description and Diagnosis

Dementia is a group of symptoms including loss of memory, judgment, language, and other cognitive (mental) function caused by the death of neurons (nerve cells) in the brain. It may also include changes in behavior, personality, and motor functions. There is commonly a loss of memory and the skills. The changes can be severe enough to seriously disrupt the individual's ability to carry out activities of daily living. These changes can be due to medical conditions such as Alzheimer's disease or a stroke (vascular dementia) or because of repeated blows to the head (in football players and boxers). Of the various types of dementia, Alzheimer's disease causes the most complications.

Dementia involves more than memory loss. It also involves decline in intellectual function, including difficulties with language, simple calculations, planning and judgment, and abstract reasoning. While dementia is not caused by aging, it is quite common in older individuals. It results from infections, brain diseases, tumors, and injuries to or biochemical changes within the brain. It should be noted that the term "dementia" has been replaced by "neurocognitive disorder" in DSM-5. The reason is that while dementia is most associated with cognitive impairment in the elderly, the term "neurocognitive disorder" is widely used and often preferred for conditions affecting younger individuals, such as impairment due to traumatic brain injury or HIV infection (American Psychiatric Association, 2013).

There are several types of dementia. Following are brief descriptions of the more common types.

Alzheimer's disease. Alzheimer's disease is the sixth leading cause of death in the United States and the fifth leading cause of death for persons 65 years of age and older. Between 60% and 90% and more of dementias are estimated to be of this type. Before the age of 70, about 10% of adults are diagnosed with the disorder. That figure rises to at least 25% after ago 70. Women are more likely than are men to develop this disease, in part because they tend to live longer (American Psychiatric Association, 2013).

Vascular dementia. This type is also called multi-infarct dementia because it involves changes in blood vessels in the brain. It is the second most common cause of dementia after Alzheimer's disease. Within three months following a stroke, between 20% and 30% of individuals are diagnosed with this type. It is more common in men than in women (American Psychiatric Association, 2013). Risk factors for it include high blood pressure, diabetes, a history of smoking, and heart disease.

Dementia with Lewy bodies. Dementia with Lewy bodies is probably the next most common form of dementia after vascular dementia. Lewy bodies are chemical substances in damaged nerve cells in the brain that cause or complicate dementia. Because the relationship between Lewy bodies in various types of dementia is not well understood, exact statistics for this type are unclear. Yet it is estimated that up to 30.5% of all dementias are of this type (American Psychiatric Association, 2013).

Other dementias. There are several other less common types of dementia. These include frontal lobe dementia, Pick's disease, Huntington disease,

Parkinson's disease, HIV infection, and head trauma. Repeated head trauma in those playing contact sports in high school and college is now considered a risk factor for developing dementia in later life. These other dementias may account for about 10% of all dementias.

Treatment

The primary goals of treating dementias are to preserve functioning and independence, and maintain quality of life, as much as possible. Specific treatment of dementia is based on its type and the particular case. In some types, cognitive function can be improved but not corrected. In some cases, dementia respond better to treatment than others. For example, treating high blood pressure in someone with the vascular dementia type can lead to considerable improvement in memory and cognitive functioning. In contrast, those in the advanced-stage Alzheimer's type may experience little or no improvement. However, in all cases, appropriate care and support is always helpful and should be extended. Medication and cognitive behavior therapy interventions are additional interventions.

Medications that target the symptoms of dementia include Cognex, Aricept, Exelon, Reminyl, and Namenda. Cognitive behavior therapy (CBT) interventions may be used to reduce the frequency or severity of problem behaviors such as aggression or socially inappropriate behavior. CBT is particularly useful in identifying and modifying the situations that trigger problem behaviors, which can be effective.

Len Sperry, MD, PhD

See also: Aricept (Donepezil); Cognitive Behavior Therapy; Dementia; Namenda (Memantine)

Further Reading

American Psychiatric Association. *Diagnostic and Statistical Manual of Mental Disorders*, 5th ed. Arlington, VA: American Psychiatric Association, 2013.

Burns, Alistair, and Bengt Winblad, eds. *Severe Dementia.* New York, NY: John Wiley & Sons, 2006.

Doraiswamy, P. Murali, Lisa Gwyther, and Tina Adler. *The Alzheimer's Action Plan: What You Need to Know—and What You Can Do—about Memory Problems, from Prevention to Early Intervention and Care.* New York, NY: St. Martin's Press, 2009.

Mace, Nancy, and Peter V. Ravins. *The 36-Hour Day: A Family Guide to Caring for People with Alzheimer Disease, Other Dementias, and Memory Loss in Later Life*, 5th ed. Baltimore, MD: The Johns Hopkins University Press, 2012.

Depakote (Divalproex Sodium)

Depakote is a prescribed medication for the treatment and prevention of seizures. Its generic name is divalproex sodium.

Definitions

- **Absence seizures** are ones characterized by abrupt, short-term lack of conscious activity along with behaviors such as eye rolls, blank stares, and lip movements. It is also referred to as petit mal seizures.

- **Antiseizure medications** are a group of prescription drugs used to treat epilepsy as well as burning, stabbing, and shooting pain. It is also called anticonvulsant medications.

- **Epilepsy** is a medical condition involving episodes of irregular electrical discharge within the brain that causes impairment or loss of consciousness, followed by convulsions.

- **Seizure** is a sudden convulsion or uncontrolled discharge of nerve cells that may spread to other cells throughout the brain.

- **Tonic-clonic seizures** are ones that involve the entire body and are accompanied by muscle contractions, rigidity, and unconsciousness. It is also referred to as grand mal or generalized seizures.

- **Trigeminal neuralgia** is a disorder of the trigeminal nerve which causes severe facial pain.

Description

Depakote is one of the antiseizure medications. It is effective in the treatment of epilepsy, particularly in preventing simple and complex absence seizures and tonic-clonic seizures. Depakote is also used to treat the manic phase of bipolar disorder in adults, to prevent migraines in adults, and to reduce the pain of trigeminal neuralgia. It is effective in the treatment of epilepsy and in preventing absence seizures, mixed, and tonic-clonic (grand mal) seizures. Depakote is also used to treat the manic phase of bipolar disorder in adults, to prevent migraines in adults, and to reduce the pain of trigeminal neuralgia.

Its generic names are divalproex sodium, sodium valproate, and valproic acid. Depakote contains the same medication as Depakene except that it is coated to reduce some of its gastrointestinal side effects. Depakote is believed to work by increasing the levels of gamma-aminobutyric acid (GABA), which is an inhibitory neurotransmitter. That means that as GABA levels increase in the brain neurons or nerve cells, these cells are less likely to become activated or fire. The results are that seizure activity decreases, manic behavior is curbed, and the frequency of migraine headache is decreased.

Precautions and Side Effects

Because Depakote can interfere with blood clotting, blood tests should be done before starting the medication and at intervals throughout its use. Depakote use can increase the risk of birth defects when taken during pregnancy. Women who take Depakote should not breast-feed, since it can pass into the breast milk. Depakote causes drowsiness and impairs alertness in some individuals, so care must be taken in driving and using machinery until they determine how the drug affects them. The sedative effects are increased in the presence of alcohol, so it should be avoided when taking Depakote.

Common side effects of Depakote are mild stomach cramps, change in menstrual cycle, diarrhea, loss of hair, indigestion, change in appetite, nausea and vomiting, and trembling in the hands and arms. Such side effects tend to resolve with time. Another common side effect is weight gain. Those taking Depakote should be on a balanced, low-fat diet coupled with an increase in physical activity to counter this side effect.

Len Sperry, MD, PhD

See also: Bipolar Disorder; Seizures

Further Reading

Devinsky, Orrin. *Epilepsy: Patient and Family Guide*, 3rd ed. New York, NY: Demos Medical, 2007.

Diamond, Seymour, and Merle Lea Diamond. *A Patient's Guide to Headache and Migraine*, 2nd ed. Newtown, PA: Handbooks in Health Care, 2009.

Kuzniecky, Ruben, ed. *Epilepsy 101: The Ultimate Guide for Patients and Families*. Leona, NJ: Medicus Press, 2009.

Tatum, William O., Peter W. Kaplan, and Pierre Jallon. *Epilepsy A to Z: A Concise Encyclopedia*, 2nd ed. New York, NY: Demos Medical, 2009.

Dependent Personality Disorder

Dependent personality disorder is a mental disorder characterized by a pattern of submissiveness, a lack of self-confidence, and an excessive need to be taken care of by others.

Definitions

- **Assertiveness training** is a behavior change method for increasing self-esteem and self-expression in intimidating interpersonal situations.

- *Diagnostic and Statistical Manual of Mental Disorders* is the handbook mental health professionals use to diagnose mental disorders. The current edition (fifth) is known as DSM-5.

- **Personality disorder** is a long-standing pattern of maladaptive (problematic) behavior, thoughts, and emotions that deviates from the accepted norms of an individual's culture.

- **Psychotherapy** is a psychological method for achieving desired changes in thinking, feeling, and behavior. It is also called therapeutic counseling.

Description and Diagnosis

The dependent personality disorder is a personality disorder characterized by a pervasive pattern of dependent and submissive behaviors. Individuals with this disorder are excessively passive, insecure, and isolated, and become overly dependent on others. Because of their fear of rejection and abandonment, they go to great lengths to secure and maintain relationships. Individuals with this disorder see themselves as inadequate and helpless. As a result they relinquish personal responsibility and put their fate in the hands of others to protect and take care of them. While at first acceptable, this dependent behavior can become controlling and may even appear hostile. This disorder is more common in females (2:1 females to males). In females, the dependent style often takes the form of submissiveness. In males, the dependent style is more likely to be autocratic, so that the husband and boss depends on his wife and secretary to perform basic tasks which he himself cannot accomplish. Whatever the case, this disorder can lead to anxiety and depression when the dependent relationship is threatened.

The clinical presentation of the dependent personality disorder is characterized by the following: behavioral style, interpersonal style, thinking style, and feeling style. Individuals' behavioral and interpersonal styles are characterized by docility, passivity, and non-assertiveness. In interpersonal relations, they tend to be pleasing, self-sacrificing, clinging, and constantly requiring others' reassurance. Their reliance on others leads to a subtle demand that others assume responsibility for major areas of their lives. Their thinking style of dependent personalities is characterized by suggestibility. Also, they tend to minimize difficulties, and because of their naiveté are easily persuadable and easily taken advantage of. Their feeling style is characterized by insecurity and anxiousness. Because they lack self-confidence, they may experience considerable discomfort at being alone. They may be preoccupied with the fear of abandonment and disapproval of others. Their mood tends to be one of anxiety or fearfulness.

The cause of this disorder is not well understood. However, these individuals tend to have characteristic view of themselves, the world, and others, and a basic life strategy. They view themselves as inadequate and self-effacing. They tend to view the world and others as caretakers since they do not believe they can care for themselves. Accordingly, their basic life strategy and pattern is to cling and rely on others to care for them. In turn, they respond by being pleasing and willing to do whatever others want.

According to the *Diagnostic and Statistical Manual of Mental Disorders, Fifth Edition*, individuals can be diagnosed with this disorder if they exhibit a pervasive need to be cared for and cling to others because of their fear of separation. They constantly seek the advice and reassurance of others when making decisions. More than anything, they want others to take responsibility for most major areas of their lives. Not surprisingly, they seldom express disagreement with others for fear they will lose their support and approval. Because they lack confidence in their own judgment and ability, they have difficulty starting projects and doing things on their own. These individuals will even engage in actions that are difficult and unpleasant in order to receive support and caring from others. Because of unrealistic fears of being unable to take care of themselves, they feel helpless or uncomfortable when faced with being alone. When a close relationship is about to end, they immediately seek out another caring and supportive relationship. Finally, they become preoccupied with fears of being left to take care of themselves (American Psychiatric Association, 2013).

Treatment

The clinical treatment of this disorder usually involves psychotherapy. In general, the long-range goal of psychotherapy with a dependent personality is to increase the individual's sense of independence and ability to function interdependently. At other times, the therapist may need to settle for a more modest goal, that is, helping the individual become a "healthier" dependent personality. Treatment strategies typically include challenging the individual's limiting beliefs about personal inadequacy and learning ways in which to increase assertiveness in communicating with others. Assertiveness training is commonly used to achieve this. A variety of methods can be used to increase self-reliance. Among these are providing these individuals with directives and opportunities for making decisions, being alone, and taking responsibility for their own well-being.

Len Sperry, MD, PhD

See also: Personality Disorders; Psychotherapy

Further Reading

American Psychiatric Association. *Diagnostic and Statistical Manual of Mental Disorders*, 5th ed. Arlington, VA: American Psychiatric Association, 2013.

Bornstein, Robert F. *The Dependent Personality*. New York, NY: The Guilford Press, 1993.

Dobbert, Duane L. *Understanding Personality Disorders: An Introduction*. Lanham, MD: Rowman & Littlefield, 2011.

Sperry, Len. *Handbook of Diagnosis and Treatment of the DSM-5 Personality Disorders*, 3rd ed. New York, NY: Routledge, 2016.

Depersonalization/Derealization Disorder

Depersonalization/derealization disorder is a mental disorder characterized by symptoms of depersonalization, derealization, or both.

Definitions

- **Antianxiety medications** are prescribed drugs that relieve anxiety symptoms. They are also called anxiolytics or tranquilizers.

- **Antidepressants** are prescription medications used to treat depression and depressive symptoms.

- **Cognitive behavior therapy** is a type of psychotherapy that focuses on maladaptive (faulty) behaviors, emotions, and thoughts. It is also called CBT.

- **Depersonalization** is a mental state of detachment or a sense of being "outside" oneself or body and observing one's actions or thoughts.

- **Derealization** is a mental state characterized by a sense that one is out of touch with one's surroundings, as if in a dream.

- **Dissociative disorders** are a group of mental disorders characterized by a disturbance of self, memory, awareness, or consciousness and which cause impaired functioning.

- **DSM-5** stands for the *Diagnostic and Statistical Manual of Mental Disorders, Fifth Edition*, which is a diagnostic system used by professionals to identify mental disorders with specific diagnostic criteria.

- **Psychotherapy** is a psychological method for achieving desired changes in thinking, feeling, and behavior. It is also called therapeutic counseling.

- **Psychotic disorder** is a severe mental condition in which an individual loses touch with reality. Symptoms can include hallucinations (hearing or seeing things that are not there), delusions (fixed false beliefs that persist despite contrary evidence), and disordered thinking.

Description and Diagnosis

Depersonalization/derealization disorder is one of the dissociative disorders in DSM-5. It is characterized by the experience of being out of touch with oneself and/or one's immediate surroundings. The symptom of depersonalization relates to an individual's perceptions about his or her physical body or mind, while derealization relates to an individual's surroundings. Individuals presenting with this disorder may express that they feel as if they are in a dream, that things around them seem as if they are artificial, that they are having an out-of-body experience, or that they feel as if they are an automated robot. It is also likely that an individual may have difficulty describing his or her symptoms. This disorder was previously called "depersonalization disorder" but was changed to include the symptom of derealization as it is now considered to result from the same cause.

Many individuals will experience short-term (from hours to several days) depersonalization or derealization symptoms sometime during their lifetime. Most common is daydreaming. However, longer-term manifestation that is diagnosable as this disorder is rare, affecting less than 2% of the population. This disorder occurs equally as often in both males and females. In most cases, the cause of this disorder is not known. However, childhood trauma, severe stress, and the ingestion of hallucinogenic drugs are known to cause this disorder. Typically, this disorder manifests around age 16 and almost always prior to age 25 (American Psychiatric Association, 2013).

To be diagnosed with this disorder, individuals must experience persistent or recurrent depersonalization and/or derealization. Individuals must still be able to think logically about what is in fact reality and what is only a thought or perception; this is called reality testing. If they cannot discern what is real and what is not, then clinicians must consider the psychotic disorders for diagnosis. In addition, if an individual is over age 40, medical conditions must be carefully ruled out as it is extremely rare for such late onset. For some who experience this disorder, it may have a sudden onset with continuous symptoms while others may have only intermittent episodes (American Psychiatric Association, 2013).

The exact cause of this disorder is not well understood. Nevertheless, it is believed to be linked to an imbalance of neurotransmitters (brain chemicals) that make a brain vulnerable to fear and severe stress. Other likely causes include experiencing abuse or observing violence toward a family member. It might also include severe stress or trauma associated with a car accident.

Treatment

Treatment for depersonalization/derealization disorder may include both medications and psychotherapy. Commonly used medications include both antianxiety medication and antidepressants. Various psychotherapy approaches can be used. The most is cognitive behavior therapy.

Jeremy Connelly, MEd, and Len Sperry, MD, PhD

See also: Antianxiety Medication; Antidepressant Medications; Cognitive Behavior Therapy; *Diagnostic and Statistical Manual of Mental Disorders* (DSM); Dissociative Disorders; Psychotherapy; Schizophrenia

Further Reading

American Psychiatric Association, *Diagnostic and Statistical Manual of Mental Disorders*, 5th ed. Arlington, VA: American Psychiatric Association, 2013.

David, Anthony S., Dawn Baker, Emma Lawrence, Mauricio Sierra, Nick Medford, and Elaine Hunter. *Overcoming Depersonalization and Feelings of Unreality: A Self-Help Guide Using Cognitive Behavioral Therapy Techniques*. London, UK: Robinson, 2007.

Neziroglu, Fugen, and Katharine Donnelly. *Overcoming Depersonalization Disorder: A Mindfulness and Acceptance Guide to Conquering Feelings of Numbness and Unreality*. Oakland, CA: New Harbinger, 2012.

Deplin (Methyl Folate)

Deplin is a prescription remedy that is usually taken with a prescription antidepressant medication to more effectively treat symptoms of depression. Its generic name is methyl folate.

Definitions

- **Antidepressant medications** are prescription drugs that are primarily used to treat depression and depressive disorders. They are known as antidepressants.

- **Blood–brain barrier** is a specialized layer of cells around the blood vessels of the brain controlling which substances can pass from the circulatory system into the brain.

- **Folate** is a B vitamin which is needed to maintain cell growth and brain function. Deficiencies are associated with depression and result from diet, illness, aging, and some medications. The synthetic form of it is called folic acid.

- **Genetic variations** (single nucleotide polymorphisms) can predict an individual's response to certain drugs, susceptibility to environmental factors such as toxins, and risk of developing particular diseases.

- **Medical food** is a therapeutic substance administered under the supervision of a physician. It is intended for the specific dietary management of a medical condition, such as depression.

- **Methyl folate** is the active form of folate which helps in producing mood-regulating neurotransmitters. The risk of depression is higher in those with genetic variations that reduce the ability to make L-methyl folate.

- **Personalized medicine** is medical practice that uses information about an individual's unique genetic makeup and environment to customize medical care to the individual's unique needs.

Description

Deplin is a prescribed medical food (remedy) containing methyl folate, the active form of folate, which is a B vitamin. Unlike folic acid, methyl folate crosses the blood–brain barrier where it helps balance the neurotransmitters (chemical messengers) that affect mood (serotonin, norepinephrine, and dopamine). Deplin provides the necessary nutritional support so the brain can produce sufficient levels of the needed neurotransmitters to balance mood. In this novel form of treatment, Deplin is used in addition to (augmentation) an antidepressant. The way in which Deplin works differs from that of antidepressants. For example, a selective serotonin reuptake inhibitor (SSRI) antidepressant like Paxil works by slowing the "reuptake" of serotonin, making it available longer to the brain. But this SSRI may not work for long, or at all, if the brain is not producing sufficient quantities of serotonin (or other neurotransmitters) in the first place. This may explain why only 30% of those prescribed their first antidepressant get well (achieve remission) and why up to 50% of all those taking antidepressants never reach remission of their depression. Research shows that those with low levels of methyl folate are six times as likely to fail to respond to antidepressants only as those with normal levels. The reason for this appears to be genetic variations that reduce the individual's ability to make methyl folate. Taking folic acid does not have the same effect since only methyl folate crosses the blood–brain barrier. Initial research showed that an SSRI antidepressant augmented with Deplin more than doubled the response rates of an SSRI antidepressant augmented by a placebo (14.6% vs. 32.3%). Deplin reflects a shift that is beginning to occur in the practice of medicine. Customizing medication and other medical and preventive care is the basis for what is being called "personalized medicine."

Precautions and Side Effects

The rate of side effects reported by those who were given Deplin with an antidepressant at the beginning of therapy was similar to the rate of side effects reported by those who took only an antidepressant. But only a half of those who were on Deplin and an antidepressant stopped their therapy due to side effects. This means that those on Deplin and an antidepressant responded to the "main effects" (their depression improved) while "side effects" were not present or less bothersome. In terms of side effects, Deplin was not linked to weight gain, insomnia (difficulty sleeping), or sexual dysfunction. Since Deplin is relatively new, research on it is currently limited.

Len Sperry, MD, PhD

See also: Depression; Personalized Medicine; Serotonin

Further Reading

Breuning, Loretta G. *Meet Your Happy Chemicals: Dopamine, Endorphin, Oxytocin, Serotonin.* Seattle, WA: CreateSpace, 2012.

Dunbar, Katherine Read, ed. *Antidepressants.* Farmington Hills, MI: Greenhaven Press, 2006.

O'Connor, Richard. *Undoing Depression: What Therapy Doesn't Teach You and Medication Can't Give You,* 2nd ed. New York, NY: Little, Brown, 2010.

Stahl, Stephen M. *Antidepressants.* New York, NY: Cambridge University Press, 2009.

Stargrove, Mitchell Bebel, Jonathan Treasure, and Dwight McKee. *Herb, Nutrient, and Drug Interactions: Clinical Implications and Therapeutic Strategies.* St. Louis, MO: Mosby, 2007.

Depression and Depressive Disorders

Depression is an emotional state characterized by feelings of sadness, low self-esteem, guilt, or reduced ability to enjoy life. It is not considered a mental disorder unless it significantly disrupts the individual's daily functioning.

Definitions

- **Bipolar disorders** are a group of mental disorders characterized by changes in mood and in energy (e.g., being highly irritable and impulsive while not needing sleep). These include bipolar I disorder, bipolar II disorder, and cyclothymic disorder.

- **Cognitive behavior therapy** is a type of psychotherapy that focuses on maladaptive (problematic) behaviors, emotions, and thoughts. It is also called CBT.

- **Depressive disorders** are a group of mental disorders characterized by a sad or irritable mood and cognitive and physical changes that significantly disrupt the individual's daily functioning. It includes major depressive disorder, persistent depressive disorder, disruptive mood dysregulation, and premenstrual dysphoric disorder.

- **Premenstrual syndrome** is a medical condition in which cramps, breast tenderness, bloating, irritability, and depression occur prior to a woman's menstrual period and subside after it.

- **SSRI** stands for selective serotonin reuptake inhibitors. They are a class of antidepressant medications that work by blocking the reabsorption of serotonin in nerve cells and raising its level in the brain resulting in symptom reduction.

Description

"Depression" is the general name for a group of mental conditions known as depressive disorders. Most individuals experience depressive symptoms (feeling down or blue) at some point in their lives. When these symptoms are mild and short lived, they are considered a normal emotional reaction. However, when they are more severe and significantly affect daily functioning, they are considered a depressive disorder. Depressive disorders are mental conditions that require medical and psychological treatment.

Depressive disorders are widespread and are a leading cause of disability in the world. Commonly recognized symptoms of the various types of depressive disorders are recurring feelings of sadness and guilt, sleep problems, changes in appetite, decreased energy, irritability, poor concentration, hopelessness, and thoughts of death or suicide. If only these "down" symptoms are experienced, the diagnosis is likely to be a (unipolar) depressive disorder. But if the depressed periods alternate with extreme "up" periods, the individual may have a bipolar disorder.

Depression is one of the leading causes of disability in the United States. According to National Institute of Mental Health, approximately 9.5% of adult Americans have some type of depressive disorder. One out of every four college students has some type of diagnosable mental illness. Even elementary school students have been diagnosed with depressive symptoms. Women experience depression at a rate of nearly twice that of men. Internationally, depression is estimated to become the second most common health problem in the world by 2020.

The following depressive disorders are briefly described here. They are major depressive disorder, persistent depressive disorder, disruptive mood dysregulation, and premenstrual dysphoric disorder.

Major Depressive Disorder

Major depressive disorder is also called major depression. In this disorder individuals experience episodes of sad mood or anhedonia (loss of interest or pleasure) that last longer than two weeks. These episodes are marked with five or more symptoms, and they significantly disrupt their everyday function (American Psychiatric Association, 2013). Individuals may also have thoughts of self-harm. This disorder is quite different from bereavement or a grief reaction associated with the death of a loved one. Some with this disorder may experience a single episode of severe depression in their lifetimes. For many others, recurrent episodes of such depression will occur throughout their lives.

Persistent Depressive Disorder

Persistent depressive disorder was previously called dysthymic disorder. It is a new diagnosis in DSM-5 that consolidates major depressive disorder and dysthymic disorder (American Psychiatric Association, 2013). Persistent depressive disorder is characterized by a depressed mood that lasts for at least two years and other depressive symptoms. While the symptoms tend to be less severe than those in major depressive disorder, they cause significant disruptions in the individual daily functioning. For many individuals, this disorder is a lifelong condition.

Disruptive Mood Dysregulation Disorder

Disruptive mood dysregulation disorder is a diagnosis for children between the ages of 6 and 18 years. It is characterized by severe and persistent irritability resulting in temper tantrums and persistent anger or irritability between the tantrums. Both interfere with children's ability to function at home, in school, or with their friends. Prior to DSM-5, many with this symptom pattern were likely to be labeled as "bipolar children." Some of these children were diagnosed with bipolar disorder even though they seldom met all the symptoms and criteria. In fact, few will go on to develop bipolar disorder as adults. Rather, children with chronic irritability are more likely to develop depressive and/or anxiety disorders when they become adults (American Psychiatric Association, 2013).

Premenstrual Dysphoric Disorder

Premenstrual dysphoric disorder is a severe form of premenstrual syndrome in which mood swings, depression, irritability, or anxiety significantly disrupts everyday functioning. Both premenstrual syndrome and premenstrual dysphoric disorder have physical and emotional symptoms. However, premenstrual dysphoric disorder causes extreme mood shifts that can disrupt the individual's work and relationships. In both the syndrome and disorder, symptoms typically begin 7 to 10 days before the menstrual period starts and continue for the first few days of the period. Both can cause fatigue, bloating, breast tenderness, and changes in sleep and eating patterns. However, in the disorder at least one of the following emotional or behavioral symptoms stands out: extreme moodiness, marked irritability or anger, overwhelming sadness or hopelessness, or extreme anxiety or tension.

The cause of these depressive disorders is not clearly understood. Yet they appear to have some genetic, biochemical, and environmental factors that cause or worsen these disorders. Genetic imbalances in neurotransmitters (brain chemicals) and hormones are likely causes. There are also various environmental factors that are involved. These include stressful environments, certain medical conditions, and precipitating events such as the loss of a job or relationship. Alcohol and drug use and prescribed medications that alter brain chemistry can also be causes.

Treatment

Treatment of these depressive disorders depends on the type of disorder and the specific case. Those with mild forms of a disorder may respond fully to cognitive behavior therapy (CBT) or other form of psychotherapy and not require medication. Others with moderate or severe forms of a disorder may require the combination of antidepressant medication like the SSRIs and therapy. Medication can provide relatively rapid relief from the symptoms of depression. CBT can help by changing the individual's patterns of thinking or behaving that resulted in the depressive episode.

Len Sperry, MD, PhD

See also: Bipolar Disorders; Cognitive Behavior Therapy; Disruptive Mood Dysregulation Disorder; Major Depressive Disorder; Persistent Depressive Disorder; Premenstrual Dysphoric Disorder

Further Reading

American Psychiatric Association. *Diagnostic and Statistical Manual of Mental Disorders*, 5th ed. Arlington, VA: American Psychiatric Association Press, 2013.

Finnerty, Todd. *Disruptive Mood Dysregulation Disorder (DMDD), ADHD and the Bipolar Child under DSM-5: A Concise Guide for Parents and Professionals.* PsychContinuingEd.com, 2013.

Huston, James E., and Lani C. Fujitsubo. *PMDD: A Guide to Coping with Premenstrual Dysphoric Disorder.* Oakland, CA: New Harbinger Publications, 2002.

Knaus, William J., and Albert Ellis. *The Cognitive Behavioral Workbook for Depression*, 2nd ed. Oakland, CA: New Harbinger Publications, 2012.

National Institute of Mental Health, *Statistics.* Washington, DC: National Institute of Mental Health. http://www.nimh.nih.gov/statistics/index.shtml.

Noonan, Susan J., Timothy J. Petersen, Jonathan E. Alpert, and Andrew A. Nierenberg. *Managing Your Depression: What You Can Do to Feel Better.* Baltimore, MD: Johns Hopkins Press Health Book, 2013.

Papolos, Demitri. *The Bipolar Child: The Definitive and Reassuring Guide to Childhood's Most Misunderstood Disorder*, 3rd ed. New York, NY: Broadway Books, 2008.

Depression in Youth

Depression in youth can significantly interfere with a child's or teen's mood and behavior often resulting in sadness, loneliness, and inactivity.

Definition

- **Depression** is an emotional state characterized by feelings of sadness, low self-esteem, guilt, or reduced ability to enjoy life. It is not considered a mental disorder unless it significantly disrupts one's daily functioning.

Description

Depression in children and adolescents is classified as an internalizing disorder. This means that it takes place largely within the child's mind and doesn't produce external behaviors such as hyperactivity or aggression. Clinical depression in youth can be differentiated from the more normal phases of sadness and anxiety associated with development, especially in the teenage years. Unfortunately, it is often not recognized because it can be difficult to identify. If depression in children and teens is left untreated, it can lead to self-destructive behaviors, such as cutting or even suicide.

It has been estimated that as many as 2%–8% of youth may experience major depressive disorder. Researchers tend to think that the numbers for teens are higher than that. Some research says as many as 20% of adolescents may experience major depression at some point before the end of high school.

Causes and Symptoms

The causes of depression in children and teens are varied. Studies have indicated that everything from genetics to environmental factors can play a role. It is generally agreed that there is a strong link between the presence of stressors and the development of depression. Sadly, there can be a cycle of stressful events that happen to a child who experiences depression. Life stressors lead to depression and depression leads to even more feelings of stress. But some children handle their experiences of stress more easily, while others suffer from depression.

Without dismissing biological causes and genetics, it is clear that depression is often a multigenerational reaction to stressors. In other words, in some instances it is a learned behavior or a set of problematic reactions to stimuli in the lives of the depressed person. Problematic personal judgments in combination with negative social interactions can set the framework for depression in youth.

The symptoms of depression in youth are similar to those of depression in general. They include emotional issues such as intense feelings of sadness, low expression of emotion, and irritability. Other symptoms to look for as signs of depression are lack of sleep, unhealthy eating habits, and risky or injurious behaviors. Symptom includes talking about or acting on suicidal thoughts. In addition to these symptoms, others include a child having low self-esteem, focusing on negative or bad things, and distancing from friends and others.

Diagnosis and Prognosis

Traditionally, the diagnosis of depression in young people depends on the observations of parents and teachers. However, beginning in the late 1970s several self-reporting tools were developed. These tests refined the ability to detect depression based on a child's own reporting of his or her symptoms. The success of these tools, examples of which are the Children's Depression Inventory and the Kids Schedule for Affective Disorders and Schizophrenia in School-Age Children, highlights the importance of educating children and teens on how to recognize the symptoms and seek help for depression.

With early treatment for depression in youth, the prognosis is positive. This is usually most successful with counseling that involves the family and, in some cases, medication to help alleviate symptoms in children with depression. The longer treatment is delayed, the more challenging it will be to provide effective interventions.

Treatment

Cognitive behavior therapy is a preferred method of treatment for depression in youth. It contains a range of activities and approaches, including related therapies like rational-emotive therapy, attribution retraining, learned optimism, and journal writing. Some of these are ways of beginning to reframe the emotional issues for children and teens. This helps them to learn new ways of understanding and counteract their depressive thoughts and behaviors. Getting involved in positive and fun activities, especially ones that involve physical movement, is another effective method for combatting depression.

In some cases, psychiatric drugs are used for children and teens who suffer from depression. Medication to help treat depression in youth can be used either as a temporary measure or on a long-term basis. The combination of psychotherapy and medication is a common approach to treatment.

Alexandra Cunningham, PhD, and William M. Cunningham, MA

See also: Children's Depression Inventory; Depression and Depressive Disorders

Further Reading

Merrell, Kenneth W. *Helping Students Overcome Depression and Anxiety: A Practical Guide.* New York, NY: Guilford Publications, 2013.

Reivich, Karen, Jane E. Gillham, Tara M. Chaplin, and Martin E. P. Seligman. "From Helplessness to Optimism: The Role of Resilience in Treating and Preventing Depression in Youth." In *Handbook of Resilience in Children*, edited by Sam Goldstein and Robert B. Brooks, pp. 201–214. New York, NY: Springer, 2013.

Sperry, Len, ed. *Family Assessment: Contemporary and Cutting-Edge Strategies.* New York, NY: Routledge, 2012.

Depressive Personality Disorder

Depressive personality disorder is a mental disorder characterized by a persistent and lifelong pattern of pessimism, unhappiness, low self-esteem, and guilt. It is also known as melancholic personality disorder.

Definitions

- **Antidepressants** are prescribed medications that are primarily used to treat depression and depressive disorders and sometimes depressive personality disorder.

- **Cognitive behavior therapy** is a type of psychotherapy that focuses on maladaptive (faulty) behaviors, emotions, and thoughts. It is also called CBT.

- **Depression** is a sad mood or emotional state that is characterized by feelings of low self-worth or guilt and a reduced ability to enjoy life. Unless it greatly disrupts an individual's daily functioning, it is not considered a mental disorder.

- **Depressive disorders** are a group of mental disorders characterized by a sad or irritable mood and cognitive and physical changes that significantly disrupt an individual's daily functioning. These disorders include major depressive disorder and persistent depressive disorder.

- **Hypomanic personality disorder** is a mental disorder characterized by an enduring pattern of hypomania that shapes cognition, attitudes, and identity. This pattern predictably shapes such individuals' behavior and relationships with others.

- **Persistent depressive disorder** is a depressive disorder characterized by a chronic, depressed mood lasting for more than two years. It was previously called dysthymic disorder.

- **Personality disorder** is a long-standing pattern of maladaptive (problematic) behavior, thoughts, and emotions that deviates from the accepted norms of an individual's culture.

Description and Diagnosis

Depressive personality disorder is a persistent and pervasive pattern of pessimism, unhappiness, low self-esteem, and guilt that begins in early adulthood and occurs in a variety of contexts. Depressive personality disorder occurs before, during, and after other depressive disorders, making it a distinct diagnosis. Individuals with this disorder are marked by characteristic pessimism. They appear depressed, dejected, and joyless which can be disheartening to others. While they can suffer from mood swings, they are more often unhappy and melancholic. They are also overly critical and judgmental of others and constantly feel guilty and worthless.

Depressive personality disorder is listed among the personality disorders in the *Psychodynamic Diagnostic Manual*. It is described as the converse or polar opposite of the hypomanic personality disorder. Interestingly, depressive personality disorder was not listed with the other personality disorders in the *Diagnostic and Statistical Manual of Mental Disorders, Fourth Edition, Text Revision* (DSM-IV-TR). Nevertheless, it was listed in its Appendix B as a diagnosis worthy of further study, along with research criteria.

The DSM-IV-TR provides the following research criteria for depressive personality disorder. The moods of individuals with this disorder tend to be dominated by dejection, gloominess, cheerlessness, joylessness, and unhappiness. Their self-view is that of inadequacy, worthlessness, and low self-esteem. They tend to be critical, blaming and self-derogatory, brooding, and given to worry. They are also pessimistic and prone to feelings of guilt and remorse. In addition, they are negative, critical, and judgmental toward others.

As with most other personality disorders, there is no known cause for the depressive personality disorder. However, a variety of factors may be causative. These include inherited traits, early childhood experiences, and a predisposition toward pessimism. It appears that individuals with this disorder are more likely to develop persistent depressive disorder than those with other personality disorders or depressive disorders.

Treatment

Treatment depends on the severity of the condition. Psychotherapy, particularly, cognitive behavior therapy, appears to be beneficial in treating mild and moderate forms of this disorder. Medications, particularly antidepressants, may be helpful in treating the symptoms of depression of this disorder. Medication may be combined with psychotherapy for moderate to severe forms of the disorder.

Len Sperry, MD, PhD

See also: Antidepressant Medications; Cognitive Behavior Therapy; Depressive Disorders; Hypomanic Personality Disorder

Further Reading

American Psychiatric Association. *Diagnostic and Statistical Manual of Mental Disorders*, 4th ed, *text revision*. Washington, DC: American Psychiatric Association, 2000.

PDM Task Force. *Psychodynamic Diagnostic Manual*. Silver Spring, MD: Alliance of Psychoanalytic Organizations, 2006.

Detoxification

Detoxification is the process of safely removing addictive drugs from an individual's body.

Definitions

- **Addiction** is a chronic disease of the brain, which involves compulsive and uncontrolled pursuit of reward or relief with substance use or other compulsive behaviors.

- **Anxiety** is a negative emotional state characterized by feelings of nervousness, worry, and apprehension about imagined danger.

- **Benzodiazepines** are a class of drugs that slow the nervous system and are prescribed to relieve nervousness and tension, to induce sleep, and to treat other symptoms. They are highly addictive.

- **Recovery** is a series of steps an individual takes to improve his or her wellness and health while living a self-directed life and striving to reach his or her highest potential.

- **Seizure** is an episode of abnormal electrical activity in the brain that results in changes in the brain and in behavior.

Description

Detoxification is the process of removing toxic substances (e.g., drugs, alcohol, mind-altering chemicals) from an individual's body, usually, under the care of a physician. Individuals who use drugs or alcohol can develop a physical dependence over time. Abruptly stopping the use of alcohol and drugs can result in significant withdrawal symptoms. It is extremely important for an individual with an addiction who is going through the detoxification process to be observed and treated by a health-care professional, as several drugs can result in life-threatening situations. For example, an individual who consumes alcohol or benzodiazepines on a daily basis can have a seizure if the individual abruptly stops using the substance on his or her own. Often, an individual will be prescribed a medication while being treated for detoxification so that he or she is more comfortable and also that he or she does not experience a seizure.

When an individual becomes physically dependent on drugs or alcohol, the individual may experience severe withdrawal symptoms when he or she stops using. Depending on the drug being abused, symptoms will vary. For example, an individual who is withdrawing (detoxifying) from heavy use of alcohol may experience increased heart rate, difficulty sleeping, anxiety, shaking, and seizures. An individual who is withdrawing from benzodiazepines may experience difficulty sleeping, muscle cramps, irritability, restlessness, seizures, and even death. The first step to recovery for individuals with addiction is detoxification.

Treatment

Treatment for detoxification is designed to remove toxins that are left in the body. An individual can go through the process of detoxification at several facilities (e.g., private clinics, addiction clinics, and mental health centers). An individual can also participate in an inpatient or outpatient treatment program for detoxification. This option is very beneficial because medical staff closely observes individuals. Furthermore, individuals are more likely prevented from using alcohol or drugs in an inpatient or outpatient program. Typically, the detoxification process can take less time when participating in an inpatient or outpatient treatment program.

Elizabeth Smith Kelsey, PhD, and
Len Sperry, MD, PhD

See also: Addiction; Benzodiazepines; Detoxification Interventions; Recovery; Seizures

Further Reading

Baker, Sidney M. *Detoxification and Healing: The Optimal Health*. New York, NY: McGraw Hill, 2003.

Junger, Alejandro. *Clean: The Revolutionary Program to Restore the Body's Natural Ability to Heal Itself*. New York, NY: HarperCollins, 2012.

Page, Linda R. *Detoxification: All You Need to Know to Recharge, Renew, and Rejuvenate Your Body, Mind, and Spirit*. Carmel Valley, CA: Traditional Wisdom, 1999.

Detoxification Interventions

Detoxification interventions are of three types: medical, social, and a blending of the medical and social models of detoxification.

Definitions

- **Detoxification** is the process of safely removing addictive drugs from an individual's body.

- **Methadone** is a drug that reduces symptoms of withdrawal for people addicted to other drugs.

- **Recovery** is a series of steps an individual takes to improve his or her wellness and health while living a self-directed life and striving to reach his or her highest potential.

- **Withdrawal** is the unpleasant and potentially life-threatening physiological changes that occur due to the discontinuation of certain drugs after prolonged regular use.

Description

When a person suffers from physical or mental impairment because of ingesting substances that are in the long term poisonous to the body, detoxification may be necessary before any other means can be used that will help improve his or her life situation. Everyone is exposed to toxic or poisonous elements during his or her life. Through the lymph, circulatory and digestive systems, particularly the liver, kidneys, and stomach, the body naturally detoxifies itself. Urination and bowel movements are two ways in which this naturally occurs. Special detoxification treatments become necessary when the body's natural processes can no longer handle the amount of dangerous substances in the body and become overwhelmed.

In substance abuse treatment settings, detoxification is seen as a necessary precursor to other courses of treatment. It is considered the first step in recovery. Until the patient has removed the effects of toxic substances from his or her body, it is considered difficult, if not impossible, to deal with the psychological and psychosocial aspects of his or her problems. Medically supervised detoxification from drugs and alcohol is the safest way to achieve this goal. But this approach is relatively recent. It was not until 1958 that the American Medical Association (AMA) declared alcoholism was a disease. Until

then, alcoholism and drug addictions were considered a moral or legal problem. They were not considered valid medical conditions that required medical intervention. By the 1970s more humane treatment of people with addictions was becoming the norm, for those suffering not only from alcoholism but also from drug addiction and other activities deemed chronic if not lethal.

There are two traditional models of detoxification: a medical model and a social model. The major differences between the two are that the medical model uses physicians, nursing staff, and medication to assist people through the sometimes fatal and painful withdrawal stages of detoxification. Those who prefer the social model do not see the need for medication or routine medical care. They choose to conduct detoxification in a nonmedical setting that relies on the presence of caring people, professional and otherwise, to help the person through the difficult process of detoxification.

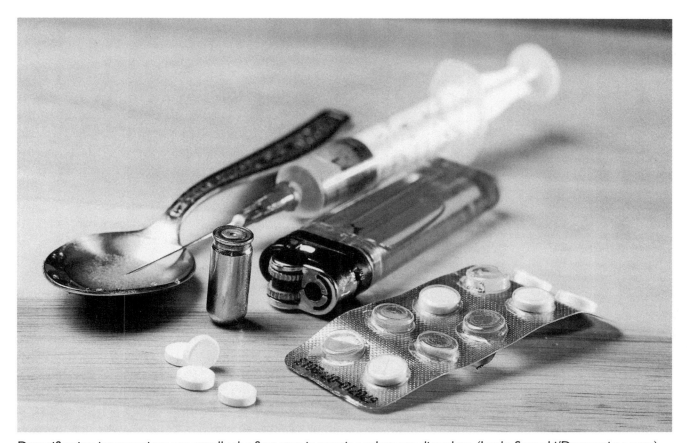

Detoxification interventions are usually the first step in treating substance disorders. (Ivaylo Sarayski/Dreamstime.com)

Today a blend of these two intervention models is often used, with nonmedical people monitoring psychological withdrawal symptoms and professional medical people addressing the symptoms of physical withdrawal and detoxification. Inpatient treatment protocols have become more sophisticated and complex often involving the use of multiple drugs, such as methadone, to aid in the process. Three of the most dangerous drugs to detox from are heroin, benzodiazepines, and alcohol. These drugs are currently considered the most dangerous due to detox side effects, including seizures, strokes, and even death.

Most medical professionals working with substance-dependent clients discourage detoxification without medical supervision. The AMA continues to maintain that substance dependence is a disease, and it encourages physicians and other clinicians, health organizations, and policy makers to base all their activities on this premise. For mental health professionals, reliance on detoxification remains a necessary first step toward effective psychological treatment.

Alexandra Cunningham, PhD

See also: Addiction Counseling; Detoxification

Further Reading

Breggin, Peter R. *Psychiatric Drug Withdrawal: A Guide for Prescribers, Therapists, Patients and Their Families.* New York, NY: Springer, 2012.

Center for Substance Abuse Treatment. "Detoxification and Substance Abuse Treatment. Treatment Improvement Protocol (TIP) Series." Substance Abuse and Mental Health Services Administration (US), 2006.

Developmental Coordination Disorder

Developmental coordination disorder (DCD) is defined as a significant impairment in the development of motor coordination that interferes with the ability to learn or to conduct the activities of daily life.

Definition

- **Developmental** relates to growth and the ability to learn new things, especially in regard to the gradual learning and maturing process in children.

Description

Although it is clear that children develop at different rates, poor motor coordination is recognized as a developmental problem. Sometimes children exhibit clumsiness or delays in activities such as crawling, walking, or dressing themselves. The term "developmental coordination disorder" refers to the difficulty in movement skills affecting children that is not due to intellectual, sensory, or neurological impairment. A key feature of DCD is difficulty in learning and performing everyday tasks at home, school, and play environments. It can affect as many as 6% of children who are between 5 and 11 years of age (National Institutes of Health, 2014). Occasionally, lack of coordination persists through adolescence and adulthood. This affects such things as handwriting or fine motor skills required for assembling puzzles or playing ball.

There has been confusion in the area of DCD because experts like pediatricians, neurologists, educators, and occupational and physical therapists saw the condition from their own points of view and found it hard to find a unified perspective. The condition was often called developmental dyspraxia, apraxia, or ataxia. By 1994 there was general agreement on the name "developmental coordination disorder." It describes a condition of significant problems in the development of motor coordination. The motor issues need to be distinct from medical conditions such as cerebral palsy or muscular dystrophy or even pervasive developmental disorder.

Causes and Symptoms

It is suspected that children with a history of prenatal or perinatal difficulties exhibit a higher incidence of developmental coordination disorder. The problems experienced by children with DCD are usually a result of problems in the brain's receptor system due to physical damage. Children with DCD may have a wide range of dysfunctions. These dysfunctions are often grouped into the areas of gross motor, fine motor, and psychosocial. Recently, the systems model has suggested a complex interaction among various levels of the central nervous system. This usually results in impairments in such related areas as proprioception, motor programming, and the sequencing of muscle activities. These can appear in children as clumsiness walking, problems with their peers, or issues with handwriting. These problems can affect the ability to learn and to manage daily activities.

Diagnosis and Prognosis

In diagnosing DCD, it is important to distinguish it from problems or disorders that may have overlapping or similar symptoms. These disorders include cerebral palsy, mental retardation, pervasive developmental disorder, and attention-deficit hyperactivity disorder. Those children who score below the 15th percentile on standardized tests of motor skills and having an IQ score above 69 would qualify for a diagnosis of DCD (National Institutes of Health, 2014). Research in DCD has emphasized the motor and academic outcomes of children rather than the long-term emotional and behavioral consequences of the disorder.

There are two schools of thought on the persistence of DCD. One view holds that DCD is largely confined to childhood and that most children eventually learn or outgrow it. This approach may take longer and much more effort to acquire sufficient motor skills but it usually happens. Another view is that improvement of DCD symptoms is not simply a matter of aging and that it continues to be a motor and a social problem in adolescence. Evidence of its effects can also be found in some adults who suffered from DCD.

Treatment

Current treatment focuses on helping children improve their motor and psychosocial challenges. Task-specific intervention is one of many approaches designed to improve the motor performance of children and young adults with motor learning difficulties. Among them are physical therapy, sensory integration, the process-oriented treatment approach, and perceptual motor training. It should be noted that there are studies which show that children who have received perceptual motor training have demonstrated motor improvements equal to or greater than those of children who have received either sensory integration therapy or process-oriented treatment.

Alexandra Cunningham, PhD, and William M. Cunningham, MA

See also: Developmental Disabilities; Specific Learning Disorder

Further Reading

American Psychiatric Association. *Diagnostic and Statistical Manual of Mental Disorders, DSM-IV-TR.* Washington, DC: Author, 2000.

Cermak, Sharon A., and Dawne Larkin. *Developmental Coordination Disorder.* Del Mar, CA: Thomson Learning, 2001.

National Institutes of Health. "Developmental Coordination Disorder." MedlinePlus. Accessed January 30, 2014. http://www.nlm.nih.gov/medlineplus/ency/article/001533.htm.

Developmental Disabilities

Developmental disabilities are conditions that restrict normal growth and activities whether physically, psychologically, educationally, or emotionally.

Definitions

- **Developmental** relates to growth and the ability to learn new things, especially in regard to the gradual learning and maturing process in children.

- **Disability** means a physical or mental condition that limits a person's movement, sense perception, or participation in normal physical or mental activities.

Description

Developmental disabilities usually begin during pregnancy, childbirth, or early infancy. The term also includes disabilities that may happen later due to injury, infection, or a variety of other factors. Whatever the source, they often impact daily functioning and therefore can become a challenge that may last a lifetime.

Not surprisingly many disabilities are overlapping; for example, a person with attention-deficit hyperactivity disorder may not do well in school, while a deaf person may experience specific emotional challenges in social interactions. "Developmental disabilities" is an umbrella term that describes a broad range of impairments that affect the growth and abilities of individuals in physical, learning, language, or behavior areas.

Developmental disabilities occur fairly evenly among all racial, ethnic, and socioeconomic groups. Despite this even distribution, some factors for increased risk and poorer prognosis are associated with the resources, education, and cultural norms of the parents. Recent estimates in the United States show that about one in six, or around 15% of children aged 3 through 17 years have one or more developmental disabilities, although levels of severity differ greatly (Centers for Disease Control and Prevention, 2013). According to the Centers for Disease Control, developmental disabilities include autism spectrum disorders, cerebral palsy, hearing/vision loss or impairment, intellectual disability, and learning disability.

Causes and Symptoms

Most developmental disabilities seem to be caused by a complex mix of factors. Some of the key factors include genetics, parental health, and other behaviors. These include smoking and drinking during pregnancy, complications during the birthing process, infections the mother might have during pregnancy or the baby might develop very early in life, and exposure of the mother or child to high levels of environmental toxins. An example of such toxins is lead. For some developmental disabilities, the cause is easy to pinpoint, but for many other conditions, the causes are not clear.

At least 25% of hearing loss among babies is due to maternal infections during pregnancy, complications after birth, and head trauma. Some of the most common known causes of intellectual disability include fetal alcohol syndrome and genetic and chromosomal conditions, such as Down syndrome and Fragile X syndrome. In certain cases infections during pregnancy, such as an infection passed from animals to humans, can cause a developmental disability. Children who have a sibling or parent with an autism spectrum disorder are at a higher risk of also having an autism spectrum disorder. Low birth weight, premature birth, multiple births, and infections during pregnancy are associated with an increased risk for many developmental disabilities. Untreated newborn jaundice can cause a type of brain damage known as kernicterus. Children with this brain damage are more likely to have cerebral palsy, hearing and vision problems, and problems with their teeth. Early detection and treatment of newborn jaundice can prevent brain damage.

Diagnosis and Prognosis

Parents are normally the best monitors and observers of the development of their children. If certain expected developmental milestones like smiling, interacting, talking, and walking are not reached within the expected range, then medical advice should be sought. Often the medical professional will join the parents in monitoring any perceived developmental delays or problems. If problems persist, the child should undergo developmental screening and evaluations to determine if the child's skills and abilities are on track, delayed, or not present. The earlier the diagnosis is made, the greater the opportunity for help and improvement.

Treatment

If a child exhibits developmental delays, it is important to get help as soon as possible. Early identification and intervention can have a significant impact on a child's ability to learn new skills. In addition, early intervention can reduce the need for later more costly interventions over a longer period of time.

People with developmental disabilities have physical, educational, or emotional deficits that require attention and help. Federal and state laws protect all those who are formally identified as having developmental disorders from discrimination. It is important for children and adults with disabilities to have access to health care and health programs in order to live as fully as they can, to stay well, and to be socially active.

Health-care professionals are aware that conditions such as asthma, gastrointestinal symptoms, eczema and skin allergies, and migraine headaches have been found to be more common among children with developmental disabilities. Thus, it is especially important for children with developmental disabilities to see a health-care provider regularly. Many communities have independent living centers that are nonprofit, community-based agencies that help people with disabilities achieve and maintain self-sufficient lives within the community. Services offered include advocacy, information and referral, independent living skills training, and peer counseling.

Alexandra Cunningham, PhD

See also: Autism Spectrum Disorders; Down Syndrome

Further Reading

Centers for Disease Control and Prevention. "Developmental Disabilities—Facts about Developmental Disabilities." Accessed September 19, 2013. http://www.cdc.gov/ncbddd/developmentaldisabilities/facts.html.

Greenspan, Stanley I., Serena Wieder, and Robin Simmons. *The Child with Special Needs: Encouraging Intellectual and Emotional Growth*. Reading, MA: Addison Wesley Longman, 1998.

National Institutes of Health. "Eunice Kennedy Shriver." National Institute of Child Health and Human Development. Accessed January 4, 2014. http://www.nichd.nih.gov/Pages/index.aspx.

Dexedrine (Dextroamphetamine)

Dexedrine is a prescription medication used to treat attention-deficit hyperactivity disorder (ADHD) and narcolepsy. Its generic name is dextroamphetamine.

Definitions

- **Attention-deficit hyperactivity disorder** is a disorder characterized by significant problems with attention, hyperactivity, or acting impulsively that are not appropriate for an individual's age.

- **Narcolepsy** is a condition of daytime sleepiness in which uncontrollable sleep attacks interfere with normal functioning.

- **Stimulants** are a class of drugs that increase brain activity and produce a sense of alertness, euphoria, endurance, and productivity

or suppress appetite. Examples are cocaine, amphetamines, and Ritalin.

- **Tourette's syndrome** is an inherited disorder characterized by tics (involuntary movements or vocalizations). Tics are preceded by a felt tension that is relieved after the tic is performed.

Description

Dexedrine belongs to the class of medications known as stimulants. Dexedrine is used to treat poor concentration and impulse control problems common in ADHD, and to treat narcolepsy. ADHD is believed to be caused by a decrease in norepinephrine levels. Dexedrine appears to work by increasing norepinephrine and dopamine levels in the brain. The result in an increase in attention, concentration, appetite, energy level, judgment, memory, and impulse control. Dexedrine is also a standard treatment for narcolepsy. Dexedrine is available in a combination pill with the drug amphetamine (Adderall). The choice of using Dexedrine alone or in combination with other medications depends on the individual's health history.

Precautions and Side Effects

Dexedrine can be a habit-forming medication and should not be used for long periods or at higher doses than prescribed. It should not be used in those with a history of alcohol or substance abuse. Since it can lower seizure threshold, it is not appropriate for use by those with a seizure disorder. Dexedrine should not be used by those with glaucoma (high pressure in the eye), Tourette's syndrome, or a family history of Tourette's since it can worsen tics. Similarly, it should not be used by those taking or have taken a monoamine oxidase inhibitor (MAOI) within the past 14 days. It must be used with caution by those with hyperthyroidism, high blood pressure, liver function impairment, kidney function impairment, and heart conditions, and by those with bipolar disorder since it can trigger mania. Dexedrine causes a withdrawal syndrome when stopped abruptly, so it should be tapered off gradually when discontinuing it. Dexedrine may be unsafe for use during pregnancy and breast-feeding, and its use is not recommended.

Common side effects of Dexedrine include stomach pain, nausea, loss of appetite, dizziness, insomnia, anxiety, restlessness, euphoria, headache, weight loss, changes in blood pressure and heart rate, palpitations, tremor, dry mouth, unpleasant taste, diarrhea or constipation, visual disturbances, impotence, and sexual dysfunction. Growth retardation in children can occur with prolonged use. Side effects that need medical attention include suicidal thoughts, confusion, chest pain, or heart palpitations, shortness of breath, restlessness, hallucinations (seeing or hearing, things that are not really there), fainting, tics, and seizures.

Dexedrine can increase, decrease, or alter the effects of other medications taken with it. Such interacting medications include antidepressant medications such as MAOIs, selective serotonin reuptake inhibitors like Prozac and Paxil, and tricyclics such as Tofranil. Effexor can cause greater-than-expected weight loss when used with Dexedrine. Antacids and the glaucoma and diuretic drug acetazolamide decrease the excretion of Dexedrine from the body and may cause toxic levels to accumulate. Many herbal supplements may also interact with Dexedrine and cause toxicity, including ginseng and green tea.

Len Sperry, MD, PhD

See also: Attention-Deficit Hyperactivity Disorder; Bipolar Disorder; Tourette's Syndrome

Further Reading

Barkley, Russell A. *Taking Charge of ADHD: The Complete, Authoritative Guide for Parents*, 3rd ed. New York, NY: Guilford Press, 2013.

Chandler, Chris. *The Science of ADHD: A Guide for Parents and Professionals*. New York, NY: Wiley-Blackwell, 2011.

Preston, John D., John H. O'Neal, and Mary C. Talaga. *Handbook of Clinical Psychopharmacology for Therapists*, 7th ed. Oakland, CA: New Harbinger, 2013.

DHEA (Dehydroepiandrosterone)

DHEA is a hormone used for increasing cognitive functioning and slowing the progression of Alzheimer's disease and some medical conditions. Its technical name is dehydroepiandrosterone.

Definitions

- **Adrenal insufficiency** exits when the adrenal glands do not produce sufficient epinephrine, norepinephrine, cortisol, aldosterone, and corticosterone. Addison's disease can result from it.

- **Hormone** is a chemical messenger that regulates such bodily functions as growth, development, metabolism, reproduction, and mood.

Description

DHEA is produced naturally by the adrenal glands. It has a number of uses, including increasing cognitive performance; slowing the progression of Parkinson's disease and Alzheimer's disease, adrenal insufficiency, depression, systemic lupus erythematosus (lupus), and erectile dysfunction; and improving sexuality and well-being. DHEA is also used to increase muscle mass, strength, and energy, but it is banned by the National Collegiate Athletic Association. The body converts DHEA into male and female sex hormones, such as estrogen and testosterone.

DHEA is also available as a nutritional supplement made from a substance found in soy and wild yams. Because of concerns about false claims, these supplements were taken off the U.S. market in 1985. But it was reintroduced after the Dietary Supplement Health and Education Act was passed in 1994. DHEA levels in the body begin to decrease after age 30 and may be low in those with anorexia, end-stage kidney disease, type 2 diabetes, AIDS, and adrenal insufficiency, and in the critically ill. DHEA levels may also be depleted by a number of medications, including insulin, corticosteroids, opiates, and Danocrine. While evidence supports the short-term use of DHEA in the treatment of adrenal insufficiency, depression, and lupus, there is concern about its long-term use. Because DHEA can elevate levels of androgens and estrogens in the body, it could increase the risk of prostate, breast, ovarian, and other hormone-sensitive cancers. Therefore, it is not recommended for regular use without medical supervision. DHEA is being investigated and may eventually be approved by the Food and Drug Administration as a prescription drug for treating systemic lupus erythematosus and improving bone mineral density in women with lupus who are taking steroid drugs for treatment. Clinical trials are being conducted on DHEA with anxiety disorder, schizophrenia, and schizoaffective disorder. Information on participation in a clinical trial is available at the website of the NIH Clinical center, http://www.cc.nih.gov.ezproxy.fau.edu/participate.

Precautions and Side Effects

Because DHEA is a hormone it should be used under medical supervision, particularly those with or at risk for mood and psychotic disorders. Children and pregnant or breast-feeding women should not use it. Since it may alter liver function, those with liver disease should not use it. DHEA supplements may alter the levels estrogen and testosterone, which can increase the risk of hormone-sensitive cancers such as breast, prostate, and ovarian cancer. Those taking DHEA supplements may develop blood clots, so people with clotting disorders, heart disease, and a history of stroke should avoid DHEA supplements. DHEA supplements can affect the levels of other hormones, such as insulin and thyroid hormone, and also affect cholesterol levels. Those with diabetes, high cholesterol, thyroid disorders, Cushing's disease, and other hormonal disorders should be particularly cautious.

Common side effects of DHEA supplements include acne, insomnia, fatigue, oily skin, abdominal pain, hair loss, nasal congestion, irregular heartbeats, and heart palpitations. Since DHEA supplements may influence the production of male and female hormones, facial hair growth and a deepening of the voice may occur in women. Men may develop male pattern baldness, aggressiveness, high blood pressure, breast enlargement, and shrinkage of the testicles.

DHEA supplements may interfere with the effectiveness of antipsychotic medications such as Thorazine and Compazine. It may increase the effects of AZT (HIV medication), barbiturates, oral contraceptives, and benzodiazepines, such as Halcion, Xanax, and Valium.

Len Sperry, MD, PhD

See also: Alzheimer's Disease

Further Reading

Dasgupta, Amitava, and Catherine A. Hammett-Stabler, eds. *Herbal Supplements: Efficacy, Toxicity, Interactions with Western Drugs, and Effects on Clinical Laboratory Tests.* Hoboken, NJ: Wiley, 2011.

PDR for Herbal Medicines. Montvale, NJ: Thompson, 2007.

Watson, Ronald Ross, ed. *DHEA in Human Health and Aging.* Boca Raton, FL: CRC Press, 2011.

Diagnosis

Diagnosis is the process of identifying and labeling a medical or psychiatric disorder.

Definitions

- **Case conceptualization** is a method and strategy for obtaining and organizing information, understanding and explaining maladaptive patterns, focusing treatment, anticipating challenges, and preparing for termination.

- **Clinical assessment** is the formal process of collecting clinical data to establish a diagnosis, to develop a case conceptualization, and to plan treatment.

- ***Diagnostic and Statistical Manual of Mental Disorders*** is the handbook mental health professionals use to diagnose mental disorders. The current edition (fifth) is known as DSM-5.

- **Mental status examination** is a clinical evaluation of an individual's appearance, orientation, behavior, mood and affect, speech, thinking, perception, cognition, insight, and judgment.

- **Psychiatric diagnosis** is a form of diagnosis based on the identification and labeling of mental disorder based on meeting diagnostic criteria matching a particular disorder.

Description

Diagnosis is a form of clinical assessment for the identification and labeling of a medical or psychiatric condition or disorder based on its signs and symptoms.

Clinical assessment has at least three goals. The first is to establish a psychiatric diagnosis based on *Diagnostic and Statistical Manual of Mental Disorders* (DSM) criteria. The second is to develop a case conceptualization. The third is to plan treatment based on the diagnosis and case conceptualization. Of these three, establishing a psychiatric diagnosis is the first and, some would say, the most important step in clinical assessment.

Developments and Current Status

A psychiatric diagnosis is arrived at by comparing specific symptoms and impairment against the criteria for a given clinical disorder. Psychiatrists, psychologists, and mental health counselors diagnose psychiatric (mental) disorders using the criteria listed in the *Diagnostic and Statistical Manual of Mental Disorders* (DSM). The DSM is a reference work consulted by these and other clinicians, including social workers, couples and family therapists, medical and nursing students, and pastoral counselors.

The psychiatric diagnosis is based on a psychiatric evaluation (clinical assessment) that includes both psychiatric interview and observational data. Typically, a psychiatric interview includes questioning the individual about the reason for the diagnostic evaluation (clinical assessment); history of the present illness including symptoms, severity, and length of time involved; past psychiatric history; and developmental, psychosocial, and educational history. Additional data often includes information about health history and use of prescribed medications, alcohol, and street drugs. If the individual is unable or unwilling to provide such information, collateral information is sought. Information to better understand the individual's present condition and past history comes from relatives, friends, or available medical and psychiatric records.

An essential element of the psychiatric evaluation is a mental status examination, which is an assessment of the individual's overall level of functioning at the time of the evaluation. Psychological tests that the examiner thinks are necessary to establish or rule out a specific diagnosis may be undertaken.

A diagnosis is used to establish a prognosis (prediction of response to treatment) for the individual and to foster communication among health-care professionals involved in the individual's care. Furthermore, a formal DSM diagnosis may be required by insurers to pay for treatment services.

Len Sperry, MD, PhD

See also: Behavioral Assessment; *Diagnostic and Statistical Manual of Mental Disorders* (DSM); Mental Status Examination

Further Reading

American Psychiatric Association. *Diagnostic and Statistical Manual of Mental Disorders*, 5th ed, *DSM-5*. Washington, DC: American Psychiatric Publishing, 2013.

Frances, Allen. *Essentials of Psychiatric Diagnosis: Responding to the Challenge of DSM-5*. New York, NY: Guilford Press, 2013.

North, Carol, and Sean Yutzy. *Goodwin and Guze's Psychiatric Diagnosis*. New York, NY: Oxford University Press, 2010.

Diagnostic and Statistical Manual of Mental Disorders (DSM)

The *Diagnostic and Statistical Manual of Mental Disorders* is a diagnostic classification framework that characterizes mental disorders with specific diagnostic criteria.

Definitions

- **Mental disorder** is a mental or behavioral pattern or anomaly that causes either distress or an impaired ability to function in daily life. It is also known as a mental illness or psychiatric disorder.

- **Phenomenological** refers to a method of classification that emphasizes externally observable phenomena and descriptions rather than their underlying nature or origin.

Description

The *Diagnostic and Statistical Manual of Mental Disorders* (DSM) provides a common language and standard criteria for the classification of mental disorders.

The DSM is used in the United States as well as in other countries. It is used by clinicians, researchers, drug regulation agencies, insurance companies, the pharmaceutical industry, and policy makers. DSM is published by the American Psychiatric Association. Two other diagnostic manuals are the *International Statistical Classification of Diseases and Related Health Problems* (ICD) published by the World Health Organization and the *Psychodynamic Diagnostic Manual* published by the Alliance of Psychoanalytic Organizations. The stated purpose of the DSM is threefold: to provide a useful guide to clinical practice, to facilitate research and improve communication among clinicians and researchers, and to serve as an educational tool for teaching psychopathology.

Developments and Current Status

The origins of the DSM are in census and psychiatric hospital statistics, and from a United States Army and Veterans Administration (VA) manual. The DSM was substantially revised in 1980. The six revisions since its first publication in 1952 incrementally added to the number of mental disorders while removing those no longer considered to be mental disorders. The last major revision is DSM-5 in 2013. While the DSM is the official diagnostic system for mental disorders in the United States, it is also used widely in Europe and other parts of the world. Throughout its history, the DSM coding system is designed to correspond with the codes used in the ICD, although not all codes may match at all times because the two publications are not revised synchronously. The following is a brief description of all the DSM manuals from the beginning through DSM-5.

DSM-I. In 1952 DSM was published by the American Psychiatric Association. It listed 106 diagnostic categories and was merely 130 pages long. In 1949, the World Health Organization published the sixth revision of the *International Statistical Classification of Diseases* (ICD), which included a section on mental disorders for the first time. Soon afterward, the APA Committee on Nomenclature and Statistics was tasked with developing a diagnostic manual for use in the United States. It based this manual on the structure and conceptual framework of "Medical 203" of the VA system and ICD nomenclature. Many passages of text were identical to those in Medical 203. DSM-I

included several categories of personality disturbance, neurosis, psychosis, and acute and psychophysiological reactions.

DSM-II. In 1968 DSM-II was published and listed 182 diagnostic categories. It was 134 pages long. It was remarkably similar to the DSM-I. It appeared prior to ICD-9, which was published in 1975. While the designation "reaction" was dropped, the term "neurosis" was retained. Both the DSM-I and the DSM-II reflected the predominant psychodynamic view. However, both included biological perspectives and concepts from a descriptive system of classification. Symptoms were not specified in detail for specific disorders. Many were seen as reflections of broad underlying conflicts or maladaptive reactions to life problems, rooted in a distinction between neurosis and psychosis (roughly, anxiety/depression broadly in touch with reality, or hallucinations/delusions appearing disconnected from reality). Sociological and biological knowledge was incorporated, in a model that did not emphasize a clear boundary between normality and abnormality. The idea that personality disorders did not involve emotional distress was discarded.

DSM-III. In 1980 DSM-III was published and listed 265 diagnostic categories. The original purpose of this revision was to make the DSM nomenclature consistent with the then current version of ICD. Another purpose was to improve the uniformity and validity of psychiatric diagnosis, and to standardize diagnostic practices. The establishment of these criteria was an attempt to facilitate the pharmaceutical regulatory process. The psychodynamic view was abandoned, in favor of a phenomenological (descriptive) model. Mental disorders were conceptualized as a clinically significant behavioral or psychological syndrome. The personality disorders were placed on axis II along with mental retardation. Besides the expansion of diagnostic categories, the most notable difference that would greatly impact clinical practice was the addition of a multiaxial system. This means an individual is evaluated on five axes or dimensions, each representing a different aspect of functioning. Axes I and II refer to types of psychological or psychiatric disorders, while Axes III through V represent general medical conditions, psychosocial and environmental problems, and a global assessment of functioning, respectively.

DSM-III-R. In 1987 the DSM-III-R was published as a revision of DSM-III. Six categories were deleted while others were added. Controversial diagnoses such as premenstrual dysphoric disorder and masochistic personality disorder were considered and discarded. "Sexual orientation disturbance" was also removed and was largely subsumed under "sexual disorder not otherwise specified," which can include "persistent and marked distress about one's sexual orientation." Altogether, DSM-III-R contained 292 diagnoses and was 567 pages long. Further efforts were made for the diagnoses to be purely descriptive.

DSM-IV. In 1994, DSM-IV was published with 297 disorders. Revisions were based on research reviewed by work groups and results from multicenter field trials relating diagnoses to clinical practice. A major change from previous versions was the inclusion of a clinical significance criterion to almost half of all the categories, which required symptoms cause clinically significant distress or impairment in social, occupational, or other important areas of functioning. Some personality disorder diagnoses were deleted or moved to the appendix.

DSM-IV-TR. In 2000, a text revision of the DSM-IV, known as the DSM-IV-TR, was published. The diagnostic categories and the vast majority of the specific criteria for diagnosis were unchanged. The text sections giving extra information on each diagnosis were updated, as were some of the diagnostic codes to maintain consistency with the ICD.

DSM-5. In 2013, DSM-5 was published. It includes the same number of disorders as in DSM-IV. A number of changes in structure as well as content were made since the last edition. The most obvious is that the multiaxial system has been removed. The five Axes (I, II, III, IV, V) had been the focal point of DSM since it was introduced in 1978 with DSM-III. DSM-5 now documents diagnoses in a nonaxial manner, which combines the former Axes I, II, and III with separate notations for psychosocial and contextual factors (formerly Axis IV) and disability (formerly Axis V). Other changes involve the addition of some new diagnoses, the removal of others, and revision of criteria for several disorders. These changes will align DSM-5 with the World Health Organization's International Classification of Diseases, eleventh edition (ICD-11). They are expected to foster improved communication and common use of diagnoses across disorders. DSM-5 is comprised of three sections. The first section describes how to use the updated manual. The second section describes the diagnostic categories. The third section includes cultural formulations and diagnostic conditions that are yet considered formal disorders.

Overall, three main changes are evident in the various editions of DSM. First, there has been a clear shift from defining mental disorders by their causes toward defining disorders as clusters of symptoms. Second, there is a coordination of diagnoses with the ICD. Third, there has been increased use of field trials and statistical analysis in evaluating the adequacy of diagnostic terms and criteria.

Len Sperry, MD, PhD

See also: Psychodynamic Diagnostic Manual (PDM)

Further Reading

American Psychiatric Association. Diagnostic and Statistical Manual of Mental Disorders, 5th ed, DSM-5. Arlington, VA: Author, 2013.

Borch-Jacobsen, Mikkel. Making Minds and Madness: From Hysteria to Depression. Cambridge, UK: Cambridge University Press, 2009.

PDM Task Force. Psychodynamic Diagnostic Manual. Silver Spring, MD: Alliance of Psychoanalytic Organizations, 2006.

Regier, Darrel A., ed. The Conceptual Evolution of DSM-5. Washington, DC: American Psychiatric Publishing, 2011.

Dialectical Behavior Therapy (DBT)

Dialectical behavior therapy is a type of cognitive behavior therapy (CBT) which focuses on coping with stress, regulating emotions, and improving relationships. It is also known as DBT.

Definitions

- **Behavior therapy** is a psychotherapy approach that focuses on identifying and changing maladaptive behaviors.

- **Cognitive behavior therapy** is a psychotherapy approach that focuses on maladaptive (faulty) behaviors, emotions, and thoughts.

- **Cognitive restructuring** is psychotherapy technique for replacing maladaptive thought patterns with more constructive thoughts and beliefs.

- **Cognitive therapy** is a type of cognitive behavior therapy that focuses on identifying and changing distorted thinking patterns.

- **Dialectic** is a form of discussion that resolves differences between two views rather than concluding that only one is true.

- **Schemas** are core beliefs or assumptions about one's self and the world.

- **Schema therapy** is a type of cognitive behavior therapy that focuses on identifying and changing maladaptive schemas.

Description

Dialectical behavior therapy (DBT) is a type of CBT that focuses on learning skills to cope with stress, regulate emotions, and improve relationships. DBT is an outgrowth of behavior therapy in that both focus on behavioral deficits and emotional excesses (inability to regulate emotions). Like CBT, DBT emphasizes a collaborative relationship between client and therapist. Both utilize learning principles, analyze triggers and environmental prompts, explore schemas and emotions, and utilize homework. In addition, recognize the importance of empathic responding.

Unlike traditional CBT, DBT emphasizes emotion regulation more than maladaptive (problematic) beliefs and schemas. Cognitively oriented CBT insists that dysfunctional feelings and behaviors are due to maladaptive beliefs and schemas that produce consistently biased judgments and cognitive errors. Instead, DBT focuses on how maladaptive schemas are initially formed. It explores schemas and the underlying dialectic conflicts that produced them rather than using cognitive restructuring to change them. DBT therapists attempt to connect clients' maladaptive beliefs

to underlying affect and need, and then assist them to reinterpret their belief systems based on greater awareness of their feelings and needs.

The core strategies in DBT are "validation" and "problem solving." DBT attempts to validate clients' behavior and demonstrate an understanding of their difficulties and suffering. Problem solving focuses on the establishment of necessary skills. DBT has four primary treatment modes: individual therapy, skills training in a group, telephone contact, and therapist consultation. Following an initial period of pretreatment involving assessment, commitment, and orientation to therapy, DBT focused on the specific targets for that stage, which are arranged in a definite hierarchy of relative importance. These include decreasing suicidal behaviors, decreasing therapy-interfering behaviors, decreasing behaviors that interfere with the quality of life, increasing behavioral skills, decreasing behaviors related to post-traumatic stress, improving self-esteem, and attaining individual targets negotiated with the client.

Developments and Current Status

DBT was developed for the treatment of borderline personality disorder by American psychologist Marsha Linehan (1943–). Linehan developed this approach after finding that traditional psychotherapeutic approaches were ineffective in treating suicidal individuals with borderline personality disorder. She focused her approach on skills training because these individuals had considerable skill deficits. She also found that skills training was best accomplished in weekly didactic groups. These groups use a step-by-step format to teach four sets of skills. These skill sets are core mindfulness, interpersonal effectiveness, emotion regulation, and distress tolerance.

Core mindfulness. This is the ability to take control of one's mind rather than being controlled by it. Mindfulness focuses one's attention by a process of observing, describing, and participating from a nonjudgmental perspective. This allows for more objective, effective, and meaningful experiences in the present moment.

Interpersonal effectiveness. This is the ability to communicate and express oneself effectively while understanding and remaining committed to one's goals and self-respect. It includes being able to ask for what one needs, say no, and cope with interpersonal conflict. Skills training includes assertive communication, interpersonal problem solving, and negotiation.

Emotion regulation. This is the ability to regulate your emotions by understanding the relationship between thoughts, feelings, body sensations, and behaviors. It also includes awareness of one's vulnerabilities and how they affect one's emotional states. These include inadequate sleep, misuse of medications, lack of exercise, and not incorporating positive experiences in daily life.

Distress tolerance. This is the ability to get through a difficult time without making the situation worse. Being able to tolerate distress (painful emotions) reduces the likelihood of engaging in self-destructive behaviors. Distress tolerance teaches the use of distraction, radical acceptance, and evaluating pros/cons as alternatives.

Research indicates that DBT is most effectively accomplished in an inpatient, partial hospitalization or residential treatment setting rather than in outpatient and private practice. DBT is best implemented with a treatment team in which one therapist provides skills training and another provides individual therapy. This is best accomplished when other therapists can provide a consultation function and when all therapists have access to a therapist consultation group for support.

More recently, DBT has been modified and extended for use with other personality disorders as well as Axis I or symptom disorders such as mood disorders, anxiety disorders, eating disorders, and substance disorders. DBT is an outgrowth of behavior therapy but is less cognitive than traditional CBT since DBT assumes that cognitions are less important than affect regulation. DBT has been adapted for private practice settings. It is recommended that the skill training component be best provided by another therapist; it is not absolutely necessary. Also, private practice clinicians using DBT would do well to have access to a psychotherapy consultant if involvement in a therapist consultation group is not possible.

Len Sperry, MD, PhD

See also: Behavior Therapy; Cognitive Behavior Therapy; Cognitive Therapy; Schema-Focused Therapy

Further Reading

Linehan, Marsha M. *Cognitive-Behavioral Treatment of Borderline Personality Disorder.* New York, NY: Guilford Press, 1993.

Linehan, Marsha M. *Skills Training Manual for Treating Borderline Personality Disorder.* New York, NY: Guilford Press, 1993.

Sperry, Len. *Cognitive Behavior Therapy of DSM-5 Personality Disorders*, 3rd ed. New York, NY: Routledge, 2016.

Van Dijk, Sheri. *DBT Made Simple: A Step-by-Step Guide to Dialectical Behavior Therapy.* Oakland, CA: New Harbinger Publications, 2013.

Dictionary of Occupational Titles (Book)

This book source was created in 1939 by the U.S. Department of Labor as a reference list of occupations for use by those interested in or seeking job placement.

Definitions

- **Occupational information** describes useful vocational data and facts, including career descriptions, requirements, benefits, and possible compensation for students, job seekers, and business/industry professionals to assist them in navigating the world of work.

- **Occupational Information Network (O*NET)** is the online occupational website that was created in 1991 to replace the *Dictionary of Occupational Titles* (DOT) print publication.

Description

The *Dictionary of Occupational Titles* (DOT) was published by the U.S. Department of Labor in 1939 to offer job seekers, employers, and career advisors with a comprehensive list of occupations and facts related to those. Containing over 17,000 vocational titles and descriptions, this first edition categorized jobs as skilled, semiskilled, or unskilled. The first edition of the DOT was also used to properly place World War II veterans in careers commensurate with their skills on their return. Second, third, and fourth editions of the DOT were published in 1949, 1965, and 1977, respectively.

Supplements to the fourth edition followed periodically to update the list of job categories and modify the skills required (e.g., technology related) and to notify readers of changes in workforce demand. A final update occurred in 1991. Soon after, the DOT was replaced by an online source, the Occupational Information Network, or O*NET. This website provides a comprehensive, up-to-date guide for students, trainees, workers, and employers to gather vocational information. Though it now contains only 13,000 job categories, fewer than the DOT had in 1939, these categories are now organized under occupational umbrellas, making it easier for searchers to scan through related fields of interest. The O*NET system houses a variety of useful sources, including the *Dictionary of Occupational Titles*, the *Directory of Occupational Titles*, and the *Occupational Job Outlook*. There are multiple ways to search the O*NET system, including sorting by job category, description, skills, interests, and/or work values.

Impact (Psychological Influence)

O*NET is readily used by career counselors and advisors as a valuable reference tool to help assess client's work values, interests, and aptitudes and assist in finding proper placement. Given O*NET's wide range of search capabilities and the vast amount of information it contains, it is a popular site for those seeking employment or those looking to attract good employees. The system is updated on a biannual basis to allow for the most current information to be obtained by users.

Melissa A. Mariani, PhD

See also: Career Assessment; Career Counseling; Career Development; Occupational Information

Further Reading

Farr, J. Michael, Laverne L. Ludden, and U.S. Department of Labor. *O-Net Dictionary of Occupational Titles: Based on Information Obtained from the U.S. Department of Labor and Other Sources*, 4th ed. St. Paul, MN: JIST Publishing, 2007.

*O*NET Online*. National Center for O*NET Development. Accessed February 18, 2014. http://www.onet online.org/.

Peterson, Norman G., Michael D. Mumford, Walter C. Borman, P. Richard Jeanneret, and Edwin A. Fleishman. *An Occupational Information System for the 21st Century: The Development of O*NET*. Washington, DC: American Psychological Association, 1999.

Disability and Disability Evaluation

Disability is a physical or mental impairment that substantially limits one or more of the major life activities of an individual. Disability evaluation is a formal determination of the degree of a physical, mental, or emotional disability.

Definitions

- **Americans with Disabilities Act (ADA)** is a civil rights law intended to protect against discrimination based on disability. It was originally signed in 1990 and amended in 2008.

- **Disability** is any restriction or lack (resulting from an impairment) of ability to perform an activity in the manner or within the range considered normal for a human being.

- **Handicap** is a disadvantage for a given individual that limits or prevents the fulfillment of a role that is normal.

- **Impairment** is any loss or abnormality of psychological, physiological, or anatomical structure or function.

Description

In the United States disability has been legally defined in the Americans with Disabilities Act. Disability is a physical or mental impairment that substantially limits one or more of the major life activities of an individual. Major life activities include self-care, full range of movement, communication, vision, hearing, working, learning, and social relating. Disability can be caused by congenital (birth related), traumatic (accidental), or other factors, and vary widely in severity. They may be temporary or permanent, correctable, or irreversible. Physical disabilities include blindness, deafness, deformity, muscular and nervous disorders, paralysis, and loss of limbs. Mental disabilities are of two types: mental illness and mental retardation.

The terms "impairment," "disability," and "handicap" are often used synonymously. However, there are technical distinctions and different meanings for these terms. The most commonly accepted definitions are those of the World Health Organization in "The International Classification of Impairments, Disabilities, and Health." Basically, "impairment" refers to a problem with a structure or organ of the body, whereas "disability" is a functional limitation with regard to a particular activity. In contrast, "handicap" refers to a disadvantage in filling a role in life related to an individual's peer group. As already noted, disabilities can be correctable. Thus, an individual may not be able to walk because of an impairment of mobility (movement) such as paralysis. However, if this individual uses a wheelchair and is able to perform daily activities, then the impairment is presumably limited.

Developments and Current Status

The presence or absence of diagnosis of disability is essential in determining whether an individual meets the eligibility criteria for Social Security. It is also used to determine eligibility for benefits and income under disability insurance and for workmen's compensation benefits. A disability evaluation is the formal assessment procedure used in making this determination.

A mental disability evaluation examination is usually performed by a psychologist or psychiatrist. Intelligence testing and/or memory testing is commonly used when the alleged disability is due to learning disabilities, inability to read or write, a stroke, organic brain disorders, accident, or mental retardation A psychiatric evaluation and mental status examination is used when the alleged disability is due to personality disorder, an anxiety or mood disorder, or schizophrenia.

The physician or psychologist who performs the examination sends a written report to a specified Social Security board, a disability insurer, or a workman's compensation board. The report contains an opinion about the examinee's capacity to remember and understand instructions and to deal with supervisors and coworkers, and with work and life stresses. Based on this input, the board or insurer determines the disability and its extent.

Len Sperry, MD, PhD

See also: Americans with Disabilities Act (ADA)

Further Reading

Flanagan, Steven, Herbert H. Zaretsky, and Alex Moroz. *Medical Aspects of Disability: A Handbook for the Rehabilitation Professional*, 4th ed. New York, NY: Springer, 2011.

Klein, Stanley D., and John D. Kemp, eds. *Reflections from a Different Journey: What Adults with Disabilities Wish All Parents Knew*, 2nd ed. New York, NY: McGraw Hill, 2011.

Nielsen, Kim E. *A Disability History of the United States*. Boston, MA: Beacon Press, 2013.

World Health Organization. *The International Classification of Functioning, Disability and Health*. Geneva, Switzerland, 2001. http://www.who.int/classifications/icf/en/.

Disinhibited Social Engagement Disorder

Disinhibited social engagement disorder is a mental disorder in children characterized by an overly familiar and culturally inappropriate behavior with strangers.

Definitions

- **Attachment** is the emotional bond between children and caregivers that provides a secure (healthy) base from which children are able to safely explore their environment and relate to others.

- **Cognitive behavior therapy** is a type of psychotherapy that focuses on maladaptive (faulty) behaviors, emotions, and thoughts.

- **Fetal alcohol syndrome** is a medical condition characterized by birth defects and learning and behavioral problems in children resulting from the mother's alcohol use during pregnancy.

- **Post-traumatic stress disorder** is a mental disorder characterized by nightmares, emotional numbing, and recurrent flashbacks of a traumatic event that an individual experienced or witnessed.

- **Reactive attachment disorder** is a mental disorder characterized by disturbed and developmentally inappropriate social relatedness.

- **Trauma- and stressor-related disorders** are a group of mental disorders characterized by exposure to a traumatic or stressful event. These include post-traumatic stress disorder, reactive attachment disorder, and disinhibited social engagement disorder.

Description and Diagnosis

Disinhibited social engagement disorder is one of the trauma- and stressor-related disorders. This disorder is characterized by a pattern of behavior that is culturally inappropriate and overly familiar with relative strangers. Such behavior violates ordinary social customs and cultural boundaries. In some ways, this disorder is the mirror opposite of reactive attachment disorder. Whereas children with reactive attachment disorder cannot easily relate to individuals they know, those with disinhibited social engagement disorder relate indiscriminately to individuals they do not know. They show little anxiety and no distrust of those strangers as they engage in culturally inappropriate physical contact and displays of affection. These children tend to be happy and affectionate around strangers. They may or may not be this way with their parents or caregivers. Strangers may view these children as clingy. However, they are likely to become emotionally sensitive and anxious if strangers seem to reject their affection.

According to the *Diagnostic and Statistical Manual of Mental Disorders, Fifth Edition*, children can be diagnosed with this disorder if they exhibit a pattern of behavior in which they seek out attention and contact with unfamiliar adults. They show a noticeable and concerning familiarity with strangers, such as inappropriate verbal and physical interactions. They may go off with strangers without hesitation. They may also not be aware of their caregiver in these unfamiliar settings. Their pattern of social neglect is evident by repeated changes in the primary caregiver or limited opportunities to form developmentally appropriate connections

with caregivers. Finally, this diagnosis can be made if the child is at least nine months of age (American Psychiatric Association, 2013).

The cause of this disorder is not well understood. However, social neglect is often present in the first few months of life in children diagnosed with this disorder (American Psychiatric Association, 2013). Children may respond to such limited displays of caring by actively seeking other sources of security and nurture. Then, having learned that parents or caretakers cannot be depended upon to care for and protect them, they look for others who might meet their needs and attempt to engage them in a friendly or overly friendly manner. Besides such neglect, repeated changes in the primary caregiver and limited opportunities to form appropriate connections and secure (healthy) attachments with caregivers may also be factors that contribute to the development of this disorder. There may also be a biological bases for this disorder. The indiscriminate social behavior seen in disinhibited social engagement disorder is also noted in some other disorders. These include cases of fetal alcohol syndrome even where there is no history of social neglect.

Treatment

The treatment of this disorder usually involves psychological interventions. The active involvement of the child's primary caregiver is essential. Establishing a sense of safety and security between the child and the caregiver is the first goal of treatment. Once such trust and consistency is formed, the child is less likely to seek comfort from strangers. Caregivers are then taught how to help their child set interpersonal boundaries. Cognitive behavior therapy can help in reducing stress and negative emotions associated with caring for a child with this disorder.

Len Sperry, MD, PhD

See also: Attachment Styles; Cognitive Behavior Therapy; Reactive Attachment Disorder

Further Reading

American Psychiatric Association. *Diagnostic and Statistical Manual of Mental Disorders*, 5th ed. Arlington, VA: American Psychiatric Association, 2013.

Cain, Catherine Swanson. *Attachment Disorders: Treatment Strategies for Traumatized Children*. New York, NY: Jason Aronson, Inc., 2006.

Parritz, Robin Hornik, and Michael F. Troy. *Disorders of Childhood: Development and Psychopathology*, 2nd ed. Belmont, CA: Wadsworth Publishing, 2014.

Disruptive, Impulse-Control, and Conduct Disorders

Disruptive, impulse-control, and conduct disorders are a group of mental disorders characterized by a lack of self-control.

Definitions

- **Attention-deficit/hyperactivity disorder** is a mental disorder characterized by difficulty focusing as well as being overly active. It is commonly referred to as ADHD.

- **DSM-5** stands for the *Diagnostic and Statistical Manual of Mental Disorders, Fifth Edition*, which is a diagnostic system used by professionals to identify mental disorders with specific diagnostic criteria.

- **Family therapy** is a method of therapy that seeks to create change by improving the relationships and rules of the family.

- **Personality disorders** is a long-standing pattern of maladaptive (problematic) behavior, thoughts, and emotions that deviates from the accepted norms of an individual's culture.

- **Psychotherapy** is a psychological method for achieving desired changes in thinking, feeling, and behavior. It is also called therapeutic counseling.

Description

Disruptive, impulse-control, and conduct disorders are a category of mental disorders that are characterized by the inability to regulate one's behavior, emotional responses, or both. This group of disorders includes oppositional defiant disorder, intermittent explosive disorder, and conduct disorder. A key factor that differentiates this group of disorders from disorders is that individuals with this group of disorders act in a way that violates the rights of others or social rules. The prevalence of these disorders varies, but as a rule, they tend to affect males more frequently than females (American Psychiatric Association, 2013). It is important to note that many of the symptoms of these disorders appear in the course of normal childhood development. Therefore, the occasional occurrence of some symptoms does not necessarily mean that an individual has, or will develop, one of these disorders. This group of disorders also includes antisocial personality disorder. However, that disorder is listed primarily as a personality disorder in DSM-5. A brief description of these DSM-5 disorders follows.

Conduct disorder. It is characterized by a pattern of behavior that violates the rights of others. This disorder represents a pattern of symptoms that is dominated by a lack of behavioral regulation. This disorder is one of the most severe of this category. Individuals with this disorder may exhibit a pattern of hurting other people and animals, and destroying property. Some individuals with this disorder may also lack guilt about their actions or empathy toward others. To be diagnosed with this disorder, an individual must exhibit a number of symptoms that may include fighting (with or without a weapon), bullying, torturing animals, sexual assault, purposefully destroying property, breaking into someone's home or vehicle, theft, sneaking out of his or her home, and skipping school. Prevalence of this disorder is estimated to be approximately 4% of the population (American Psychiatric Association, 2013). For some, this disorder manifests in childhood; for others, it may manifest in adolescence or adulthood. For those who develop this disorder as a child, their outcome is often worse than for those who develop it later. Treatment for this disorder may include psychotherapy, family therapy, and medication.

Kleptomania. It is characterized by impulsive stealing. The principal difference between kleptomania and thievery is that individuals with this disorder steal because they are excited by it or feel tension that is released when stealing, whereas thievery involves stealing for monetary gain. The prevalence if this disorder is rare, affecting less than 1% of the population (American Psychiatric Association, 2013). However, this disorder is associated with up to 25% of individuals who shoplift. For an individual to be diagnosed with this disorder, he or she must demonstrate a pattern of stealing that is not for monetary gain. The individual must experience a tension that is released by stealing followed by pleasure (American Psychiatric Association, 2013). Treatment for this disorder typically involves psychotherapy.

Intermittent explosive disorder. It is characterized by a pattern of behavioral outburst cause by an inability to regulate one's emotions and impulses. This disorder represents a pattern of symptoms that are not dominated by either an inability to regulate one's behavior or emptions but approximately divided between the two. One of the common features of this disorder is aggression toward others. This aggression may be physical or verbal and far exceeds that which is normal for the individual's age or the situation where it is expressed. Most often, there is little or no provocation preceding the outburst. For this diagnosis to apply, the individual must exhibit a pattern of aggression that does not result in harm to others or property, which occurs at least twice a week for three consecutive months. However, if the consequences of the individual's actions are more severe and others or property is harmed, only three outbursts in a given year are required. Also, the individual must be at least six years of age and the aggression cannot have been preplanned and excessive. The prevalence of this disorder is estimated to be 2.7% (American Psychiatric Association, 2013). This disorder usually begins in late childhood but may affect people well into middle age. Treatment for this disorder may include psychotherapy, family therapy, and medication.

Oppositional defiant disorder. It is characterized by a pattern of irritability, moodiness, or defiance. This disorder represents a pattern of symptoms dominated by a lack of emotional regulation. This disorder is not to be confused with the otherwise normal childhood mood fluctuations or argumentativeness. The key differentiator is that these symptoms are persistent. For this diagnosis to apply, the individual must exhibit a number of symptoms to suggest that he or she is angry, temperamental, purposefully annoying, blaming, argumentative, or spiteful. Most important, the individual must demonstrate this with someone who is not a sibling and for at least six months. In addition, the individual must demonstrate these symptoms at least once a week or more, depending on age (American Psychiatric Association, 2013). Like all disorders, the social and cultural setting of the child is important to consider when making a diagnosis. The prevalence of this disorder is estimated to be 3.3% (American Psychiatric Association, 2013). The disorder is most likely to manifest prior to grade school. Individuals who experience this disorder may later develop conduct disorder and may be a greater risk for developing other mental disorders. Also, it is common for individuals suffering from this disorder to also have ADHD. Treatment for this disorder may include psychotherapy, family therapy, and medication.

Pyromania. It is characterized by multiple episodes of starting fires. Individuals who experience this disorder not only set fires but also are obsessed or fascinated by fire. The prevalence of this disorder as a standalone diagnosis is very rare, affecting less than one-third of 1% of the population (American Psychiatric Association, 2013). However, it does co-occur more frequently with other disorders. For someone to be diagnosable with this disorder, the individual must intentionally set multiple fires. The individual must experience emotional excitement, relief, or pleasure associated with setting the fire and the aftermath. Also, the individual must not have a cause or motive to set fires aside from his or her own interest or fascination in fire itself, such as in the case of criminal arson (American Psychiatric Association, 2013). As this disorder is often one of multiple disorders that occur in an individual, treatment varies depending on the other diagnosis but will typically involve psychotherapy aimed at changing the beliefs and behaviors surrounding fire.

Jeremy Connelly, MEd, and Len Sperry, MD, PhD

See also: Antisocial Personality Disorder; Attention-Deficit Hyperactivity Disorder; Conduct Disorder; *Diagnostic and Statistical Manual of Mental Disorders* (DSM); Family Therapy; Intermittent Explosive Disorder; Kleptomania; Oppositional Defiant Disorder (ODD); Personality Disorders; Psychotherapy; Pyromania

Further Reading

American Psychiatric Association. *Diagnostic and Statistical Manual of Mental Disorders*, 5th ed. Arlington, VA: American Psychiatric Association, 2013.

Bernstein, Neil. *Treating the Unmanageable Adolescent: A Guide to Oppositional Defiant and Conduct Disorders*. Lanham, MD: Rowman & Littlefield, 1996.

Grant, John. *Impulse Control Disorders: A Clinicians Guide to Understanding and Treating Behavioral Addictions*. New York, NY: W.W. Norton, 2008.

Disruptive Mood Dysregulation Disorder

Disruptive mood dysregulation disorder is a mental disorder in children characterized by a severe and frequent temper tantrums that interfere with daily functioning.

Definitions

- **Bipolar and related Disorders** are a group of mental disorders characterized by changes in mood and in energy (e.g., being highly irritable and impulsive while not needing sleep). These disorders include bipolar I disorder, bipolar II disorder, and cyclothymic disorder.

- **Depression** is an emotional state characterized by feelings of sadness, low self-esteem, guilt, or reduced ability to enjoy life. It is not considered a mental disorder unless it significantly disrupts one's daily functioning.

- **Depressive disorders** are a group of mental disorders characterized by a sad or irritable mood and cognitive and physical changes that significantly disrupt the individual's daily functioning. These disorders include major depressive disorder, persistent depressive disorder, disruptive mood dysregulation, and premenstrual dysphoric disorder.

- **Dysregulation** is a problem with the control of physical or emotional functions.

- **Temper tantrums** are disruptive behaviors or emotional outbursts displayed in response to unmet needs or desires.

Description and Diagnosis

Disruptive mood dysregulation disorder is one of a group of depressive disorders. It is characterized by severe and persistent irritability resulting in temper tantrums and persistent anger or irritability between the tantrums. Both interfere with children's ability to function at home, in school, or with their friends. Prior to DSM-5, many with this symptom pattern were likely to be labeled as "bipolar children." Some of these children were diagnosed with bipolar disorder even though they seldom met all the symptoms and criteria. Research suggests that most will not go on to develop bipolar disorder as adults. Instead, children with chronic irritability are more likely to develop depressive and/or anxiety disorders when they become adults (American Psychiatric Association, 2013).

In terms of mood symptoms, children with this disorder can be irritable, upset, or moody from time to time. They may switch rapidly from irritable, easily annoyed, and angry mood states to silly, goofy, and giddy states of elation. They can experience periods of sadness almost every day. During adolescence this may be demonstrated by suicidal thoughts and behaviors. Often these children are very bright and capable but are greatly challenged by this disorder.

Occasional temper tantrums are a normal part of growing up. However, when children are continually irritable or angry or when temper tantrums are frequent, intense, and ongoing, it may suggest this depressive disorder. Such individuals (6 to 18 years of age) are probably fighting off depression or at least fighting to overcome imagined burdens. While anxiety reflects the individual's awareness of a burden to overcome, expressed frustration, irritability, and anger reflect the individual's efforts to react against and reach some resolution.

According to the *Diagnostic and Statistical Manual of Mental Disorders, Fifth Edition*, individuals can be diagnosed with this disorder if they exhibit chronic irritability that contributes to recurrent frustrations and temper outbursts. These outbursts occur more than three times per week and their moods between temper outbursts are persistently irritable or angry. The symptoms have been present for at least a year and the irritability and temper has been expressed across at least two settings, such as at home, school, or work, and contribute to significant functional disruption in those environments. This diagnosis can be given only to those between the ages of 6 and 18. Finally, this disorder cannot have been caused by a substance, medication, or a medical condition or other mental disorder (American Psychiatric Association, 2013).

The cause of this disorder is not well understood. It may be that genetic, environmental, and temperamental (personality) factors are operative (American Psychiatric Association, 2013). Because it is a mood disorder it is likely that it could result from a combination of biological predispositions and environmental conditions. It can run in families suggesting a genetic basis, or it can be a result of stressful environments in which the child lives. It may also be that a recent death in the family, a divorce, or relocation is a factor. Some children have neurological disorders like migraine headaches that may account for their persistent irritability. Or, their mood dysregulation may be associated with early psychological trauma and abuse.

As with other mood and conduct disorders in children, diagnosis is often delayed or mistaken for other conditions. Before a correct diagnosis is made, other diagnoses can be given. These include attention-deficit hyperactivity disorder, obsessive-compulsive disorder, depression, separation anxiety disorder, oppositional defiant disorder, and other conduct disorders. Even after the disruptive mood dysregulation disorder diagnosis is given, many children continue to be diagnosed with one or more of these diagnoses as well. Therefore, children with it and other diagnoses should be comprehensively evaluated and treated for these issues.

Treatment

Effective treatment of this disorder is individualized to the needs of the particular child and family. It usually includes individual therapy. Consulting with the child's family and school are usually necessary and helpful. Parents of children with this disorder need to fully understand it. For this reason, the therapist might meet with parents and assist them in dealing more effectively with their child or adolescent. Parents and teachers are helped to analyze the triggers and the purpose of their tantrums. They learn that when these disruptions longer serve a useful purpose, children can learn alternative ways of getting their needs met and relating in a healthier way with peer and family members. It may also be necessary for family therapy to address the family behaviors that promote the disruptive behaviors. Depending on the age of the child, medication may be prescribed. Medication, such as Ritalin and Risperdal, has been used to reduce impulsivity and irritability.

Len Sperry, MD, PhD, and
Alexandra Cunningham, PhD

See also: Bipolar Disorder; Conduct Disorder; Depression; Oppositional Defiant Disorder (ODD); Risperdal (Risperidone); Ritalin (Methylphenidate)

Further Reading

American Psychiatric Association. *Diagnostic and Statistical Manual of Mental Disorders*, 5th ed. Arlington, VA: American Psychiatric Association, 2013.

Finnerty, Todd. *Disruptive Mood Dysregulation Disorder (DMDD), ADHD and the Bipolar Child under DSM-5: A Concise Guide for Parents and Professionals*. PsychContinuingEd.com, 2013.

Greene, Ross W. *The Explosive Child: A New Approach for Understanding and Parenting Easily Frustrated, Chronically Inflexible Children*. New York, NY: HarperCollins, 2001.

Papolos, Demitri. *The Bipolar Child: The Definitive and Reassuring Guide to Childhood's Most Misunderstood Disorder*, 3rd ed. New York, NY: Broadway Books, 2008.

Dissociative Amnesia

Dissociative amnesia is a dissociative disorder characterized by the inability to remember important personal information beyond what could be explained by normal forgetfulness. It is also known as psychogenic amnesia.

Definitions

- **Amnesia** is the inability to recall past events or retain new information. It usually occurs as a result of physical or psychological trauma.

- **Depersonalization** is a mental state of detachment or a sense of being "outside" oneself and observing one's actions or thoughts.

- **Dissociation** is a psychological process in which individuals experience being disconnected from their sensory experience, sense of self (identity), or personal history.

- **Dissociative disorders** are a group of mental disorders characterized by a disturbance of self, memory, awareness, or consciousness and which cause impaired functioning.

- **Dissociative fugue** is a dissociative disorder characterized by a temporary loss of personal identity, moving to a new location, and assuming a new identity.

- **Dissociative identity disorder** is a dissociative disorder characterized by having more than one distinct identity. Previously it was referred as multiple personality disorder.

- **Post-traumatic stress disorder** is a mental disorder characterized by unwanted recollections or a reexperiencing of a traumatic event with arousal symptoms.

Description and Diagnosis

Dissociative amnesia is a dissociative disorder in which the characteristic feature is the sudden and temporary loss of ability to recall important personal information. This disorder is usually a reaction to experiencing or witnessing a traumatic event or violent crime. The loss of memory can involve information about a specific topic or memories of the immediate or distant past. It is too extensive to be explained by ordinary forgetfulness, and it cannot be due to a head injury, alcohol-induced blackouts, seizure disorder, or electroconvulsive therapy. Unlike the common portrayal of amnesia in television shows and movies, dissociative amnesia rarely involves a total loss of recall.

A hallmark of this disorder is its rapid onset and rapid recovery. In contrast, recovery of amnesia from organic or medical causes is gradual and is rarely complete. These memories are not actually lost. Rather, they are buried but are not readily accessible. However, they can resurface spontaneously or be accessed in psychotherapy. Individuals with dissociative amnesia may develop depersonalization as part of the disorder, but do not experience a change in identity, which is characteristic of dissociative fugue disorder. The incidence of dissociative amnesia increases during stressful or traumatic times, such as during a war or after a natural disaster. The likelihood of developing this disorder is quite rare in the United States. It is found in only 1.0% of American adult males and 2.6% of adult females (American Psychiatric Association, 2013).

According to the *Diagnostic and Statistical Manual of Mental Disorders, Fifth Edition*, individuals can be diagnosed with this disorder if they are unable to recall important information that is autobiographical in nature. This loss of memory can involve information about a specific topic or memories from the immediate or distant past such as traumatic or stressful events. It can include a loss of knowledge about one's identity or loss of previous knowledge about the world. Besides displaying such symptoms, the individual's functioning is also greatly affected in job, social, or other areas of life. This memory loss cannot be due to substance use, seizures, head injury, or other mental disorders like post-traumatic stress disorder, dissociative identity disorder, or neurological disorder (American Psychiatric Association, 2013).

The cause of this disorder is exposure to an overwhelming stressor such as combat, sexual assault, accidents, natural disasters, and extreme conflict or emotional stress (American Psychiatric Association, 2013). Genetics may also have a role since this disorder tends to run in families.

Treatment

Treatment begins with a comprehensive assessment of the triggering event, current stressors, medical history, psychiatric history and treatment, history of alcohol and substance use, and history of trauma and abuse. Referral for a medical evaluation may be needed to rule out physical trauma, neurological conditions, and drug-induced causes. Treatment of amnesia depends on the root cause of amnesia. Psychotherapy can be helpful for amnesia caused by emotional trauma. The goal is to safely express and process painful lost memories. It may also involve developing new coping skills, improving relationships, and restoring functioning.

Providing a supportive environment may be sufficient for spontaneous resolution to occur.

Len Sperry, MD, PhD

See also: Amnesia; Dissociation; Dissociative Identity Disorder; Post-Traumatic Stress Disorder (PTSD)

Further Reading

American Psychiatric Association. *Diagnostic and Statistical Manual of Mental Disorders*, 5th ed. Arlington, VA: American Psychiatric Association, 2013.

Boon, Suzette. *Coping with Trauma-Related Dissociation: Skills Training for Patients and Therapists.* New York, NY: W.W. Norton, 2011.

Papanicolaou, Andrew C. *The Amnesias: A Clinical Textbook of Memory Disorders.* New York, NY: Oxford University Press, 2006.

Dissociative Disorders

Dissociative disorders are a group of mental disorders characterized by a disturbance of self, memory, awareness, or consciousness and which cause impaired functioning.

Definitions

- **Antianxiety** medications are prescribed drugs that relieve anxiety symptoms. They are also called anxiolytics or tranquilizers.

- **Antidepressants** are prescription medications used to treat depression and depressive symptoms.

- **Cognitive behavior therapy** is a type of psychotherapy that focuses on maladaptive (faulty) behaviors, emotions, and thoughts. It is also called CBT.

- **Dissociation** is a psychological process in which individuals experience being disconnected or detached from their sensory experience, sense of self (identity), or personal history.

- **Dissociative fugue** is a dissociative disorder characterized by a temporary loss of personal identity, moving to a new location, and assuming a new identity.

- **DSM-5** stands for the *Diagnostic and Statistical Manual of Mental Disorders, Fifth Edition*, which is a diagnostic system used by professionals to identify mental disorders with specific diagnostic criteria.

- **Hypnotherapy** is the use of hypnosis to help an individual change his or her beliefs, attitudes, or patterns through suggestion while the individual is in an altered state (hypnotized).

- **Psychotherapy** is a psychological method for achieving desired changes in thinking, feeling, and behavior. It is also called therapeutic counseling.

- **Psychotic disorder** is a severe mental condition in which an individual loses touch with reality. Symptoms can include hallucinations (hearing or seeing things that are not there), delusions (fixed false beliefs that persist despite contrary evidence), and disordered thinking.

Description

Dissociative disorders are a group of DSM-5 mental disorders that includes dissociative identity disorders, dissociative amnesia, depersonalization/derealization disorder, and other specified dissociative disorder. The central features of these disorders are relatively severe dissociative symptoms and impairment of functioning. Dissociation is a detachment from reality. When individuals suffer from dissociative symptoms, they experience being removed or detached from reality. Dissociative symptoms are numerous and vary significantly in severity. Daydreaming is a non-pathological form of it, while depersonalization (sense that the self is unreal) is a pathological form of dissociation.

Mild dissociation experiences include dreaming or being mad at one's dog when he or she has had a bad day at work. These experiences are not nearly as severe as the experience of one of the dissociative disorders. In addition, these symptoms usually have a rapid onset and are distressing. It is important to note that the dissociative disorders are different from the psychotic disorders whereby individuals can no longer separate what is real and what is not, as in the case of hallucinations. What follows is a brief description of the four DSM-5 dissociative disorders.

Dissociative identity disorder. This disorder is characterized by an individual having two or more distinct personalities or identities. Often, an individual suffering from this disorder functions as if each identity was a completely different, independent person. When one identity is being expressed, the individual will often not recall what the alternate identity has done. Some who suffer from this disorder maintain a "possessed" personality where a demon or spirit overtakes them. There is variance in the obviousness of the change in personality. For some, there is a dramatic shift between personalities; for others, the change is subtle. Prevalence of this disorder is estimated to be 1.5% and to affect slightly more males than females (American Psychiatric Association, 2013). One of the most important aspects of this disorder is that individuals suffering from it have a very high probability of suicide. Abuse and traumatic events in childhood are associated with the manifestation of this disorder. The vast majority of cases do not resolve on their own and need highly skilled treatment. Treatment of this disorder requires some form of psychotherapy. This disorder was formerly called multiple personality disorder.

Dissociative amnesia. Dissociative amnesia is a dissociative disorder characterized by the inability to remember important personal information beyond what could be explained by normal forgetfulness. The information that cannot be recalled may be isolated to a specific period of time. Often, the event that cannot be recalled is of a stressful or traumatic nature. In other cases, individuals may suffer a complete loss of life history. This disorder is sometimes accompanied by dissociative fugue. It is found in only 1.0% of adult males and less than 3% of adult females (American Psychiatric Association, 2013). Treatment for this disorder will most likely incorporate psychotherapy, as there are no medications shown to be effective with this disorder. In addition, hypnotherapy may be used. This disorder is also known as psychogenic amnesia.

Depersonalization/derealization disorder. Depersonalization/derealization disorder is a dissociative disorder characterized by a symptom of either detachment, a sense of being "outside" oneself or observing one's actions or thoughts (depersonalization), detachment from a sense of one's surroundings, or both (derealization). Although relatively severe depersonalization/derealization is represented as a disorder, mild symptoms such as daydreams may manifest in otherwise normal-functioning individuals for short durations. The principal difference between normal experience and a qualifying disorder is the distress experienced by the individual and the duration of the symptoms. This disorder is most often caused by medical conditions or the ingestions of illicit drugs but may also be caused by extreme stress and trauma. It is relatively rare, occurring in less than 2% of the population (American Psychiatric Association, 2013). Treatment for this disorder may include both medications and psychotherapy.

Other specified dissociative disorder. This disorder is characterized by dissociative symptoms that cause substantial distress or impairment but do not fit the necessary criteria of the preceding disorders. This disorder is best understood as a grouping of four specific subtypes. These subtypes include chronic but relatively mild dissociative symptoms related to one's identity, loss of identity due to intense and prolonged coercion such as that which takes place in a cult. Others are short-term dissociative symptoms lasting less than one month as a result of a traumatic event, and significant and unusual loss of awareness related to one's environment. The prevalence of this disorder is unknown as it represents a newly established disorder in the DSM-5 (American Psychiatric Association, 2013). Like the other dissociative disorders, treatment may include both medication and psychotherapy. However, the psychotherapy of each subtype will be focused in the particular subtype.

Jeremy Connelly, MEd, and Len Sperry, MD, PhD

See also: Antianxiety Medication; Antidepressant Medications; Cognitive Behavior Therapy; *Diagnostic and Statistical Manual of Mental Disorders* (DSM); Dissociation; Dissociative Fugue; Dissociative Identity Disorder; Psychotherapy; Psychotic Disorders

Further Reading

American Psychiatric Association. *Diagnostic and Statistical Manual of Mental Disorders*, 5th ed. Arlington, VA: American Psychiatric Association, 2013.

Biever, John, and Maryann Karinch. *The Wandering Mind: Understanding Dissociation, from Daydreams to Disorder.* Lanham, MD: Rowman & Littlefield, 2012.

Chu, James. *Rebuilding Lives: Treating Complex PTSD and Dissociative Disorders,* 2nd ed. Hoboken, NJ: John Wiley & Sons, 2011.

Dell, Paul, and John O'Neil. *Dissociation and the Dissociative Disorders: DSM-5 and Beyond.* New York, NY: Routledge, 2009.

Dissociative Identity Disorder

Dissociative identity disorder is a mental disorder characterized by having more than one distinct identity or personality. Previously this disorder was known as multiple personality disorder.

Definitions

- **Amnesia** is the inability to recall past events or retain new information. It usually occurs as a result of physical or psychological trauma.

- **Borderline personality disorder** is a mental disorder characterized by a pattern of instability in interpersonal relationships, self-image, affects, self-harm, and a high degree of impulsivity.

- **Dissociate and dissociation** is a detachment from reality. Daydreaming is a non-pathological form of it, while depersonalization (a sense that the self is unreal) and dissociative identity disorder are pathological forms of dissociation.

- **Dissociative disorders** are a group of mental disorders characterized by a disturbance of self, memory, awareness, or consciousness and which cause impaired functioning.

Description and Diagnosis

Dissociative identity disorder is one of the class of dissociative disorders characterized by the presence of two or more distinct alter egos (identities) within the same individual. Each alter ego is dominant at a particular time. Each alter helps the individual to cope with and meet the individual's needs. Because there can be 10 or more alters within the individual, it can be difficult to detect and diagnose the disorder early in its course. It may take six or more years of psychological treatment before the proper diagnosis of dissociative identity disorder is made. Because of the waxing and waning character of this disorder and the innumerable permutations of symptoms, the individual may present differently on different occasions. Accordingly, such individuals may receive many diagnoses.

Those with this disorder usually enter psychotherapy for various concerns ranging from anxiety to sleep disorders. In the course of treatment these individuals may complain of new concerns like the sudden onset of dizziness, difficulty finding their parked car, indecision about small matters, or denial of actions that were observed by others. On further investigation, a different alter ego emerges or is discovered in the course of treatment. Other symptoms of this disorder include auditory hallucinations, amnesia, and sudden mood swings. In fact, depression is one the most common of this disorder. The diagnosis of borderline personality disorder is also common, particularly in those who are lower functioning and engage in self-harmful behaviors.

This disorder usually begins in early childhood, although it is usually diagnosed between the ages of late adolescence and early middle age. In their late 50s, many with this disorder identify with one of their more resilient alters. The likelihood of developing dissociative identity disorder is small among adults in the United States, with 1.6% being males and 1.4% females (American Psychiatric Association, 2013).

According to the *Diagnostic and Statistical Manual of Mental Disorders, Fifth Edition,* individuals can be diagnosed with this disorder if they exhibit a disruption of identity, which involves the presence of two or more distinct identities. As a result of this disruption the individual experiences altered affect, behavior, memory, consciousness, sensory motor functioning, or overall perception. These symptoms may be reported by the individual or observed by others. Memory impairment regarding important personal information, recall of daily events, and recall of traumatic events also occur in this disorder. Besides the individual displaying such symptoms, the individual's functioning is also greatly affected, including job, relationships, or other areas of life. Furthermore, the disorder cannot be caused by a medication, substance use, or medical condition, such as seizures. Lastly, the disturbance is also not a part of any cultural or religious practices (American Psychiatric Association, 2013).

The cause of this disorder is usually severe and repeated trauma in childhood. It may involve severe emotional, physical, or sexual abuse, neglect, natural disaster, terrorism, war, or the loss of a parent. To survive extreme stress, these individuals dissociate (separate) the thoughts, feelings, and memories of this traumatic experiences from conscious awareness. Approximately 90% of clients living with this disorder have experienced a repeated and severe history of physical and/or sexual abuse as children (American Psychiatric Association, 2013).

Treatment

The ultimate goal of treatment of this disorder is the integration of all alters into a single personality. While this disorder is not very common, some with this disorder experience an integration of their various alters without treatment. For the rest, focused psychotherapy is the primary treatment strategy. The treatment of this disorder tends to be long, demanding, and painful. The initial goal is to establish a trusting relationship, while the intermediate goal is to maximize the individual's functioning. However, some degree of conflict-free collaboration among the various alters may be the only realistic goal for some individuals. Currently, treatment places less emphasis on processing past trauma and more emphasis on improving functioning and helping individuals live more meaningful lives. Generally, medications have limited value in treating this disorder. But they can useful in treating symptoms such as depression, insomnia, and panic.

Len Sperry, MD, PhD

See also: Amnesia; Borderline Personality Disorder; Dissociation

Further Reading

American Psychiatric Association. *Diagnostic and Statistical Manual of Mental Disorders*, 5th ed. Arlington, VA: American Psychiatric Association, 2013.

Boon, Suzette. *Coping with Trauma-Related Dissociation: Skills Training for Patients and Therapists*. New York, NY: W.W. Norton, 2011.

Haddock, Deborah. *The Dissociative Identity Disorder Sourcebook*. New York, NY: McGraw-Hill, 2001.

Howell, Elizabeth F. *Understanding and Treating Dissociative Identity Disorder: A Relational Approach*. New York, NY: Routledge, 2011.

Dissociative Personality Disorder

Dissociative personality disorder is mental disorder characterized by dissociation as a central personality trait.

Definitions

- **Dissociation** is a psychological process in which individuals experience being disconnected from their sensory experience, sense of self (identity), or personal history.

- **Dissociative disorders** are a group of mental disorders characterized by a disturbance of self, memory, awareness, or consciousness and which cause impaired functioning.

- **Dissociative identity disorder** is a mental disorder characterized by having more than one distinct identity or personality. Previously, it was known as multiple personality disorder.

- **DSM-5** stands for the *Diagnostic and Statistical Manual of Mental Disorders, Fifth Edition*, which is a diagnostic system used by professionals to identify mental disorders with specific diagnostic criteria.

- **Hypnosis** is a trancelike state that resembles sleep but is induced by another's suggestions that are readily accepted by the individual.

- **Personality disorder** is a long-standing pattern of maladaptive (problematic) behavior, thoughts, and emotions that deviates from the accepted norms of an individual's culture. Personality disorder reflects an individual's unique personality structure.

- **Psychoanalytic theory** is a psychological theory that explains behaviors and perceptions as the result of unconscious, sexual, and biological instincts. It was originally developed by Sigmund Freud.

- **Psychoanalytic therapy** is a form of psychotherapy that emphasizes unconscious (outside awareness) conflicts and focuses on an individual's early childhood and dreams.

- *Psychodynamic Diagnostic Manual* **(PDM)** is a diagnostic system based on psychoanalytic theory that is used by professionals to identify mental disorders with specific diagnostic criteria.

- **Self-hypnosis** is the act of hypnotizing oneself.

Description and Diagnosis

Dissociative personality disorder is a personality disorder in which an individual's dominant pattern involves dissociation. This characteristic may be expressed in many ways. For some, it may be confusion or the inability to recall a memory, while others may forget entire periods of their life. In the most severe cases, individuals may take on completely new identities or experience multiple identities. It is believed that this personality type results from early abuse by their primary caregiver.

While dissociative personality is not a diagnosis in DSM-5, it does share some characteristics of dissociative identity disorder. However, dissociative personality disorder is described in the *Psychodynamic Diagnostic Manual* (PDM). According to the PDM (2006), the dissociative personality disorder is diagnosable by the following criteria. Individuals are preoccupied with denying traumatic events. Their basic emotion is fear or anger. Their basic belief or view of themselves is that they are fragile or susceptible to frequent suffering. Their basic belief or view of others is that others are the dangerous, exploitive, oppressive, or saviors. Accordingly, they protect themselves from their belief about the world by dissociating their experience.

The exact cause of this personality disorder is not well understood. However, a variety of factors may be causative. According to the *Psychodynamic Diagnostic Manual* (2006), this disorder is commonly associated with an early history of severe and repeated physical or sexual trauma. These individuals tend to be easily hypnotized and have the capacity for self-hypnosis. Their primary way of defending themselves is to dissociate.

Treatment

Prior to treating dissociative personality disorder, it is imperative that a clinician first assess the individual for suicide risk, as individuals suffering from this disorder are prone to suicide. Psychoanalytic therapy is commonly used. Generally, treatment for this disorder is long term and relatively difficult.

Len Sperry, MD, PhD, and Jeremy Connelly, MEd

See also: Dissociative Disorders; *Diagnostic and Statistical Manual of Mental Disorders* (DSM); Personality Disorders; Psychoanalytic Theory; *Psychodynamic Diagnostic Manual* (PDM)

Further Reading

Boon, Suzette. *Coping with Trauma-Related Dissociation: Skills Training for Patients and Therapists.* New York, NY: W. W. Norton, 2011.

PDM Task Force. *Psychodynamic Diagnostic Manual (PDM).* Silver Spring, MD: Alliance of Psychoanalytic Organizations, 2006.

Divided Self, The (Book)

The Divided Self: An Existential Study in Sanity and Madness, published in 1960, is a book written by psychiatrist and psychoanalyst Ronald D. Laing about people with psychotic disorders.

Definitions

- **Antipsychotic medications** are prescription drugs used to treat psychotic disorders. They are sometimes referred to as antipsychotics or neuroleptics.

- **Psychotic** features are characteristics of psychotic disorders: delusions, hallucinations, disorganized thinking and speech, grossly disorganized or abnormal motor behavior, and negative symptoms, for example, lack of initiative and diminished emotional expression.

- **Psychotic disorder** is a severe mental disorder in which an individual loses touch with reality. Symptoms can include hallucinations (hearing or seeing things that are not there), delusions (fixed false beliefs that persist despite contrary evidence), and disordered thinking.

- **Schizophrenia** is a chronic mental disorder that affects behavior, thinking, and emotion which make distinguishing between real and unreal experiences difficult. Symptoms include hallucinations, delusions, thought and communication disturbances, and withdrawal from others.

Description

Scottish psychiatrist Ronald D. Laing (1927–1989) was one of the most prominent figures in the anti-psychiatry movement of the 1960s and 1970s. His observations led him to be very critical of the way the psychiatric community described and diagnosed insanity, especially in regard to schizophrenia. His critique called into question whether there is a clear diagnostic line between madness and sanity. In *The Divided Self*, Laing focuses specifically on schizophrenia. He claims that the disorder is largely an artificial creation of the psychiatric community that only served to label socially undesirable and misunderstood behavior. He questioned the value of antipsychotic drugs and argued that they were not the best or only treatment option for people with schizophrenia. He believed that the unreal world of schizophrenics was not simply a delusion. He described psychosis as the way that people with mental problems protect themselves from what they believe is threatening them.

Laing's insights were very heavily influenced by an existential approach to the observation of mental illness, based largely on the work of Jean Paul Sartre. His own psychological difficulties may have led him to see schizophrenia from the inside out, not just as an external observer. Laing established a therapeutic community near London to implement his ideas about how the mentally ill should be treated. In this community, drugs, or antipsychotics, were not a part of the treatment regimen. He continued to try to find ways to appreciate and learn from the world of psychotic individuals while still helping them to live at peace with the rest of society.

Impact (Psychological Influence)

Laing rose to prominence and fame quickly. He published a series of books and was criticized by the press because it believed his distinctions between the mentally ill and the sane were in many cases arbitrary, prejudiced, and potentially harmful. Partially because of

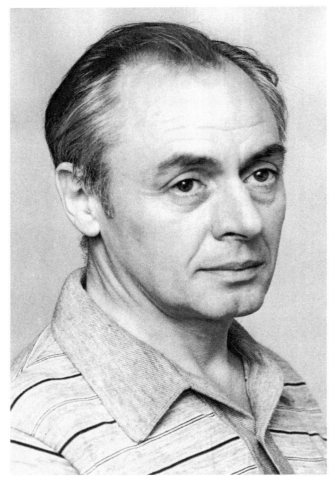

Psychiatrist and psychoanalyst Ronald D. Laing (1927–1989) discussed psychotic disorders in *The Divided Self: An Existential Study in Sanity and Madness*, published in 1960. (Ray Moreton/Keystone/Getty Images)

these criticisms and his own personal issues, his influence was short lived.

In his later work, Laing argued that psychotic individuals were sometimes more sane than other people and that psychotic experiences could have a healing dimension. With these claims he undermined his credibility with the scientific community and alienated many who thought he had gone too far. At the same time he was engaging in his own interests such as eastern spirituality and other health areas like birthing techniques. This led him farther away from psychiatry. His abuse of alcohol, from which he died in 1989, was the cause of him losing his medical license.

Recently, there has been a renewed interest in his ideas as society struggles with how to offer treatment to those suffering from psychosis. An effort to provide treatment while respecting clients' rights, their experiences, and their dignity is important to many in the psychological community. Laing's early work including *The Divided Self* is still used to challenge the health-care community to be honest and clear about treatment of psychosis in a mental health context. This important book reminds readers that caring for the mentally ill should not mean excluding them from society simply on the basis of a diagnosis or label.

Alexandra Cunningham, PhD, and
William M. Cunningham, MA

See also: Antipsychotics; Brief Psychotic Disorder; Psychosis; Schizophrenia; Shared Psychotic Disorder; Substance-Induced Psychotic Disorder

Further Reading

Broughton, John M. "The Divided Self in Adolescence." *Human Development* 24, no. 1 (1981): 13–32.

Burston, Daniel. *The Wing of Madness: The Life and Work of R.D. Laing*. Cambridge, MA: Harvard University Press, 1998.

Laing, Ronald D. *The Divided Self: An Existential Study in Sanity and Madness*. London: Penguin, 1960.

Divorce

Divorce is the dissolution or termination of a marital union.

Description

More than one-half of all American first marriages end in divorce and over a million children a year are impacted by their parent's marital breakup. The effects of divorce on children have been highly investigated by social researchers as they attempt to better understand how to help children adjust to the challenges related to divorce.

Research indicates that children of divorce (COD) are more at risk for certain psychological problems when compared to children from continuously married parents (CCMP). Possible consequences include a decline in academic achievement, increases in anger, acting out or delinquent behaviors, higher rates of depression and anxiety, decrease in psychological well-being and self-esteem, decreased quality of family functioning, feelings of being caught between parents, and decreased coping capacity. Research also indicates that compared to CCMP, adult COD are at risk for lower self-esteem and less satisfaction with life, and have more symptoms of depression and anxiety. Adult COD also report less marital happiness, more marital discord, and more thoughts of divorce, and are more likely to get divorced.

Consequences of divorce should be viewed as risk factors more so than predictions as the magnitude, or effect, of divorce is relatively moderate. Scientifically rigorous research has shown that 90% of COD reach adulthood with comparable levels of psychological well-being (levels of self-esteem, life satisfaction, happiness, and psychiatric symptoms) as CCMP. Although some children are more vulnerable and at greater risk than others, most COD adjust to divorce within a few years of the marital breakup.

Researchers have identified two factors that particularly impact the effects of divorce on psychological well-being. COD who come from high marital discord families (e.g., yelling, screaming, and violence) actually have higher post-divorce well-being when compared to CCMP. This indicates that children exposed to high levels of conflict and discord may benefit from divorce. When parents reported low levels of discord, COD were worse off than CCMP. It may be that when parents outwardly get along a divorce is more shocking and difficult to adjust to for children. The other factor

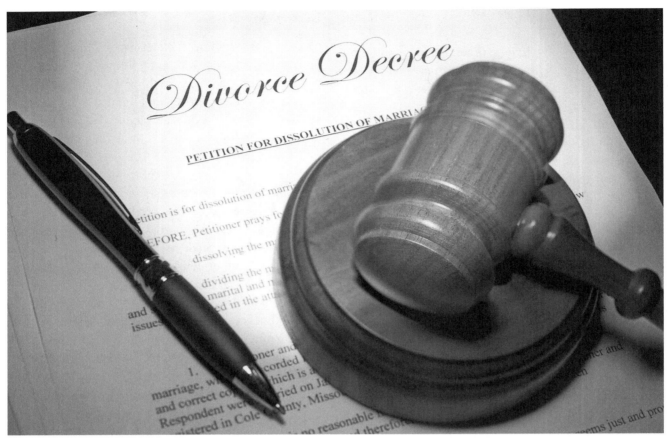

Divorce, the legal dissolution or termination of a marital union, has become common in America and many other Western nations. Divorce can have a major psychological impact on everyone involved, particularly young children. (Zimmytws/Dreamstime.com)

that impacts the effect of divorce is the number of re-marriages and re-divorce transitions of the parents. COD whose parents did not remarry had levels of psychological well-being comparable to that of CCMP. This suggests that the negative impact of divorce may be more associated with post-divorce remarriages.

Current Status

Because of the prevalence of divorce and the large numbers of children impacted by it, a substantial body of research exist. There is an increase call for investigation into the buffering effects and resiliency factors in children. Current research continues on the development of after-school programs to assist COD, and further research into impact of remarriage is needed.

Steven R. Vensel, PhD

See also: Single-Parent Families

Further Reading

Amato, Paul R. "Reconciling Divergent Perspectives: Judith Wallerstein, Quantitative Family Research, and Children of Divorce." *Family Relations* 52, no. 4 (2003): 332–339.

Emery, Robert. *The Truth about Children and Divorce: Dealing with the Emotions So You and Your Children Can Thrive.* New York, NY: Viking, 2004.

Dodo Bird Verdict

The Dodo bird verdict is the claim that all psycho-therapies are equally effective regardless of their components.

Definitions

- **Anxiety disorders** are a group of mental health disorders characterized by anxiety which tends to be intermittent instead of persistent. The group includes panic disorder, phobias, and generalized anxiety disorders.

- **Cognitive behavior therapy** is a form of psychotherapy that focuses on changing maladaptive (faulty) behaviors, emotions, and thoughts. It is also known as CBT.

- **Common factors** is the viewpoint that psychotherapy has common components or factors and that these effect change more than specific factors or techniques.

- **Psychotherapy** is a psychological method for achieving desired changes in thinking, feeling, and behavior. Psychotherapy is also called therapeutic counseling.

- **Therapeutic alliance** is a helping relationship between a psychotherapist and an individual in which they work together to effect change for the individual seeking help.

Description

The "Dodo bird verdict" is the name given to an ongoing debate in psychology. It is a controversial topic that claims that all psychotherapies produce equal outcomes regardless of their specific components. Psychologist Saul Rosenzweig (1907–2004) named the Dodo bird verdict in a 1936 article about common factors underlying competing approaches to psychotherapy. He argued that all therapy approaches were equally effective because of common factors. Rosenzweig used an illustration from Lewis Carroll's *Alice's Adventures in Wonderland* (1865) to describe the verdict. Several characters became wet and the Dodo bird has them run around the lake until they are dry. In time all get dry and he says, "Everyone has won, so all must have prizes." Rosenzweig's point is that common factors (e.g., everyone running around the lake) were more important than specific technical differences (e.g., how long or how far everyone had to run). He argued that all

therapies are winners; they all produce equally effective outcomes (e.g., everyone became dry in the end).

In his 1975 review of psychotherapy research, psychologist Lester Luborsky (1920–2009) reported that there were few significant differences in the outcomes among the different psychotherapy approaches. Since then there have been several other studies that both support and oppose the verdict. Supporters of it claim that only common factors really effect change, particularly the therapeutic alliance. This is the means by

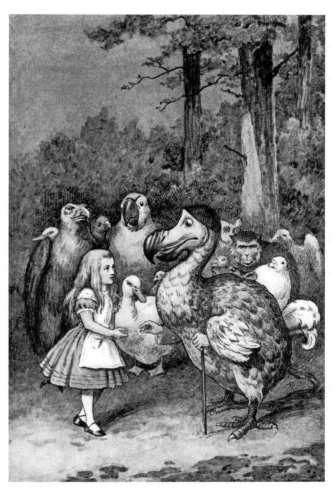

The Dodo bird verdict is the name given to an ongoing debate in psychology. Saul Rosenzweig used an illustration from Lewis Carroll's *Alice's Adventures in Wonderland* (1865) to make the point that common factors (e.g., everyone running around the lake) were more important than specific technical differences (e.g., how long or how far everyone had to run). He argued that all therapies can be equally effective, regardless of their specifics. (istockphoto.com/duncan1890)

which a therapist and an individual engage with each other and effect positive change in the individual. According to supporters, the more positive the therapeutic alliance, the better chance of improvement, regardless of the techniques used.

Critics of the Dodo bird verdict contend that specific techniques used in different therapies are more important and result in effective outcomes. Their most compelling argument is the research on cognitive behavior therapy (CBT) for anxiety disorders. CBT techniques are very effective in changing the individual's maladaptive (faulty) thoughts and behavioral patterns. The change effected results in reduction of anxiety symptoms.

Len Sperry, MD, PhD, and Elizabeth Smith Kelsey, PhD

See also: Anxiety Disorders; Cognitive Behavior Therapy; Psychotherapy

Further Reading

Luborsky, Lester , Robert Rosenthal, Louis Diguer, Tomasz P. Andrusyna, Jeffrey S. Berman, Jill T. Levitt, David A. Seligman and Elizabeth D. Krause. "The Dodo Bird Verdict Is Alive and Well-Mostly." *Clinical Psychology: Science and Practice* 9, no. 1 (2002): 2–12.

Norcross, John. *Psychotherapy Relationships That Work: Therapist Contributions and Responsiveness to Patients.* New York, NY: Oxford University Press, 2002.

Rosenzweig, Saul.. "Some Implicit Common Factors in Diverse Methods of Psychotherapy." *American Journal of Orthopsychiatry* 6, no. 3 (1936): 412–415.

Wampold, Bruce. *The Great Psychotherapy Debate: Models, Methods, and Findings.* New York, NY: Routledge, 2009.

Domestic Violence

Domestic violence takes many forms and is known by many different names, including spousal abuse, intimate partner violence, domestic abuse, domestic battery, family violence, and dating abuse. It is defined as a pattern of behavior involving abuse by one partner against the other in a relationship where it is used to gain or maintain power or control over the other. This can include physical abuse, threats, sexual abuse, emotional abuse, patterns of control, intimidation, or stalking. It can also involve endangerment of the other partner, such as kidnapping or harassment.

Description

The abused partner is referred to as the victim or survivor. Using this terminology must come with caution as it must match the mind-set of the person. For instance, a person coming for therapy or assistance may react with strong negativity to specific terms, so it is important to use the appropriate terminology. Academically there is a push toward the term "survivor" as it is found to encompass the notion of empowerment and resiliency.

Domestic violence encompasses a pattern of psychological, physical, emotional, economic, or sexual harm or threat of harm from one partner to another. This form of abuse can be a learned behavior or attitude of entitlement that can stem from a culturally supported environment. Those typically victim to this abuse are generally women and their children. However, it must be acknowledged that violence can occur in heterosexual and homosexual relationships, as well as with either a male or a female as the perpetrator or victim.

Separating from a violent relationship is often complicated for the victim and can take months or even years. This can be connected to concerns over financial safety or over fear of being alone or experiencing further harm due to past threats. The abused partner may feel trapped and may also experience denial that it won't happen again. The abused partner may also blame himself or herself for the acts of violence feeling he or she caused it by saying or acting in certain ways to upset his or her partner.

In the 1970s, Lenore Walker identified the cycle of abuse. This theory helps to explain patterns of behavior in abusive relationships. The theory focuses on the notion that once an abusive relationship is established, it is characterized by predictable patterns of abuse. This concept has been widely used and accepted in the field of domestic violence programs, education, and advocacy programs.

The cycle has four phases, and these repeat until the conflict has stopped generally by the victim or survivor leaving the relationship. The tension-building phase occurs prior to an abusive act and is generally calm phase where things seem to be peaceful. However, this will eventually lead back to difficulties and to the tension-building phase triggering the cycle to begin again.

There are four major types of intimate partner violence that are supported by research. The first is common couple violence where it occurs in a single argument and one or both partners physically attack each other. Intimate terrorism involves emotional and psychological abuse.

Violent resistance or self-defense occurs when the victim commits an act against the abusive partner. Finally, mutual violent control is a rare occurrence where both partners battle for control utilizing violent behaviors and actions.

Incidents of domestic violence can turn deadly especially when the abused partner attempts to leave the relationship. In certain cultures "honor killings" occur when it is felt that a family member has "shamed" the family. For instance, in some Middle Eastern cultures women are to adhere to certain standards such as being accompanied by male family members. If the women were to act against this notion of honor (including leaving an abusive relationship), the family's response to the perceived shame could result in that woman's death.

Current Status

Currently, one in every four women will experience domestic violence in her lifetime. It is estimated that 85% of domestic violence victims are women. Females between the ages of 20 and 24 are currently at the greatest risk of intimate partner violence. There are over 18.5 million mental health visits made each year as a result of domestic violence. However, despite these large numbers, most cases are never reported to the police.

Mindy Parsons, PhD

See also: Abuse; Child Abuse

Further Reading

Cohan, John Alan. "Honor Killings and the Cultural Defense." *California Western International Law Journal* 40 (2010): 177–252.

Eisenstat, Stephanie A., and Lundy Bancroft. "Domestic Violence." *The New England Journal of Medicine* 341 (1999): 886–892.

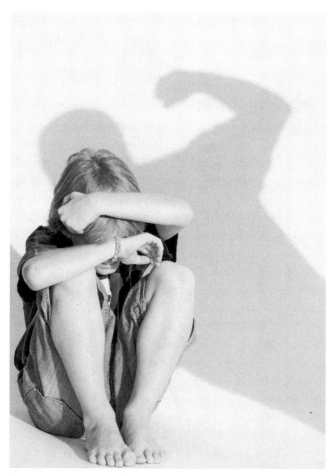

Domestic violence takes many forms and is known by many different names, including spousal abuse, intimate partner violence, domestic abuse, domestic battery, family violence, and dating abuse. In addition to potential physical harm, domestic abuse can lead victims to feel anxious, depressed, fearful, and helpless. (Godfer/Dreamstime.com)

identified by poor communication, passive aggressive behavior, and tension between the partners as well as fear of causing an outburst. The abused partner may make attempts to modify his or her behavior at this point to try and avoid triggering his or her partner. The next phase is acting out, which is where there is an active abusive incident. Following this is the reconciliation or honeymoon phase, where the abuser apologizes, ignores the incident, or gives an overabundance of affection. There are promises that it will never happen again. The abuser may make statements of desire to harm himself or herself to gain sympathy from his or her partner. The fourth part to the cycle is the

Engel, Beverly. *Breaking the Cycle of Abuse: How to Move beyond Your Past to Create an Abuse Free Future.* Hoboken, NJ: John Wiley & Sons, 2005.

Lawson, David M. *Family Violence: Explanations and Evidence-Based Clinical Practice.* Alexandria, VA: American Counseling Association, 2013.

Walker, Lenore E. *The Battered Woman.* New York, NY: Harper and Row, 1979.

Organization

National Coalition Against Domestic Violence
One Broadway, Suite B210
Denver, CO 80203
Telephone: (303) 839-1852
Fax: (303) 831-9251
E-mail: mainoffice@ncadv.org
Website: http://www.ncadv.org/

Dopamine

Dopamine is a chemical messenger in the brain that regulates attention, affect, pleasure, and coping with stress. It is involved in disorders such as addictions, depression, and schizophrenia.

Definitions

- **Blood–brain barrier** is a specialized layer of cells around the blood vessels of the brain controlling which substances can pass from the circulatory system into the brain.

- **D1–D5** are the five dopamine receptor proteins responsible for receiving the dopamine transmission or signal for a cell.

- **Mesolimbic pathway** is the "reward pathway" of the brain.

- **Nucleus accumbens** is part of the brain involved in the mesolimbic reward pathway, which receives dopamine signaling from the ventral tegmental area.

- **Parkinson's disease** is a degenerative nervous disease characterized by shuffling gain, tremors, and muscle stiffness.

- **Ventral tegmental area** produces dopamine and signals to the nucleus accumbens and the rest of the striatum.

Description

Dopamine is a neurotransmitter (chemical messenger) in the brain that transmits nerve impulses that regulates attention, concentration, movement, impulse control, affect and mood, sleep, motivation, pleasure, and coping with stress. Pleasurable experiences are associated with high dopamine levels while stress is associated with lower levels. Altered levels of dopamine can cause a range of symptoms and problems, including depression, attention-deficit hyperactivity disorder (ADHD), addictions, and schizophrenia. It also plays a prominent role in the manifestations of Parkinson's disease.

Dopamine is part of the dopamine family of neurotransmitters, which includes adrenaline and noradrenaline. All are monoamines, which means that their chemical structure includes an amino group linked with an aromatic ring. Dopamine is made from the amino acid tyrosine (its precursor) in three brain areas: the substantia nigra, the ventral tegmentum, and the arcuate nucleus. The first two areas are implicated in many mental disorders. Because dopamine cannot cross the blood–brain barrier, medical professionals cannot just give dopamine directly. Instead, they give its precursor, tyrosine, which can cross the barrier so that the brain can make dopamine on its own. There are five dopamine receptors (D1–D5) which recognize the dopamine molecule, bind to it, and transmit its signal to other cells.

A decline in dopamine (D2 receptors in the substantia nigra) is linked with Parkinson's disease. Low levels of dopamine can also result in symptoms of depression, such as a loss of pleasure or motivation. Low levels of dopamine binding to other D2 receptor are associated with social anxiety, while high levels are linked to the hypersocial behavior of those experiencing the manic phase of bipolar disorder. ADHD is also associated with problems in dopamine transmission.

In contrast, schizophrenia is linked with high dopamine levels (in the ventral tegmentum) and the symptoms of hallucinations and disturbed thinking. Interestingly, those with Parkinson's disease who take medication that raises dopamine levels too high can develop symptoms of schizophrenia, while those with schizophrenia who take medication that lowers dopamine levels can experience symptoms of Parkinson's disease.

Precautions and Side Effects

Side effects from medications that act on dopamine have been reported. More common ones are nausea, vomiting, and headache. Less common are irregular or rapid heartbeat, chest pain, dizziness, and trouble breathing.

Medications act on various dopamine receptors and increase or decrease dopamine levels. L-dopa is medication (antiparkinsonian) used in treating Parkinson's disease. It is a dopamine precursor that is synthesized into dopamine in the brain and reverses the effects of low dopamine levels. Monoamine oxidase inhibitors (MAOIs) block the activity of the enzyme that breaks down dopamine. As a result, MAOIs like Nardil and Parnate are antidepressants that increase dopamine levels. Antipsychotics are divided into two classes: typical and atypical antipsychotics that target different types of dopamine receptors. Clozaril is an atypical antipsychotic that targets the D4 receptor more strongly than the D2 receptor, while Parlodel targets D2 and is a partial inhibitor of D1. Abilify is a partial dopamine agonist (mimic), and Symmetrel is also a dopamine agonist.

Len Sperry, MD, PhD

See also: Abilify (Aripiprazole); Addictions; Depression; Schizophrenia

Further Reading

Breuning, Loretta G. *Meet Your Happy Chemicals: Dopamine, Endorphin, Oxytocin, Serotonin.* Seattle, WA: CreateSpace, 2012.

Iversen, Leslie, Susan Iversen, Stephen Dunnett, and Anders Bjorklund: *Dopamine Handbook.* New York, NY: Oxford University Press, 2010.

Stahl, Stephen M. *The Prescriber's Guide: Antipsychotics and Mood Stabilizers. Stahl's Essential Psychopharmacology.* Cambridge: Cambridge University Press, 2009.

Down Syndrome

Down syndrome is a chromosomal disorder that results in impairments of mental and physical development.

Description

Down syndrome (DS) is the most commonly occurring chromosomal condition in which children exhibit atypical physical features such as upward slanted eyes, small stature, and a deep crease in the palm of the hands. Although he was not the first to describe it, the syndrome was named after Dr. John Langdon Down, who published a detailed analysis of the condition in 1866. People with Down syndrome demonstrate a range of physical and mental impairments. According to the Centers for Disease Control, approximately 1 out of 691 children born in the United States is diagnosed with Down syndrome. Many people with DS have an intellectual deficit, or mental retardation, on a range from mild to severe. According to the National Down Syndrome Society, the average IQ score of a young adult with DS is approximately 50 while the national average is 100.

Through genetic testing, it is possible to identify Down syndrome at birth or before birth through prenatal testing such as amniocentesis. Prenatal testing can often lead to a decision on the part of the parents to terminate the pregnancy. The ability to identify the syndrome prenatally and terminate pregnancy is a controversial issue among the DS community.

Causes and Symptoms

Down syndrome is the most common chromosome abnormality in humans. Typically, human beings have cells that contain 23 pairs of chromosomes, half from each parent. When a person's cells show the presence of all or part of a third copy of chromosome 21, he or she has DS.

People with Down syndrome can be recognized due to certain abnormal physical characteristics. These include a short and wide physique, weak muscles, an upward slant to the eyes, and a deep crease across the center of the palm. These physical features vary from person to person. Individuals with DS can also experience conditions such as heart disease, celiac disease, and orthopedic conditions, which require medical supervision and care.

In childhood it is typical for individuals with Down syndrome to have a delay in speech development.

People with DS often demonstrate some degree of mental retardation. Often fine motor skills are also slow to develop. The development of gross motor skills affects some children who might not master walking until the age of four years.

Diagnosis and Prognosis

Genetic testing allows physicians to diagnose Down syndrome prenatally and at birth. Down syndrome is diagnosed through genetic tests that identify an extra copy of chromosome 21. Due to prenatal testing, many pregnancies end in early termination.

Decades ago the life expectancy for those with DS was nine years old. Over the last several decades, medical and educational interventions have substantially increased the prognosis for people with DS. Today people with DS typically live to 50 years of age or more.

People with Down syndrome have an elevated risk of developing several medical conditions. Commonly occurring medical diagnosis include heart disease, immune system problems, and seizure disorders. Complications with DS and these conditions increase the risk of premature death for these individuals. Regular checkups with a physician are highly recommended for people with DS.

Treatment

Treatment for Down syndrome is based on an analysis of each person's physical and intellectual challenges. Early childhood intervention through therapy and educational program is proven most effective. Preschool programs for children with Down syndrome will typically address all aspects of physical, occupational and speech therapies.

It is not only early childhood interventions and education which help. Also important is continued screening for physical and psychological issues that could affect life expectancy. Seeking appropriate medical treatment is important. In addition to medical interventions, it is helpful for people with Down syndrome to live in a supportive family or residential environment. The opportunity for vocational training can add immeasurably to the productivity, length, and quality of life for people with DS.

In the past, children with Down syndrome often received only basic, home-based education. Currently many DS children are integrated into the regular educational curriculum. For those who are not placed in regular education, specialized educational opportunities are available. Some students with DS graduate from high school and some go to college.

It has been found that education and opportunities to learn increase independence and self-care and improve quality of life. In the United States, there are increasing opportunities for participating in postsecondary education. Many adults with Down syndrome are able to work in the community, while others require a more sheltered work environment.

Alexandra Cunningham, PhD, and William M. Cunningham, MA

See also: Developmental Disabilities; Mental Retardation

Further Reading

"Learning About Down Syndrome." National Human Genome Research Institute. Last modified May 15, 2013. Accessed June 13, 2013. http://www.genome.gov/19517824.

Moran, Julie. "Aging and Down Syndrome: A Health and Well-Being Guidebook." National Down Syndrome Society. Accessed April 4, 2013.

Wiseman, Frances K., Kate A. Alford, Victor L. J. Tybulewicz, and Elizabeth M. C. Fisher. "Down Syndrome-Recent Progress and Future Prospects." *Journal of Human Molecular Genetics* 18 (2009): 75–83.

Dreams and Dream Interpretations

Dreams can range from the absurd and disjointed to exciting or even terrifying. But figuring out what dreams mean is often subject to intense debate. Still, the interpretation of dreams has long been used in therapy for promoting personal change. It is defined as the process of assigning meaning to dreams and is used broadly across many theoretical orientations. It is a therapeutic approach that offers considerable flexibility in integrating theory and techniques to interpret a client's dreams.

Dream interpretation is thought to offer insight into a person's innermost longings, ability to problem solve, ability to adapt, and overall approach to creative self-expression. Many believe that the content of a person's dreams is directly correlated to his or her waking life, as well as the level of psychological functioning. Dreams offer a therapist insightful information about a client's personality traits, as well as potential clinical challenges.

Sigmund Freud, who wrote *The Interpretation of Dreams*, was among the first to show a strong interest in interpreting the dreams of his patients. He suggested that dreams were related to wish fulfillment. He also believed that the content of the dream is connected to the unconscious wishes of the dreamer.

Freud identified four elements to dream interpretation, which he referred to as "dream work." The four elements include condensation, displacement, symbolization, and secondary revision. Condensation represents the multitude of ideas and concepts that are represented in a single dream and the information is condensed into a single thought or image. Displacement is the element that disguises the emotional meaning of the content. Symbolization censors the repressed ideas contained in the dream by including objects that are symbols of the content. Secondary revision is the final stage of the process. Freud suggested that strange elements are reorganized to make the dream understandable.

Carl Jung agreed with some points made by Freud. However, Jung did not share Freud's view that dreams are an expression of wish fulfillment. Jung instead believed that dreams were a way of revealing the personal and collective unconscious. He suggested that dreams were a way of compensating for less developed aspects of a person's psyche. Later research showed that personality that a person possesses in waking life is the same or similar to those expressed in dreams.

Dream interpretation as part of therapy is approached in a four-step process. It starts by reviewing all the images that were part of the dream. The client narrates the dream completely prior to the therapist asking any questions. The next step includes the therapist asking clarifying questions about the dream, including the client's affect, what the client saw, heard, or touched. Mining for this type of information helps uncover the feelings and sensations that were part of the dream. The third step attempts to revive the dream and the associate feelings by placing the client in a relaxed state. The therapist then helps the client relive the experiences of his or her dream. The key of this third step is to narrow in on any images that were particularly vivid for the dreamer. The fourth and final stage of dream interpretation has the therapist linking the experiences of the dream to other areas of the client's life and then integrating the experiences with the client's history and present life experiences.

Dream interpretation, however, lacks a unified and established methodology. The science and scientific support of dream interpretation is lacking. For instance, if one were to search what dreaming of fire means, one source indicates it represents a cleansing or punishment, whereas another source says it is connected with anger or a new beginning. While there are some similarities, these ideas are vague and differ enough that there is conflicting support of the meaning of this dream.

Dream interpretation has grown in popularity since the 1970s. Today, many bookstores have a wide collection of books available about the meaning of dreams, including dream dictionaries, symbol guides, and tips for interpreting and understanding dreams. However, the popularity tends to be more with the general public than with researchers in the mental health field. In fact, some researchers feel that dream interpretation is a neglected technique in contemporary treatment; however, others argue that there is not enough evidence to support using this as a treatment modality.

Mindy Parsons, PhD

See also: Freud, Sigmund (1856–1939); Jung, Carl (1875–1961); Jungian Therapy; Psychoanalysis

Further Reading
Freud, Sigmund. *The Interpretation of Dreams*. New York: Macmillan, 1915.

Frieden, Ken. *Freud's Dream of Interpretation*. New York: State University of New York Press, 1990.

Grinstein, Alexander. *Freud's Rules of Dream Interpretation*. New York: International Universities Press, 1983.

Hindman Miller, Gustavus. *Ten Thousand Dreams Interpreted, or What's in a Dream: A Scientific and Practical Exposition*. New York: M. A. Donohue & Company, 1931.

Means, John R., Jay R. Palmatier, Gregory L. Wilson, J. Scott Hickey, M. Joan Hess-Homeier, and C. Sue Hickey. "Dream Interpretation." *Psychotherapy* 23 (1986): 448–452.

Dreikurs, Rudolf (1897–1972)

Rudolf Dreikurs, MD, was an American psychiatrist and educator known for advancing Adlerian psychology through his writings and professional publications.

Description

Rudolf Dreikurs, MD (1897–1972), was an American psychiatrist and educator who advanced the theory and practice of Adlerian psychology, created by Alfred Adler (1870–1937). This approach to psychology understands individuals as social beings with a need to belong and strive for significance. It is also known as Individual Psychology. Dreikurs was a student and eventually close colleague of Alfred Adler. After Adler's death in 1937, Dreikurs went on to promote the use of Individual Psychology around the world.

Among his many contributions to the theory of Individual Psychology, he described a model of misbehavior and suggested that children "act out" when they experience a lack of belonging to a particular group or in their family. When a child misbehaves, he or she is acting from one of four "mistaken goals": attention seeking, power, revenge, or assumed inadequacy. Attention seeking is when a child keeps others busy through various behaviors to seek attention. The power goal is when a child seeks power to feel in control and a sense of belonging. The revenge goal is when a child seeks to get even or to retaliate for a previously perceived wrong doing of another person. The assumed inadequacy goal is when a child gives up to be left alone so that others will expect little from the child. Dreikurs worked with children by helping them enhance their cooperation and belonging skills by empowering them feel that they are valuable contributors to a classroom or family.

In 1952, Dreikurs founded the North American Society of Adlerian Psychology, of which he was an active leader of the society up until his death in 1972. He wrote many books that expanded the theory and practice of Adlerian psychology. He also founded the Alfred Adler Institute in 1952, which is now called Adler University, in Chicago, Illinois.

Jon Sperry, PhD, and Len Sperry, MD, PhD

See also: Adler, Alfred (1870–1937); Early Recollections; Individual Psychology; Lifestyle and Lifestyle Convictions

Further Reading

Dreikurs, Rudolf. *The Challenge of Marriage*. Philadelphia, PA: Taylor & Francis Group, 1998.

Dreikurs, Rudolf. *The Challenge of Parenthood*. New York, NY: Duell, Sloan and Peirce, 1958.

Dreikurs, Rudolf, and Loren Grey. *Logical Consequences: A New Approach to Discipline*. New York, NY: Meredith Press, 1968.

Terner, Janet, and W. L. Pew. *The Courage to Be Imperfect: The Life and Work of Rudolf Dreikurs*. New York, NY: Hawthorn Books, 1978.

Drug Culture

Drug culture is a description for those people, groups, or communities where the use of drugs is a key element of daily life and social relationships.

Definitions

- **Alcohol use disorder** is a mental disorder involving a pattern of alcohol use which leads to significant problems for the user.

- **Benzodiazepines** are a class of drugs that slow the nervous system and are prescribed to relieve nervousness and tension, to induce sleep, and to treat other symptoms. They are highly addictive.

- **Opioids** are a group of drugs that reduce pain. They are highly addictive and include both prescription drugs like Percocet and illegal drugs like heroin.

- **Psychoactive** is a drug or substance that has a significant effect on mental processes. There are five groups of psychoactive drugs: opioids, stimulants, depressants, hallucinogens, and cannabis.

- **Psychotropic medications** are prescribed drugs that affect thinking, feeling, and behavior. They include antipsychotic, antianxiety, antidepressant, and antimanic medications.

- **Stimulant** is a drug that increases brain activity and produces a sense of alertness, euphoria, endurance, and productivity, or suppresses appetite. Examples are cocaine, amphetamines, and Ritalin.

- **Substance abuse** involves the use of substances (drugs or alcohol) in amounts or with methods that are harmful.

Description

Drugs, which can be defined as behavior-altering chemicals, have played a part in the history of most civilizations. There are several kinds of drugs, including alcohol, stimulants, opioids, benzodiazepines, cannabis, and psychoactives. Over time drugs have been used as parts of religious rituals, as well as for medicinal purposes and entertainment, escape, or recreation.

Culture can be defined as learned behavior based on a combination of shared customs, language, and beliefs. Subcultures share traits with the dominant culture but distinguish themselves with different customs, ideas, and practices. Some subcultures form as a result of a positive response to problems in the larger culture, and some are negative reactions against the values of the dominant culture. The drug culture can be viewed as a result of both negative and positive responses to the issues in the larger culture.

Drug cultures are examples of subcultures built around the idea that drugs, especially illegal drugs, are an important part of the human experience. Drug cultures are often associated with other sociological minority classifications such as race, poverty, or youth. Since society at large ostracizes and punishes the use of illegal drugs, the basis for conflict between the larger society and the drug culture is inevitable.

Current Status and Impact (Psychological Influence)

Drugs cause internal chemical changes in the body whether the intention of their use is medically beneficial or recreationally damaging. The dilemma that society and the medical community face is how to draw a sensible line between medically beneficial and dangerous drugs. In addition to this issue, many people are concerned about the overuse and dependence both of medically beneficial and of dangerous drugs for those who use them.

Not all drugs are illegal. Legal drugs include alcohol, prescription medications, and some mood-altering drugs depending on location. In the United States approximately two-thirds of the population drink alcohol. It is worth noting that for a decade in the 1920s, America tried to outlaw alcohol as an illegal drug during a period called prohibition. Prohibition had negative social and legal implications but was an attempt to prohibit the use of this addictive substance.

Another legal drug is nicotine. About 20% of people in the United States report using nicotine regularly, and it is a highly addictive drug. Other highly addictive drugs that people are dependent on are legally prescribed medications traditionally used to treat disorders such as depression or anxiety. The variety of mood-altering drugs that are available from multiple sources grows each year. The demand in the market for these products, distributed both legally and illegally, contributes to this growth.

Even though legal drugs cause both social and health problems, the appeal of the drug culture has always been illegal drugs. It is estimated that about 10% of people in the United States use illegal drugs regularly and many more have experimented with them at some point in their lives. It is estimated that millions of Americans are dependent on the use of illegal drugs such as heroin and cocaine.

Perhaps nothing illustrates the mystique surrounding illegal drugs better than two famous works of art. The first is a novel and later film written by Hunter S. Thompson in 1971, called *Fear and Loathing in Las Vegas*. The film's subtitle is *A Savage Journey to the Heart of the American Dream* and gave the sense of the love/hate relationship that Americans have with illegal drugs and the glamorization of their role. Another, more recent portrayal of drug culture is the Martin Scorsese film *The Wolf of Wall Street*. In this film, the presence of illegal drugs highlights the drug culture of the wealthy and successful. The use of high-class drugs and partying was a large part of the financial and social status of the characters in this film and is a reflection of the drug culture for the rich during the 1980s and beyond.

The government and society in general are unsure of how to handle drugs and the drug culture. It seems clear that the issue is important, but it does not seem to have a simple solution. Legalization or decriminalization of drug use is gaining government clearance for substances such as cannabis in many locations across the globe. But some have cited both health and moral problems with the legalization of formerly illegal drugs. It is reported that as many as 25% of adolescents, between the ages of 16 and 17, are estimated to have used marijuana. The use of medical and recreational marijuana was first made legal in states like California, Colorado, and Washington. Many expect that this trend will grow, with more states legalizing its use.

Drug campaigns, such as the "Just Say No" approach of the 1980s, have not been effective in reducing the use of drugs or formation of drug subcultures. Many issues still exist, such as how to distinguish between medical and recreational use of drugs or decriminalizing possession of drugs for private use. Prevention programs such as improving substance abuse education and treatments have been in place for decades with varied impact. The drug culture is in frequent conflict with policy makers and authorities, like the Drug Enforcement Authority. Despite efforts to eradicate legal and illegal drug use and abuse, drug cultures persist and provide opportunities for those who engage or believe in the use of personal or medical drug use.

Alexandra Cunningham, PhD, and William M. Cunningham, MA

See also: Prescription Drug Abuse; Psychedelic Drugs

Further Reading

Aldridge, Judith, Fiona Measham, and Lisa Williams. *Illegal Leisure Revisited: Changing Patterns of Alcohol and Drug use in Adolescents and Young Adults.* New York, NY: Routledge, 2011.

Brake, Michael. *The Sociology of Youth Culture and Youth Subcultures: Sex, Drugs and Rock 'n' Roll?* New York, NY: Routledge, 2013.

DuPont, Robert L. "Prescription Drug Abuse: An Epidemic Dilemma." *Journal of Psychoactive Drugs* 42, no. 2 (2010): 127–132.

Drug Dependence

Drug dependence is a mental condition characterized by physical dependence. It is similar to but different from addiction.

Definitions

- **Addiction** is a chronic disease of the brain which involves compulsive and uncontrolled pursuit of reward or relief with substance use or other compulsive behaviors.

- **Alcohol use disorder** is a mental disorder involving a pattern of alcohol use which leads to significant problems for the user.

- **Cannabis use disorder** is a mental disorder characterized by cannabis (marijuana) use which leads to significant problems for the user.

- *Diagnostic and Statistical Manual of Mental Disorders* is the handbook mental health professionals use to diagnose mental disorders. The current edition (fifth) is known as DSM-5.

- **Physical dependence** refers to physical changes in the body that result in tolerance and withdrawal symptoms when drug use is discontinued.

- **Psychological dependence** refers to the loss of control over the intense urges to use a substance at the expense of adverse (harmful) consequences.

- **Stimulant use disorder** is a mental disorder that is characterized by the use of stimulants, which leads to significant problems for the user. It includes amphetamine and cocaine.

- **Substance-related and addictive disorders** are a group of mental disorders that include substance disorders characterized by physiological dependence, drug-seeking behavior, tolerance, and social withdrawal. This group also includes the non-substance disorder of gambling.

- **Tolerance** is the phenomenon in which the body requires increased amounts of the substance to achieve the desired effect.

- **Withdrawal** is the unpleasant and potentially life-threatening physiological changes that occur due to the discontinuation of certain drugs after prolonged regular use.

Description

Drug dependence is a mental condition characterized by the symptoms of physical dependence (tolerance and withdrawal) following the use of a drug or alcohol. In everyday language, the term "drug dependence" is used interchangeably with addiction. While both share some common features, there are also significant differences. Their technical meaning tends to differentiate them. For instance, the term "dependence" is used by many researchers and professionals to describe physical dependence following use of drugs or alcohol. Physical dependence is also observed with certain prescribed medications, such as antidepressants. On the other hand, addiction is characterized by psychological dependence, although there may also be some physical dependence. However, the physical changes associated with drug withdrawal are distinct from the loss of control over the intense urges that is associated with addiction. In short, psychological dependence refers to impaired control over drinking or drug use, while physical dependence refers to tolerance and withdrawal symptoms.

Until recently, the *Diagnostic and Statistical Manual of Mental Disorders* has added to the confusion by its inconsistent use of the terms "addiction" and "dependence" to describe alcohol and drug problems. DSM-5 resolved that confusion by eliminating the category of drug (substance) dependence entirely. Now, the compulsive drug-seeking behavior of addiction is differentiated from the normal responses of tolerance and withdrawal experienced by some when using prescribed medications. While drug (substance) dependence had been considered a mental disorder in previous editions of *Diagnostic and Statistical Manual of Mental Disorders* (DSM), it is no longer considered a disorder in DSM-5.

However, DSM-5 does describe several substance-related and addictive disorders. These include alcohol use disorder, cannabis use disorder, and stimulant use disorder. To make such diagnoses, it must be evident that there is impaired control over the use of the substance or addictive behavior and that it significantly disrupts the lives of the user. Currently, the causes of these disorders are not well understood. However, there are probably multiple causative factors. These may include biological or genetic history, psychological traits and coping skills, and environmental factors such as parent's use of substances and peer influence.

Len Sperry, MD, PhD, and Jon Sperry, PhD

See also: Addiction; Alcohol Use Disorder; Cannabis Use Disorder; Stimulant Use Disorder; Substance-Related and Addictive Disorders

Further Reading

American Psychiatric Association. *Diagnostic and Statistical Manual of Mental Disorders*, 5th ed. Arlington, VA: American Psychiatric Association Press, 2013.

Miller, William, and Richard Muñoz. *Controlling Your Drinking*. New York, NY: Guilford Press, 2005.

Miller, William, and Stephen Rollnick. *Motivational Interviewing: Preparing People for Change*, 2nd ed. New York, NY: Guilford Press, 2002.

Drug Enforcement Administration (DEA)

The Drug Enforcement Administration is a federal law enforcement agency that enforces controlled substances laws and regulations. It is also called the DEA.

Definitions

- **Benzodiazepines** are a class of drugs that slow the nervous system and are prescribed to relieve nervousness and tension, to induce sleep, and to treat other symptoms. They are highly addictive.

- **Controlled substances** are a drug or chemical whose use, manufacture, and possession laws are regulated by the federal government.

These can be illegal substances or prescription medication.

- **Controlled Substances Act** was passed into law in 1973 to regulate the importation, manufacture, possession, and use of certain substances.

- **Illicit drugs** are illegal drugs that have no medical use and are often used for their ability to distort an individual's mental process.

- **Opioids** are a group of drugs that reduce pain. They are highly addictive and include both prescription drugs like Percocet and illegal drugs like heroin.

- **Psychoactive** is a drug or substance that has a significant effect on mental processes. There are five groups of psychoactive drugs: opioids, stimulants, depressants, hallucinogens, and cannabis.

- **Psychotropic medications** are prescribed drugs that affect thinking, feeling, and behavior. They include antipsychotic, antianxiety, antidepressant, and antimanic medications.

- **War on Drugs** refers to the national campaign against drug abuse, which was popularized during the early 1970s following a speech by President Richard Nixon in which he publicly declared drug abuse as "public enemy number one."

Description

The Drug Enforcement Administration (DEA) is a law enforcement agency under the U.S. Department of Justice that enforces controlled substances laws and regulations. Its goal is to reduce illegal drug use and drug trafficking in the United States. The DEA enforces the Controlled Substances Act. It regulates and monitors the growing, manufacture, and distribution of controlled substances and illicit substances. Controlled substances are often abused and used for nonmedical purposes. Psychotropic medications such as opioids and benzodiazepines have medical purposes, but they are also used for nonmedical purposes. Many

psychoactive substances have medical purposes, but many psychoactive substances are used by individuals to experience the "high."

In response to increasing drug trade and related crimes, President Richard Nixon declared an all-out global war on the drug menace. It became known as the War on Drugs. The Drug Enforcement Administration was initiated on July 1, 1973, and signed into effect by President Richard Nixon. The DEA is led by an Administrator of Drug Enforcement, who is appointed by the president of the United States. The creation of this federal agency was to prevent illicit drug trafficking based on the growing concerns about the availability of drugs in the United States.

Impact (Psychological Influence)

Though the DEA began with just 1,470 special agents and a budget of less than $75 million, the agency has grown considerably now, staffing some 5,000 agents and operating on a budget of over $2 billion. Over the past several decades the agency has improved its operations and influence by adding new divisions and incorporating advancements in technology. DEA efforts have increased in recent years in response to the drastic rise in oxycodone, Xanax, and other prescription drugs resulting from the pill mill and pain clinic epidemics. Efforts have also focused on black market drugs, including crack cocaine, heroine, Ecstasy, and steroids. Most recently, the DEA has been in the middle of the national controversy over the possible legalization of medical marijuana.

Jon Sperry, PhD, Len Sperry, MD, PhD, and Melissa Mariani, PhD

See also: Barbiturates; Benzodiazepines; Detoxification; Drug Dependence

Further Reading

Greene, Meg, and Arthur Meier Schlesinger Jr. *The Drug Enforcement Administration* (*U.S. Government: How It Works*). Open Library: Chelsea House Publishing, 2011.

Newton, Michael. *Drug Enforcement Administration* (*Law Enforcement Agencies*). Open Library: Chelsea House Publishing, 2000.

United States Drug Enforcement Administration—U.S. Department of Justice. "DEA History." 2014. Accessed

June 10, 2014. http://www.justice.gov/dea/about/history.shtml.

United States Drug Enforcement Administration. "DEA Mission Statement." 2014. Accessed September 20, 2014. http://www.justice.gov/dea/about/mission.shtml.

U.S. Department of Justice Drug Enforcement Administration. "Office of Diversion Control." 2014. Accessed September 20, 2014. http://www.deadiversion.usdoj.gov/index.html.

DSM

See Diagnostic and Statistical Manual of Mental Disorders (DSM)

Dual Diagnosis

Dual diagnosis is the co-occurrence of a mental disorder and a substance-related disorder.

Definitions

- **Biopsychosocial** refers to the interrelationship of biological, psychological, and social factors.

- **Co-occurrence** means that two things are happening at the same time.

- **Comorbid** refers to the occurrence of two or more disorders in the same person that can start at the same time or one after the other.

- **DSM-5** is the abbreviation for the *Diagnostic and Statistical Manual of Mental Disorders, Fifth Edition*, which is the handbook mental health professionals use to diagnose mental disorders.

- **Motivational interviewing** is a five-stage model used by clinicians to help clients with substance abuse problems become motivated to change. The five stages are pre-contemplation, contemplation, preparation, action, and maintenance.

- **Substance-related disorders** are a class of DSM-5 disorders characterized by the use of one or more substances that lead to significant distress or disruption of daily life. Alcohol and cannabis (marijuana) are examples of these disorders.

Description

Dual diagnosis is the co-occurrence of a mental disorder and a substance disorder. Either disorder can occur first, but one does not necessarily cause the other. Both mental and substance disorders are influenced by biopsychosocial factors. Genetic factors play a role in an individual's susceptibility to both. Substance use may result in the expression of symptoms in individuals predisposed to a mental disorder. From a psychological standpoint, it may be that those with a mental disorder use substances to make themselves feel better. Environmental factors such as physical, emotional, and sexual abuse can also play a role. When an individual begins using drugs, this drug use may change brain functioning in a manner that increases the possibility of a disorder.

The term "dual diagnosis" was originally used by researchers and practitioners during the mid-1980s. During this time, several initiatives began the integration of mental health and substance abuse services to overcome the problems associated with single treatment efforts. Traditionally, patients with co-occurring disorders received mental health care and substance abuse services from two different practitioners in two different locations. This sequential treatment approach made it difficult for patients to receive comprehensive care, to access care, and to integrate information from different practitioners.

A dual diagnosis is correlated with multiple problems such as relapse, frequent hospitalization, depression, suicidality, imprisonment, homelessness, and interpersonal difficulties. Individuals with dual diagnoses have higher rates of symptoms, hospitalization, housing problems, and dysfunction than individuals diagnosed with a single disorder. Furthermore, treatment costs are higher among people with dual diagnoses compared to those with a single diagnosis. Those with comorbid disorders are more susceptible to dropping out of outpatient treatment and are frequent users of hospital and emergency services. To increase treatment outcomes, dual diagnosis treatment facilities integrate mental health interventions and substance abuse interventions within one program. Interventions for both mental illness and substance abuse require long-term efforts that work to stabilize, educate, and promote self-management. A team approach of mental health and substance treatment practitioners working together can greatly improve care and reduce treatment costs. Comprehensive treatment programs offer individual, group, and family counseling; psychiatric services; medication monitoring; psychoeducation; case management; and outreach services. Individuals with mental disorder are frequently unaware that they have a substance abuse problem and may not be motivated to seek treatment. Motivational interviewing is useful to help individuals gain awareness, develop motivation, and elicit behavior change. Unless treatment is successful, the presence of dual diagnosis greatly reduces individuals' ability to live within and contribute to their community.

Len Sperry, MD, PhD, and Christina Ladd, PhD

See also: Comorbidity; Substance Abuse Treatment

Further Reading

American Psychiatric Association. *Diagnostic and Statistical Manual of Mental Disorders*, 5th ed. Arlington, VA: American Psychiatric Association, 2013.

Evans, Katie, and Michael J. Sullivan. *Counseling the Mentally Ill Substance Abuser*. New York, NY: The Guildford Press, 2000.

National Institute on Drug Abuse. "Comorbidity: Addiction and Other Mental Disorders." 2011. Accessed September 11, 2014. http://www.drugabuse.gov/sites/default/files/comorbidity.pdf.

Ortman, Dennis. *The Dual Diagnosis Recovery Sourcebook: A Physical, Mental, and Spiritual Approach to Addiction with an Emotional Disorder*. Lincolnwood, Illinois: Lowell House, 2001.

Dyslexia

Dyslexia is the impairment that affects a person's ability to read written language with the speed and ability of others.

Description

Dyslexia is another term for specific learning disorder for people who have trouble with reading. Some researchers suggest that 15% of the general population have dyslexia. The diagnosis is not related to intelligence, vision, or other learning disorders. It is estimated that 80% of all individuals diagnosed with learning disorders have a form of dyslexia.

Dyslexia impairs an individual's ability to easily recognize and understand written information. Even though reading is a challenge for these people, some with dyslexia experience an increase in their thinking and visualization abilities. Although most children with dyslexia are identified when they go to school, there are some whose condition is not fully diagnosed until adulthood. Identifying it can be complicated because children with the diagnosis have normal vision and intelligence.

Causes and Symptoms

Although difficulties with reading can arise from different sources, dyslexia is distinct since it is caused by neurological deficits. This means that there are similar brain differences among those with dyslexia. Researchers have identified that these differences are usually located in the temporal processing center of the brain.

There are many common symptoms of dyslexia. Symptoms include delayed letter recognition and difficulty in rhyming and listing words that begin with the same sound. These children can also be slow to learn letter sounds and read slowly. Often the recognition of words is affected and therefore the child can be reluctant to read. If a child exhibits one or more of these symptoms, it does not necessarily mean that the child has dyslexia. A thorough evaluation is needed to determine if a child has dyslexia and not some other problem which leads to difficulties in reading.

Although dyslexia mainly affects a person's ability to read and understand information, it can also impair language expression. It can also be linked to and complicated by other disorders, such as attention-deficit disorder and mathematics disorder. Dyslexia and IQ are not related since intelligence develops separately from reading.

Diagnosis and Prognosis

The diagnosis of dyslexia is now officially called specified learning disorder, with deficiency in reading. In order to qualify for this diagnosis, a person is required to have trouble with identifying and understanding written words. This can include problems such as poor fluid reading and frequent spelling mistakes. Dyslexia is usually recognized during the early years of school as children struggle to learn to read. People with dyslexia can learn to read with good comprehension, but it generally takes them longer to read than others. They may also perform more slowly at related tasks such as spelling and sorting words.

Treatment

In order to help people with dyslexia with their reading difficulties, different supports can be put into place. Therapy and educational supports aim at helping children work through visual and auditory processing of words. Usually these supports are most effective when used in childhood while the brain is still developing. It is important to note that there is no cure for dyslexia. It's a lifelong condition caused by inherited traits that affect how your brain works. However, most children with dyslexia can succeed in school with tutoring or a specialized education program. Emotional support also plays an important role in helping people adjust to the difficulties they experience. The use of relaxation and anxiety-reducing strategies benefits people with dyslexia, who experience stress as a result of the disorder.

Alexandra Cunningham, PhD

See also: Reading Disorder; Specific Learning Disorder

Further Reading

American Psychiatric Association. *Diagnostic and Statistical Manual of Mental Disorders*, 5th ed. Alexandria, VA: American Psychiatric Association, 2013.

Shaywitz, Sally. *Overcoming Dyslexia: A New and Complete Science-Based Program for Reading Problems at Any Level*. New York, NY: First Vintage Books, 2005.

Dyspareunia

Dyspareunia is a mental disorder characterized by genital pain during sexual intercourse.

Definitions

- **Cognitive behavior therapy** is a type of psychotherapy that focuses on maladaptive (problematic) behaviors, emotions, and thoughts. It is also called CBT.

- **DSM** stands for the *Diagnostic and Statistical Manual of Mental Disorders*, which is a diagnostic system used by professionals to identify mental disorders with specific diagnostic criteria. The current edition is DSM-5.

- **Exposure** is a cognitive behavior therapy intervention (method) in which an individual is exposed to a feared object or situation. It is also referred to as flooding.

- **Genito-pelvic pain/penetration disorder** is a mental disorder in women characterized by persistent fear, pain, or difficulty with vaginal intercourse. Previously this disorder was referred to as dyspareunia and vaginismus.

- **Pelvic floor muscle training** involves a series of exercises designed to strengthen the muscles of the pelvic floor. These exercises are used to treat problems with urine leakage, bowel control, and pelvic pain.

- **Psychotherapy** is a psychological method for achieving desired changes in thinking, feeling, and behavior. It is also called therapy or therapeutic counseling.

- **Sexual dysfunctions disorders** are a group of mental disorders characterized by significant difficulty in responding sexually or experiencing sexual pleasure. They include delayed ejaculation, female organismic disorder, and genito-pelvic pain penetration disorder.

- **Systematic desensitization** is form of cognitive behavior therapy that gradually exposes individuals to their phobia (fear) while remaining calm and relaxed.

- **Vaginismus** is the inability to allow vaginal penetration because of anxiety and fear of pain that results in vaginal spasm.

Description and Diagnosis

Dyspareunia was a sexual disorder in DSM-IV-TR but is not listed as such in DSM-5. It is characterized by genital pain during sexual intercourse. This pain is experienced during intercourse, but for some, it may be experienced either before or after. While it is experienced in males and females, it is more common in females. This disorder has been combined with vaginismus in the current DSM-5 in the diagnosis of genito-pelvic pain/penetration disorder. These two disorders were combined in DSM-5 because it was difficult for clinicians to distinguish between these two disorders and because they commonly occurred together.

According to the *Diagnostic and Statistical Manual of Mental Disorders, Fourth Edition, Text Revision*, an individual may be diagnosed with this disorder if he or she experiences repeated pain accompanying intercourse. As with most mental disorders, these symptoms must cause the individual distress. The pain cannot be better explained by an alternative cause such as a lack of lubrication, medical condition, or substance use. This disorder may be present for an individual's entire life, or it may begin after a period of normal sexual functioning. Symptoms may occur in a particular circumstance or in all situations involving intercourse (American Psychiatric Association, 2000).

The cause of this disorder is unclear. It is believed that sexual abuse, body-image issues, relationship issues, religious beliefs, and a history of vaginal infection may contribute to the manifestation of this disorder. However, for the majority of individuals, a combination of psychological, physiological, and social factors are likely to be present. For this reason, it is important for a clinician to be diligent in his or her assessment of this disorder.

Treatment

Treatment includes a comprehensive medical evaluation to identify any medical condition that might cause dyspareunia. If one is found, then medical treatment is appropriate. If no such cause is identified, it is usually treated with a combination of physical therapy and psychotherapy. Physical therapy is necessary to help the individual learn how to train and control pelvic floor muscles. The most common form of psychotherapy for this disorder is cognitive behavior therapy (CBT). CBT is used to reduce fear, anxiety, and pain. It emphasizes systematic desensitization and exposure techniques. If trauma issues are involved, it would also address them or refer for specialized treatment.

Len Sperry, MD, PhD, and
Jeremy Connelly, MEd

See also: Cognitive Behavior Therapy; *Diagnostic and Statistical Manual of Mental Disorders* (DSM); Exposure Therapy; Genito-pelvic Pain/Penetration Disorder; Psychotherapy; Sexual Dysfunctions; Specific Phobia; Vaginismus

Further Reading

American Psychiatric Association. *Diagnostic and Statistical Manual of Mental Disorders*, 4th ed, *text revision*. Washington, DC: American Psychiatric Association, 2000.

American Psychiatric Association. *Diagnostic and Statistical Manual of Mental Disorders*, 5th ed. Arlington, VA: American Psychiatric Association, 2013.

Leiblum, Sandra. *Principles and Practice of Sex Therapy*, 4th ed. New York, NY: The Guilford Press, 2007.

Wincze, John, and Michael Carey. *Sexual Dysfunction: A Guide for Assessment and Treatment*, 2nd ed. New York, NY: The Guilford Press, 2001.

E

Early Recollections

Early recollections is a personality test that analyzes single-incident memories from childhood.

Definitions

- **Adlerian therapy** is a psychotherapy approach developed by Alfred Adler that emphasizes the individual's life style. Connectedness with others (belonging), meeting the life tasks, and contributions to society (social interest) are considered the hallmarks of mental health.

- **Inferiority complex** is a behavioral manifestation of a subjective feeling of inferiority.

- **Inferiority feeling** is the emotional reaction to a self-appraisal of deficiency that is subjective, global, and judgmental.

- **Life style** refers to one's attitudes and convictions about belonging and finding a place in the world.

- **Life style convictions** are the attitudes and beliefs that direct an individual's sense of belonging.

- **Life tasks** are the main challenges (work, love, and friendship) that life presents to all individuals.

- **Private logic** are convictions that run counter to social interest and fail to foster a constructive sense of belonging with others.

- **Projective technique** is a psychological test in which an individual's responses to ambiguous stimuli like are analyzed to determine underlying personality traits, feelings, or attitudes.

- **Safeguarding mechanisms** are the behaviors of attitudes that individuals select to evade responsibility and not meet the life tasks. Safeguarding mechanisms are called defense mechanism by other approaches.

- **Social interest** refers to the behaviors and attitudes that display an individual's sense of belonging, concern for, and contributions to the community.

Description

Early recollections (ERs) are a projective technique in which early memories are used to identify an individual's life style convictions and other personality dynamics. Research indicates that memories are not identical simulations of the past but are stories shaped by one's current view of others, the world, and ourselves. As a result, the gathering of ERs can be used as a projective technique that indicates one's strengths, goals, lines of movement, fears, worries, and other relevant psychological data. ERs provide a rapid, accurate, and cost-effective personality assessment that has similar reliability and validity to other personality tests. ERs are typically elicited by a counselor or psychotherapist both to assess the client's life style convictions and personality and to monitor change in the course of therapy.

Developments and Current Status

Alfred Adler (1870–1937) was a Viennese physician who developed Adlerian therapy. In his earliest writings, he emphasized the clinical value of understanding the individual's life story. Adler viewed it as the story that an individual repeats to himself or herself to warn or to comfort himself or herself. It helps the individual focus on his or her goals. Based on past experiences, this story prepares the individual to meet the future with a ready-made, already-tested style of action. Adler called this story or narrative the "life style." It is important to distinguish life style from the contemporary uses of the word "lifestyle" as in "lifestyles of the rich and famous." Life style and its related life style convictions specify the individual's subjective view of oneself, others, and the world.

An individual's life style develops based on childhood experiences and perceptions of those experiences. ERs are those single incidents from childhood in which the individual reconstitutes in present experience as mental pictures or as focused sensory memories. They are understood dynamically; that is, the act of recollecting and re-remembering is a present activity. Historical accuracy is of no concern with these recollections. Rather, ERs, as understood in Adlerian therapy, mirror presently held convictions, evaluations, attitudes, and biases. In such memories, the level of activity or passivity of an individual is very likely to predict how the individual will respond to present and future circumstances. For example, in a series of memories, an individual who passively accepts unfavorable circumstances in his or her memories is likely to respond in a similar passive way in present life situations. In contrast, an individual who acts to improve circumstances in a series of memories is likely to respond in an active way in present life situations.

Individuals develop four life style convictions: a self-view—the convictions one has about who one is; a self-ideal—the convictions of what one should be or are obliged to be to have a place; a world view—one's picture of the world or convictions about the not self and what the world demands of the individual; and one's ethical convictions—a personal moral code. When there is conflict between the self-concept and the ideal, inferiority feelings develop. It is important to note feelings of inferiority are not considered abnormal. However, when the individual begins to act inferior rather than feel inferior, the individual expresses an "inferiority complex." Thus, while the inferiority feeling is universal and normal, the inferiority complex reflects the discouragement of a limited segment of our society and is usually abnormal.

One of the main tools Adlerian therapists use to assess how an individual is functioning is a life style assessment. The goal of the life style assessment is to explore the individual's perceptions of his or her childhood experiences to discover the influence those perceptions have on the individual's current functioning. Basic to life style assessment is the elicitation of ERs.

The basic technique of eliciting ERs begins by asking the individual to think back before the age of 10 and to verbally share the earliest memory that comes to mind. It is essential that the focuses are on experiences occurring before the age of 10. Ten years is considered the age at which a child develops the ability to record events in chronological sequence. Then, the individual is asked to describe the memory as if it were a video recording with a beginning, middle, and end, and that has a feeling associated with it. The therapist writes down the memory using as many of the individual's words as possible. Then, the therapist asks the individual to freeze a certain scene or frame of the most vivid part of that memory and describe that frame. The individual is then asked to indicate his or her feeling or feelings about that vivid scene. Next, the individual is asked to indicate his or her thought or thoughts about that vivid scene.

Usually a minimum of three ERs are collected. From these, the therapist looks for themes. These themes usually offer valuable insight into the individual's presenting problem or concern. There are many ways to interpret themes from ERs. One way of interpretation is to notice who is and who is not included in the ERs, who else may be present in the ERs, and the extent of details that are included and what is emphasized. Overall, ERs provide a quick, accurate, and clinically useful assessment of an individual's personality dynamics, particularly life style convictions.

Len Sperry, MD, PhD

See also: Adler, Alfred (1870–1937); Adlerian Therapy

Further Reading

Carlson, Jon, Richard E. Watts, and Michael Maniacci. *Adlerian Therapy: Theory and Practice*. Washington, DC: American Psychological Association Books, 2006.

Clark, Arthur J. *Early Recollections: Theory and Practice in Counseling and Psychotherapy*. New York, NY: Brunner-Routledge, 2002.

Mosak, Harold H., and Robert Di Pietro. *Early Recollections: Interpretative Method and Application*. New York, NY: Routledge, 2006.

Orgler, Herta. *Alfred Adler: the Man and His Work*. New York, NY: Capricorn Books, 1963.

Eating Disorders

Eating and feeding disorders are a group of extreme and potentially life-threatening beliefs, feelings, and behaviors about personal weight and food consumption.

Definitions

- **Binge eating** or bingeing is an out-of-control eating episode in which an abnormally large amount of food is ingested in a short period of time.

- **Compensatory** behaviors include self-induced vomiting, use of laxative or diuretics, fasting, and excessive exercise.

- **Diuretics** are substances that elevate the rate of urination and water loss.

- **Laxatives** are drugs, medications, or substances that stimulate the evacuation of the bowels.

- **Low weight** is weight that is less than minimally expected for age and height.

- **Purging** is to clear the stomach and/or the intestines of material by the use of laxatives, diuretics, or self-induced vomiting.

Description

Feeding and eating disorders (FEDs) are a group of psychological disorders characterized by impaired eating habits and abnormal perception of one's weight.

FEDs have serious health consequences and are potentially life threatening. Anorexia, bulimia, and binge eating are the most commonly known FEDs but are not the only FEDs listed in the *Diagnostic and Statistical Manual of Mental Disorders* (DSM-5).

Causes and Symptoms

Anorexia nervosa is characterized by self-starvation and excessive weight loss. Approximately 90%–95% of people diagnosed with anorexia are females. Symptoms include low body weight, inadequate food intake to maintain weight, an extreme fear of gaining weight or becoming overweight, disturbed perceptions of body image, and an inability to recognize the seriousness of the behaviors. People suffering from anorexia are overly preoccupied with weight, food, fat and calorie intake, and dieting. Sufferers often develop food rituals such as arranging food on their plate or eating foods only in a specific order. They may make excuses to avoid mealtimes or situations where food may be consumed and make frequent reference to feeling fat or overweight. In spite of extreme thinness, sufferers perceive themselves as overweight. Self-starvation is the essential component of anorexia and as such has significant and serious health consequences, including muscle loss, reduced bone density, severe dehydration, kidney failure, weakness, fatigue, low blood pressure, slow heart rate, loss of hair, loss of menstrual cycle, and death. Anorexia is one of the most lethal mental health disorders, with 5%–20% of people suffering with anorexia dying from complications associated with starvation.

Avoidant/restrictive food intake disorder is similar to anorexia, but food aversion is not related to a disturbance of body image. Food is avoided for a variety of reasons such as lack of interest in eating; dislike or aversion to certain food characteristics such as the smell, color, or texture; and fear of negative consequences of eating, such as choking or vomiting. Avoidant/restrictive food disorder is more prevalent in children than in adults and is equally common in males and females.

Bulimia nervosa is characterized by a sense of out-of-control binge eating and engaging in excessive behaviors in order to compensate for the amount of food ingested. Compensatory behaviors include self-induced vomiting, abuse of laxatives or diuretics, excessive and extreme exercise. Health consequences include damage to the digestive system; dehydration and electrolyte imbalances; inflammation and damage to the esophagus from frequent vomiting; tooth decay from stomach acids; and in rare cases stomach rupture. Approximately 1%–2% of the U.S. population suffers from bulimia, with 80% being female.

Binge eating disorder is similar to bulimia, but individuals do not engage in the compensatory behaviors associated with bulimia. Symptoms include a sense of out-of-control eating, eating alone due to shame, feelings of guilt, and shame over binging. Health consequences are less severe than bulimia and include high blood pressure, heart disease, diabetes, and weight gain. Approximately 1%–5% of the population suffers from binge eating disorder, with 60% being female.

Other eating disorders recognized in the DSM-5 include pica disorder, which is characterized by eating of nonfood items, and rumination disorder, which is characterized by regurgitating previously swallowed food to be re-chewed, re-swallowed, or spit out. Prevalence data for pica and rumination disorder is inconclusive.

Factors contributing to the development of food eating disorders include a complex combination of interpersonal, social, behavioral, biological, and psychological dynamics. Interpersonal and psychological issues include low self-esteem, feelings of inadequacy, lack of control, and an inability to express emotions. Social factors may include peer pressure to look thin, being ridiculed over one's appearance, and being bullied or being physically, emotionally, or sexually abused. Family dynamics also play a role in the development of FEDs. Current research is investigating the role of biological and genetic factors in the development of FEDs.

Prognosis

Psychologists, counselors, clinical social workers, psychiatrists, medical physicians, and nutritionists treat food eating disorders. A combination of psychotherapy and group counseling provided simultaneously with medical and nutritional interventions is the most effective form of treatment. Counseling addresses the underlying psychological, interpersonal, social, cultural, and family dynamics that contribute to the eating disorder. Medical and nutritional professionals monitor, guide, and equip clients in recovery, leading to healthier food-related behaviors. When FEDs become severe, intensive inpatient treatment may be necessary.

The National Eating Disorders Association (NEDA), founded in 2001, is a leading nonprofit prevention and advocacy organization that assists individuals and families better understand FEDs. The NEDA maintains an extensive online web presence. FEDs are complex and serious health conditions that develop in a variety of ways. FEDs are treatable, with full recovery possible with professional intervention.

Steven R. Vensel, PhD

See also: Anorexia Nervosa; Binge Eating Disorder; Bulimia Nervosa

Further Reading

American Psychiatric Association. *Diagnostic and Statistical Manual of Mental Disorders*, 5th ed. Arlington, VA: American Psychiatric Association Press, 2013.

Maine, Margo, William N. Davis, and Jane Shure, eds. *Effective Clinical Practice in the Treatment of Eating Disorders: The Heart of the Matter.* New York, NY: Routledge, 2009.

Maine, Margo, and Joe Kelly. *The Body Myth: Adult Women and the Pressure to Be Perfect.* Hoboken, NJ: Wiley, 2005.

National Eating Disorders Association. "Who We Are." Accessed March 12, 2014. http://www.nationaleatingdisorders.org/who-we-are.

Thompson, J. Kevin, and Linda Smolak, eds. *Body Image, Eating Disorders, and Obesity in Youth: Assessment, Prevention, and Treatment*, 2nd ed. Washington, DC: APA, 2009.

Thompson, J. Kevin. *Body Image, Eating Disorders, and Obesity: An Integrative Guide for Assessment and Treatment.* Washington, DC: APA, 2003.

Economic and Financial Stress

Economic and financial stress is often a response to trying unsuccessfully to balance outgoing money for bills and earning enough income. It is a common challenge that many face in an attempt to meet personal and family financial obligations. In times of economic decline, such as a recession, many Americans blame the economy for the majority of stress they experience. Numerous studies have found a strong link between economic and financial stress and an increased rate of mental health issues. Economic downturns, such as the Great Depression or the U.S. recession that began in 2007 and lasted well into 2013, were linked to increased rates of psychological disorders, including depression, suicide, substance abuse, domestic violence, and antisocial behavior. Among the most significant factors in the onset of mental health are job loss and underemployment, both of which have been connected to depression and substance abuse.

Definition

- **Economic and financial stress** is the physical and emotional response to external events that affect an individual and/or his or her family's economic stability. It can be triggered by the loss of a job or home or any change in economic status or stability.

Economic and financial stress is a common occurrence for many during a bad economy, but the problem is a chronic one for those living near or below the poverty line. Many individuals become frustrated by the high prices associated with groceries, gas, and other necessities. Unemployment has plagued many Americans, causing devastation and financial ruin for families all over the country. Financial and economic stress is often experienced when working on budgets, paying bills, worrying about saving money for emergencies, or being able to afford necessary items. Financial and economic stress can also be influenced by an attempt to maintain social status.

There are different emotional and physical responses to economic and financial stress. Some individuals may have difficulty sleeping, experience weight gain or loss, or develop symptoms of anxiety, such as panic attacks.

Throughout U.S. history, there have been several major turns in the economy that have brought on great stress, frustration, and concern for many. The loss of jobs, income, and even homes can often lead to significant mental distress. There is also concern that this form of stress can have a large effect on four key mental health concerns: major depression and anxiety disorders, suicide, substance abuse, and violent behavior. There is a higher rate of suicide among those who are unemployed.

Current Status

One of the most common causes of economic and financial stress among young adults has to do with being overwhelmed by college loan debt. Not only do these young adults leave college with hefty student loans, many have a difficult time finding work in their respective fields or at adequate salaries, which only adds to their inability to pay back the loans. This, in turn, has hurt other industries, as this generation is not spending money on cars, homes, or building families and instead are working simply to make loan payments. Economic and financial stress has also led many young adults to remain living with their parents after college graduation and for some even after starting families.

Mindy Parsons, PhD

See also: Domestic Violence; Homelessness; Poverty and Mental Illness

Further Reading

Dashiff, Carol, Wendy DiMicco, Beverly Myers, and Kathy Sheppard. "Poverty and Adolescent Mental Health." *Journal of Child and Adolescent Psychiatric Nursing* 22 (2009): 23–32.

Goldman-Mellor, Sidra J., Katherine B. Saxton, and Ralph C. Catalano. "Economic Contraction and Mental Health: A Review of the Evidence, 1990–2009." *International Journal of Mental Health* 39 (2010): 6–31.

Kuruvilla, A., and K. S. Jacob. "Poverty, Social Stress and Mental Health." *Indian Journal of Medical Research* 126 (2007): 273–278.

Ecstasy (MDMA or 3,4-Methylenedioxy-Methamphetamine)

Ecstasy is a synthetic, psychoactive drug—known as MDMA—which produces stimulant and hallucinogenic effects.

Definitions

- **Catecholamines** are a group of neurotransmitters released by the brain in response to acute stress. These include dopamine, norepinephrine, and epinephrine.

- **Dopamine** is a chemical messenger in the brain that transmits nerve impulses that regulate attention, concentration, emotion, movement, impulse control, and judgment.

- **Neurotransmitters** are a group of chemical messengers in the brain that messages to other nerve cells. Common neurotransmitters include acetylcholine, dopamine, norepinephrine, and serotonin.

- **Norepinephrine** is a chemical messenger in the brain that serves to transmit nerve impulses that regulate attention and power the "fight-flight" stress response. As such, it causes constriction of blood vessels. It is also called noradrenaline. Serotonin is a chemical messenger in the brain that serves to transmit nerve impulses that regulate mood in terms of calmness, happiness, pain, sexuality, and sleep. Low levels are associated with depression and compulsivity.

Description

Ecstasy is the popular name for the synthetic, psychoactive drug MDMA. It is known as a club drug and has several street names, including Adam, B-bombs, bean, Blue Nile, clarity, crystal, decadence, disco biscuit, E, essence, Eve, go, hug drug, Iboga, love drug, molly, morning shot, pollutants, Rolls Royce, Snackies, speed for lovers, sweeties, wheels, X, and XTC. It is chemically similar to methamphetamine and to mescaline. Ecstasy acts both as a stimulant and as a psychedelic, producing an energizing effect as well as distortions in time and perception and enhanced enjoyment from tactile experiences. Ecstasy exerts its primary effects in the brain on neurons that use the neurotransmitter serotonin to communicate with other neurons. Serotonin is central in regulating mood, aggression, sexual activity, sleep, and

sensitivity to pain. Most users take ecstasy orally. Users also sometimes inhale or inject it. Although ecstasy is available as a capsule or a powder, it is usually sold in tablet form.

Ecstasy is absorbed quickly after being ingested and can be detected in the blood within 30 minutes. While its peak effects occur in 60 to 90 minutes, the main effects last three to five hours. Women are more sensitive to ecstasy than men and are more likely to experience an optimal effect of the drug at a lower dose, proportional to weight, than men. Most users of ecstasy are white teenagers and young adults from middle- and upper-class households. According to the National Survey on Drug Use and Health in 2010, an estimated 695,000 Americans had used Ecstasy within the past month, and almost 1 million Americans report using it for the first time. Marijuana, alcohol, and cocaine are commonly used with ecstasy.

Ecstasy was first synthesized in 1912 by Merck, the pharmaceutical giant, which patented it in 1914. The name "ecstasy" was coined in the early 1980s to increase the market for the drug. Ecstasy became popular as a club drug and was often sold in nightclubs and bars. By the mid-1980s the U.S. Drug Enforcement Administration banned ecstasy. Currently, it is classified as a Schedule I drug, meaning it has high potential for abuse and no currently accepted medical value.

Precautions and Side Effects

Recently, an herbal version of ecstasy has been widely available. Although those who take herbal ecstasy believe it to be a legal, safe alternative to ecstasy, there are reports of numerous adverse effects, including severe reactions such as high blood pressure, seizures, heart attacks, strokes, and death. Ecstasy in the form of MDMA causes the release of dopamine, serotonin, and norepinephrine. Research shows that chronic use of MDMA causes brain damage by destroying neurons that release serotonin resulting in memory problems that persist for at least two weeks after stopping use of the drug. Long-term effects of ecstasy use may result in shrinkage of the hippocampus, resulting in cognitive impairment. Other research has found that the use of this drug damages neurons that regulate dopamine resulting in tremors, unsteady gait, and paralysis, which are symptoms of Parkinson's disease. Exposure to MDMA during pregnancy is associated with learning deficits that last into adulthood.

While most users report intensely pleasurable experiences after taking ecstasy, about 25% of users also report undesirable experiences. Short-term adverse reactions that have been reported include dilated pupils, unusual sensitivity to bright light, headache, sweating, increased heart rate, tooth grinding, spasms of the jaw muscle, loss of appetite, nausea, muscle aches, fatigue, dizziness, vertigo, thirst, numbness, tingling skin, retention of urine, staggering gait, unsteadiness, tics, tremors, restlessness, agitation, paranoia, and nystagmus. Diving a car under the influence of ecstasy is unsafe. The depletion of serotonin seems to cause "midweek blues," which is the lethargy, concentration and memory problems, and depressed mood that many ecstasy users experience for a few days after taking the drug. Finally, ecstasy users tend to develop tolerance to the drug with repeated use. Novice users may take one or two tablets per session, whereas experienced users may need to take three or more tablets to achieve the same effect. Heavy users sometimes binge use, either by taking several tablets simultaneously or by repeatedly taking tablets during a single session that may last up to 48 hours.

Len Sperry, MD, PhD

See also: Drug Enforcement Administration (DEA)

Further Reading

Erickson, Carlton K. *Addiction Essentials: The Go-to Guide for Clinicians and Patients.* New York, NY: W.W. Norton, 2011.

Holland, Julie, ed. *Ecstasy: The Complete Guide. Kindle Edition.* Rochester, VT: Park Street Press, 2010.

Iversen, Leslie. *Speed, Ecstasy, Ritalin: The Science of Amphetamines.* Oxford: Oxford University Press, 2006.

Effexor (Venlafaxine)

Effexor is a prescribed antidepressant medication used to treat depression and generalized anxiety disorder. Its generic name is venlafaxine.

Definitions

- **Neuroleptic malignant syndrome** is a potentially fatal condition resulting from combining medications and characterized by severe muscle rigidity (stiffening), fever, sweating, high blood pressure, delirium, and sometimes coma.

- **Norepinephrine** is a neurotransmitter (chemical messenger) in the brain believed to regulate mood.

- **Selective serotonin norepinephrine reuptake inhibitors (SNRI)** are medications that act on and increase the levels of serotonin and norepinephrine in the brain that influences mood. They differ from selective serotonin reuptake inhibitors which act only on serotonin.

- **Serotonin** is a neurotransmitter (chemical messenger) in the brain believed to regulate attention, mood, and powers the "fight-flight" stress response.

- **Serotonin syndrome** is a serious medication reaction resulting from an excess of serotonin in the brain. It occurs when a number of medications that increase serotonin are taken together. Symptoms include high blood pressure, high fever, headache, delirium, shock, and coma.

Description

Effexor is in the class of antidepressant medication known as serotonin and norepinephrine reuptake inhibitors (SNRIs). It is primarily used to treat depression and generalized anxiety disorder. Effexor has also been used to treat obsessive-compulsive disorder and irritable bowel syndrome. Effexor has actions common to both the tricyclic antidepressants, such as Tofranil and Elavil, and the selective serotonin reuptake inhibitors (SSRIs), such as Prozac, Zoloft, and Paxil. Effexor is thought to work by increasing the levels of the neurotransmitters (chemical messengers) in the brain.

Precautions and Side Effects

Those taking Effexor should be monitored closely for insomnia, anxiety, mania, significant weight loss, and seizures. Its use should also be monitored in children and adults up to age 24 because they are at an increased risk of developing suicidal thoughts. Caution should also be exercised when prescribing Effexor to those with impaired liver or kidney function, those over age 60, children, individuals with known bipolar disorder or a history of seizures, and those with diabetes. Care should be taken to weigh the risks and benefits of Effexor in women who are or wish to become pregnant, as well as in breast-feeding mothers. Those with diabetes should monitor their blood or urine sugar carefully, since Effexor can affect blood sugar. Alcohol should not be used while taking Effexor. Care must be taken in driving, operating machinery, or participating in hazardous activities when taking this medication. Effexor use should not be stopped abruptly since it can cause withdrawal symptoms (serotonin discontinuation syndrome).

Some common side effects with Effexor use include nausea, drowsiness, dizziness, dry mouth, constipation, loss of appetite, blurred vision, nervousness, trouble sleeping, unusual sweating, and yawning. Like other SNRIs sexual side effects are relatively common in Effexor. These include impotence and decreased sex drive.

Effexor interacts with a number of other medications. Dangerously high blood pressure has resulted from the combination of Effexor and monoamine oxidase inhibitors like Nardil or Parnate. Effexor also interacts with Desyrel, Meridia, and Imitrex and may cause a condition known as neuroleptic malignant syndrome. Those taking blood thinners, including aspirin, are at risk for increased bleeding when taking Effexor. The sedative effects (drowsiness) of Effexor are increased by other central nervous system depressants such as alcohol, sedatives, sleeping medications, or other medications used for mental disorders such as schizophrenia.

Len Sperry, MD, PhD

See also: Antidepressants; Depression; Generalized Anxiety Disorder

Further Reading

Dunbar, Katherine Read, ed. *Antidepressants*. Farmington Hills, MI: Greenhaven Press, 2006.

O'Connor, Richard. *Undoing Depression: What Therapy Doesn't Teach You and Medication Can't Give You*, 2nd ed. New York, NY: Little, Brown, 2010.

Preston, John D., John H. O'Neal, and Mary C. Talaga. *Handbook of Clinical Psychopharmacology for Therapists*, 7th ed. Oakland, CA: New Harbinger, 2013.

Stahl, Stephen M. *Antidepressants*. New York, NY: Cambridge University Press, 2009.

Ego and the Mechanisms of Defense, The (Book)

Child psychoanalyst Anna Freud's most popular work, *The Ego and the Mechanisms of Defense*, discusses how human defense mechanisms protect the psyche from states of stress and anxiety.

Definitions

- **Anna Freud**, daughter of Sigmund Freud, is best known as the founder of child psychoanalysis, developer of ego psychology, and author of *The Ego and the Mechanisms of Defense*.

- **Defense mechanisms** are unconscious, maladaptive coping strategies that people use to prevent unpleasant feelings and experiences.

- **Ego psychology** is a formal theory of psychoanalytic thought based on Freud's structural model of the id, ego, and superego and their related functions.

Description

Considered the founding text in ego psychology and child psychoanalysis, *The Ego and the Mechanisms of Defense*, written by Anna Freud (1895–1982), was first published in German in Vienna in 1936. Due to its popularity it was translated into English soon after, two years before Sigmund Freud's death. It has since been updated/revised. *The Ego and the Mechanisms of Defense* is the publication that Anna, the youngest of Freud's six children, is best known for. She is also the only one of Freud's children to make her own mark in the area of psychoanalysis, credited as the founder of child psychoanalysis. Beginning her professional career as a schoolteacher, Anna gained firsthand knowledge of children and adolescents. However, after undergoing psychoanalysis with her father, her interests in the field peaked, leading to her eventual professional transition.

The Ego and the Mechanisms of Defense discusses the individual ego's defense reactions that arise from conflicts among the id, ego, and superego. Human beings tend to react in a variety of ways in an attempt to alleviate feelings of anxiety and stress. These *defense mechanisms* are unconscious coping strategies that people use to prevent themselves from experiencing unpleasant feelings or situations. Defense mechanisms, though they can result in both positive and negative consequences, are viewed as maladaptive as they attempt to distort, deny, or manipulate reality. Anna Freud listed 10 defense mechanisms based on her father's works: (1) repression, (2) regression, (3) reaction formation, (4) isolation, (5) undoing, (6) projection, (7) introjection, (8) turning against one's own person, (9) reversal into the opposite, and (10) sublimation/displacement; but she went on to hone this list to five main ones in her later research (repression, regression, projection, reaction formation, and sublimation).

Impact (Psychological Influence)

The Ego and the Mechanisms of Defense is considered a classic contribution to psychoanalytic psychology. This seminal text provided the foundations of child psychoanalysis as Freud included several clinical illustrations from analysis with children and adolescents. The book remains a staple used in modern-day child psychology courses.

Melissa A. Mariani, PhD

See also: Defense Mechanisms; Freud, Anna (1895–1982); Freud, Sigmund (1856–1939)

Further Reading

Freud, Anna. *The Ego and the Mechanisms of Defense: The Writings of Anna Freud* (Revised edition). Madison, CT: International Universities Press. 1979.

Sandler, Joseph, and Anna Freud. *The Analysis of Defense: The Ego and the Mechanisms of Defense Revisited*. Madison, CT: International Universities Press. 1985.

Ego Depletion

"Ego depletion" is the term used to describe the temporary exhaustion of self-control.

Definitions

- **Psychoanalytic theory** is a psychological theory that explains behaviors and perceptions as the result of unconscious, sexual, and biological instincts. This is the original theory of Sigmund Freud.

- **Self-control** is the capacity for self-discipline. Some use this term interchangeably with willpower.

- **Willpower** is the ability to resist a short-term temptation in order to achieve a long-term goal. It also involves the ability to delay gratification. Some use this term interchangeably with self-control.

Description

"Ego depletion" is a term used to describe significant expenditure of the mental energy required for self-control or willpower. The depletion of this resource affects the individual's capacities for further self-control. An example of this is when an individual deliberately forgoes a tasty but unhealthy breakfast but later succumbs to the temptation for a sweet roll and coffee later in the morning. The term "ego depletion" was coined by the American psychologist Roy Baumeister (1953–). He credits Freud and psychoanalytic theory, particularly the concepts of ego and psychic or mental energy. Baumeister considers willpower to be like a muscle. A specific muscle has a given amount of energy to do work and it can be used up slowly or rapidly in a given amount of time. The more work a muscle does in a single action, the more energy is used and the less is available for further action.

As a muscle's energy may be used slowly over many small actions or quickly in fewer large actions, so too can an individual's ability to exert the willpower decrease with his or her choices. That is because individuals have only a limited amount of mental energy that they may utilize in a given amount of time. As individuals use this energy for self-control, they deplete this energy and have less available for the next action. Furthermore, the more difficult a given decision is, the more mental energy is required to act on the decision. Also like muscles, ego depletion is a temporary state. As time lapses between willpower act, the energy used from previous acts is slowly replaced. When it is overused its energy is depleted. So too with self-control. When willpower is overused, an individual's capacity for self-control is reduced because of ego depletion. Baumeister's research shows that ego depletion is linked to depletion of blood glucose (sugar) levels. More specifically, ego depletion causes a slowdown in regions of the brain associated with self-control. In short, ego depletion results in slower brain functioning, which subsequently diminishes willpower. At the same time, it also increases cravings for food, alcohol, drugs, and other forbidden desires. In addition, ego depletion increases the intensity of feelings, particularly negative or unpleasant ones. Fortunately, there are strategies for increasing willpower and decreasing ego depletion.

Len Sperry, MD, PhD, and
Jeremy Connelly, MEd

See also: Psychoanalytic Theory; Willpower

Further Reading

Baumeister, Roy, and John Tierney. *Willpower: Rediscovering the Greatest Human Strength*. New York, NY: Penguin, 2011.

McGonigal, Kelly. *The Willpower Instinct: How Self-Control Works, Why It Matters, and What You Can Do to Get More of It*. New York, NY: Avery/Penguin Group, 2012.

Ego Development

"Ego development" refers to the psychological concept of the ego and the nature of its development across the human lifespan.

Description

The ego is the internal process that allows a person to make sense of the world around him or her and have a distinct personality from all others. It is the lens though which all experiences are captured. The ego is the person within the human body.

The most prominent conceptualization of ego is that of Jane Loevinger (Loevinger, 1976). Loevinger theorizes that the ego is a holistic construct that unifies the personality into a single whole. The ego develops a frame of reference within a person that integrates all of a person's experiences into an understanding of the world and how to live in it. Loevinger referred to the ego as the "master trait" that organizes our experiences and shapes how we make meaning, develop a worldview, and gain a sense of self. The ego changes on one's experiences, so it is always developing. It was important to Loevinger to develop an understanding of the concept of ego based on research. She developed the Washington University Sentence Completion Test, which is the primary measurement of ego development.

Loevinger describes four domains that are woven together to form the ego. The first is *character development* that incorporates impulse control and moral development. The second domain is *cognitive style* that includes conceptual complexity and cognitive development. The third is *interpersonal style* that defines our attitudes toward relationships and other people. The forth domain is *conscious preoccupations*, which are the focus of the most dominant conscious thoughts and behaviors. The focus of our thoughts and behaviors changes over time and can include focusing on getting our needs met, or conformity to rules, and many other foci depending on one's age and experiences.

Loevinger theorized that the ego develops in stages and each stage is built on the previous stage. Each stage represents a restructuring of the self and greater awareness of self, others, personal autonomy, and responsibility. Loevinger proposed nine stages of ego development.

(1) Presocial and symbiotic stage. This is early infancy with exclusive focus on gratification of immediate needs and attachment to mother. There is no language at this stage. No conceptualization of others or self.

(2) Impulsive stage. Asserting a growing sense of self, demanding, impulsive, dependent, a focus on bodily feelings, and age-appropriate sexuality and aggression. Dichotomous thinking, that is, categorizes experiences as either good or bad/nice to me or mean to me.

(3) Self-protective stage. Beginning to develop self-control, complaining, blaming; focus on not getting caught and learning rules and externalizing blame.

(4) Conformist stage. Beginning to conform to social norms and rules, invested in belonging, black and white thinking, cognitive simplicity, and moralistic. Belonging to and gaining approval of group is most valued.

(5) Self-aware. Increasing but limited self-awareness; self-critical and beginning to become aware of inner feelings about self and others; beginning to reflect on God, death, relationships, and health.

(6) Conscientious. Rules are internalized, responsible, self-critical, reflective, and empathic; true conceptual complexity, able to discern patterns, and can see the broader social perspective; guilt triggered by hurting others and morality is based on principles.

(7) Individualistic. Increasing sense of individuality, recognition of individual differences, and emotional dependence; awareness of inner conflicts without need to resolve; value relationships over achievements; unique expression of self.

(8) Autonomous. Respectful of autonomy of self and others. Relationships are understood as emotionally interdependent rather than dependent or independent; high toleration for ambiguity and conceptual complexity; able to cope with inner conflicts between needs and duties. Deepening self-acceptance results in self-fulfillment valued over achievement.

(9) Integrated. A rare stage to attain. Empathic and wise with a full sense of identity and self-actualization; at peace with self and seeks to further understand and fulfill potential intrinsic nature; reconciled to one's destiny.

Current Status

Ego development will continue to be a focus of inquiry as social researchers seek to further understand human relationships, needs, and challenges.

Steven R. Vensel, PhD

See also: Ego Psychology

Further Reading

Loevinger, Jane. "Construct Validity of the Sentence Completion Test of Ego Development." *Applied Psychological Measurement* 3 (1979): 281–311.

Loevinger, Jane. *Ego Development*. San Francisco, CA: Jossey-Bass, 1976.

Loevinger, Jane. "On Ego Development and the Structure of Personality." *Developmental Review* 3 (1983): 339–350.

Manners, John, and Kevin Durkin. "A Critical Review of the Validity of Ego Development Theory and Its Measurements." *Journal of Personality Assessment* 77, no. 3 (2001): 541–567.

Ego Psychology

Ego psychology is a form of psychoanalysis. It is based on Freud's model of the mind and the role of the ego in managing competing demands.

Definitions

- **Defense mechanisms** are strategies for self-protection against anxiety and other negative emotions that accompany stress.

- **Ego depletion** is the term used to describe the temporary exhaustion of self-control. It is also known as willpower depletion.

- **Object relations** is a form of psychoanalytic psychology which explains the essential need for close relationship. The attempted fulfillment of this need through mental representations of self and others is believed to determine one's motivations and behaviors.

- **Oedipus complex** is the desire for sexual involvement with the parent of the opposite sex and a concurrent sense of rivalry with the parent of the same sex. Freud considered the complex a critical stage in normal developmental.

- **Psychoanalysis** is a theory of human behavior and a form of therapy based on psychoanalytic theory. In psychoanalysis clients are encouraged to talk freely about personal experiences, particularly their early childhood and dreams. It was initially developed by Sigmund Freud.

- **Psychoanalytic psychology** is a psychological theory that explains behaviors and perceptions as the result of unconscious, sexual, and biological instincts. It was originally developed by Sigmund Freud.

- **Psychotic disorder** is a severe mental condition in which an individual loses touch with reality. Symptoms can include hallucinations, delusions, and disordered thinking.

- **Subconscious** is the part of the conscious mind which consists of information that is not in awareness unless attention is directed to it. It is also called the preconscious.

- **Unconscious** is the part of the conscious mind which consists of the primitive, instinctual wishes and information that operates without awareness and over which one does not have active control.

Description

Ego psychology is a form of psychoanalysis. It is based on Sigmund Freud's (1856–1939) theory about how the human mind is structured. According to Freud, the mind is divided into three parts: the id, the ego, and the superego. Each of these parts has specific functions and develops at different times during childhood. The id (German for "it") is the primitive instinctual drive. It is present at birth and is concerned with gratification and pleasure. The id operates under what Freud called the "pleasure principle." It is considered to be irrational because it is not based on reality. The ego (Greek for "I") develops between six and eight months after birth. One function of the ego is to manage the impulses of the id in rational, socially acceptable ways. The final part of the mind to develop is the superego. This occurs in the first few years of life and is the result of the resolution of the Oedipus complex. The superego is responsible for an individual's notion of right and wrong. It is concerned with morality and rules. The superego reflects the beliefs and values of a child's caregivers, usually parents. Like the id, the superego is also irrational. Freud further separated the mind into conscious and unconscious realms. He described three levels of human consciousness. At the surface (or top level) is the conscious; just below this is the preconscious or subconscious, and at the very bottom is the unconscious. The id and superego operate outside of individuals' awareness in the subconscious. The ego is both conscious and subconscious, with some material held in the preconscious memory. According to Freud, there are different layers. One of the main goals of psychoanalysis is to make individuals aware of their subconscious thoughts and drives in order to change their behavior.

The ego must balance the competing demands of the id, the superego, and society in general. According to ego psychology, personality is determined by the way in which an individual's ego manages the conflicting pressures of the id and the superego. The ego has many functions with which to accomplish this task. Some of these are reality testing, impulse control, object relations, and defense mechanisms. Reality testing is the ability to distinguish what is happening in one's own mind from the outside world. This function allows individuals to see themselves as separate from their environments and respond to various stimuli in appropriate ways. Those who experience symptoms of psychotic disorders such as hallucinations or delusions are unable to do this. Impulse control is the ability to hold back urges without acting on them. For example, the primitive instinctual drive may prompt an individual to assault someone who cuts him or her off in traffic. The healthy ego will inhibit this behavior and satisfy the urge in more acceptable ways. Those with impulse control disorders and addictions are said to have poor ego functioning in this area. Object relations refers to the way individuals perceive themselves and others. This is based on childhood development and early experiences with others. Finally, defense mechanisms are a primary way in which the ego manages the competing demands of the id and superego. A defense is an unconscious effort to protect individuals from unacceptable or uncomfortable feelings. Some of these are considered primitive, while others are more sophisticated and mature. Splitting is an example of an immature defense mechanism. It occurs when others are considered all good or all bad, with no middle ground. Humor is an example of a mature defense mechanism.

George Stoupas, MS, and Len Sperry, MD, PhD

See also: Defense Mechanisms; Ego Depletion; Ego Development; Object Relations Theory; Psychoanalysis; Psychoanalytic Theory; Psychotic Disorder; Subconscious

Further Reading

Freud, Anna. *The Ego and the Mechanisms of Defense*. London: Karnac Books, 1993.

Freud, Sigmund. *The Ego and the Id: The Standard Edition*. New York, NY: W.W. Norton, 1990.

Hartmann, Heinz. *Ego Psychology and the Problem of Adaptation*. New York, NY: International Universities Press, 1964.

Elavil (Amitriptyline)

Elavil is a prescription antidepressant medication used to treat various forms of depression and some forms of pain. Its generic name is amitriptyline.

Definitions

- **Neuroleptic malignant syndrome** is a rare and life-threatening complication of antipsychotic medication use. The syndrome is characterized by high fever, muscle rigidity, changed mental status, or changes in book pressure.

- **Selective serotonin reuptake inhibitors** are a class of antidepressant medications that work by blocking the reabsorption of serotonin in nerve cells and raising its level in the brain.

- **Tricyclic antidepressants** are an older class of antidepressants called tricyclic because of their three-ring chemical structure.

Description

Elavil is in the class of medications known as tricyclic antidepressants. Elavil and the other tricyclics are thought to work by blocking reabsorption of neurotransmitters (chemicals messengers), particularly serotonin. They have long been used to treat depressive disorders but have largely been replaced by the selective serotonin reuptake inhibitors. Elavil is sometimes prescribed for various types of chronic pain, including cancer pain and neuropathic pain (nerves), and to prevent migraine headaches. Since it is usually given at bedtime, it also promotes sleep.

Precautions and Side Effects

Elavil should not be stopped abruptly. Instead, the dose should be decreased gradually and then discontinued. Headache, nausea, and a worsening of original symptoms are likely if it is stopped abruptly. Individuals may need to stop this medication before surgery. Children and adults up to age 24 are at an increased risk of developing suicidal thoughts or behaviors when they first begin taking Elavil and other antidepressants. Those taking the monoamine oxidase inhibitors (MAOIs) like Parnate or Nardil should not combine it with Elavil. Elavil should be used with caution in those with glaucoma, seizures, urinary retention, overactive thyroid, poor liver or kidney function, alcoholism, asthma, digestive disorders, enlarged prostate, seizures, or heart disease. Since fetal deformities have been reported with taking this drug during pregnancy, women should discuss the risks and benefits of Elavil with their doctors. Breast-feeding should be avoided while using Elavil.

Common mild side effects of Elavil can include drowsiness, dizziness, dry mouth, blurred vision, constipation, weight gain, or trouble urinating. More serious but uncommon side effects include easy bruising, persistent heartburn, shaking, mask-like facial expressions, muscle spasms, severe stomach pain, decreased sexual desire, impotence, or painful breasts. Medical attention should be sought for these rare but serious side effects: black stools, vomit that looks like coffee grounds, severe dizziness, fast and irregular heartbeat, fainting, or seizures. Elavil occasionally causes a very serious condition called neuroleptic malignant syndrome.

Elavil may decrease the therapeutic effective of some medications used to treat high blood pressure. It should not be taken with other antidepressants, particularly MAOIs, or with Ritalin. It should not be taken with Tagamet or Neo-Synephrine or other over-the-counter medications without checking with one's doctor. Those taking Elavil should avoid the natural remedies like St. John's wort and belladonna. Because black tea can decrease the absorption of this medication, Elavil should be taken at least two hours before or after drinking such tea.

Len Sperry, MD, PhD

See also: Antidepressants; Depression

Further Reading

Dunbar, Katherine Read, ed. *Antidepressants*. Farmington Hills, MI: Greenhaven Press, 2006.

O'Connor, Richard. *Undoing Depression: What Therapy Doesn't Teach You and Medication Can't Give You*, 2nd ed. New York, NY: Little, Brown, 2010.

Stahl, Stephen M. *Antidepressants*. New York, NY: Cambridge University Press, 2009.

Stargrove, Mitchell Bebel, et al. *Herb, Nutrient, and Drug Interactions: Clinical Implications and Therapeutic Strategies*. St. Louis, MO: Mosby, 2007.

Elder Abuse

Elder abuse is the physical, sexual, or emotional abuse of an elderly individual, usually one who is disabled or frail. It is also called senior abuse.

Definitions

- **Abandonment** involves the desertion of a vulnerable elder by anyone who has assumed the responsibility for care or custody of that individual.

- **Emotional abuse** involves inflicting mental pain, anguish, or distress on an elder person through verbal or nonverbal acts.

- **Exploitation** involves illegal taking, misuse, or concealment of funds, property, or assets of a vulnerable elder.

- **Neglect** involves refusal or failure by those responsible to provide food, shelter, health care or protection for a vulnerable elder.

- **Physical abuse** involves inflicting, or threatening to inflict, physical pain or injury on a vulnerable elder or depriving the elder of a basic need.

- **Sexual abuse** involves nonconsensual sexual contact of any kind, coercing an elder to witness sexual behaviors.

Description

Elder abuse is harm or abuse of individuals over the age of 65. It is a crime that all health-care and social service professionals are mandated to report. It can involve abandonment, emotional abuse, exploitation, neglect, physical abuse, or sexual abuse. It is not uncommon for an elder to experience more than one type of mistreatment at the same or different times. For example, someone who financially exploits an elder may also neglect to provide appropriate care in the form of food, medication, or shelter. There are two categories of elder abuse. One is domestic elder abuse, which is committed by someone with whom the elder has a special relationship such as a spouse or child. The other is institutional abuse, which is committed by a caregiver obliged to provide care and protection in a residential facility such as an assisted living facility (nursing home) or group home. The National Center on Elder Abuse (NCEA) reported that in 2013 nearly 6 million cases of elder abuse were reported.

The typical victim of elder abuse is a 75-year-old Caucasian female who lives with an adult child on whom she depends. Those with Alzheimer's disease or other types of dementias are twice as likely to be abused. This often occurs because of unsettling personality changes in these individuals. Demented elderly can be exasperating due to their memory loss, incontinence (loss of bladder control), and frequent aggressive behavior. Such factors are extremely taxing on caretakers. The result can be full-blown elder abuse and the resulting shame. The NCEA predicts that elder abuse will continue to rise. Among the many factors supporting this prediction is that the elderly and their adult children are expected to spend increasingly more time together. Because of increasing life expectancy, adult children can expect to spend more time taking care of their aging parents than their parents took care of them! The child might have been at home for the first 18 to 20 years of life. However, with elders living into their late 80s and early 90s, an adult child might have to take responsibility for a parent over 65 for 25 or more years. Elder abuse may be one of the most distressing and difficult situations that adult children will face in their lives.

Len Sperry, MD, PhD

See also: Abuse; Neglect; Sexual Abuse

Further Reading

Brandl, Bonnie, Carmel Bitondo Dyer, Candace J. Heisler, Joanne Marlatt Otto, Lori A. Stiegel, and Randolph W. Thomas. *Elder Abuse Detection and Intervention: A Collaborative Approach*. New York, NY: Springer, 2006.

Payne, Brian K. *Crime and Elder Abuse: An Integrated Perspective*, 3rd ed. Springfield, IL: Charles C. Thomas Publishers, 2011.

The National Center on Elder Abuse (NCEA). "Elder Abuse." Accessed. July 11, 2015. http://www.ncea .aoa.gov.

Electroconvulsive Therapy (ECT)

Electroconvulsive therapy (ECT) is a medical intervention for severe mental disorders in which seizures are induced with an electrical impulse. It is also referred to as shock treatment or electroshock therapy.

Definitions

- **Amnesia** is a disturbance of memory characterized by partial or total inability to recall past experiences. It can result from trauma or from medication or electroconvulsive therapy.

- **Epilepsy** is a neurological disorder characterized by periodic loss of consciousness with or without convulsions. It is caused by brain damage, or the cause may be unknown.

- **Metrazol** is a synthetic stimulant pharmaceutical used to produce electrical stimulation in the brain and induce seizures.

- **Seizure** is uncontrolled electrical activity in the brain which can produce convulsions (spasms), loss of consciousness, amnesia, or physical symptoms depending on its cause and the area of the brain affected.

- **Therapeutic clonic seizure** is a type of seizure in which an individual loses consciousness and has convulsions characterized by repetitive, jerking (clonic) movements.

Description

Electroconvulsive therapy is a medical intervention for the treatment of major depression and severe mental disorders in individuals who have not responded to other treatments. ECT is administered by placing electrodes on one or both sides of the head and passing a brief electrical impulse through the brain. This procedure is performed while the individual is under anesthesia. Its purpose is to induce a therapeutic clonic seizure that lasts for about 15 seconds. The expected benefit is that the individual's symptoms may remit. How ECT works is unknown, but there are a number of theories for explaining its effectiveness. One theory suggests that ECT causes an alteration of neurotransmitters (chemical messengers) in the brain that results in increased mood and energy. Another theory suggests that ECT modifies stress hormone regulation in the brain, resulting in positive outcomes. Treatment outcomes can be influenced by the placement of electrodes, frequency and duration of the treatments, and the electrical voltage or waveform of the shock.

Development and Current Status

Constance Pascal (1877–1937), a French psychiatrist, introduced the term "shock." Previously the term "shock" had been used in medicine to imply a combination of low body temperature (hypothermia) and low blood pressure (hypotension). In 1926, she wrote a book titled *Le Traitement Desmaladies Mentales Par Les Chocs*. In that book Pascal theorized that psychopathology was due to mental shock. Therefore, to treat mental illness and restore healthy functioning of the brain, she argued that the brain and body must be shocked back into balance. She believed that this could be achieved through the injection of gold, insulin, or vaccines. A year later, psychiatrists began experimenting with injecting large doses of insulin to induce a form of shock. This research was further developed by Manfred Sakel (1900–1957) and the result was termed "insulin coma therapy" (ICT). ICT was the first type of shock therapy.

Ladislas Meduna (1896–1964) was a psychiatrist who believed that seizures were an essential component of effective shock therapy. His theory was based on his studies of biopsies of human brain tissues from individuals with epilepsy and major mental disorders. Seizures often occur in comas and both are forms of shock. Meduna began injecting camphor and Metrazol to induce seizures. Meduna went on to work with Ugo Cerletti (1877–1963) of the Rome University psychiatry clinic. Cerletti suggested using electricity instead of Metrazol to induce seizures. Cerletti and a colleague Lucio Bini (1908–1964) are credited with inventing ECT in 1938.

ECT is a controversial treatment modality. The main concern is whether its benefits outweigh risks, which include brain damage and memory loss. Peter Breggin (1936–), an American psychiatrist, is one of the most vocal critic of ECT. He believes ECT causes closed head injury and advocates for replacing it, as well as psychiatric medications, with more humanistic approaches like psychotherapy and education. Although advancements in research and technology have rendered ECT a safe procedure, the controversy still exists. Because of such concerns, ECT is rarely used as the first attempted intervention.

Today, ECT is used primarily to treat chronic mental conditions where other interventions have failed. Vagus nerve stimulation (VNS) and transcranial magnetic stimulation (TMS) are modern variations of ECT. Both VNS and TMS are more precise methods of inducing seizures.

Len Sperry, MD, PhD, and Layven Reguero, MEd

See also: Depression; Seizures

Further Reading

Breggin, Peter R. *Brain-Disabling Treatments in Psychiatry: Drugs, Electroshock and the Psychopharmaceutical Complex*, 2nd ed. New York, NY: Springer, 2008.

Kivler, Carol A. *Will I Ever Be the Same Again? Transforming the Face of ECT*. Timonium, MD: Three Gem Publishing, 2011.

Mankad, Mehul V., John L. Beyer, Richard D. Weiner, and Andrew D. Krystal. *Clinical Manual of Electroconvulsive Therapy*. Arlington, VA: American Psychiatric Publishing, Inc., 2010.

Shorter, Edward, and David Healy. *Shock Therapy: A History of Electroconvulsive Treatment in Mental Illness*. Piscataway, NJ: Rutgers University Press, 2007.

Electroencephalography (EEG)

Electroencephalography is a medical diagnostic test that records electrical activity on the scalp to evaluate various brain functions and psychological disorders. It is also known as the brain wave test.

Definitions

- **Computed tomography** is a medical diagnostic test in which computer-processed X-rays produce tomographs (cross-sectional images) of body areas.

- **Encephalitis** is an inflammation of the brain.

- **Epilepsy** is a neurological disorder characterized by recurrent seizures with or without a loss of consciousness.

- **Fast Fourier transform** is a mathematical process used in EEG analysis to investigate the composition of an EEG signal.

- **Magnetic resonance imaging** is a medical diagnostic test which uses electromagnetic radiation and a strong magnetic field to produce detailed images of the brain and internal organs.

Description

An electroencephalogram (EEG) is a neurological test for recording electrical activity of the brain. Electrodes are placed in a standard pattern on the individual's scalp. The electrodes are then connected to a recording device. This device makes a continuous graphic record of the individual's brain activity (brain waves) on a strip of recording paper or computer screen. This graphic record is called an EEG. If the display is computerized, it is called a digital EEG. Usually, the EEG takes about one hour to administer. However, long-term EEG monitoring is often used for diagnosis of seizure disorders or sleep disorders.

The EEG is a useful tool in the diagnosis and management of epilepsy and other seizure disorders. Also, the EEG is a useful test in making or confirming the diagnosis of stroke, brain tumors, encephalitis, and sleep disorders. It can also determine brain status and brain death. A quantitative version of the EEG (qEEG) produces a brain map that can increase the test's diagnostic value. The qEEG involves modifying the EEG signals with a computer using the fast Fourier transform algorithm. The result is displayed on a schematic map of the head to form a topographic image. This brain map is particularly useful in the diagnosis of Alzheimer's disease and mild closed-head injuries. It can also identify areas of the brain with abnormally slow activity and differentiate between early dementia (increased slowing) and uncomplicated depression (no slowing). The qEEG is also known as BEAM (brain electrical activity mapping).

Developments and Current Status

In 1924, the German psychiatrist Hans Berger (1873–1941) recorded the first human EEG. Since that time the use of this neurological test has greatly expanded because of refinements such as BEAM and magnetoencephalograph (MEG). MEG measures both the individual's electrical field and activity and the associated magnetic field. This magnetic field is detected with a biomagnetometer and recorded as an MEG. Data provided by it is quite different from that provided by computed tomography and or magnetic resonance imaging. Both of these brain imaging instruments provide still images of the brain. These images are useful in providing structural and anatomical information. In contrast, MEG provides information on the brain in real time. It is used to map cognitive functions such as speech, memory, attention, and consciousness. MEG also provides surgeons with real-time computer-generated images of lesions (tumors) essential in planning surgery.

Len Sperry, MD, PhD

See also: Magnetic Resonance Imaging (MRI); Single-Photon Emission Computed Tomography (SPECT)

Further Reading

Daube, J. R., and R. Devin. *Clinical Neurophysiology*, 3rd ed. New York, NY: Oxford University Press, 2009.

Ebersole, J. S., and T. A. Pedley. *Current Practice of Clinical Electroencephalography*, 3rd ed. Philadelphia, PA: Lippincott Williams & Wilkins, 2003.

KidsHealth.org. "EEG (Electroencephalography)." September 2008. http://kidshealth.org/parent/system/medical/eeg.html.

Rowan, A. J., and E. Tolunsky. *Primer of EEG*. London: Elsevier, 2003.

Electronic Communication

"Electronic communication" refers to communicating through the use of electronic media such as computers, cellular phones, fax machines, or other devices using e-mail, voice mail, texting, instant messaging, and/or video conferencing. Electronic communication is any type of communicating that is based on electricity; it is also referred to as computer-mediated communication (CMC).

Definitions

- **Computer-mediated communication (CMC)** describes the electronic means of communicating via the Internet including e-mailing, text messaging, social networking, and video conferencing.

- **Electronic messaging** is the sending and receiving of an e-mail, instant message, or text message from a computer, cellular phone, or electronic tablet.

- **Transmission** is the act of sending a message in the form of text, picture, or video or other information from a given source.

Description

Electronic communication describes the sending and receiving of information through the use of various types of electronic media. These vehicles for communication include television, radio, desktop computers, cellular phones or other handheld devices, fax machines, gaming consoles, and/or electronic tablets. Use of electronic media differs from static, or print, media in that it is interactive. People use several types of electronic

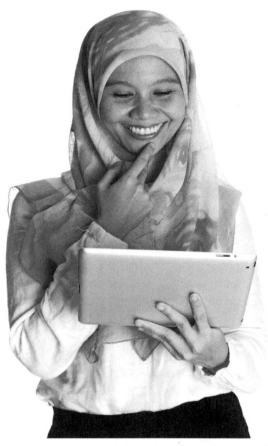

Electronic communication describes the sending and receiving of information through the use of various types of electronic media. While such communication has brought the world closer together than ever before, it can also lead to misunderstandings and can be used to commit harmful acts such as cyberbullying. (Akulamatiau/Dreamstime.com)

communication, such as e-mail, text messaging, social networking, and video conferencing. Electronic means of communication has drastically increased over the past few decades with advances in technology. Prior to these advancements, communication was limited to what a person could see and hear in front of him or her or how far the person was able to physically travel to transport that information via land, sea, or air. However, the development of the World Wide Web and the Internet has changed that, making it possible for people to communicate with one another regardless of their proximity. It also permits communication to happen almost instantaneously. Using these means, people are able to communicate greater amounts of information more quickly and cost effectively, over greater distances, and to larger numbers of people. This form of communication affords users with both personal and professional benefits.

Electronic communication allows people to transmit various types of media (text, pictures, sound, video) into a single message. This can greatly enhance the communication experience and provide a richer context to the information being sent. However, studies indicate that approximately 60%–90% of information is communicated nonverbally. Effective communication thus relies on both the content of the message and the intent of the sender of that message. Therefore, the sender must be clear in determining both in order for the message to be received accurately. Experts have argued that no form of electronic communication can replace the traditional, face-to-face experience.

The foundation for electronic modes of communication began in the late 19th century with Thomas Edison and direct current electricity. The next invention that significantly impacted this movement was the telegraph and the use of Morse Code. Alexander Graham Bell's invention of the telephone soon followed. Next came transmitting messages via radio waves, which was a popular means because of its ease and cost effectiveness. The first computer was developed in the early 1940s and drastically changed the way people communicate. Developments in this media then exploded in the 1970s and 1980s with companies like IBM, Microsoft, and Macintosh. The National Science Foundation also created the basis of the Internet in the late 1980s. The 1990s on into the 21st century has seen much expansion in modes of electronic communication, with cellular phones, tablets, and the use of social networking.

Impact (Psychological Influence)

Reports indicate that over 70% of all communication nowadays is communicated electronically. While this type of communication is on the rise, many people are not adequately trained in its use and this can lead to miscommunication and error, which can be problematic in social settings and business dealings. Adolescents, teens, and young adults in particular are subgroups that are using electronic means of communicating at high rates. Technology statistics from the PEW Internet and American Life Project indicated that

71% of teens own a cell phone, 94% utilize the Internet (with more than half using it daily), 58% have a profile on a social networking site, and 26% maintain a personal web page. Determining which types of interactions can be communicated effectively using electronic means and what should be done via phone call or face-to-face is imperative.

Melissa A. Mariani, PhD

See also: Cyberbullying; Facebooking; Sexting; Social Media

Further Reading

Campbell, Richard, Christopher R. Martin, and Bettina Fabos. *Media and Culture: Mass Communication in a Digital Age*, 9th ed. Orange, CA: Bedford/St. Martin's, 2013.

Hanson, Ralph E. Mass Communication: *Living in a Media World*, 4th ed. Thousand Oaks, CA: CQ Press, 2013.

Lengel, Laura, Alice Tomic, and Crispin Thurlow. *Computer Mediated Communication*, 1st ed. Thousand Oaks, CA: Sage, 2004.

Pew Internet and American Life Project. "Demographics of Internet Users." Accessed July 15, 2013. http://www.pew Internet.org/trends/User_Demo_Jan_2009.htm.

Ellis, Albert (1913–2007)

Albert Ellis was an American psychologist who developed rational emotive behavioral therapy.

Description

Albert Ellis was an influential American psychologist and author. He began his career as a sexologist before pioneering the development of rational emotive behavior therapy (REBT), a form of psychotherapy that focuses on disputing irrational thoughts, beliefs, and expectations. It evolved from rational therapy and rational emotive therapy. Disputation is a therapeutic technique consisting of a series of questions asked by the therapist to guide a client away from irrational beliefs and toward more helpful and healthy thought patterns. Designed to help people actively overcome challenges and live more fulfilled lives, REBT grew from a fringe school of thought to become a major philosophy and practice. A prolific writer and active social commentator, Ellis continually advocated the use of intention-based REBT therapy for changing patient behavior and beliefs in a variety of personal and social situations.

A charismatic and influential psychotherapist, Albert Ellis significantly shifted the course of his chosen profession over the course of his lifetime. Originally a proponent of traditional psychoanalysis, his expertise in sex and sexual practices, and his personal behavior modifications led him to create rational emotive behavior therapy in the late 1950s. Part of the cognitive-based therapy family, REBT is a hands-on, engaged system for helping patients identify and modify their beliefs to allow for more healthy/rational thoughts and greater personal well-being.

Immensely popular with the general public through his best-selling self-help books, Ellis's approach was initially viewed as little more than a provocative, fringe-element challenge by his peers. They criticized his directive and confrontational methods, which were in sharp contrast to the general practices of the day. Yet Ellis's models of treatment became increasingly accepted because it worked—often quite quickly—in the lives of his clients. Over his 60-year career, his work moved to the mainstream and permanently altered the modern therapeutic landscape. By the 1980s, he was universally viewed as one of the profession's most influential figures along with Sigmund Freud and Carl Rogers, winning many national and international achievement awards.

Credited with more than 800 scientific papers and some 80 full-length books, Albert Ellis was an outspoken voice for change with the psychoanalytic community. However, his voice was not universally welcomed, as his theories were a sharp departure from the methods that dominated the 1950s when he began publishing his REBT works. Profane, provocative, directive, and confrontational, Ellis was also considered warm, funny, and deeply committed to helping his clients improve their lives.

Born into a poor family, Ellis was a shy and sickly child with distant parents. He was frequently hospitalized but used his early challenges to test coping methods that became the foundations of his REBT practice. For example, he challenged himself to talk to 100 unknown females to get over his fear of rejection, and through this and other behavior-changing

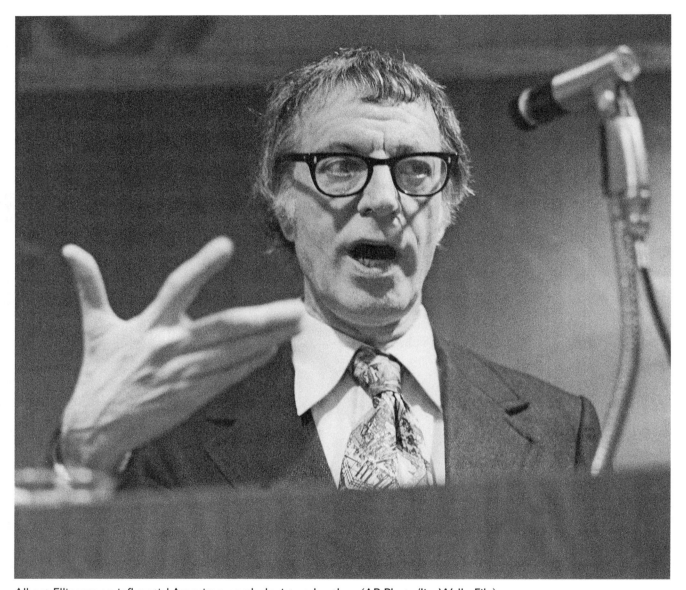

Albert Ellis was an influential American psychologist and author. (AP Photo/Jim Wells, File)

experiments he developed an early interest in counseling philosophies.

Still, he traveled a circuitous path to psychotherapy, trying his hand at business and writing fiction before turning to the field. Early on, he focused on human sexuality, partnering with Kinsey and publishing several notable books, including the influential *Sex without Guilt* in 1958. This gave him early recognition as a pioneering thinker in the American sexual revolution of the 1960s and provided him with valuable experience using cognitive interventions to shift both belief and behavior.

These experiences, coupled with his childhood behavior modification experiments, led him to challenge the dominant psychoanalytical practices of the 1950s and 1960s, which were nondirective and passive when dealing with clients. In sharp contrast, Ellis favored a directive, intentional approach designed to challenge and lead clients to a more rational and healthy way of thinking and living.

This approach contained several practices that were considered groundbreaking at the time but are now widely accepted. For example, Ellis promoted scientific and outcome-based testing of psychoanalytic approaches to evaluate their true effectiveness with different client populations. He assigned homework to reinforce sessions, insisting that learning did not happen solely in the therapeutic environment. Multiple approaches beyond talk therapy were encouraged, including anything that pushed the client to change, such as group sessions, hypnotherapy, imagery, and singing.

While his peers were shocked, his clients praised him for getting results in their lives. His ABC-DE framework allowed the therapist and client together to challenge thought patterns and recognize "irrational" beliefs that were holding the client back from desired achievements. During his weekly Friday night workshops held at his New York institute, he demonstrated his approach with volunteers in front of a live audience, beginning in 1965 and continuing until his death. Despite publishing a mountainous amount of literature, traveling and speaking globally, marrying three times, and running multiple institutes dedicated to his theories, it is estimated he personally conducted over 300,000 therapeutic sessions before his death in 2007.

Ellis's status as an influencer has not diminished since his death. His REBT theories continue to shape modern psychotherapeutic practice, with his research actively carried on by his widow, Debbie Joffe Ellis, and the Albert Ellis Institute in New York. While other types of cognitive behavior therapy, a form of psychotherapy that focuses on changing maladaptive (faulty) behaviors, emotions, and thoughts, are perhaps now more widespread, there is no denying that elements of his REBT teachings paved the way.

Even outside of the psychoanalytic community, his plain-English self-help books remain on shelves around the world, enduringly popular and continuously encouraging the general public to adopt his tenets of rational living.

Mindy Parsons, PhD, Len Sperry, MD, PhD, and George Stoupas, MS

See also: Cognitive Behavior Therapy; Psychoanalysis; Rational Emotive Behavior Therapy (REBT)

Further Reading

American Psychological Association. "Albert Ellis Obituary." *American Psychology* 64, no. 3 (2009): 215–216.

Backx, Wouter. "Views on REBT, Past, Present, and Future: Albert Ellis' Contribution to the Field." *Journal of Rational-Emotive Cognitive-Behavior Therapy* 29 (2011): 263–271.

Bernard, Michael E. "Albert Ellis: Unsung Hero of Positive Psychology." *The Journal of Positive Psychology: Dedicated to Furthering Research and Promoting Good Practice* 5, no. 4 (2010): 302–310.

DiGuiseppe, Raymond. "Reflection on My 32 Years with Albert Ellis." *Journal of Rational-Emotive Cognitive-Behavior Therapy* 29 (2011): 220–227.

Eckstein, Daniel, and Debbe Joffe Ellis, "Al Ellis: Up Close and Personal." *The Family Journal* 19 (2011): 407.

Ellis, Albert. *All Out!: An Autobiography.* New York, NY: Prometheus Books, 2009.

Ellis, Albert. "Being a Therapist." *Psychiatric Times* 7 (2012).

Haggbloom, Steven. "The 100 Most Eminent Psychologists of the 20th Century." *Review of General Psychology* 6, no. 2 (2002): 139–152.

Organization

The Albert Ellis Institute
145 East 32nd Street
New York, NY 10016
Telephone: (212) 535-0822
Fax: (212) 249-3582
E-mail: info@albertellis.org
Website: www.albertellis.org

Emotional Intelligence

Emotional intelligence is the ability to identify and make sense of one's own emotions and the emotions of others. It is also known as EQ.

Definitions

- **Countertransference** refers to the feelings evoked within a clinician during psychotherapy. Unless recognized and dealt with, these feelings can interfere with treatment.

- **Hard-wired** means genetically determined.

- **Psychotherapy** is a psychological method for achieving desired changes in thinking, feeling, and behavior. It is also called therapy and therapeutic counseling.

- **Transference** refers to the feelings evoked within a client during therapy with a mental health practitioner. Feelings the client has, or had, for someone else are directed toward the therapist.

Description

Emotional intelligence (EQ) is the capacity to recognize, understand, and manage personal emotions and to identify and respond to the emotions of others. It influences how individuals think, behave, interact with others, and make decisions. Emotional intelligence is different from intelligence (IQ), which is the capacity to learn, reason, and problem solve. Intelligence remains relatively stable throughout life, whereas emotional intelligence can be learned and developed.

The term "emotional intelligence" was originally used in 1964 by Michael Beldoch (1931–) in the book *The Communication of Emotional Meaning*. The term became better known because of psychologist Daniel Goleman's (1946–) best-selling book *Emotional Intelligence—Why It Can Matter More Than IQ*, published in 1995. Goleman contends that emotional intelligence is equally important, if not more important than IQ. Positive emotions influence an individual to perceive positive events as more likely to arise in the future. The opposite is true of negative emotions. They influence an individual to perceive negative events as more likely to happen. In other words, different emotions lead to different thoughts, perceptions, expectations, and behaviors. Individuals with the ability to express, understand, and manage their emotions are better able to estimate the likelihood of a future event and the possibilities associated with it. They are also better able to attend to internal and external events and regulate their mood to effectively cope with situations.

The human brain is hard-wired so that emotions have an advantage over thoughts. Whenever an individual touches, tastes, smells, sees, or hears something, electrical signals are sent to the brain. Before getting to the part of the brain where logic and reason takes place, these signals travel through the limbic system. The limbic system is where emotions are created and experienced. Therefore, events are first experienced emotionally, and then thoughts follow. Humans do not have control over emotional experiences but do have control over the thoughts that occur afterward. Awareness of emotions allows for control over the type of response chosen once feelings are experienced. The way an individual responds to emotions is influenced by his or her personal history.

Emotional intelligence is equally important for therapists as it is for their clients. How a therapist responds to personal feelings that arise (countertransference) during a therapy session can influence the outcome of treatment. Similarly, how a client responds to personal feelings toward the practitioner (transference) will impact the therapeutic process and achievement of treatment goals.

Emotional intelligence requires four sets of personal and interpersonal skills. They are self-awareness, social awareness, self-management, and relationship management skills. Self-awareness is the ability to assess one's own emotions and understand personal patterns of responding to situations. Social awareness is the ability to identify and understand other individuals' emotions. Self-management is the ability to regulate personal emotions and choose appropriate behaviors. Finally, relationship management is the ability to have awareness of one's own emotions and the emotions of others and to use this awareness to develop and maintain interpersonal relations. Practice of these skills is necessary to develop the emotional capacity to effectively cope with internal and external stimuli. Emotional intelligence is particularly helpful in dealing with stressful events that have the potential to negatively impact physical and mental well-being.

Len Sperry, MD, PhD, and Christina Ladd, PhD

See also: Emotionally Focused Psychotherapy; Positive Psychology

Further Reading

Beldoch, M. "Sensitivity to Expression of Emotional Meaning in Three Modes of Communication." In *The Communication of Emotional Meaning*, edited by J. R. Davitz et al., pp. 31–42. New York, NY: McGraw-Hill, 1964.

Bradberry, Travis, and Jean Greaves. *Emotional Intelligence 2.0*. San Diego, CA: TalentSmart, 2009.

Goleman, Dan. *Emotional Intelligence*. New York, NY: Bantam Books, 1995.

Emotionally Focused Psychotherapy

Emotionally focused psychotherapy is a psychotherapy approach for increasing awareness, understanding, and ability to manage emotional experiences. It is also known as EFT.

Definitions

- **Adaptive** means having the ability to adjust to a circumstance.

- **Arriving** means to get to the place where emotions can be identified and understood.

- **Emotion coach** refers to the role of the therapist in emotionally focused psychotherapy. The emotion coach collaborates with an individual, couple, or family to assist in the development of emotional awareness, acceptance, and understanding. The emotion coach is the facilitator of emotional change.

- **Emotional intelligence** is the ability to recognize, understand, and manage personal emotions and to identify and respond to the emotions of others. It influences how individuals think, behave, interact with others, and make decisions.

- **Leaving** refers to moving away from the emotions originally arrived at toward transformation of those emotions.

- **Maladaptive** refers to the inability to adjust to a circumstance.

- **Psychotherapy** is a psychological method for achieving desired changes in thinking, feeling, and behavior. It is also called therapy and therapeutic counseling.

Description

Emotionally focused is a form of couple's therapy that assists in the expression and restructuring of emotional responses. It helps couples change maladaptive emotional reactions toward each other to more adaptive responses that strengthen the relationship. EFT is also used with individuals and families. EFT views emotions as the fundamental element in development of the self. Emotions have adaptive and maladaptive functions. They are instrumental in helping individuals adapt and respond to their environment. They are biological functions that assist in the appraisal of situations, others, and one's self. Emotions communicate goals, regulate personal interactions, and influence decisions. Since emotions are significantly influenced by past experiences, they can be negative reactions to events. However, expression of emotions can assist individuals in changing negative responses.

Emotion-focused psychotherapy subscribes to "bottom-up processing" to assist in changing negative emotional responses. This requires an individual to develop awareness and keep track of physical sensations that arise in the body. Any thoughts that arise are ignored, while physical signals are felt in the fullest until they subside or are appropriately identified. An emotion coach collaborates with an individual to assist in developing awareness and understanding of emotional experiences. Together they identify alternative emotional responses. A supportive, safe, and accepting environment promotes openness and positive interactive experiences that provide emotional comfort. The goal is to identify bodily sensations and feelings, develop adaptive emotional responses, and enhance emotional intelligence. Individuals who have emotional intelligence have awareness and understanding of their own emotions and the emotions of others. They also have the ability to manage their emotions in a way that enhances well-being.

There are two phases in emotionally focused psychotherapy, arriving and leaving. In phase one, the emotions coach guides the individual to "arrive" at his or her emotions by (1) developing awareness of his or her emotions; (2) feeling, accepting, and managing his or her emotions, (3) describing his or her feelings with words to promote problem solving, and (4) helping the individual develop the ability to determine if his or her emotional responses are congruent with his or her feelings. If they are not, helping them assess the main feelings they are experiencing can be very therapeutic.

Phase two involves learning how to change maladaptive emotional responses in order to "leave" the emotions the individual initially arrived at. The·

emotions coach assists the individual to move forward by helping him or her (1) decide if an emotion is adaptive and should be reinforced or maladaptive and needs to be transformed, (2) identity the thoughts associated with maladaptive emotions, (3) identify and use adaptive emotional responses, and (4) dispute negative thoughts associated with negative emotions and replace them with positive thoughts. The emotions coach plays an instrumental role in helping the individual to develop an awareness and acceptance of his or her emotions. The emotions coach also guides the individual through the process of transforming negative emotional responses into healthy and adaptive emotional responses.

Developments and Current Status

Emotionally focused psychotherapy was developed by Susan Johnson (n.d.) and Leslie Greenberg (1945–) in the 1980s. Initially, it was Johnson who discovered that couples with problems remained caught in dysfunction due to negative emotional interactions. She used attachment theory as the foundational element for emotionally focused psychotherapy. Attachment theory describes how individuals in relationships react to a perceived hurt, separation, or threat.

Emotionally focused psychotherapy is considered one of the most scientifically confirmed therapy treatments in the domain of couples therapy. It integrates components of person-centered, experiential, gestalt, and existential therapy with several theories such as modern emotion, cognitive, attachment, narrative, interpersonal, and psychodynamic theory. It works to improve emotional, psychological, physical, and relationship closeness. Emotionally focused psychotherapy has also been scientifically proven in the treatment of depression. It is gaining recognition in the treatment of other disorders such as trauma, anxiety, and eating disorders.

Len Sperry, MD, PhD, and Christina Ladd, PhD

See also: Couples Therapy; Emotional Intelligence; Family Therapy; Psychotherapy

Further Reading

Angus, Lynne E., and Greenberg, Leslie S. *Working with Narrative in Emotion-Focused Therapy: Changing Stories, Healing Lives*. Washington, DC: American Psychological Association, 2011.

Greenberg, Leslie S. *Emotion Focused Therapy (Theories of Psychotherapy)*. Washington, DC: American Psychological Association, 2011.

Johnson, Susan M. *Creating Connections: The Practice of Emotionally Focused Couples Therapy*, 2nd ed. New York, NY: Brunner/Mazel, 2004.

Johnson, Susan M., and Leslie S. Greenberg. "Emotionally Focused Marital Therapy: An Overview." *Psychotherapy: Theory, Research, Practice, Training* 24, no. 3 (1987): 552–560.

Empirically Supported Treatment

Empirically supported treatments are therapeutic interventions (techniques) that research demonstrates to be effective in facilitating therapeutic change. It is also known as evidence-based treatments.

Definitions

- **Accountability** is the expectation or requirement to conduct evaluations and report performance information.

- **Benchmark** is a standard by which a product or clinical activity can be measured or evaluated.

- **Evidence-based practice** is a form of practice that is based on the integration of the best research evidence with clinical experience and client values.

- **Health Maintenance Organization** is an organization that provides or arranges managed care.

- **Managed care** is a system of health care that controls costs by placing limits on physicians' fees and by restricting access to certain medical procedures and providers.

- **Practice** is a method or process used to accomplish a goal or objective.

- **Psychotherapy** is a psychological method for achieving desired changes in thinking, feeling, and behavior. It is also called therapeutic counseling.

- **Randomized controlled trial** is a research design in which participants are assigned randomly (by chance) to an experimental treatment or one that receives a comparison treatment or placebo.

Description

Empirically supported treatments (ESTs) are health-care practices that utilize scientific evidence to defend their use. EST refers to therapeutic interventions demonstrated to be useful in randomized controlled trials or their equivalents. This means that evidence-based treatments have been proven to produce therapeutic change in the controlled contexts of scientific research. These research findings are the evidence that supports the use of certain treatments instead of alternative treatment options.

EST is similar to the concept of best practices. Both aim to increase accountability of health-care practices. EST is also similar to but different from evidence-based practice (EBP). EBP may include ESTs, but it is larger in scope than treatments. EBP involves specific interventions (practices) used to bring about therapeutic change. However, EBPs do not have the scientific support of ESTs. More specifically, to merit that designation, ESTs demonstrated that they are (1) superior to a placebo treatment in two or more randomized controlled studies, (2) equivalent to a well-established treatment in several rigorous and independent controlled studies, or (3) effective in a large series of single-case controlled studies. At the present time ESTs are performed with treatment manuals that specify how the intervention is to be conducted.

Development and Current Status

Prior to the 1990s, there were no specific guidelines for either clinicians or consumers regarding which treatments to select for which conditions. This changed in 1993, when a task force appointed within the American Psychological Association developed a set of criteria for "empirically validated treatments." Later these came to be known as ESTs. These treatments have been proven to produce therapeutic change in controlled contexts of scientific research. There has been considerable controversy about ESTs. Some believe that the controlled context of scientific research cannot be replicated in clinical practice. Others contend that the results of scientific study are generalizable to clinical contexts. For the past two decades this debate has been fueled by the increasing expectation for accountability. Increasingly, medical and psychological practice has become more accountable and evidence based. Division 12 of the American Psychological Association (APA) provides a list of treatments that are empirically supported for use with specific health needs. APA also provides the scientific standards for defining treatment effectiveness.

Resources for health-care interventions are limited. This fact has created an effort to conduct medical and psychological practice in the most efficient manner possible. EST attempts to achieve get the best results for less money and in the shortest amount of time. Modern use of ESTs has its roots in Health Maintenance Organizations. Managed care was established to increase the efficiency and cost effectiveness of health care. ESTs can and do have a critical role in managed care. Managed care encourages and often requires health-care professionals to incorporate ESTs as well as EBPs into the health-care process.

Len Sperry, MD, PhD, and Layven Reguero, MEd

See also: Evidence-Based Practice; Managed Care

Further Reading

Berberich, Deborah A. *Out of the Rabbit Hole: Breaking the Cycle of Addiction: Evidence-Based Treatment for Adolescents with Co-occurring Disorders.* Bloomington, IN: Xlibris Publishers, 2013.

Christopherson, Edward R., and Susan Mortweet Vanscoyoc. *Treatments That Work with Children: Empirically Supported Strategies for Managing Childhood Problems,* 2nd ed. Washington, DC: American Psychological Association, 2013.

O'Donohue, William T., and Jane E. Fisher. *Cognitive Behavior Therapy: Applying Empirically Supported Techniques in Your Practice,* 2nd ed. New York, NY: John Wiley & Sons, 2009.

Sobel, Stephen V. *Successful Psychopharmacology: Evidence Based Treatment Solutions for Achieving Remission.* New York, NY: W.W. Norton, 2012.

Encopresis Disorder

Encopresis disorder is a mental disorder characterized by the voluntary or involuntary passage of stools in a child who has already been toilet trained.

Definitions

- **Behavioral modification** is a treatment approach that replaces undesirable behaviors with more desirable ones through positive or negative reinforcement.

- **Conduct disorder** is a mental disorder characterized by repetitive and persistent pattern of behavior in which the basic rights of others, societal norms, or rules are violated.

- **Constipation** refers to bowel movements that are infrequent and difficult to pass.

- **DSM-5** stands for the *Diagnostic and Statistical Manual of Mental Disorders, Fifth Edition*, which is a diagnostic system used by professionals to identify mental disorders with specific diagnostic criteria.

- **Elimination disorders** are a group of DSM-5 disorders characterized by the inappropriate elimination of feces or urine. They include enuresis and encopresis.

- **Incontinence** is the inability to control the release of feces or urine.

- **Laxative** is a medication that helps an individual to have a bowel movement.

- **Oppositional defiant disorder** is a mental disorder in the DSM-5 that is characterized by a pattern of angry and irritable mood, argumentative and defiant behavior, and vindictiveness.

- **Psychotherapy** is a psychological method for achieving desired changes in thinking, feeling, and behavior. It is also called therapeutic counseling.

- **Sexual abuse** involves nonconsensual sexual contact of any kind, coercing an elder to witness sexual behaviors.

- **Specifiers** are extensions to a diagnosis that further clarifies the course, severity, or type of features of a disorder or illness.

Description and Diagnosis

Encopresis is one of the DSM-5 elimination disorders. The core feature of encopresis involves an individual repeatedly having bowel movements in inappropriate places after an age when bowel control is normally expected (e.g., on the floor or in the clothing). Encopresis is also referred to as fecal incontinence and soiling. After the age of four years, a child is expected to be toilet trained. After the age of four, if a child is repeatedly having bowel movements regularly and over a period of months in inappropriate places, the child may be diagnosed with encopresis. Encopresis is more prevalent among males and approximately 1% of five-year-olds have this disorder (American Psychiatric Association, 2013).

This disorder may be intentional but is more often involuntary. When fecal incontinence is clearly intentional, features of conduct disorder and oppositional defiant disorder may be present. These disorders include problems with self-control of emotions and behaviors (e.g., being angry, resentful, intimidating others, and violating social norms). Sexual abuse may also be a contributing factor in voluntary encopresis. An individual with voluntary incontinence has control over where and when he or she will have a bowel movement. The individual chooses to have a bowel movement in inappropriate places. Older children may choose to smear feces or hide feces in their home. Younger children with encopresis may act out as a result of a power struggle with their caretaker. When fecal incontinence is involuntary, an individual has no control over bowel movements. Involuntary incontinence usually results from withholding feces, resulting in constipation. As the feces continues to build up in the large intestine, leakage will most likely occur in the individual's clothing. This may cause a child or individual to feel shameful and avoid social situations. The amount of impairment may depend on the child's self-esteem; bullying and teasing by peers; and the rejection, anger, and consequences of the caretaker. Nearly 95% of encopresis is due to involuntary incontinence (American Psychiatric Association, 2013).

According to the *Diagnostic and Statistical Manual of Mental Disorders, Fifth Edition*, individuals can be diagnosed with this disorder if they have repeated passage of stools in inappropriate places, whether the act is involuntary or intentional. The individual must be at least four years of age (or at an equivalent developmental level) and at least one such event must occur each month for a period of at least three months. Repeated passage of feces in inappropriate places must not be attributable to the physiological effects of a substance (e.g., laxatives) or another medical condition except through the process involving constipation. In addition to the DSM-5 criteria needed to make the diagnosis of encopresis, there are two specifiers that must be included to make this diagnosis. The diagnosis of encopresis can specify whether the disorder is with constipation and an overflow of incontinence. This specifier is made by a physical examination or by history and there is evidence of constipation. Alternatively, the diagnosis of encopresis can specify whether the disorder is without constipation and an overflow of incontinence by history or physical examination (American Psychiatric Association, 2013).

The most common cause of encopresis is long-term constipation. Constipation may occur for several reasons, including stress, low fiber diet, not drinking enough water, lack of exercise, and changes in bathroom routines (e.g., using a bathroom that is not your own). Physical problems associated with the intestine's inability to move stool may be another cause of encopresis. Another causal factor of encopresis may involve emotional issues. A child may develop a fear or frustration related to toilet training. This may be attributed to premature toilet training and stressful events in the child's life (e.g., parents divorcing, relocation of residences, the birth of a new child). In some instances, a child may simply refuse to use the toilet.

Treatment

There are several treatments available for those with encopresis. Addressing the cause of the constipation usually treats involuntary encopresis. Treatment can include adding more fiber to the individual's diet, short-term use of a laxative, and increasing the amount of water intake. Involuntary incontinence usually ceases once constipation is resolved. The treatment used for voluntary encopresis will depend on the cause of the disorder. Often scheduling toilet times and praising and rewarding a child for using the toilet may be helpful and eliminate encopresis. Psychotherapy, using behavioral modification, is another form of treatment that has been found to be effective. With proper treatment, prognosis for encopresis is relatively high due to the majority of cases being involuntary.

Len Sperry, MD, PhD, and Elizabeth Smith Kelsey, PhD

See also: Conduct Disorder; *Diagnostic and Statistical Manual of Mental Disorders* (DSM); Oppositional Defiant Disorder (ODD); Psychotherapy; Sexual Abuse

Further Reading

American Psychiatric Association. *Diagnostic and Statistical Manual of Mental Disorders*, 5th ed. Arlington, VA: American Psychiatric Association, 2013.

Christopherson, Edward R., and Patrick C. Friman. *Elimination Disorders in Children and Adolescents, in the Series Advances in Psychotherapy, Evidenced-Based Practice*. Cambridge, MA: Hogrefe Publishing, 2010.

Schaefer, Charles E. *Childhood Encopresis and Enuresis: Causes and Therapy*. Northvale, NJ: Jason Aronson, 1993.

Enuresis

"Enuresis" is a term for involuntary urination, most frequently experienced as bed-wetting, which affects children and adolescents between the ages of 5 and 17.

Description

Enuresis, the involuntary voiding of urine, is a medical condition most commonly diagnosed in children. There are three subtypes of enuresis. Nocturnal enuresis, or nighttime bed-wetting, is the most common form of enuresis and is more common in boys than in girls. Diurnal enuresis is daytime wetting, which is more common in girls than boys. The third type of enuresis is a combination of nocturnal and diurnal enuresis.

Causes and Symptoms

The term "enuresis" describes a specific medical condition and diagnosis. It is important to note that although enuresis has a psychological medical code, children who suffer from enuresis are not considered to be suffering from psychological problems. In order to be diagnosed with enuresis, a person has to have occurrences of involuntary wetting at least twice a week for three months. The individual must be older than the age of anticipated bladder control, usually five years old. The wetting is not due to a general medical condition. "Primary enuresis" refers to children who have never gained control of their bladder. "Secondary enuresis" refers to children who have been successful at bladder control for at least six months but revert to wetting due to stress.

There is no clear etiology or identified cause of enuresis, but many theories exist. Urinary control is part of the maturing process and nighttime bladder control is the last to develop. Nocturnal enuresis (NE) is by far the most common form of enuresis and has received the most attention from researchers and medical professionals. Genetics may be a factor in NE, as children who have one parent who were bed wetters are 43% more likely to develop NE. Children with both parents who were bed wetters are 77% more likely to develop NE compared to children whose parents did not suffer from NE. Other theories have been proposed to explain NE, such as children who have small bladders, who are deep sleepers, or who have received improper toilet training. However, none of these theories have resulted in any conclusive evidence as to the cause of NE. Researchers agree that there are many factors leading to enuresis.

Prognosis

The percentage of the population with enuresis changes with age. Approximately 20% of five-year-olds have monthly bed-wetting episodes. Bed-wetting decreases to 10% of children aged six years, and of these cases approximately 15% gain bladder control each year. By age 15, 1%–3% of teenagers experience nighttime bed-wetting. From ages four to six the number of boys and girls diagnosed is about equal, with boys increasing in ratio with age. By age 11 there are approximately twice as many boys as girls suffering from NE.

Enuresis is often a cause of great stress for families and children. Bed-wetting is associated with low self-esteem in children, which improves as the condition is overcome. An unfortunate but common parental response is to punish or shame a child for bed-wetting. Studies indicate that children rarely wet the bed intentionally, and punitive parental responses are ineffective and often make the condition worse. The most effective treatment is to allow the child to mature as virtually all children outgrow bed-wetting. Other strategies to control NE include the use of bed-wetting alarms which make a loud sound when moisture is detected in order to associate the feeling of a full bladder with waking up. Use of diaper-type underwear made specifically for sleeping has been very helpful in reducing family and child stress.

Enuresis is a common and stressful problem for many children, adolescents, and their families. Developing a positive approach that avoids shaming is an important consideration in helping a child outgrow enuresis.

Steven R. Vensel, PhD

See also: Encopresis Disorder

Further Reading

Christophersen, Edward, and Patrick Friman. *Elimination Disorders in Children and Adolescents.* Cambridge: Hogrefe, 2010.

Cossio, Sissi. "Enuresis." *Southern Medical Journal* 95, no. 2 (2002): 183–187.

Envy and Gratitude (Book)

Envy and Gratitude is a now famous monograph written by the well-known psychoanalyst Melanie Klein (1882–1960) and published just three years before her death.

Description

In this controversial work, Klein theorized that even infants are torn between the struggle for goodness or destructiveness, which she defined as gratitude and envy. A controversial and important work, Melanie Klein's *Envy and Gratitude* was first published in 1957 at the end of her career. Since its first publishing, this both highly acclaimed and criticized monograph has become a topic of debate and study for psychoanalysts and feminists alike.

Envy and Gratitude explores Klein's theory about how infants are torn between the two grounding emotions of the human experience—envy and gratitude. As Klein described it, infants struggle with a primary envy. Therefore, infants must fight a constant battle between the two forces of envy and gratitude, between the "life and death instincts" that all humans face. Largely theoretical in nature, Klein's views on infant psychosis in *Envy and Gratitude* led to what is now known as the Kleinian Theory in clinical practice.

Unlike other psychoanalysts before her, Klein believed the primal feelings of envy or gratitude are present at the beginning of life. Drawing on her extensive experience with children and developmental psychosis, Klein theorized that a mother's breast is the first source of this primal feeling of envy or gratitude. In *Envy and Gratitude*, she describes how a mother's breast plays a central role in the developmental psyche of infants. As Klein explains it, an infant experiences satisfaction and gratitude by nursing on a mother's breast—the central object of the infant's world. In the same way, an infant feels denied and experiences envy when a mother's breast is taken away.

When *Envy and Gratitude* was first released in 1957, many psychoanalysts criticized Klein's "wild analytic approach." However, Klein also drew high praise from psychoanalysts all over the world for her bold views. At her death three years after publishing *Envy and Gratitude*, Klein was described as "second only to Freud in overall importance to both the science and art of psychoanalysis."

Impact (Psychological Influence)

In the 50th anniversary year of *Envy and Gratitude*, a group of psychoanalysts published *Envy and Gratitude Revisited*. This collection of 14 critical essays examines how Klein's views on envy in the original *Envy and Gratitude* have influenced the work of contemporary mental health professionals. Each of these 14 psychoanalysts presented his or her own reflections on Klein's original work. These authors also gave their own theories of how envy relates to a host of diverse topics, including narcissism, compulsion, jealously, greed, and gender issues. Even 50 years later, Melanie Klein's timeless work continues to make a significant contribution to the psychoanalytic world. Other notable works by Klein include *Love, Guilt and Reparation: And Other Works 1921–1945, The Psychoanalysis of Children, Envy and Gratitude*, and *Narrative of a Child Analysis*.

Mindy Parsons, PhD

See also: Klein, Melanie (1882–1960); Object Relations Theory; Psychoanalysis

Future Reading

Carter, Linda, and Marcus West, eds. Book reviews. *Envy and Gratitude Revisited*, edited by Priscilla Roth and Alessandra Lemma. London: International Psychoanalytical Association. *Journal of Analytical Psychology* 54 (2009): 143–153.

Etchegoyen, R. Horacio, and Clara R. Nemas. "Salieri's Dilemma: A Counterpoint between Envy and Appreciation." *International Journal of Psychoanalysis* 84 (2003): 45–58.

Henry, Astrid. "Enviously Grateful, Gratefully Envious: The Dynamics of General Relationships in U.S. Feminism." *Women's Studies Quarterly* 34, no. 3/4 (Fall/Winter 2006): 140–153.

Klein, Melanie. *Envy and Gratitude and Other Works*. New York: Free Press, 2002.

Mason, Albert. "Images in Psychiatry: Melanie Klein (1882–1960)." *American Journal of Psychiatry* 160 (2003): 2.

Roth, Priscilla, and Alessandra Lemma. Book review. *Envy and Gratitude Revisited*, edited by Priscilla Roth and Alessandra Lemma. *Journal of the American Psychoanalytic Association* 57 (2009): 1002.

Envy and Jealousy

Envy and jealousy are generally considered negative emotions associated with a person's desire to have something or someone that someone else already has and not having it feels like a threat to the person's sense of self.

Description

Envy and jealousy stem from a negative comparison to what someone else has. Envy and jealousy can be over a way of thinking, feeling, or acting or with a tangible item, such as clothes, car, home, and spouse. It includes a resentful awareness of an advantage enjoyed by another joined with a desire to possess the same advantage.

These two highly negative emotions are often a response to an individual's belief that someone else has some type of advantage of him or her. These negative emotions can lead to negative self-thoughts by focusing on what others may have or who they may be with. Envy can sometimes be connected to depression and low self-esteem and, when left unchecked, may escalate to destructive or even violent behavior.

Although from childhood people learn that direct expressions of envy and jealousy can be dangerous, some people find themselves consumed by comparisons. Comparison leads to stress and can depress and divide people. Envy can end up ruining relationships and lives, as well as being highly destructive in the workplace.

While most Americans tend to think they are beyond class distinctions, Gallup Polls have disproved this assertion. Social class is only one example of social comparison. People compare to evaluate themselves and hope to improve their own self-esteem and status. However, just the opposite is often a result from engaging in such exercises. These thoughts and emotions can end up angering or humiliating the person who focuses on comparisons, and especially those who have more than he or she does.

Envy and jealousy are synonymous and often are used interchangeably. While they are related, it is important to note the differences between envy and jealousy. Envy is seeing that someone has something or someone that the individual feels the person does not deserve, while jealousy also expresses disappointment.

Jealousy and envy date back in written history to the Bible and the story of Adam and Eve's sons, Cain and Abel. Cain and Abel both gave offerings to God, but Cain's was rejected while Abel's was received. It is believed that in a jealous rage Cain killed his brother Abel.

Envy and jealously are sometimes seen with narcissistic personality disorder. Many individuals who have this form of personality disorder believe that others are envious of them. It is important for a narcissist to feel superior to others. Envy and jealousy have also been associated with borderline personality disorder.

Current Status

Envy and jealousy have often been associated with the color green in English-speaking cultures. Terms such as the "green eyed monster" and "green with envy" have been frequently used popular expressions. The media has played on this with the candy green M&M's by portraying others as being envious of her. This is also seen in the Disney classic Snow White where the Evil Queen is envious of Snow White's youth and beauty. She is so overcome with jealousy that she tries to end Snow White's life.

Mindy Parsons, PhD

See also: Borderline Personality Disorder; Narcissistic Personality Disorder

Further Reading

Anderson, Robert E. "Envy and Jealousy." *American Journal of Psychotherapy* 56 (2002): 455–479.

Fiske, Susan T. "Envy Up, Scorn Down: How Comparison Divides Us." *American Psychologist* 65, no. 8 (2010): 698–706.

Nauta, Rein. "Cain and Abel: Violence, Shame and Jealousy." *Pastoral Psychology* 58 (2009): 65–71.

Epigenetics

Epigenetics is the study of changes in genes that do not involve alteration of the genetic code.

Definitions

- **DNA** is short for deoxyribonucleic acid. It is a molecule found in all living organisms which contains the blueprints that dictate growth and functioning.

- **DNA methylation** is an epigenetic mechanism used by cells to regulate gene expression.

- **Epi** is a prefix used to mean above, over or in addition to.

- **Epigenesis** refers to the series of developmental processes an organism goes through. Environmental factors (i.e., diet, weather) can greatly influence this process.

- **Gene expression** is the process by which information from a gene is used to make proteins.

- **Genes** are the carriers of the genetic code present in each cell.

- **Genetic code** is the sequence of nucleotides in DNA or RNA that is the biochemical basis of heredity (inherited traits).

- **Genetics** is the scientific study of genes and heredity. It focuses on how living things inherit traits from parents.

- **Genotype** is one's genetic makeup and the potential for unique traits or characteristics to develop.

- **Nucleotides** are the molecular subunits of the nucleic acids, DNA and RNA. Nucleotides transport energy inside a cell.

- **Phenotype** refers to the observable traits of an organism, such as size, shape, color, and behavior. Phenotype is determined by a combination of gene expression and environmental factors and their interaction.

- **Proteins** are nutrients used as energy sources (calories) by the body. They are essential components of muscle, skin, and bones.

- **RNA** is short for ribonucleic acid. It is a group of molecules found in all living organisms that work together to transfer genetic information from DNA to proteins in the cell. RNA play a significant role in the expression of genes.

Description

Epigenetics is the study of factors that influence genetic expression but are not part of the DNA (or gene) sequence. These factors impact the growth and development of all organisms. Development is shaped by the interaction between genes and the environment. Epigenetic traits occur in addition to, or on top of, genetic traits. Epigenetic processes have the potential to change when, and if, particular genes are activated but do not have any impact on the order of the nucleotides contained in a DNA molecule. Nucleotides are the foundational components of DNA and RNA (nucleic acids). Epigenetic changes can also activate or suppress protein molecules related with DNA. These molecular activities influence the expression of genes that an organism needs to function.

The term "epigenetics" was originally coined by C. H. Waddington (1905–1975) in 1942 when he combined the words "epigenesis" and "genetics." Waddington worked in the scientific fields of biology and genetics and believed that both fields should be united. He hypothesized that genes interact with environmental influences to create a particular phenotype. The term "epigenetics" has also been used in the field of psychology. Erik Erikson (1902–1994) used the word in his 1968 book *Identity: Youth and Crisis*. Erikson believed that an individual's personality is developed during his or her progression through eight psychosocial stages. Movement through these stages is significantly impacted by environmental factors.

Epigenetic modifications are affected by stress, nutrition, and self-care during pregnancy. After birth, early developmental (life) experiences have the potential to trigger epigenetic changes that impact the brain, physiology, and behavior. For example, abuse, neglect, and separation from the primary caregiver can result in changes in DNA methylation and gene expression. Epigenetic changes have the potential to affect an individual's ability to respond and adapt to life experiences that occur early in the developmental process.

Len Sperry, MD, PhD, and
Christina Ladd, PhD

See also: Brain; Erikson, Erik (1902–1994); Psychosocial Development, Stages of

Further Reading

Cameron, Noel, and Barry Bogin. *Human Growth and Development*. New York, NY: Academic Press, 2012.

Erikson, Erik. *Identity: Youth and Crisis.* New York, NY: W.W. Norton, 1968.

Francis, Richard C. *Epigenetics: How Environment Shapes Our Genes.* New York, NY: W.W. Norton, 2012.

Erectile Disorder

Erectile disorder is a mental disorder characterized by the inability to achieve or maintain erections during sexual activities with a partner. It is also known as impotence.

Definitions

- **Acquired erectile disorder** means sexual difficulties began occurring after a period of normal sexual functioning.

- *Diagnostic and Statistical Manual of Mental Disorders* is the handbook mental health professionals use to diagnose mental disorders. The current edition (fifth) is known as DSM-5.

- **Lifelong erectile disorder** means sexual difficulties have been reoccurring since the first sexual encounter.

- **Sexual dysfunction disorders** are a group of mental disorders characterized by significant difficulty in the ability to respond sexually or to experience sexual pleasure. Disorders include delayed ejaculation, female organismic disorder, and genito-pelvic pain/penetration disorder.

Description and Diagnosis

Erectile disorder is one of the DSM-5 sexual dysfunction disorders characterized by failure to attain or keep penile erection or rigidity when engaging in sexual activities with another person. A thorough medical and sexual history is required to determine how long the problem has been occurring. Additional information regarding relationship, partner, personal, cultural, and medical factors must be obtained.

The occurrence of this disorder is higher among men over the age of 50. Around 40%–50% of men aged 60 to 70 and older experience erectile disorder. Approximately 13%–21% of men between the ages of 40 and 50 report occasional erectile difficulties. Approximately 2% of men younger than 40 to 50 years experience significant problems with erections. Although 20% of men are afraid they will have difficulty obtaining and maintaining an erection during their first sexual encounter, only 8% actually experience a problem (American Psychiatric Association, 2013). As a man ages, the probability of experiencing erectile disorder increases.

According to the *Diagnostic and Statistical Manual of Mental Disorders, Fifth Edition*, individuals can be diagnosed with this disorder if they experience several symptoms during most sexual encounters, approximately 75%–100% of the time. The problem must occur for a period of at least six months and cause the individual a great deal of distress. The disorder is not the result of mental illness, relationship difficulties, substance abuse, medication side effects, a medical condition, or other stressors. The problem might be situational where the individual might experience erectile disorder only with particular partners, in particular situations, or with specific forms of stimulation. Conversely, the problem might be general in nature, which would indicate it is not attributable to a particular person, situation, or type of stimulation. The problem may have first occurred when the individual initially became sexually active (lifelong) or after a history of normal sexual performance (acquired) (American Psychiatric Association, 2013).

The cause of this disorder may be attributed to physical and/or psychological influences. Acquired erectile disorder tends to be ongoing and is associated with biological factors such as heart disease, diabetes, and neurological disorders. Lifelong erectile disorder tends to be intermittent and is associated with psychological factors such as anxiety or use of drugs or alcohol.

Treatment

Erectile disorder is treated with medication, lifestyle changes, or psychological treatment depending on the type. For acquired erectile disorder, the first step in treatment is to obtain a medical exam to diagnose and treat underlying health or lifestyle problems that may be contributing to the sexual dysfunction. Then any psychological issues contributing to the sexual problem may be addressed. The lifelong type is typically treatable with psychological treatment interventions. It is used to reduce anxiety and address relationship concerns or other stressors that may influence erectile issues. Both types may also be treated with prescribed medications.

Christina Ladd, PhD, Jon Sperry, PhD, and Len Sperry, MD, PhD

See also: Sexual Dysfunctions

Further Reading

American Psychiatric Association. *Diagnostic and Statistical Manual of Mental Disorders*, 5th ed. Arlington, VA: American Psychiatric Association Press, 2013.

Mayo Clinic. 2014. "Erectile Dysfunction." Accessed September 22, 2014. http://www.mayoclinic.org/search/search-results?q=erectile%20dysfunction.

McCarthy, Barry, and Michael E. Metz. *Coping with Erectile Dysfunction: How to Regain Confidence and Enjoy Great Sex*. Oakland, CA: New Harbinger, 2004.

PubMed Health. 2013. "Erection Problems." Accessed September 22, 2014. http://www.ncbi.nlm.nih.gov/pubmedhealth/PMH0003650/.

Shamloul, Randy, and Anthony J. Bella. *Erectile Dysfunction*. Princeton, NJ: Biota Publishing, 2014.

Erickson, Milton (1901–1980)

Milton Erickson was an American psychiatrist best known for his pioneering work in clinical hypnosis and family therapy.

Description

Milton Hyland Erickson was born in Aurum, Nevada, on December 5, 1901, and grew up on a farm in Lowell, Wisconsin, with eight siblings. As a child Erickson suffered from dyslexia, was color blind, and tone deaf. At age 17 Erickson contracted the viral infection of polio and was so severely paralyzed that doctors informed his parents that his death was imminent. Although he survived the polio attack, he was left paralyzed and unable to speak. For months all he could move was his eyes. Observing his family members for hours on end he became vividly aware of the significance of nonverbal communication. He noticed that body language, tone of voice, and other nonverbal expressions often contradicted what people were saying to him. He observed that people could say "yes" but really mean "no" at the same time. During his long recovery Erickson also began to concentrate on "body memories" of muscle movement and was eventually able to regain the ability to talk and use his arms. Erickson developed keen insights into human behavior through these experiences and became very interested in the unconscious mind and hypnosis, a psychological technique used to induce a trance state. When the mind is in a trance, it is an altered mental state of consciousness in which a person experiences heightened concentration with a greater ability to block out distractions.

No longer having the strength required to be a farmer like his father Erickson decided to enroll in college. Intending to build up his strength in order to have the health and endurance needed for his studies, Erickson embarked alone on a thousand-mile canoe trip. At first Erickson was able to swim only a few feet and was unable to pull his canoe out of the water. By the end of the trip he was able to swim over a mile and could walk with the use of a cane. Erickson graduated from the University of Wisconsin School of Medicine in 1928 as a medical doctor with a degree in psychology.

After graduating from medical school as a psychiatrist, Erickson worked in psychiatric hospitals and earned a reputation in the psychiatric community for his work in hypnosis. While at Wayne County Hospital in Michigan as director of Psychiatric Research and Training, Erickson conducted extensive research in the therapeutic value of hypnosis. His final medical appointment was as clinical director of the Arizona State Hospital. Erickson retired from hospital work in 1948 due to the progressive effects of polio. In spite of being in constant pain and struggling with the progressive loss of mobility Erickson remained extremely active in teaching, writing, and private practice. He was an associate editor for a medical journal, *Diseases of the Nervous System*, was a consultant to the U.S. government during World War II studying the effects of propaganda and the psychology of the enemy, and provided hypnosis to the U.S. Olympic Rifle Team who went on

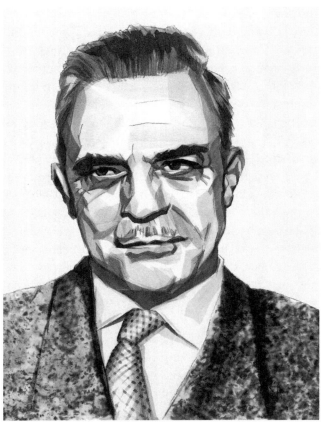

Milton Erickson was an American psychiatrist best known for his pioneering work in clinical hypnosis and family therapy. (Jan Rieckhoff/ullstein bild via Getty Images)

deep in thought while driving or waiting in line or being lost in a book are examples of trance. Erickson used the naturally occurring trance states clients would be in. He also developed verbal and nonverbal techniques to induce trance in clients. Clients did not have to be consciously aware of the message for the intervention to have an effect. For instance, instead of talking directly and consciously about bed-wetting to a 12-year-old boy struggling with that problem, Erickson used the metaphor of how to throw a baseball. Explaining about the muscle control and timing needed to throw a ball communicated to the child's subconscious mind what would be needed to stay dry during the night. Erickson also brought greater flexibility to the use of hypnosis and believed that clients were able to find their own unique solutions rather than imposing them on the client.

Milton Erickson revolutionized the practice of hypnosis and became known as the world's leading hypnotherapist. Many of his psychotherapeutic strategies have been adopted into mainstream psychotherapies and family therapy. Erickson traveled and lectured extensively; he was a prolific writer authoring several books and over 140 scholarly articles before his death on March 25, 1980.

Steven R. Vensel, PhD

See also: Hypnotherapy

Further Reading

Erickson, Betty Alice, and Bradford Keeney, eds. *Milton H. Erickson, M.D.: An American Healer* (*Profiles in Healing Series*). Philadelphia, PA: Ringing Rocks Press, 2006.

Havens, Ronald A. *The Wisdom of Milton H. Erickson. The Complete Volume.* Carmarthen, Wales, UK: Crown House, 2003.

Milton H. Erickson Foundation. "Dr. Milton H. Erickson." Accessed April 12, 2014. http://erickson-foundation.org/about/erickson/.

Rosen, Sidney, ed. *My Voice Will Go with You. The Teaching Tales of Milton H. Erickson.* New York, NY: W.W. Norton, 1982.

to beat the Russians for the first time. Erickson was the founding president of the American Society for Clinical Hypnosis and established the *American Journal of Clinical Hypnosis*, serving as editor for 10 years.

Erickson is best known for his unique and pioneering approach to hypnosis, which differed from traditional forms of hypnosis in use at the time. Traditional hypnosis was direct and authoritative, but Erickson's approach was flexible, accommodating, and less direct. Eventually becoming known as Ericksonian hypnosis, Erickson believed that the unconscious mind was always at work, always listening, could be influenced, and contained all of the necessary resources to bring about positive change. He frequently used the imagination, stories, jokes, riddles, and metaphor to communicate to a client's unconscious mind. He believed that trance states are an everyday common experience that most people are not aware of when they are in a trance state. Being

Erikson, Erik (1902–1994)

Erik Erikson was a German American psychologist best known for his theories of psychosocial developmental, identity formation, and creating the phrase "identity crisis." He is listed in the top 20 most eminent psychologist of the 20th century.

Description

Erik Erikson was born Erik Salomonsen in Frankfurt, Germany, on June 15, 1902. His mother, Karla Abrahamsen, was Danish and came from a prominent Jewish family in Copenhagen, Denmark. Karla was married to Waldemar Salomonsen but was not living with him when she became pregnant with Erik. Erikson never knew his birth father, or his mother's first husband, and details of his birth were concealed from him during childhood due to his birth coming from an extramarital relationship. Erikson was adopted by Karla's second husband, physician Theodor Homberger, and was raised believing that Homberger was his birth father. When Erikson learned the truth of his birth history, he was left with a sense of confusion over who he really was. Erikson was frequently teased by his temple school classmates for being "Nordic" because he was tall with blond hair and blue eyes, which added to his identity confusion. In grammar school he was teased for being Jewish. These childhood experiences led to a lifelong interest in how personal identity is formed and how individuals figure out who they are.

After high school Erikson traveled throughout Europe before entering and graduating from art school. In Vienna, Austria, Erikson taught children of American parents who had come for Freudian psychoanalytic training. During this time he met Anna Freud, Sigmund Freud's daughter, and received psychoanalysis from her. His experience with Freud and analysis resulted in a deep sense of personal growth and eventually led him to become an analyst himself. Erikson trained at the Vienna Psychoanalytic Institute. He also studied the Montessori method, an educational approach that focused on a child's natural self-constructed psychological, physical, and social development. While teaching in Vienna he met Joan Serson, a Canadian dance instructor teaching at the same school as Erikson. They were married in 1930. When the Nazis came to power in Germany, Erikson emigrated to Denmark. In 1933 he moved to the United States where he changed his name from Erik Homberger to Erik H. Erikson.

Erikson held teaching positions in several universities, including Harvard Medical School and the University of California at Berkeley. While at Berkeley he began his research into childhood and development by studying the cultural and childrearing practices of the Lakota and Yurok Indian tribes. He also held positions in hospitals, institutes, and child guidance centers as well as maintaining a private practice. During his career he published a number of books addressing theories of identity and development. His books included *Childhood and Society* (1950), *Identity: Youth and Crisis* (1968), and *Life History and the Historical Moment* (1975). His book *Gandhi's Truth* (1969) won a Pulitzer Prize and the U.S. National Book Award in Philosophy and Religion.

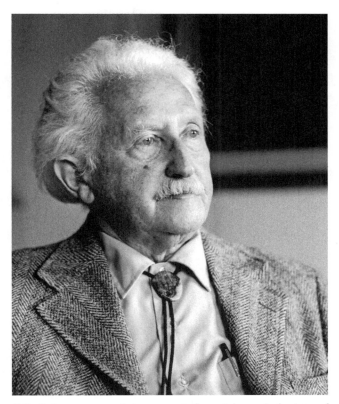

Erik Erikson, one of the most influential psychologists of the 20th century, was best known for his theories of psychosocial development and identity formation. He coined the phrase "identity crisis." (Ted Streshinsky/Corbis)

Impact (Psychological Influence)

Stages of psychosocial development. Erikson is best known for his theory of the eight stages of psychosocial development. Although trained in Freudian psychoanalytic theory, Erikson rejected Freud's deterministic beliefs that personality is developed in the context of unconscious aggressive and sexual instincts in childhood. Erikson believed that the environment in which a child developed was essential in the development of self-awareness and identity. Erikson taught that people develop throughout their lifespan and are impacted by social, biological, and psychological factors. As people move through life, they are faced with age-specific challenges and tasks that must be mastered in order for a healthy identify to form. Once a positive identity is formed in one stage, they are able to move to the next stage. When a person is unable to cope with a particular stage, he or she develops a poor self-image which has a negative impact on subsequent stages of development. Erikson identified eight stages of development: Trust versus Mistrust (birth to 1 year old), Autonomy versus Shame and Doubt (1 to 2 years old), Initiative versus Guilt (3 to 5 years old), Industry versus Inferiority (6 to 11 years old), Identity versus Role Confusion (adolescence), Intimacy versus Isolation (early adulthood), Generativity versus Stagnation (middle adulthood), and Integrity versus Despair (later life).

Identity crisis. Erikson coined the phrase "identity crisis" as a description of what can occur during adolescence when physical, sexual, and cognitive growth is at a maximum. An identity crisis is a time of deep reflection and analysis of oneself as an individual develops a separate and unique self-image and identity from that of his or her parents. It is a time during which an adolescent unifies all that he or she is in terms of temperament, giftedness, body type, abilities, strengths, and weaknesses. Included in this emergent identity is an appreciation of the many possibilities open to the individual, including the development of personal values, roles, occupational choices, friendships, and sexuality. Successful resolution of the crisis is influenced by the successful resolution of previous stages.

Erik Erikson made significant contributions to the fields of child development, psychology, psychotherapy, and theories of human development. Erikson was an influential and pioneering psychoanalyst whose groundbreaking and original developmental theories continue to be taught throughout the psychological, child development, and mental health professions.

Steven R. Vensel, PhD

See also: Psychosocial Development, Stages of

Further Reading

Coles, Robert. *The Erik Erikson Reader.* New York, NY: W.W. Norton, 2000.

Erikson, Erik H. *Childhood and Society.* New York, NY: W.W. Norton, 1980.

Erikson, Erik H. *Identity and the Life Cycle.* New York, NY: W.W. Norton, 1980.

Friedman, Lawrence J., and Robert Coles. *Identity's Architect: A Biography of Erik H. Erikson.* New York, NY: Scribner, 1999.

Haggbloom, Steven, Renee Warnick, Jason E. Warnick, Vinessa K. Jones, Gary L. Yarbrough, Tenea M. Russell, Chris M. Borecky, Reagan McGahhey, John L. Powell III, Jamie Beavers, and Emmanuelle Monte. "The 100 Most Eminent Psychologists of the 20th Century." *Review of General Psychology* 6, no. 2 (2002): 139–152.

Ethics in Mental Health Practice

Ethics in mental health practice is the moral, legal, and value-based system that guides professional thinking, decisions, and behavior.

Definitions

- **American Counseling Association** is the professional organization for the counseling specialties, including school counseling, clinical mental health counseling, career counseling, and rehabilitation professional counselors.

- **Involuntary hospitalization** is the legal process whereby individuals are placed in inpatient mental health treatment against their will.

- **Law** is the collection of rules that govern the behavior of individuals in a community, state, or country.

- **Morality** is the perception of correct and proper behavior, often based on culture or religion.

- **Values** are principles that govern virtuous behavior. When values are lived or put in action, they are known as virtues.

Description

Ethics guide professional thinking and behavior. It determines how mental health professionals make decisions and conceptualize situations. While ethics is commonly thought of as "doing the right thing," it is much more complex. Ethics in mental health practice may refer to morality, values, or rules and laws. There are two main types of ethical practice. Mandatory ethics refers to complying with the minimum standards of professional behavior dictated by the law. This is simply following the rules. By contrast, aspirational ethics is the highest form of ethical thinking and behavior. This involves not just following the rules but understanding the principles behind them and striving to embody them in practice.

There are six principles that form the basis for ethical professional practice. These principles guide ethical thinking and behavior. They are autonomy, nonmaleficence, beneficence, justice, fidelity, and veracity. Autonomy is the freedom of clients to choose their own direction. Mental health professionals guided by this ethical principle do not force particular treatments or decisions on clients. "Nonmaleficence" means doing no harm to others. This principle prohibits professionals from doing anything that would hurt clients. Such actions may include improper diagnosis or exploitation. "Beneficence" refers to increasing the well-being and good of others. It requires that professionals act to improve their clients' lives. The ethical principle of justice is being fair and giving equally to others. This includes all individuals regardless of age, sex, race, ethnicity, disability, socioeconomic status, culture, or other characteristic. "Fidelity" refers to being trustworthy and keeping promises to clients. This is necessary for an effective therapeutic relationship. Finally, "veracity" means truthfulness. Mental health professionals must be open about client rights, risks of treatment, and other factors so clients are well informed.

All professional mental health organizations have their own specific codes of ethics. These provide guidance on how professionals should behave and they set forth specific expectations. For example, the Code of Ethics of the American Counseling Association provides guidelines for counselors on topics ranging from confidentiality to social media. These codes also instruct professionals on how to resolve ethical dilemmas. Unethical activity by mental health professionals may include inappropriate relationships with clients, use of improper treatments, or fraud. Many unethical activities are also illegal, such as billing an insurance company for services that were not provided. However, not all unethical activities are illegal. Engaging in a sexual relationship with an adult client is considered unethical but legal. The consequences for unethical professional practice range from mandated supplemental training and supervision to loss of license. These consequences are typically decided by the organization responsible for issuing and overseeing professional licenses.

In mental health practice, there are often conflicts between different ethical principles For example, a counselor who operates from the principle of beneficence may encourage a client to assert himself or herself to an abusive family member. The intention may be to increase self-esteem and practice healthy communication skills. However, this may result in harm to this client if his or her assertiveness leads to intensified abuse. In this case, the principle of nonmaleficence may have been violated. Another ethical dilemma is presented by the practice of involuntary hospitalization. In this situation, individuals' right to make their own decisions (autonomy) is taken away because they are deemed unable to care for themselves. This practice may be justified on the grounds that it protects the client from harm (beneficence).

Len Sperry, MD, PhD, and George Stoupas, MS

See also: American Counseling Association (ACA); Involuntary Hospitalization

Further Reading

Herlihy, Barbara, and Gerald Corey. *ACA Ethical Standards Casebook*, 6th ed. Alexandria, VA: American Counseling Association, 2006.

Sperry, Len. *The Ethical and Professional Practice of Psychotherapy and Counseling*. Boston, MA: Allyn & Bacon, 2007.

Wheeler, Anne Marie, and Burt Bertram. *The Counselor and the Law: A Guide to Legal and Ethical Practice*, 6th ed. Alexandria, VA: American Counseling Association, 2012.

Ethnicity

"Ethnicity" refers to a shared distinctive culture based on region of the world, language, religion, and lifestyle.

Description

Our individual identity, our understanding of the world, and the way we act are all heavily influenced by our personal history, including our ethnicity. Ethnicity is usually defined by shared cultural practices, including language, customs, religion, food, and celebrations of life. People of the same ethnicity often celebrate events such as birth, marriage, and death in a similar way. Ethnicity is not race nor is it a nationality. Race usually refers to a person's physical appearance, such as skin color, eye color, hair color, and bone structure. Nationality is defined by citizenship in a country and many nations are comprised of different ethnic groups. For example, in the United States there are citizens who come from many different ethnic backgrounds.

Ethnic identity plays a large part in the development of human identity. It is the principal way that people identify themselves with others. It gives individuals a sense of belonging to a particular cultural group. For example, many U.S. citizens with origins in Latin America often identify themselves as Hispanic. People who identify themselves as Hispanic are likely fragmented into smaller groups depending on country of origin and even region or dialect of origin within certain countries.

Current Status and Impact (Psychological Influence)

The values of the ethnic culture in which someone is raised have a big influence on personal ways of thinking and behaving. This especially applies to physical health and self-care. Ethnicity influences the extent to which we can tolerate both physical and psychological pain. This reality provides a challenge for health-care professionals who need to take into account ethnic and multicultural aspects in the treatment of each client.

The influence of ethnicity also plays a role in keeping people in predetermined social and economic classes. Lack of access to education and resources may mean that people consume foods that are not nourishing, and this may result in diets high in saturated fat, cholesterol, and carbohydrates. This can in turn lead to chronic health conditions such as diabetes, high blood pressure, and stress.

Many ethnic groups have inherited beliefs and patterns of behavior which may increase their health risks. They may believe that preventive interventions, such as mammograms or colonoscopies, are invasive or indecent. They may believe that seeing a therapist or a counselor means a person is either mentally ill or morally weak. Health-care professionals need to be sensitive to the role that ethnicity can play in the knowledge, acceptance, and use of medical diagnosis, procedures, or interventions.

Ethnicity and culture are also extremely important factors in the field of caregiving. Cultural biases may lead to the conclusion that someone from the community should be a caregiver who does not have the skills to do it well. Ethnicity can help determine not only the quality and complexity of the caregiving but also the way that caregivers do or do not recognize the stress they are under and the kind of coping mechanisms they use to help them do their work effectively.

Alexandra Cunningham, PhD, and
William M. Cunningham, MA

See also: Immigration, Psychological Factors of; Multicultural Counseling; Prejudice; Racial Identity Development; Social Justice Counseling

Further Reading

Chin, Jean Lau. *The Psychology of Prejudice and Discrimination: A Revised and Condensed Edition (Race and Ethnicity in Psychology)*. Santa Barbara, CA: Praeger, 2009.

Lips, Hilary. *A New Psychology of Women: Gender, Culture and Ethnicity*. Long Grove, IL: Waveland Press, 2010.

McGoldrick, Monica, Joe Giordano, and Nydia Garcia-Preto. *Ethnicity and Family Therapy*. New York, NY: The Guilford Press, 2005.

Evening Primrose Oil

Evening primrose oil is a natural remedy used for skin conditions such as eczema as well as various other medical conditions.

Definitions

- **Antioxidants** are substances that protect the body from damaging reactive oxygen molecules in the body. These reactive oxygen molecules are thought to play a role in the aging process and the development of degenerative disease.

- **Prostaglandins** are a group of unsaturated fatty acids involved in the contraction of smooth muscle, control of inflammation, and other body processes.

Description

Evening primrose oil comes from the seed of the evening primrose plant. It is used as a dietary supplement by alternative medical practitioners to relieve the discomfort of symptoms associated with premenstrual syndrome (PMS), eczema, sunburn, fibrocystic breast disease, arthritis, diabetes, and osteoporosis. Other uses are irritable bowel syndrome, peptic ulcer disease, multiple sclerosis, nerve damage related to diabetes, cancer, high cholesterol, heart disease, Alzheimer's disease, and chronic fatigue syndrome. It has been used in children for attention-deficit hyperactivity disorder. Women use it for PMS, breast pain, and hot flashes. However, clinical studies have shown it to be effective in treating breast pain and osteoporosis. While there is some evidence that it can reduce the symptoms of PMS, Alzheimer's disease, and attention-deficit hyperactivity disorder, clinical trials have yet to establish its efficacy in these conditions. Evening primrose oil is believed to work because it is a source of essential fatty acids (EFAs). EFAs regulate pain and inflammation and help produce hormone-like substances such as prostaglandins. Evening primrose oil is thought to work by stimulating anti-inflammatory prostaglandins, which helps reduce inflammation and relieve various symptoms.

Precautions and Side Effects

Evening primrose oil should not be given to patients with epilepsy, and medical supervision is needed if used in children. Evening primrose oil has few reported side effects. Those reported are nausea, headache, and

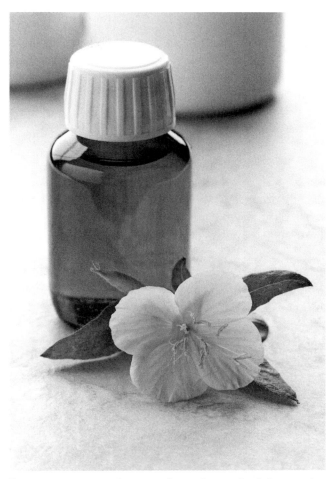

Evening primrose oil comes from the seed of the evening primrose plant. It is used as a dietary supplement. Proponents claim that it can ease symptoms associated with Alzheimer's disease and attention-deficit hyperactivity disorder (ADHD), among many other conditions. (Pipa100/Dreamstime.com)

loose stools. Rarely, bruising of the skin is reported. Evening primrose oil should not be used with Neurontin, Dilantin, or other anticonvulsant medications, since it can lower the threshold for seizures. While other significant drug interactions have yet to be reported, those taking evening primrose oil would do well to mention this to their physicians.

Len Sperry, MD, PhD

See also: Neurontin (Gabapentin)

Further Reading

Dasgupta, Amitava, and Catherine A. Hammett-Stabler, eds. *Herbal Supplements: Efficacy, Toxicity, Interactions with Western Drugs, and Effects on Clinical Labora-tory Tests.* Hoboken, NJ: Wiley, 2011.

PDR for Herbal Medicines. Montvale, NJ: Thompson, 2007.

Stargrove, Mitchell Bebel, Jonathan Treasure, and and Dwight McKee. *Herb, Nutrient, and Drug Interactions: Clinical Implications and Therapeutic Strategies.* St. Louis, MO: Mosby, 2007.

Sutton, Amy L., ed. *Complementary and Alternative Medicine Sourcebook.* Detroit, MI: Omnigraphics, 2010.

Everything You Always Wanted to Know about Sex (but Were Afraid to Ask) (Book and Movie)

Everything You Always Wanted to Know about Sex (but Were Afraid to Ask) is a sex manual that was published in 1969 by David Reuben.

Description

The 1960s was an era of social change. This was a period of time that included a sexual revolution. Sex became news and people started talking about sexual experiences and sexual practices more openly than before. Two factors helped create this change. First, the birth-control pill was introduced, which helped women prevent pregnancy after sex. The second was the publication of a groundbreaking study of human sexual responses in 1965 by scientists William H. Masters and Virginia Johnson.

In a time where sex was being revolutionized, people were interested in learning more. Psychiatrist Dr. David Reuben wrote and published the book *Everything You Always Wanted to Know about Sex (but Were Afraid to Ask).* The book was aimed at giving a good amount of information about sexuality in an interesting and informative way. Even in the revolutionary atmosphere of the 1960s, the content of the book was still shocking to many. This was because of its honest discussion of sex acts, sexual positions, and group sex. The book is also detailed and provides good information on male and female sexual anatomy. It quickly became a national and international best seller.

In that same year director and filmmaker Woody Allen produced a movie with the same name. The film contained scenarios based roughly around the content of the book. But it also aimed at highlighting the funny side of some of the basic sexual practices it described. The movie was also a success, both commercially and critically.

Impact (Psychological Influence)

There are some significant cultural impacts associated with the book *Everything You Always Wanted to Know about Sex (but Were Afraid to Ask).* It was one of the most popular nonfiction books of its era in the United States and internationally. Its openness and material had a profound effect on sex education and changed cultural attitudes toward sex. Despite the initial shock of some people, the book was successful and had many imitators. One such work was *The Joy of Sex,* an illustrated manual published in 1972. Reuben's book helped support and encourage new ways that people wrote, thought, and talked about sex.

Due to the spread of sexually transmitted diseases and HIV/AIDS in the1980s and 1990s, critiques of the book emerged. Some believed it did not address the psychological effects of the social and moral changes it supported. In addition, the book presented information only on heterosexual relations. The book was not overtly negative to other viewpoints; it just did not include them. The book also received criticism for being overly optimistic about sexual relations and about sexual identity itself. It was revised and republished in 1999 to address some of these issues.

Alexandra Cunningham, PhD, and William M. Cunningham, MA

See also: Conjoint Sexual Therapy

Further Reading

Buehler, Stephanie. *What Every Mental Health Professional Needs to Know about Sex.* New York, NY: Springer, 2013.

Reuben, David. *Everything You Always Wanted to Know about Sex: But Were Afraid to Ask.* New York, NY: HarperCollins, 1999.

Evidence-Based Practice

Evidence-based practice (EBP) is a form of practice that is based on the integration of the best research evidence with clinical expertise and client values.

Definitions

- **Accountability** is the expectation or requirement to conduct evaluations and report performance information.

- **Best practice** is a method that has consistently shown results superior to those achieved with other means, and that is used as a benchmark.

- **Empirically supported treatments** are therapeutic interventions that research demonstrates to be effective in facilitating therapeutic change.

- **Health Maintenance Organization** (HMO) is an organization that provides or arranges managed care.

- **Managed care** is a system of health care that controls costs by placing limits on physicians' fees and by restricting access to certain medical procedures and providers.

- **Practice** is a method or process used to accomplish a goal or objective.

- **Psychotherapy** is a psychological method for achieving desired changes in thinking, feeling, and behavior. It is also called therapeutic counseling.

- **Randomized controlled trial** is a research design in which participants are assigned randomly (by chance) to an experimental treatment or one that receives a comparison treatment or placebo. It is also known as randomized clinical trials.

- **Treatment** is a technique used to promote health and well-being, often implemented after a diagnosis is formulated.

Description

Evidence-based practice is similar to the concept of best practices. Both aim to increase accountability of health-care practices. EBP in psychotherapy integrates the findings of scientific research with clinician expertise and client needs and preferences (values).

"Evidence-based practice" refers to the therapeutic process a psychotherapist chooses, when those choices are informed by research evidence.

Evidence-based practice is similar to but different from empirically supported treatments (ESTs). EBP may include ESTs, but it is larger in scope than treatments. EBP involves specific interventions (practices) used to bring about therapeutic change. More specifically, to merit that designation, ESTs demonstrated that they are (1) superior to a placebo treatment in two or more randomized controlled studies, (2) equivalent to a well-established treatment in several rigorous and independent controlled studies, or (3) effective in a large series of single-case controlled studies. Clearly, the extent of research support for EBP is significantly less than that for ESTs.

Development and Current Status

Prior to the 1990s, there were no specific guidelines for either clinicians or consumers regarding which treatments to select for which conditions. In 1993, a task force of the American Psychological Association developed a set of criteria for "empirically validated treatments." Later these treatment came to be known as ESTs. However, there has been considerable controversy about ESTs. Some believe that the controlled context of scientific research cannot be replicated in clinical practice. Others contend that the results of scientific study are generalizable to clinical contexts. For the past two decades this debate has been fueled by the increasing expectation for accountability. Increasingly, medical and psychological practice has become more accountable and evidence based. In response, many have championed EBP as an alternative to ESTs.

EBP is a form of practice informed by scientific research. It also includes clinical judgment and client values. EBP in medicine was defined by the Institute of Medicine (2001) as "the integration of best research evidence with clinical expertise and patient values." The American Psychological Association (2005) modified that definition as "the integration of the best available research with clinical expertise in the context of patient characteristics, culture and preferences." The challenge for the clinician is to plan and implement treatment that balances all three: research, clinical expertise, and client characteristics. This challenge is very real as reimbursement for non-EBP clinical services is less likely. Insurance companies are increasingly demanding that clinicians provide evidence for the empirical basis underlying treatment as a condition for reimbursement for services. This fact has created an effort to conduct medical and psychological practice in the most efficient manner possible. EBP is largely about the effort to get the best results for less money and in the shortest amount of time. While EBP was not officially introduced until the 1990s, the effort was largely inspired in the 1970s with the implementation of Health Maintenance Organizations (HMOs). HMOs were the first federally legislated form of managed care. Managed care was established to increase the efficiency and cost effectiveness of health care. EBP can and does have a critical role in managed care.

EBP is about making informed choices in clinical practice to increase the probability of therapeutic outcomes. It increases consistency in therapy and assists in making the best possible therapeutic choice. EBP is largely based on clinician intuition as a result of several factors: there is an absence of research available for many practice concerns; every client has unique characteristics, values, and preferences; and the clinical expertise of the clinician effects therapeutic outcomes in a unique way. Clinical decision making is a very real challenge that is rendered more consistent and effective through the use of EBP.

Len Sperry, MD, PhD, and
Layven Reguero, MEd

See also: Best Practices; Empirically Supported Treatment; Managed Care

Further Reading

American Psychological Association. *Report of the 2005 Presidential Task Force on Evidence-Based Practice.* Washington, DC: Author. (2005).

Christopherson, Edward R., and Susan Mortweet Vanscoyoc. *Treatments That Work with Children: Empirically Supported Strategies for Managing Childhood Problems,* 2nd ed. Washington, DC: American Psychological Association, 2013.

Institute of Medicine. *Crossing the Quality Chasm: A New Health System for the 21st Century.* Washington, DC: National Academy Press, 2001.

Muran, Cristopher J., and Jacques P. Barber, eds. *The Therapeutic Alliance: An Evidence-Based Guide to Practice.* New York, NY: The Guilford Press, 2010.

O'Donohue, William T., and Jane E. Fisher. *Cognitive Behavior Therapy: Applying Empirically Supported Techniques in Your Practice,* 2nd ed. New York, NY: John Wiley & Sons, 2009.

Rubin, Allen, and Jennifer Bellamy. *Practitioner's Guide to Using Research for Evidence-Based Practice,* 2nd ed. Hoboken, NJ: John Wiley & Sons, 2012.

Evil

In the psychological sense, "evil" refers to the capacity of a human being or group of human beings, who appear to be ordinarily good people, to transform and begin acting in ways that are intentionally harmful, cruel, or abusive.

Definitions

- **"Banality of evil"** is a phrase used by political theorist Hannah Arendt to describe the mindless actions of high-ranking Nazi figure Adolf Eichmann, an unremarkable figure who engaged in atrocious crimes against countless numbers of Jews for senseless reasons.

- **"Lucifer Effect"** is a term coined by psychologist Philip Zimbardo as a result of his Stanford Prison Experiment to explain how ordinary, decent people were capable of inflicting harm and abuse on others when the situation perpetuated it.

- **Obedience studies** ("Milgram's Experiments"), led by psychologist Stanley Milgram during the early 1960s, articulated the salience of real or perceived authority at influencing a human being's thoughts, values, and actions.

- **Stanford Prison Experiment,** conducted by a team of psychologists at Stanford University in 1971, evidenced how powerful situational factors could be in changing individual thoughts, feelings, attitudes, and behaviors.

Description

People have been interested in the concept of evil for centuries. Theologians, philosophers, and psychologists alike have questioned how evil develops as well as its effect on human behavior, relationships, and on society as a whole. Debate has ensued regarding both biological and environmental factors that contribute to evil. "Evil" is a negative term that describes disdainful, violent, cruel, or abusive characteristics or actions. It has a religious connotation and is historically associated with Lucifer, God's fallen angel. Originally God's favorite, most beloved angel, Lucifer fell from grace and was cast into Hell after challenging God's authority. He was then referred to as either "Satan" or the "Devil." Given this explanation, people now use the word "evil" to describe a characteristic transformation from positive to negative: good to bad, right to wrong, helpful to harmful, decent to monstrous.

Development

Psychologist Stanley Milgram's obedience studies were some of the first to reveal how normal, mentally well people could inflict severe harm (via electric shock) on innocent victims simply because they were instructed to do so. Philip Zimbardo extended on this research conducting the famous Stanford Prison Experiment in 1971. After being assessed for mental and physical health, 24 males were selected for the study. These participants, half designated guards and the other half prisoners, were placed in a mock prison environment for a period of one to two weeks. Researchers remained on site to record daily events by videotape. The "guards" were instructed to maintain order and keep the "prisoners" in line. The prisoners were subjected to a typical incarceration situation, confined three to a cell, given limited mobility and privileges, and required to follow the established rules. After just six days the experiment had to be shut down after it became apparent that the interactions among participants were getting out of control. Guards abused their power, treating prisoners in harmful, degrading, and abusive manners and the prisoners exhibited signs of acute distress and anxiety. Study findings suggested that even good, decent people could turn to evil ways if the situation encouraged it. Zimbardo termed this the "Lucifer Effect" and went onto publish a *New York Times* best seller with the same title in 2007. This launched national interest on the topic of evil, questioning what factors either promote or diminish abusive, harmful actions and allow them to perpetuate. Lessons learned from the Stanford Prison experiment have been cited in cases involving violent, abusive tactics, brainwashing, manipulation, and mind control.

Current Status and Results

Instances of human evil such as racial, gender, and sexual prejudice have been evident throughout history. Matters of war and acts of terrorism promote hated, loathing, retaliation, and retribution. In particular, heinous crimes of genocide (ethnic cleansing) articulate evil. The Holocaust in one of the most fundamental examples of pure evil. The Nazi regime was successful in annihilating millions of Jews during World War II, an unimaginable human atrocity. More recently, in 2003–2004, U.S. military personnel of the army and Central Intelligence Agency were found to have engaged in acts of abuse and torture toward Iraqi prisoners at Abu Ghraib Prison, spawning outrage, criticism, and concern.

Research investigating acts of abuse and oppression have noted that evil does not happen in a vacuum. Psychologists Thomas Carnahan and Sam McFarland suggest that creating a dynamic that perpetuates an "us" against "them" mentality may allow for evil, tyrannical acts to occur more readily. Though it was once believed that the evil characteristic appears out of thin air in normal, well-adjusted people, further investigation into the Milgram and Stanford Prison studies have revealed that participants who inflicted harm on others scored higher in aggression, authoritarianism, narcissism, and dominance and lower in empathy and altruism. Psychologists have long described a "dark triad of personality" that includes narcissism, Machiavellianism (willingness to manipulate situations or others for personal gain), and psychopathy (antisocial behavior and lack of empathy). A fourth dark trait has been added, sadism, or gaining pleasure from inflicting harm or pain on others, as a result of these studies' findings.

Melissa A. Mariani, PhD

See also: Obedience Studies; Stanford Prison Experiment

Further Reading

Baumeister, Roy F., and Aaron Beck. *Evil: Inside Human Violence and Cruelty.* New York, NY: Henry Holt, 1999.

Haslam, S. Alexander, and Stephen D. Reicher. "Beyond the Banality of Evil." *Personality and Social Psychology Bulletin* 33 (2007): 615–622.

Zimbardo, Philip G. *The Lucifer Effect: Understanding How Good People Turn Evil.* New York, NY: Random House, 2007.

Evolutionary Psychology

Evolutionary psychology (EP) is an approach to psychology that incorporates principles from evolutionary biology into an understanding of human behavior.

Definitions

- **Evolution** is a theory first proposed by Charles Darwin that states all species and organisms develop and change through the natural selection of small, inherited variations that increase the ability of the species or organism to compete, survive, and reproduce.

- **Evolutionary time** refers to an unspecified amount of time usually in the hundreds of thousands to millions of years.

- **Natural selection** is a process by which an organism or species best adapted to an environment is able to survive longer and reproduce in greater numbers, with the adaptive traits being passed down to the next generation. As the number of adapted offspring increases, there is an ever-decreasing chance for the less adapted organism to reproduce eventually resulting in the extinction of the less adaptive traits.

Description

Evolutionary psychology is not a specific method of psychotherapy but rather an approach to understanding human behavior based on the principles of evolution, adaptations, and natural selection. Evolutionary psychologists hold that EP is not a subdiscipline of psychology but rather a biologically informed framework that encompasses all fields of understanding human behavior. Psychologists agree that human behavior is the result of internal psychological mechanisms that take place within the human brain. Most fields of psychology have a perspective or theory on what the specific internal mechanisms are and how they operate. For instance, cognitive psychology explains human behavior in terms of cognitive structures (how we think) and the impact of these thoughts on feelings and behaviors. What distinguishes evolutionary psychologist from other schools of thought is the belief that the internal psychological mechanisms are actually evolutionary adaptations produced through natural selection as our ancestors lived, reproduced, and died throughout evolutionary time.

One of the major goals of EP is to identify emotional and cognitive adaptations that have evolved and which characterize the psychological nature of human beings. EP focuses almost exclusively on how the brain has evolved and how it generates emotions and behavior. According to EP, natural selection has resulted in psychological adaptations within the brain producing universal frames of meaning (true across all cultures) in how humans interpret events; experience emotion; mate and reproduce; and make meaning of other's behaviors and form social relationships, to name a few.

EP consists of several core principles that link psychology, evolutionary biology, and brain functioning. The first principle is that the brain is a physical system designed to process information and produce behavior. The brain is governed by electrochemical reactions, which function like organic neural computer circuits and which determine how it processes information. Second, the neural circuits were established through natural selection in order to solve problems. These problems were recurring and had to do with mating, parenting, social dynamics, motivation, and cognitive development. Third, most brain functions and problem solving are unconscious and involve extremely complex neural circuitry. Fourth, natural selection has produced specialized parts of the brain for solving specific types of problems. The final principle is that our modern human skulls house a Stone Age brain. The human brain has evolved over millions of years and only the smallest fraction of time has been lived in a modern society. For 10 million years natural selection has formed the human brain to solve hunter-gatherer problems of living. The modern computer age is less than 30 years old, the industrial revolution began only 200 years ago, and agriculture first appeared only about 10,000 years ago. There have not been enough generations for the brain to develop circuits adapted to our postindustrial society. Evolutionary psychologists believe that the key to understanding how the modern human mind works is to understand that it has not evolved to solve modern problems.

EP is a new approach to understanding human behavior that blends evolutionary biology and psychology to gain a deeper insight into the human mind. EP can be applied to fields such as social psychology, cognitive psychology, and personality theory.

Steven R. Vensel, PhD

See also: Epigenetics

Further Reading

Buss, David. *Evolutionary Psychology: The New Science of the Mind*, 4th ed. Upper Saddle River, NJ: Pearson, 2011.

Center for Evolutionary Psychology. "Evolutionary Psychology: A Primer." Accessed June 27, 2014. http://www.cep.ucsb.edu/primer.html.

Cosmides, Leda, and John Tooby. "Evolutionary Psychology: New Perspectives on Cognition and Motivation." *Annual Review of Psychology* 64 (2013): 201–229.

Crawford, Charles, and Dennis Kreps. *Foundations of Evolutionary Psychology*. New York, NY: Taylor & Francis, 2008.

Dunbar, Robin, Louise Barrett, and John Lycett. *Evolutionary Psychology: A Beginner's Guide*. Oxford: Oneworld, 2007.

Excoriation Disorder

Excoriation disorder is a mental disorder characterized by recurrent picking at one's own skin.

Definitions

- **Acceptant and commitment therapy** is a type of psychotherapy that helps individuals accept the difficulties that come with life. It is a form of mindfulness-based therapy. It is also known as ACT.

- **Antiseizure medications** are prescription drugs used to treat epilepsy (seizures) as well as burning, stabbing, and shooting pain. It is also called anticonvulsant medications.

- **Cognitive behavior therapy** is a form of psychotherapy that focuses on changing faulty behaviors, emotions, and thoughts. It is also known as CBT.

- **DSM-5** stands for the *Diagnostic and Statistical Manual of Mental Disorders, Fifth Edition*, which is a diagnostic system used by professionals to identify mental disorders with specific diagnostic criteria.

- **Obsessive-compulsive and related disorders** are a group of DSM-5 disorders characterized by preoccupations and repetitive behaviors. They include obsessive-compulsive disorder, hoarding disorder, and excoriation disorder.

- **Obsessive-compulsive disorder** is a mental disorder characterized by unwanted and repeated thoughts and feelings (obsessions) or behaviors that one feels driven to perform (compulsions). It is commonly referred to as OCD.

Description and Diagnosis

Excoriation (skin picking) disorder is one of the DSM-5 obsessive-compulsive and related disorders. It is characterized by the recurrent urge to pick at one's own skin, often to the extent that damage occurs. Individuals may pick for several reasons. They may pick when they are anxious or bored or during times when they aren't even aware they are picking. They may pick to cope with negative emotions (e.g., sadness, anger, and anxiety) or in response to tension and stress. When picking their skin, individuals often experience a sense of relief, which may be followed with feelings of guilt and shame.

The most common sites that individuals pick are the arms, hands, and face; however, many individuals pick from many different sites on the body. Individuals with this disorder pick at pimples, scabs, and even healthy skin. Most pick their skin with their fingernails, while others may use pins or tweezers and others even bite their skin. Some individuals may search for a particular kind of scab to pick and may examine, play with, and even eat the skin after it has been pulled. Some individuals spend several hours a day picking their skin, and this can lead to significant distress in their life, particularly with occupational, social, or other areas of functioning. For example, students may miss school and have difficulty studying and completing assignments because of skin picking.

Individuals with this disorder often feel a sense of loss of control and embarrassment. Individuals usually pick their skin in private or sometimes in front of family members. Individuals may avoid social situations as well as going out in public due to the shame of skin picking. Most individuals with this disorder hide their scars and lesions by concealing it with makeup or wearing clothing that hides the area of skin that has been damaged. Skin picking can be very severe and lead to tissue damage, scarring, infection, and life-threatening conditions. Infections may require antibiotic treatment and in some cases may require surgery. Excoriation is more common among females and may present at any age, although it is most common during the onset of puberty (American Psychiatric Association, 2013).

According to the *Diagnostic and Statistical Manual of Mental Disorders, Fifth Edition*, individuals can be diagnosed with this disorder if they have engaged in recurrent picking of their own skin resulting in skin lesions. Individuals must have had repeated attempts to decrease or stop picking. This behavior must cause significant distress or impairment in social, occupational, or other areas of functioning. Distress with this disorder refers to a loss of control, shame, and embarrassment. Significant impairment with this behavior includes several areas of functioning, such as social, educational, occupational, and leisure. The skin picking behavior cannot be a result of any physiological effects of a substance or another medical condition. Skin picking behavior cannot be better explained by symptoms of any other mental disorder (American Psychiatric Association, 2013).

The exact causes of this disorder are unknown. Environmental factors may play a role in excoriation disorder. For example, individuals who grew up in families who engaged in and witnessed skin picking may be more prone to developing this disorder. Biological factors may also play a role. For example, the disorder is passed down from parents to children. Another possible cause of excoriation disorder may be a coping mechanism for individuals to deal with turmoil and stress within them, and these individuals have an impaired stress response. Skin picking behavior may also result from repressed rage felt by overbearing parents. These individuals often have other psychological symptoms, like anxiety and depression. Excoriation disorder is more common in individuals with obsessive-compulsive disorder (OCD). Excoriation disorder and OCD share several of the same features. For example, individuals with skin picking disorder will pick their skin over and again, often in response to recurrent thoughts or urges to pick their skin. OCD is also characterized by urges to engage in repetitive behaviors (rituals) in response to recurrent thoughts and impulses.

Treatment

Treatment for this disorder typically involves psychotherapy and medication. Cognitive behavior therapy (CBT) has been found to help individuals with skin picking disorder. The goal of CBT is to have an individual focus on and change his or her thoughts and behaviors. Acceptance and commitment therapy (ACT) has also been shown to be effective. ACT theorizes that greater well-being can be attained by overcoming negative thoughts and feelings. The goal of ACT is to have an individual look at his or her character traits and behaviors that will assist in reducing avoidant coping styles. ACT also focuses on individuals making a commitment to behavior changes. Some antidepressant medications (e.g., SSRIs, such as Prozac) are often prescribed and are effective in treating this disorder. Antiseizure medicines, such as Lamictal, are also being used for this disorder.

Len Sperry, MD, PhD, and
Elizabeth Smith Kelsey, PhD

See also: Acceptance and Commitment Therapy; Cognitive Behavior Therapy; *Diagnostic and Statistical Manual of Mental Disorders* (DSM); Obsessive-Compulsive Disorder

Further Reading

American Psychiatric Association. *Diagnostic and Statistical Manual of Mental Disorders*, 5th ed. Arlington, VA: American Psychiatric Association, 2013.

Grant, Jon E., Dan J. Stein, Douglas W. Woods, and Nancy J. Keuthen. *Trichotillomania, Skin Picking, and Other Body-Focused Repetitive Behaviors*. Arlington, VA: American Psychiatric Association Press, 2011.

Penzel, Fred. *Obsessive-Compulsive Disorders: A Complete Guide to Getting Well and Staying Well*. New York, NY: Oxford University Press, 2000.

Executive Functions

Executive functions are high-level cognitive abilities such as planning, organizing, reasoning, decision making, and problem solving that influence more basic abilities such as attention, memory, and motor skills.

Definitions

- **Attention-deficit hyperactivity disorder** is a disorder of the nervous system characterized by inattention, hyperactivity, and impulsiveness.

- **Autism spectrum disorders** are disorders with impaired ability to communicate and interact socially and with repetitive behaviors or restricted interests (e.g., autism and Asperger's syndrome).

- **Learning disabilities** are disorder characterized by difficulty with skills such as reading or writing in individuals with normal intelligence.

- **Tourette's syndrome** is a disorder of the nervous system, characterized by a variable expression of tics (unwanted movements and noises).

Description

Executive functions are the cognitive process that regulates an individual's ability to organize thoughts and activities, prioritize tasks, manage time efficiently, and make decisions. Those with executive function problems are likely to have difficulty planning a project, difficulty anticipating how much time a project will take to complete, trouble communicating details in an organized, sequential manner, difficulty with the mental strategies involved in memorization and retrieving information from memory, trouble initiating activities or tasks, or difficulty retaining information while doing something with it, such as remembering a phone number while dialing. Impairment of executive function is noted in a range of disorders, including attention-deficit/hyperactivity disorder, autism spectrum disorders, Tourette's syndrome, and learning disabilities.

Developments and Current Status

In the 1980s, the American psychologist Michael Posner (1936–) and his colleagues influenced recent research into executive functions. He identified a separate "executive" branch of cognitive function responsible for focusing attention. Because individuals with deficits in executive functioning have difficulty with learning in school and job performance, the assessment of executive function is common. There is no single test or battery (series) of tests that identifies all aspects of executive function. For that reason, psychologists and learning disorder specialists use various tests. Some of the most common are the Wisconsin Card Sorting Test, the Stroop Color and Word Test, and the Color-Word Interference Test.

Wisconsin card sorting test. This test measures the ability to shift cognitive strategies in response to changing environmental contingencies as well as the ability to develop and maintain an appropriate problem-solving strategy across changing stimulus conditions. It consists of 128 response cards and 4 stimulus cards that depict figures of varying forms, colors, or numbers of figures.

Stroop color and word test. This test is used to assess cognitive flexibility in the sense of ability to inhibit a more automatic verbal response (reading color words) in order to generate a conflicting response of naming the dissonant ink colors.

Color-word interference test. This test assesses cognitive flexibility by requiring the test-taker to inhibit reading words standing for colors while naming the colors themselves. It then asks the test-taker to switch back and forth between naming the dissonant (wrong) ink color and reading the conflicting word.

Len Sperry, MD, PhD

See also: Autism; Learning Disorders; Neuropsychological Tests

Further Reading

Anderson, Vicki, Rani Jacobs, and Peter J. Anderson. *Executive Functions and the Frontal Lobes: A Lifespan Perspective.* New York, NY: Psychology Press, 2008.

Grant, Igor, and Kenneth M. Adams, eds. *Neuropsychological Assessment of Neuropsychiatric and Neuromedical Disorders.* Oxford: Oxford University Press, 2009.

Spreen, Otfried, Esther Strauss, and Elisabeth M. S. Sherman. *A Compendium of Neuropsychological Tests: Administration, Norms, and Commentary.* Oxford: Oxford University Press, 2006.

Exhibitionistic Disorder

Exhibitionistic disorder is a mental health disorder that is characterized by the exposure of one's genitals to others in order to gain sexual satisfaction.

Definitions

- **Antiandrogens** are medications that block male sex hormones.

- **Aversion therapy** is a form of psychotherapy that focuses on reducing or avoiding an undesirable pattern in an individual by conditioning that individual to associate the behavior with an undesirable stimulus.

- **Cognitive behavior therapy** is a form of psychotherapy that focuses on changing maladaptive (faulty) behaviors, emotions, and thoughts. It is also known as CBT.

- **DSM-5** stands for the *Diagnostic and Statistical Manual of Mental Disorders, Fifth Edition*, which is a diagnostic system used by professionals to identify mental disorders with specific diagnostic criteria.

- **Hormones** are chemical substances produced in the body that control and regulate the activity of certain cells or organs.

- **Impulse control** is the degree to which an individual can control the impulse to act or the desire for immediate gratification.

- **Paraphilia** is a sexual disorder in which individuals can only become aroused by inappropriate object, actions, or fantasies.

- **Paraphilic disorders** are a group of DSM-5 mental disorders characterized by unusual sexual preferences and behaviors that are distressing or detrimental to one's self or others. They include exhibitionistic disorder, pedophilic disorder, and fetishistic disorder.

- **Selective serotonin reuptake inhibitors** are the most commonly prescribed antidepressant medication because they generally have few side effects.

- **Serotonin** is a chemical messenger in the brain that regulates learning, sleep, mood, and appetite. It is involved in disorders such as depression and anxiety.

- **Social skills training** is a treatment method that assists individuals to learn specific skills that   are missing or those that will compensate for the missing ones.

- **Specifiers** are extensions to a diagnosis that further clarifies the course, severity, or type of features of a disorder or illness.

- **Testosterone** is a hormone that influences the sexual drive in both men and women.

- **Twelve-Step Program** is a self-help group whose members attempt recovery from various addictions and compulsions on a plan called the Twelve Steps.

Description and Diagnosis

Exhibitionistic disorder is one of the DSM-5 paraphilic disorders. It is characterized by the compulsion to expose one's genitals to other individuals (usually strangers) in order to gain sexual satisfaction. The exhibitionist usually does not have the intention of further sexual activity with the other individual. Some exhibitionists have a desire to shock or upset the individual, while other exhibitionists fantasize that the individual (target) will become sexually aroused by their display. In some instances, the exhibitionist masturbates while exposing himself or herself to the individual. Some symptoms associated with exhibitionistic disorder include an individual having recurrent fantasies of exposing himself or herself but rarely or never acting on the fantasies. Other individuals have difficulty controlling urges and have exposed themselves to at least three individuals. Another aspect of this disorder is impulse control.

According to the *Diagnostic and Statistical Manual of Mental Disorders, Fifth Edition*, individuals can be diagnosed with this disorder if they have intense and recurrent arousal from exposing one's genitals to an unsuspecting individual. This must occur for a period of at least six months as demonstrated by urges, behaviors, and fantasies. An individual can be diagnosed with this disorder if he or she has acted on sexual urges with a non-consenting individual. The sexual urges must cause significant distress or impairment in occupational, social, or other meaningful areas of functioning. If the individual is living in a controlled environment (e.g., institution) to restrict his or her exhibitionistic behavior, the specifier "In a controlled environment" must be included in the diagnosis. An individual who has not acted on urges with a non-consenting individual and has not had any distress or impairment for at least five years in social, occupational, or other areas of important functioning, the specifier "In full remission" must be included in the diagnosis. There are three subtypes for exhibitionistic disorder listed in the DSM-5 that are based on physical maturity, age, of the non-consenting individuals (American Psychiatric Association, 2013).

The exact cause of exhibitionistic disorder is unknown. However, there are a number of theories about its origin or cause. One theory is biological and assumes that as testosterone increases in males so does deviant sexual behaviors. Some medications are prescribed to exhibitionists in order to lower their testosterone levels. Another theory is that emotional abuse caused by growing up in a dysfunctional family poses significant risk factors in developing exhibitionist disorder. It is also thought that exhibitionists regard their mothers as rejecting them based on their different genitals. Therefore, they grow up with a desire to force women to accept them by making women look at

their genitals. Antisocial personality disorders, alcohol abuse, and pedophilic interest may be considered risk factors for exhibitionist disorder in males with exhibitionist preferences. The prevalence of exhibitionist disorder is higher in men than among women (American Psychiatric Association, 2013).

Treatment

Treatment for this disorder usually includes a combination of psychotherapy, medications, and other treatments. Several different forms of psychotherapy have been found to be effective in treating exhibitionistic disorder. In particular, cognitive behavior therapy has been found to help individuals diagnosed with exhibitionistic disorder. Individuals are encouraged to recognize irrational behaviors and to change other distorted patterns of thinking. Aversion therapy is another form of method used for treating individuals with exhibitionistic disorder. This type of therapy involves asking the individual to fantasize about specific events that led to exhibitionism. A very unpleasant scene is inserted into the events. For example, an individual might be asked to imagine an undercover agent approaching as the individual is exposing himself or herself or imagining his or her target laughing at him or her. Another treatment method that is often used for individuals with exhibitionistic disorder is social skills training. It is believed that some men develop paraphilias partly because they never developed health relationships with other individuals. The relationships may be either sexual or nonsexual. Twelve-Step Programs for sexual addicts may be another method of treatment. Exhibitionists often feel guilty and anxious about their behavior and are often helped by the social support available in Twelve-Step Programs.

Several different medications are prescribed and used to treat an individual with exhibitionistic disorder. Selective serotonin reuptake inhibitors (SSRIs) are medications often used in treating paraphilia's. SSRIs have been found to be effective because, as the levels of serotonin increase in the brain, the sex drive decreases. Female hormones (estrogen) are also used to treat individuals with exhibitionistic disorder. The hormone used in treating this disorder works by stimulating the liver, which produces a chemical that clears testosterone from the bloodstream. Antiandrogens are also used. These medications block the uptake of testosterone and reduce the blood levels of testosterone and significantly reduce repetition of the deviant behavior. Removal of the testes, surgical castration, is another treatment option for exhibitionists. This procedure reduces the levels of testosterone in the blood, thus decreasing the sex drive. This form of treatment, however, is generally used for serious sexual offenders, such as violent rapists and pedophiles.

Elizabeth Smith Kelsey, PhD, and
Len Sperry, MD, PhD

See also: Aversion Therapy; Brain; Cognitive Behavior Therapy; *Diagnostic and Statistical Manual of Mental Disorders* (DSM); Paraphilic Disorders; Serotonin; Social Skills Training; Twelve-Step Programs

Further Reading

American Psychiatric Association. *Diagnostic and Statistical Manual of Mental Disorders*, 5th ed. Arlington, VA: American Psychiatric Association, 2013.

Carnes, Patrick. *Out of the Shadows: Understanding Sexual Addiction*, 3rd ed. Center City, MN: Hazelden Publishing, 2001.

Charlton, Randolph S., and Irvin D. Yalom. *Treating Sexual Disorders*. San Francisco, CA: Jossey-Bass, 1997.

Existential Psychotherapy

Existential psychotherapy (EP) is an experiential and relationship-oriented approach to psychotherapy that focuses on meaning and the nature of the human experience.

Description

Existential psychotherapy focuses on the nature of the human condition, the capacity for self-awareness, and the freedom to choose one's own fate. Individuality, freedom, autonomy, personal responsibility, and the search for meaning are key concepts. The goals in existential counseling are to help individuals become aware of their own possibilities and to recognize that they are responsible for both positive and negative events that take place in their lives. This method of

psychotherapy is less focused on technique and more focused on understanding freedom and responsibility, meaning and meaninglessness, isolation and relationships, and living and dying. Existential psychotherapy is a philosophical approach to helping and is well suited to individuals with existential concerns such as life transitions, making sense of life, disappointments in life, discovering values, and seeking self-expression and self-fulfillment. Existential therapy can be provided in individual or group counseling sessions.

Development

Existential psychotherapy is deeply rooted in existential philosophy, which was developed over many years and was not founded by any one individual. Both 19th- and 20th-century philosophers influenced existentialism. Søren Kierkegaard (1813–1855), Friedrich Nietzsche (1844–1900), Martin Heidegger (1889–1976), and Jean-Paul Sartre (1905–1980) are some of the early philosophers who made significant contributions to the movement. More recently, contemporary existential psychotherapy has been highly influenced by the work of Viktor Frankl, Rollo May, James Bugental, Otto Frank, and Irvin Yalom. All of these therapists individually contributed to the development of existential psychotherapy.

Existential psychotherapy does not rely on any specific techniques. EP is based on the understanding and exploration of what it means to be human. The existential perspective is that human beings are in a constant state of transition and continually need to re-create and find meaning in existence. Assisting people in finding a balance between the difficulties, tragedies, and dilemmas of being human and discovering the opportunities, possibilities, and meaning in the human experience is a fundamental aspect of the approach.

The core dimensions of EP include the following: (1) People have the ability to be self-aware, which leads to greater awareness of potential, motivation, and alternatives in living. (2) People are free to choose and are responsible to shape their own destinies. (3) People must develop the courage to create their own self-identity in order to authentically relate to others. (4) People search for significance, meaning, and purpose in life, which are discovered through engagement with what is valued. (5) Anxiety is unavoidable and can lead to change. (6) Awareness of the inevitability of death provides the motivation to live life fully with meaning and significance.

Current Status

Existential psychotherapy is a here-and-now approach that focuses on what people are becoming, not on past experiences or childhood dynamics. A meaningful and authentic relationship between the client and therapist is essential with the understanding that both may be changed by the encounter. The central goal of EP is to help people become aware of their possibilities, understand their own freedom and responsibility in making choices, and identify what is keeping them from living a meaningful life.

EP is more a style and philosophy of psychotherapy than a specific model of therapy. The lack of techniques unique to EP has resulted in an approach that is difficult to research and suffers from a lack of evidence-based treatment outcomes. Other criticisms of the existential approach include its lack of training models and language and concepts that can be perceived as mystical and vague. A significant limitation to EP is the level of philosophical knowledge required of the practitioner and a deep understanding of what it means to be human.

Existential psychotherapy is a philosophical and experiential approach to helping. EP is provided through an authentic relationship that assists individuals in developing the courage to finding meaning and significance in life while facing the realities of life.

Steven R. Vensel, PhD

See also: Frankl, Viktor (1905–1997); May, Rollo (1909–1994)

Further Reading

Corey, Gerald. *Theory and Practice of Counseling and Psychotherapy*, 8th ed. Belmont, CA: Brooks/Cole, 2009.

Emmy van Deurzen. 2013. "Existential Therapy." Accessed October 7, 2013. http://www.emmyvandeurzen.com/?page_id=25.

Van Deurzen, Emmy. *Existential Counselling and Psychotherapy in Practice*, 3rd ed. London: Sage, 2012.

Expertise

Expertise is the special knowledge or skills in a particular subject area learned from experience resulting in a high level of proficiency or competency.

Definitions

- **Attitude** is the predisposition or tendency to respond positively or negatively to specific ideas, individuals, or situations.

- **Competency** is the capacity to integrate knowledge, skills, and attitudes reflected in the quality of clinical counseling practice.

- **Deliberate practice** is the effort and time devoted to reaching for objectives just beyond one's level of proficiency (skills) and using interventions to increase one's proficiency.

- **Expert** refers to one who practices with a high level of expertise or proficiency.

- **Knowledge** is information about various topics that includes definitions and explanations of processes that explain larger constructs.

- **Master therapists** are psychotherapists who are considered by fellow therapists to be "the best of the best" in terms of expertise in psychotherapy. They are also called expert therapists.

- **Psychotherapy** is a psychological method for achieving desired changes in thinking, feeling, and behavior. It is also called therapeutic counseling.

- **Reflective practice** is a process that expert therapists utilize in which they continue to learn from experiences and increase their capacity to work effectively with clients.

- **Second-order change** is long-lasting change that can be achieved in counseling when clients experience symptom or conflict reduction and long-lasting personality change.

- **Skills** are capacities that can be acquired (learned) through education and "hands-on" training.

- **10,000 hours rule** is the rule based on the research finding that at least 10,000 hours of deliberate practice are required to achieve expertise in a given occupation.

Description

"Expertise" refers to the characteristic way in which experts think and act. It distinguishes the performance of experts from the less experienced. When it comes to psychotherapy, expert therapists are also called master therapists. These individuals have an advanced ability to quickly assess situations and easily design appropriate treatment interventions. They have the ability to quickly determine when treatment interventions are not effective and can modify treatment very efficiently compared to their peers. They engage in lifelong learning and continue to learn the nuances of working with clients through additional training and reflective practice. Expert therapists have the ability to engage their clients in highly effective therapy to ultimately achieve treatment goals and effect change with their clients in a relatively short amount of time.

Psychologist Anders Ericsson (1947–) has pioneered the study of expertise. Based on his research he has proposed the 10,000 hours rule. He reports that it takes 10,000 hours for the brain to assimilate a particular skill. This 10,000 rule also applies to counselor development. The beginner or novice counselor engages in reflective and deliberate counseling practice that will lead to more advanced counseling skills, knowledge, and attitudes. It should be noted that 10,000 hours of the same practice without learning from experience does not result in expertise.

Expertise has been studied in various professions and among specific behaviors such as violinists, chess players, educators, and athletes. Experts are characterized by being highly skilled in a particular skill area. Expert or master therapists are more effective and are able to navigate the nuances of working with individuals in psychotherapy. The process of expertise begins with the beginner stage, advanced beginner, minimally competent, proficient, and finally the expert stage.

Beginning therapists possess a very limited capacity to assess, analyze, and intervene. They are overly reliant on basic principles and techniques and are rule-bound, but they are very inexperienced and need supervision. Advanced beginners possess some capacity for assessment or diagnosis, and application of interventions, but they experience difficulty generalizing this capacity to different patients and new situations. They require clinical supervision and additional training in most counseling functions. Therapists in the minimally competent developmental stage hold the capacity to function independently but with a minimal competence and minimal effectiveness. They are able to cope with and handle crises or other problems as they arise and are able to integrate theory and research in most aspects of their practice. Proficient therapists have the capacity to function independently and effectively. Their performance is guided by flexibility and a clear understanding of their clients' personalities and patterns. They are able to integrate their personal with their professional life and values. The expert or master therapist has an intuitive grasp of clinical situations and is able to very efficiency work with clients on reducing symptoms and effecting lasting change or second-order change. Therapists who function at the expert or mastery stage spend a significant amount of time in training, supervision, and reflective practice.

Expert therapists practice and display high levels of the following competencies: clinical competence, ethical competence, cultural competence, social interest, and well-being or self-care. Clinical competency is evidenced by clinical intuition and judgment shown by clinicians based on their clinical knowledge, skills, and attitudes and reflection on those experiences as they relate to the specific circumstances of a particular patient. Cultural competency is the clinicians' awareness of cultural variables in themselves and in their clients that may affect the therapeutic relationship and treatment process. Ethical sensitivity is the capacity to recognize, anticipate, and respond to the suffering and vulnerability of those receiving professional services, especially among ethical and moral aspects. Social interest is the clinician's orientation of connecting to other human beings and searching for a sense of purpose through helping others and empowering clients to enhance their own sense of social interest. Lastly, expert counselors are usually able to balance work and personal life while actively engaging in self-care practices to maintain their own emotional, social, and physical well-being.

Based on his research Thomas Skovholt (1944–) described the attributes of master therapists. He discussed qualitative research and interviews about master therapists. He identified that mastery is achieved through an ongoing effort to improve skills, being open to feedback from supervisors, seeking new knowledge through continuing education and training, and significant clinical experience, which is a given. Skovholt and Jennings identified 11 characteristics of the ideal therapist, and they suggest that master therapists possess many of these traits: master therapists are voracious learners, they use their accumulated experiences, they value cognitive complexity and ambiguity, they have emotional receptivity, they are healthy and nurture their own emotional well-being, they are aware of how their emotional health affects their work, they possess highly developed relational skills, they cultivate strong working alliances with clients, they excel in using their exceptional therapy skills, they trust their clients, and they are culturally competent (Jennings and Skovholt, 1999). These attributes were found among their qualitative research done among master therapists.

In summary, master or expert therapists demonstrate high levels of clinical, ethical, and cultural expertise, social interest, and self-care. They have significant relational skills and are able to form very effective therapeutic alliances with clients. Research identifies that mastery takes approximately 10,000 hours with deliberate and reflective practice. Master therapists are able to quickly effect long-lasting change with clients in a relatively short amount of time. Understanding traits of master therapists informs graduate counseling and psychology programs about important competencies and processes that can influence competent trainees.

Len Sperry, MD, PhD, and Jon Sperry, PhD

See also: Master Therapist; Psychotherapy

Further Reading

Dreyfus, Hubert, and Stuart Dreyfus. *Mind over Machine.* New York, NY: Free Press, 2008.
Ericsson, K. Anders, Neil Charness, Paul J. Fltovich, and Robert R. Hoffman, eds. *The Cambridge Handbook of Expertise and Expert Performance.* Cambridge: Cambridge University Press, 2006.
Jennings, Len, and Thomas Skovholt. "The Cognitive, Emotional, and Relational Characteristics of Master Therapists." *Journal of Counseling Psychology* 46 (1999): 3–11.
Skovholt, Thomas, and Len Jennings. *Master Therapists: Exploring Expertise in Therapy and Counseling.* Boston, MA: Allyn & Bacon, 2004.
Sperry, Len, and Jon Carlson. *How Master Therapists Work: Effecting Change from the First Session through the Last Session and Beyond.* New York, NY: Routledge, 2014.

Exposure Therapy

Exposure therapy is a behavior therapy intervention (method) in which a client is exposed to a feared object or situation. It is also referred to as flooding.

Definitions

- **Behavior therapy** is a psychotherapy approach that focuses on identifying and changing maladaptive behaviors. It is also referred to as behavioral therapy.

- **Classical conditioning** is an involuntary process of neurological change in response to a stimulus that causes a reaction. Classical conditioning occurs when the involuntary reaction is associated (paired) to a new unrelated stimulus causing the reaction to occur automatically when the new stimulus is present. It is also known as Pavlovian conditioning.

- **In vivo** is a Latin term that means "in the living" and signifies therapeutically that an intervention is occurring in real life, as opposed to in an imagination or in a theory.

- **Pathology** is an experience of suffering or aspect of a disease incorporating cause, development, structure, and consequences.

- **Psychotherapy** is a psychological method for achieving desired changes in thinking, feeling, and behavior. It is also called therapeutic counseling.

- **Reciprocal inhibition** is a therapeutic technique that obstructs the presence of one response through the introduction of an opposite response.

- **Relaxation training** a progressive tensing and relaxing of specific muscle groups to teach acceptance and letting go of anxious symptoms.

- **Systematic desensitization** is a form of exposure therapy that gradually exposes an individual to his or her phobia while teaching him or her to stay relaxed in the increasing presence of his or her phobia. It is also known as graduated exposure therapy.

- **Virtual reality exposure therapy** is form of exposure therapy that uses computer-generated imagery to expose a client to simulations of a dreaded object or event.

Description

Exposure therapy is a behavior therapy intervention in which the therapist intentionally exposes a client to a feared object or situation. Exposure therapy is based on the premise that confronting dreaded objects or situations results in a reduction of distress. A variety of psychotherapeutic techniques are available in exposure therapy. The basic technique utilized in exposure therapy is called in vivo exposure. In vivo exposure therapy requires that the client be exposed to his or her dreaded object or situation in real life. For example, a therapist could bring real live spiders into a counseling session with a client who suffers from arachnophobia (fear of spiders). Another form of exposure therapy is imaginal exposure, which instructs a client to imagine being in the presence of a dreaded object or situation. As in the previously given example, a client with arachnophobia would be instructed to imagine spiders or situations involving spiders. Research evidence and clinical experience suggest that imaginal exposure is not as therapeutically effective as in vivo exposure therapy. A type of imaginal exposure therapy occurs with the assistance of virtual reality technologies. As a result of advancements in computer-generated imagery, virtual reality exposure therapy can be as effective as in vivo therapy. Interoceptive exposure is a type of exposure therapy that exposes a client to sensations that typically occur with exposure to his or her feared object or situation.

If a client suffering from arachnophobia has a symptom of shortness of breath (hyperventilation) when exposed to spiders, the therapist using interoceptive exposure therapy might suggest that the client breathe through a straw or into a paper bag to expose the client to the sensation without spiders present. If the client hyperventilates on being exposed to spiders, then exposure to hyperventilation without spiders present eventually reduces or removes the fear of the symptom and often alters the involuntary response (hyperventilation) to the classically conditioned stimulus (spiders). The fear response to a particular stimulus is replaced with a relaxation response to the same stimulus.

Exposure therapy is similar to but different from systematic desensitization. Both exposure therapy and systematic desensitization are therapeutic techniques that focus on the extinction (removal) of a conditioned response. Exposure therapy (flooding) encourages a patient to confront a fear and refrain from reacting in a typical manner. There is no subtlety to exposure therapy. It is an all or nothing exposure to a phobia that teaches a patient to tolerate the distress associated with the exposure. Therapists must be trained to assist the patient through the distress that results from exposure to a phobic stimulus. In contrast, systematic desensitization trains a patient to tolerate progressive exposure to a phobia. In systematic desensitization, the therapist will work with a client to develop an exposure hierarchy, or feared situations ranked from most tolerable to least tolerable. Systematic desensitization teaches a client to stay relaxed when exposed to his or her phobia in increasing amounts over time. The gradual nature of systematic desensitization makes it a different behavioral intervention than exposure therapy. Exposure therapy floods a client with fear until the client learns that the feared outcome is not likely to occur.

While it is important in exposure therapy to expose a client to his or her fear response, care must be taken not to overwhelm the client. The clinician works closely with the client to ensure that the client does not experience overwhelming fear during the process of exposure therapy. This is a critical aspect of the intervention as the conditioned response of fear must be replaced with relaxation. Further, exposure therapy is most effective when flooding occurs daily until extinction of the response occurs. This might require therapists to assign exposure-based "homework" between weekly sessions.

Development and Current Status

Exposure therapy was introduced by Joseph Wolpe (1915–1997), a psychiatrist from South Africa, in the 1950s. Wolpe coined the term "reciprocal inhibition" to describe the process of classically conditioning an opposite response to replace an automatic reaction to a stimulus. It was believed that a reaction and its opposite reaction could not exist simultaneously in a patient. Exposure therapy is fundamentally associated with reciprocal inhibition. Reciprocal inhibition creates response prevention, which is the blocking of unwanted avoidance behaviors. Wolpe's discoveries led to treatments that briefly increase a client's experience of anxiety but eventually lead to the extinction (removal) of anxiety. During exposure it is necessary for the client to remain as relaxed as possible. Psychotherapeutic techniques of relaxation training paired with exposure are highly effective. A client quickly learns to maintain relaxation in the presence of a feared stimulus. Although exposure therapy was originated by behavior therapists, today this technique is commonly used by cognitive behavioral therapists and even by psychodynamically oriented therapists.

Len Sperry, MD, PhD, and
Layven Reguero, MEd

See also: Empirically Supported Treatment; Evidence-Based Practice; Systematic Desensitization

Further Reading

Miltenberger, Rymond G. *Behavior Modification: Principles and Procedures*, 5th ed. Belmont, CA: Wadsworth Cengage Learning, 2012.

Reinecke, Mark A. *Little Ways to Keep Calm and Carry On: Twenty Lessons for Managing Worry, Anxiety, and Fear*. Oakland, CA: New Harbinger, 2010.

Tolin, David. *Face Your Fears: A Proven Plan to Beat Anxiety, Panic, Phobias, and Obsessions*. Hoboken, NJ: John Wiley & Sons, 2012.

Wolpe, Joseph. *The Practice of Behavior Therapy*, 4th ed. New York, NY: Pergamon Press, 1990.

Expressive Arts Therapy

Expressive arts therapy is the practice of using storytelling, imagery, dance, drama, poetry, movement, music, dream work, and visual arts to help promote and encourage personal growth and healing.

Description

Expressive arts therapy is a technique using a multitude of creative mediums to complement and work with the therapeutic process. The notion of expressive arts is not grounded in a specific technique but rather as a response to human suffering. A therapist using expressive arts must be prepared to use a variety of modalities to meet the individual needs of clients. It allows for the human psyche to express itself in an authentic, nonverbal manner through images as opposed to words. These images can be done with motion, sound, action, pictures, and so forth. Many argue that people can express themselves in their truest form by utilizing these creative formats or through creative projections.

Expressive arts therapy is considered to be a relatively new approach to therapy; however, many believe it connects back to ancient traditions in healing. Each form of expressive arts therapy has its own branch as well as specific training, for example, art therapy, play therapy, and music therapy. Each of these has its own form of training and credentialing. Forms such as art therapy and music therapy have been in formal practice longer and have journals as well as organizations. Many of these have their own ethical guidelines and standards of practice that clinicians must adhere to.

Expressive arts therapy is sometimes referred to as creative arts in counseling. The art forms include auditory, written, visual, or combinations. Creative arts allows for healing both physically and mentally. In terms of counseling, creativity allows for clients to be more in tune with themselves and encourages them to invest in the process so that they can continue to grow. Using the expressive arts in counseling is considered to be a six-step process. The first step is preparation where background information and data are collected. The second step is incubation where the mind is allowed to wander from the problem at hand. The next step is ideation whereby ideas are generated using divergent thinking. This is followed by illumination where there is enlightenment. The fifth step is evaluation, which allows for critical and convergent thinking. The final step of verification is where there is a product or action.

Development and Current Status

Incorporating art into life dates back to ancient times. People would sing, dance, and tell stories all to explore life, find their place, and honor others. Healing practices of indigenous cultures centered around expressive art techniques and rituals. For example, ancient Egyptians encouraged those who were identified as mentally ill to pursue creativity and artistic interests so that in these actions their feelings could be released and they could become whole again. Expressive arts therapy is grounded in humanistic psychotherapy and systems theories.

The Expressive Therapies Program at Leslie University in Cambridge, Massachusetts, was founded in the 1970s by Shaun McNiff, Paolo Knill, Norma Canner, and their colleagues. The emphasis was on having a creative therapeutic community composed of students and faculty. In the 1980s Paolo Knill went on to develop a network of training programs in North America as well as in Europe. These training institutes now exist around the world. Courses exploring the expressive arts are also now a part of many graduate-level counseling programs.

Over the past 20 years there has been a growth in the field, resulting in separate fields of practice. Clinicians using this modality have to first understand the creative exploration process. Clinicians must understand how to be creative in using these modalities to assist clients. The other side of this is that the term "creativity" is somewhat overused. The key component is divergent thinking, which is thinking in a flexible and exploratory manner. These are associated with coping skills and positive mental health, as well as resiliency and even happiness.

Creativity or expressive arts in counseling allows for a product to be created that helps provide the client with insight that allows for change within the client. For instance, a client may be given the task of a music autobiography where he or she identifies songs that connect to various important points of his or her life.

At first the client may not realize the connection, but in processing and exploring the songs and their connections, this allows for the client to develop deeper more meaningful insights that allow for growth and healing. Creativity and the expressive arts transcend ethnicities, cultures, races, genders, and age.

Mindy Parsons, PhD

See also: Art Therapy; Dance Therapy; Music Therapy; Play Therapy; Sand Tray Therapy

Further Reading

Atkins, Sally S. *Expressive Arts Therapy: Creative Process in Art and Life.* Boone, NC: Parkway Publishers Inc., 2003.

Gladding, Samuel T. *The Creative Arts in Counseling*, 4th ed. Alexandria, VA: American Counseling Association, 2011. http://www.counseling.org.

Levine, Stephen K., and Ellen G. Levine. *Foundations of Expressive Arts Therapy: Theoretical and Clinical Perspectives.* London: Jessica Kingsley Publishers, 1999.

Organizations

American Art Therapy Association
4875 Eisenhower Ave., Suite 240
Alexandria, VA 22301
Telephone: (888) 290-0878
E-mail: info@arttherapy.org
Website: http://www.arttherapy.org/

American Dance Therapy Association
10632 Little Patuxent Parkway, Suite 108
Columbia, MD 21044
Telephone: (410) 997-4040
Fax: (410) 997-4048
E-mail: info@adta.org
Website: www.adta.org

American Music Therapy Association
8455 Colesville Road, Suite 1000
Silver Spring, MD 20910
Telephone: (301) 589-3300
Fax: (301) 589-5175
Websites: http://www.musictherapy.org/contact/; www.musictherapy.org

American Society of Group Psychotherapy and Psychodrama

301 N. Harrison Street, #508
Princeton, NJ 08540
Telephone: (609) 737-8500
Fax: (609) 737-8510
E-mail: asgpp@asgpp.org
Website: http://www.asgpp.org/

Association for Creativity in Counseling
A Division of the American Counseling Association
6101 Stevenson Ave.
Alexandria, VA 22304
Telephone: (800) 347-6647
Fax: (800) 473-2329
E-mail: webmaster@counseling.org
Website: http://www.counseling.org

Association for the Study of Dreams
1672 University Avenue
Berkeley, CA 94703
Phone/Fax: 1 (209) 724-0889
E-mail: office@asdreams.org
Website: www.asdreams.org

International Expressive Arts Therapy Association
PO Box 320399
San Francisco, CA 94132
Telephone: (415) 522-8959
E-mail: info@ieata.org
Website: www.ieata.org

North American Drama Therapy Association
1450 Western Avenue, Suite 101
Albany, NY 12203
Telephone: (888) 416-7167
Fax: (518) 463-8656
E-mail: office@nadta.org
Website: www.nadta.org

Expressive Language Disorder

Expressive language disorder is a deficit in the normal development of language used to communicate with others.

Description

The development of language follows a general pattern when there are no intellectual, developmental, sensory, or neurological disorders. Even without the presence of these diagnoses, there are some individuals who struggle with expressing themselves using language. These individuals may be diagnosed with expressive language disorder (ELD). Usually people with ELD can understand language while they are not themselves able to communicate clearly in response. In other words, their receptive skills, or ability to understand language, are better than their expressive language. Expressive language is the ability to use language effectively. These individuals demonstrate a normal range of intelligence or IQ as measured by testing.

Expressive language disorders fall into two categories. ELD can be acquired, which is usually the result of an accident or illness that causes brain damage. This could include temporary or permanent damage caused by something like a stroke. The other type of ELD is developmental, meaning that language acquisition is slower and later than usual. For an accurate diagnosis of ELD the language deficit cannot be the result of a neurological problem. The developmental type is more common in children, and the acquired type occurs more often among adults or the elderly. It is estimated that 10%–15% of children under the age of three are diagnosed with language development delays, including ELD. In more mild cases, the disorder may not be recognized until they go to school where the prevalence of ELD falls off to the 5%–7% range.

Causes and Symptoms

In the acquired type of ELD, accidents involving head injury are a common cause of the disorder. But children born into families with a history of language delays are more likely to be diagnosed with the developmental type of ELD. If factors that affect general development, such as malnutrition, exist, a child is more likely to be diagnosed with ELD.

Clinical symptoms of this disorder include limited vocabulary and fewer verbal expressions. Many also make mistakes with verb tense and have difficulty remembering new words. Children with expressive language delays do not talk as much or as often as their peers. Yet they generally understand what is said to them. For example, children with this disorder may be able to follow two-step commands but may not be able to name their body parts. ELD may manifest itself in difficulties with written language as well.

Diagnosis and Prognosis

Expressive language disorder is medically classified as speech sound disorder. ELD may be suspected when there are difficulties with academics or socialization. Medical testing should be conducted to determine whether a diagnosis of ELD is correct. Social withdrawal and co-occurring diagnoses, such as attention-deficit disorder, are commonly associated with ELD.

Unfortunately, developmental and acquired language disorders do not improve when untreated. Without intervention, the frustration that children and adults with ELD experience may lead to behavior problems. In the case of some children, they may stop attempting to learn as they reach adolescence. When concerned about language development issues, it is best to consult a speech-language pathologist to see if a diagnosis of ELD is appropriate.

Treatment

Language therapy is the best and most direct means to treat this disorder. The goal of this therapy is to use speech therapy techniques to increase the number of words and phrases a child or adult can use. Ideally a supportive community of parents, teachers, and health-care professionals should be involved in the treatment. In cases where the self-esteem of the individual has been severely affected, some counseling or psychotherapy may also be recommended.

Alexandra Cunningham, PhD, and William M. Cunningham, MA

See also: Speech Sound Disorder; Speech-Language Pathology

Further Reading

American Psychiatric Association. *Diagnostic and Statistical Manual of Mental Disorders, DSM-IV-TR*. Washington, DC: Author, 2000.

American Psychiatric Association. *Diagnostic and Statistical Manual of Mental Disorders*, 5th ed. Alexandria, VA: American Psychiatric Association, 2013.

Feit, Debbie. *The Parent's Guide to Speech and Language Problems*. New York, NY: McGraw-Hill, 2007.

Morales, Sarah. "Expressive Language Disorder." *Children's Speech Care Center*. Last modified February 6, 2012. Accessed May 20, 2013. http://www.childspeech.net/u_iv_h.html.

Extraversion and Introversion and Personality Type

"Introversion" and "extraversion" refer to two components of personality type originally developed by Swiss psychiatrist Carl G. Jung (1875–1961) and are a part of most theories of personality type.

Definition

- **Dichotomy**, or dichotomous, refers to the division of two opposing or contradictory constructs, ideas, or forces in which being high in one is to be low in the other.

Description

"Personality type" refers to a collection of personality traits and preferences that produce a consistent and predictable pattern of thinking, feeling, and behaving. Extraversion and introversion (E/I) are two components of personality type first proposed and developed by Swiss psychiatrist Carl Jung in the 1920s to explain differences in people's behaviors. Jung believed that differences in behavior were accounted for by how individuals use their minds in different ways. These differences result in reliable patterns of behavior that can be identified in order to better understand individuals. Personality type consists of several identified and labeled patterns of thinking and behaving. There are many theories of personality type, with a variety of different labels depending on the theorist and model of personality theory. Extraversion and introversion are identified patterns that virtually all personality type theories utilize in their research, including the Neo Inventories based on the Big Five factor model and the Myers–Briggs Type Indicator (MBTI).

One of the most popular and widely used instruments in understanding normal personality differences is the (MBTI). Building on Jung's theories Katharine Cook Briggs (1875–1968) and her daughter Isabel Briggs Myers (1897–1961) applied Jung's ideas to understanding psychological type and appreciating differences between people. The MBTI measures preferences based on four dichotomies, each consisting of two opposite poles. E/I represents one of the polar dichotomies where extraversion is on one end with introversion on the other and scoring high on one end corresponds with scoring low on the other. The MBTI does not measure the strength of a preference but rather the clarity of the preference. High or low scores do not mean you are highly extraverted or introverted but rather you have a clear preference for one or the other. The MBTI identifies preferences by asking respondents to choose between two dichotomous statements such as the following: do you prefer to focus on the outer world or on your own inner world?

Myers–Briggs identifies extraverts as people who focus on the outer world of people and activities; they direct their energy toward, and receive their energy from, interacting with people and activities. Extraverts prefer to communicate by talking, learn best by doing, are sociable and expressive, and take initiative in work and relationships. Extraverts are outgoing, comfortable with people and groups, have a wide range of friends, and can be impulsive. Introverts prefer the inner world of ideas, memories, and thoughts. Introverts are reflective, often seen as "reserved," comfortable with being alone, have a small group of trusted friends, and can be slow to act.

Over the past 50 years, personality researchers have identified five dimensions or domains to personality commonly referred to as "The Big Five" or the "Five Factor Model" (FFM) of personality. The Big Five has been extensively researched, with a considerable body of literature supporting the FFM. The investigations of many personality theorists, including Robert McCrae, and Paul Costa, Jr., have led to the development of the NEO Inventories, which use a lexical approach to identifying the dimensions of personality. The lexical approach recognizes that people use natural language to describe experiences. Thousands of trait adjectives (e.g., nervous, accommodating, outgoing, friendly) were scientifically analyzed in numerous research studies and led to the identification of the five personality traits that exist, in varying dimensions, in all people. The FFM differs from the MBTI in that the MBTI identifies discrete and specific "types," whereas the FFM describes people in terms of a continuous dimension. For instance, in the MBTI a person is designated as either an extravert or an introvert; in the FFM a person is located somewhere along a path between extraversion and introversion. The FFM recognizes that most people are actually "ambiverts" and display a combination of introverted and extraverted tendencies. The FFM domains of personality are neuroticism, extraversion, openness, agreeableness, and conscientiousness.

The FFM identifies extraverts as sociable, preferring large groups and gatherings. They are assertive, active, and talkative and like excitement and stimulation. They are also upbeat, optimistic, energetic, and cheerful. Introversion is not to be seen as the opposite of extraversion but rather the absence of extraverted preferences. Introverts are reserved but not unfriendly, independent rather than followers, even-paced not sluggish, and prefer to be alone but not because they are shy. Although introverts are not highly spirited, they are not unhappy or pessimistic. The FFM does not relate introspection or reflection to E/I.

Current Status and Impact (Psychological Influence)

Both the MBTI and FMM have made a considerable impact on society but in different ways. The MBTI is an extremely popular personality indicator that has been used in thousands of consumer, education, self-help, and business applications throughout the world. The MBTI has been criticized by researchers as lacking a scientific psychometric instrument and has not been utilized in scientifically rigorous personality research. The FFM and the NEO Inventories are highly regarded by researchers for their scientific and psychometric qualities and are extensively used in a vast array of personality research inquiry.

The concept of E/I has been widely accepted as a fundamental dimension of personality and embraced by both the scientific community and general population. E/I continues to be extensively researched, and many scientific articles and popular trade books have been published.

Steven R. Vensel, PhD

See also: Five-Factor Theory; Personality Tests

Further Reading

McCrae, Robert R., and Paul T. Costa Jr. *NEO Inventories Professional Manual.* Lutz, FL: PAR, 2010.

Myers, Isabel Briggs. *Introduction to Type: A Guide to Understanding Your Results on the Myers-Briggs Type Indicator*, 6th ed. Mountain View, CA: CPP, Inc., 1998.

The Myers & Briggs Foundation. "Extraversion or Introversion." Accessed August 20, 2014. http://www.myersbriggs.org/my-mbti-personality-type/mbti-basics/extraversion-or-introversion.asp.

The Myers & Briggs Foundation. "MBTI Basics." Accessed August 20, 2014. http://www.myersbriggs.org/my-mbti-personality-type/mbti-basics/.

Wilt, Joshua, and William Revelle. "Extraversion." Review of the *Handbook of Individual Differences in Social Behavior*, edited by Mark R. Leary and Rick H. Hoyle, pp. 27–45. New York, NY: Gilford Press, 2009.

Eye Movement Desensitization and Reprocessing (EMDR)

Eye movement desensitization and reprocessing (EMDR) is an effective form of psychotherapy that assists people in the alleviation of psychological, emotional, and physiological distress related to traumatic experiences and memories.

Definitions

- **Bilateral eye movement** is to look with the eyes to the right and then to the left without moving the head.

- **Desensitization** means to decrease unwarranted negative emotional response to situations or circumstances by repeated exposure to memories or triggers.

- **Reprocessing** means to rethink, reorganize, and reconsider the meaning and significance of painful events.

- **Triggers** are situations that activate memories and emotional states associated with a past traumatic event.

Description

Eye movement desensitization and reprocessing is a type of psychotherapy developed by Francine Shapiro that assists individuals heal from the emotional distress of traumatic experiences. EMDR facilitates the accessing and reprocessing of traumatic and painful memories that are causing psychological distress. EMDR is known for its unique use of eye movement during the treatment phase of psychotherapy. During treatment clients are instructed to move their eyes back and forth while thinking about the traumatic event, present triggers, and anticipated future situations. In addition to eye movement, alternate tapping of left-then-right fingers or hearing auditory tones directed at left-then-right ears can be utilized. This "dual stimulation" of memories/thoughts and physical stimulation aids in desensitizing the client to the traumatic event, thus reducing the unwanted and unwarranted emotional response. Reprocessing focuses on vivid visual images related to the memory, negative beliefs about self, related emotions and body sensations, and developing new positive beliefs. During treatment clients develop new insight and associations regarding the memories, triggers, and beliefs about the traumatic experience.

EMDR consists of eight phases of treatment. Phase one includes history taking, assessing readiness for EMDR, identifying targets for reprocessing, and the development of a treatment plan. Phase two consists of assessing client coping skills and equipping the client with methods for handling and reducing psychological stress. In phases three through six, targets are identified and processed using EMDR. Phase seven is closure and clients are instructed to journal any related material that may arise. Phase eight examines the progress made.

Development and Current Status

EMDR was developed by American psychologist Francine Shapiro (1948–) who, in 1987, was taking a walk and thinking through some personally

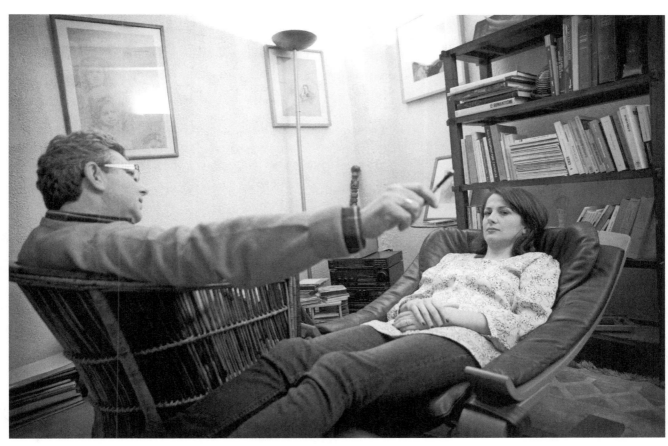

Eye movement desensitization and reprocessing is an effective form of psychotherapy that assists people in the alleviation of psychological, emotional, and physiological distress related to traumatic experiences and memories. (BSIP/UIG via Getty Images)

distressing memories. She observed that her eyes movements might be related to the decrease in the negative emotions she experienced during the walk. Over the next several years Shapiro further explored the interaction between eye movement, memories, and cognitions resulting in the development of Adaptive Information Processing (AIP) theory. The AIP model theorizes that memory networks contain related images, emotions, sensations, and thoughts related to events that take place in life. Humans have an inherent information processing system that naturally results in adaptation to these events. AIP hypothesizes that information related to traumatic events is not fully processed and the memories are stored as they were experienced at the time of the stressful event. Shapiro proposed that unprocessed stressful experiences cause distress and mental health problems such as anxiety

and post-traumatic stress disorder (PTSD). According to Shapiro EMDR alleviates the distress by processing the experiences and linking them to more adaptive information.

EMDR has been highly researched as a treatment for PTSD and has been found to be effective in the reduction of PTSD symptoms when compared to no treatment. EMDR has been found to be equivalent in outcomes to more traditional exposure therapy and cognitive behavior therapy. EMDR has been criticized as being a modification of existing exposure therapy, with the eye movements being noncritical to outcomes. Some research suggests that eye movement may not contribute to positive outcomes and other research indicates it does. The exact function of the eye movement component of EMDR is inconclusive and continues to be investigated. EMDR is also being studied in assessing the effectiveness of the method in treating a variety of mental health disorders such as phobias, anxiety, panic, and depression. EMDR is a complex psychotherapy, which utilizes numerous psychotherapeutic techniques that contribute to its effectiveness in treating trauma-related distress.

Steven R. Vensel, PhD

See also: Exposure Therapy; Post-Traumatic Stress Disorder (PTSD)

Further Reading

EMDR Institute, Inc. "What Is EMDR." Accessed March 12, 2014. http://www.emdr.com/general-information/what-is-emdr.html.

Shapiro, Francine. *EMDR as an Integrative Psychotherapy Approach; Experts of Diverse Orientations Explore the Paradigm Prism*. Washington, DC: American Psychological Association Books, 2002.

Shapiro, Francine. *Eye Movement Desensitization and Reprocessing: Basic Principles, Protocols and Procedures*, 2nd ed. New York, NY: Guilford Press, 2001.